EXPERIMENTAL ASSESSMENTS AND CLINICAL APPLICATIONS OF CONDITIONED FOOD AVERSIONS

ANNALS OF THE NEW YORK ACADEMY OF SCIENCES

Volume 443

EXPERIMENTAL ASSESSMENTS AND CLINICAL APPLICATIONS OF CONDITIONED FOOD AVERSIONS

Edited by Norman S. Braveman and Paul Bronstein

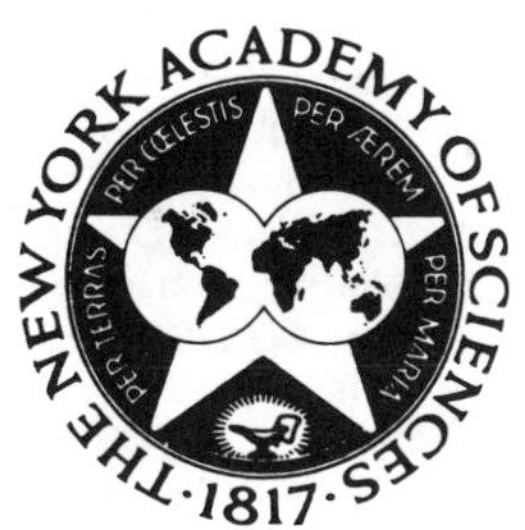

The New York Academy of Sciences
New York, New York
1985

Library of Congress Cataloging in Publication Data

Main entry under title:

Experimental assessments and clinical applications of conditioned food aversions.

(Annals of the New York Academy of Sciences, ISSN 0077-8923 : v. 443)
Papers presented at a conference held by the New York Academy of Sciences, Apr. 9–11, 1984.
Bibliography: p.
Includes index.
1. Conditioned response—Congresses. 2. Aversive stimuli—Congresses. 3. Avoidance (Psychology)—Congresses. 4. Food—Psychological aspects—Congresses.
I. Braveman, Norman S., 1941- . II. Bronstein, Paul, 1945- . III. New York Academy of Sciences. IV. Series. [DNLM: 1. Avoidance Learning—congresses. 2. Conditioning, Classical—congresses. 3. Feeding Behavior—congresses. 4. Food Preferences—congresses. 5. Taste—congresses. W1 AN626YL v. 443 / BF 319.5.A9 E96 1984]
Q11.N5 vol. 443 500s 85-10647
[QP416] [615'.73]

CCP
Printed in the United States of America
ISBN 0-89766-280-6 (Cloth)
ISBN 0-89766-281-4 (Paper)
ISSN 0077-8923

ANNALS OF THE NEW YORK ACADEMY OF SCIENCES

Volume 443
June 7, 1985

EXPERIMENTAL ASSESSMENTS AND CLINICAL APPLICATIONS OF CONDITIONED FOOD AVERSIONS[a]

Editors and Conference Organizers
NORMAN S. BRAVEMAN and PAUL BRONSTEIN

CONTENTS

[a] The papers in this volume were presented at a conference entitled Experimental Assessments and Clinical Applications of Conditioned Food Aversions, which was held by the New York Academy of Sciences on April 9–11, 1984.

Part III. Comparative Approaches to Learning, Foraging, and Toxiphobia

Part IV. Pharmacological and Toxicological Assessments Using Conditioned Food Aversion Methodology

Part V. Applications of Conditioned Food Aversion Methodology

Part VI. Conditioned Food Aversions: A Bibliography

Financial assistance received from:

- MIAMI UNIVERSITY, DEPARTMENT OF PSYCHOLOGY
- A. H. ROBINS COMPANY
- SCHERING-PLOUGH CORPORATION

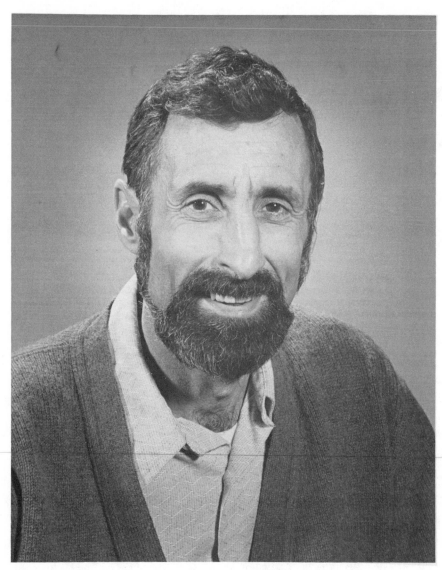

PATRICK J. CAPRETTA

Introduction

NORMAN S. BRAVEMAN[a]

Physiology of Aging Branch
National Institute on Aging
Bethesda, Maryland 20205

Conditioned food aversions (CFAs) are produced when an ingestible, usually in the form of a flavored solution, precedes or signals the onset of aversive post-ingestional consequences which, in the laboratory situation, usually results from the injection of a drug. Historically, CFAs have been viewed both as a phenomenon as well as a method. As a phenomenon the focus of research on CFAs was on what appeared to be the unique characteristics of the paradigm. Specifically, learning theorists were intrigued by the fact that the establishment of a strong CFA could be accomplished in one trial even though consumption of the ingestible and the aversive post-ingestional consequences were separated by many minutes or even hours. This was in contrast to many other learning preparations in which the to-be-associated events could, at most, be separated only by fractions of a second or not at all in order to produce conditioning.

Research on CFA as a phenomenon also focused on the fact that there seemed to be a preferential basis for associations between the taste of the ingestible and certain types of post-ingestional consequences. Traditional punishers such as electric footshock appeared to be relatively ineffective in modifying consumption of distinctively flavored substances. At the same time, however, nongustatory characteristics of these substances could be associated with electric footshock. At the same time that CFA appeared to be a special type of learning, theories of biological preparedness and concurrent interference were proposed to show that CFA learning was like other kinds of avoidance conditioning. The essential difference between CFA learning and other types of learning, however, was that in CFA learning the events to be associated had a high probability of being associated because of their evolutionary importance to the organism. These theories were, for the most part, based on data derived from the laboratory rat. When other animals (e.g., avians, reptiles, guinea pigs, and some primates) were tested it was found that CFA could also be formed to the non-taste (visual), but clearly gustatory, characteristics of ingestibles. Rather than refute the apparent evolutionary importance of CFAs, these findings tended to provide additional support for the assertion that animals appeared to be biologically prepared to form associations between eating-related cues and post-ingestional consequences.

Recent developments have seen interests shift from research on CFA as a phenomenon to its use as a method to investigate other phenomena. The reason for this shift appears to be related to the robustness of the CFA phenomenon and to the fact that pharmacologic and toxicologic agents have been used extensively to induce the post-ingestional consequences that produce CFAs. That is to say, scientists have exploited the fact that it is possible to produce very strong and long lasting CFAs in one trial. They have also found it very convenient that the timing of the events

[a] Current address: Reviews Branch, Division of Extramural Affairs, National Heart, Lung, and Blood Institute, Bethesda, MD 20205.

to be associated is not crucial in the establishment of the CFA. Moreover, the obvious similarities between the conditioned avoidance of ingestibles in the laboratory situation and those that occur in the organism's natural habitat have not been overlooked. The net result has been a burgeoning of research using CFA methodology to study the control of predation among various wild animals, to study the pharmacologic and toxicologic action of drugs and other chemical substances, to modify and control compulsive behaviors such as alcoholism, to study the central nervous system, the endocrine system and the immune system, and to study both normal and abnormal human feeding behavior.

The purposes of a conference on CFAs are several. First, we were interested in updating research advances involving CFAs both as a phenomenon and as a behavioral assay. It was felt that such an evaluation was timely because during the eight years since the first major conference on CFAs at Baylor University twice as many research papers were published as had been published in the first fifteen years of research on CFAs, attesting to the continued popularity of research in the area.

Secondly, the conference provided an opportunity to bring together, at a critical time, scientists whose research interests are broadly based but all of whom are tied together either historically or functionally by a common interest in CFA methodology. It was hoped that progress could be facilitated by the cross-fertilization of research ideas and strategies between those who are using CFA methods to study other processes and those who are studying the phenomenon itself.

Third, the conference was organized to recognize the contributions made to research involving CFA not only by the participants who presented papers but also to recognize the contributions made by Dr. Patrick J. Capretta. Pat, one of the earliest contributors to the field, died at the age of 52 on September 29, 1982 following an episodic heart arrhythmia while jogging. He had spent twenty-one of his twenty-three years in academia associated with the Psychology Department at Miami University in Oxford, Ohio. His contributions to research on CFA began in the early 1960s when he studied the modification of food preferences in chickens and rats. These experiments were among the first to recognize the importance of the relationship between the act of ingestion and the nature of the post-ingestional consequences in the effective modification of feeding behavior. Results of the studies led to what he termed a principle of stimulus relevance that guided much of the early research in the area.

Pat's interests, however, were always broader than the CFA phenomenon. The central theme that pervaded his work and that he impressed on his students was to use whatever methods were available that would allow a complete understanding of the behavior under investigation. He was most interested in understanding the influences of social, developmental, biological, and evolutionary forces on behavior. Those interests were reflected in the diversity of his own research as well as in the diversity of his students' research while they studied with him and after they began their own research programs. His own research on the feeding behavior of the tassel-eared squirrel, which occupied his attention for the last 15 years of his life, reflected not only his professional orientation but also his deep concern about and love for the environment and world in which he lived. The story is told that he became interested in this problem while walking in the woods one day. Pat observed that the squirrels would eat the bark from some trees and not from others, even though the trees appeared to him to be the same. He hypothesized that the cues guiding the feeding behavior of these animals were related in some way to the taste or odor of the bark. His research led him to a chemical analysis of the bark and related tree parts and to the discovery that indeed there were differences between the chemistry of trees selected by the squirrels and those that they did not select. Thus once again Pat introduced a technique that at the time was innovative but today has become standard for naturalistic studies of feeding behavior.

The papers that follow are expanded versions of presentations made at the conference. Although it is difficult for a written piece to capture the spontaneity of the discussions and exchange of ideas that took place, these chapters represent a thorough review and analysis of research on CFA. It is particularly interesting to note that many of the questions that stimulated research on and with CFA 20 years ago remain to be answered. What appears to have changed, however, is the willingness of scientists to adopt new strategies and methods in answering them. It will be apparent to the reader that there are also new questions that have emerged as important to an understanding of CFA as a phenomenon and a method. To those of us who knew Pat Capretta or studied with him, it is also interesting to note that many of the unanswered questions as well as some of the newer ones were questions that he posed and pondered throughout his professional career. It is truly a tribute to him that we continue to try to find the answers.

Finally, I want to thank my co-organizer and co-editor, Paul Bronstein, who shared equally in the planning and execution of the conference and in the editing of this volume. In addition, many agents and officers of the New York Academy of Sciences helped guide us through the sequence of events that led to the successful completion of this project. In particular, we are especially thankful for the aid of Dr. William Cain, who chaired the committee responsible for this conference and who worked with us from the earliest stages of the project. His insights and creative efforts were indispensible.

PART I. ASSOCIATIVE PROCESSES IN THE FORMATION OF CONDITIONED FOOD AVERSIONS

Introduction: Associative Processes in the Formation of Conditioned Food Aversions – An Emerging Functionalism?

ROBERT C. BOLLES

Department of Psychology
University of Washington
Seattle, Washington 98195

The papers in this first session are supposed to be concerned with the associative processes that underlie the conditioning of taste aversions. It is interesting, however, that none of these papers really focuses upon associative processes as such. What I think I see in all these papers instead is the somewhat surprising emergence of something like a consensus on the explanatory importance of what might be called a new functionalism. "Functionalism" is an ambiguous label, let me explain what I mean by it. The explanation is actually given rather nicely by Shettleworth. She suggests that there is a spectrum, something like a rainbow, of explanatory devices for dealing with behavior. At one end of the spectrum, at the indigo-violet end, say, there are the mechanical principles of the hard sciences. The far-blue approach deals with genes and neurons, neural transmitters, and brain areas. This is the traditional mechanistic, reductionistic way to explain psychological phenomena. At the other end, over on the far-red side of the spectrum, we have "ultimate" or function-oriented explanatory devices such as inclusive fitness and the idea of adaptation to selection pressures. Orange considers perhaps how animals solve motivational and biological problems such as getting enough to eat. Psychologists range all over the spectrum, but the part of it that belongs peculiarly to them is the yellow-green part in the middle that couches its explanations of behavior in terms of associative mechanisms, learning principles, and so on. What I see in these papers in the first session is a small subtle shift, but a very significant one, out of the green (associative mechanisms per se as a universal explanatory account of learning) toward the yellow-orange part of the spectrum, toward a much more functionalistic view, which looks at aversions and preferences in terms of motivational systems. And perhaps it is the case that people who work with conditioned taste aversions are, in general, becoming increasingly more concerned with the biological significance of the phenomenon and less concerned with mediating mechanisms. I see this trend as somewhat surprising but, from my perspective, rather gratifying.

Garcia begins his paper by making a distinction between what I would call motivational systems. He refers to a system that defends the skin, the system that, in effect, defends the animal from external physical dangers; and he has a system that defends the gut, the gastrointestinal tract. The first system *has* to be peculiarly sensitive to noises and lights and other external stimuli. (I emphasize the word "has" to bring out the functional aspects of this system. It simply will not function functionally if it does not have this bias.) And the other system *has* to be sensitive to the tastes and odors of foods, and it has to be sensitive to the consequences of ingestion. There is another differentiation: the skin-defense system is rich in responses. Indeed, the whole point of such a system is to be able to produce adaptive motor behavior when the animal is confronted by an external threat. The gut defense system, on the other hand, is impoverished in terms of its response repertoire, but it can make a great variety of changes, and some very delicate changes, in the incentive value of taste and odor stimuli. Thus Garcia describes two separate systems designed to solve two separate kinds of problems, which it presumably does through quite different kinds of mechanisms. What makes this a functionalistic approach is that the analysis begins with function. It begins with what the system is designed to do, what it must do, and what its duty is if the animal is to solve its problems. Then later there is the search for mechanisms. Thus, it is only later that Garcia began the search for mutual inhibitory mechanisms such that the activation of one system would shut down the other. That he found mutual inhibition says, once again, that these systems have functional significance.

It is perfectly clear to me that the conditioned taste aversion phenomenon, the Garcia effect, transcends pure associationism. Indeed, that was the whole point of much of the early research on conditioned taste aversions. Capretta's[7] principle of stimulus relevance, that the act of consumption must be related to the consequences of consumption in order to modify food preferences, was an expansion of the functionalist-Thorndikian principle of belongingness. Similarly, Garcia, in the bright-noisy water experiment[10] said that we have to set aside all that we know about fundamental associative principles in order to deal with this particular phenomenon. We have to forget what we have learned to believe about interstimulus intervals and the equipotentiality or intersubstitutability of stimuli. Certain kinds of motivational systems will select certain classes of stimuli that are relevant to the solution of its problems. The interstimulus interval also *has* to be relevant. The animal *has* to be able to associate events with time intervals like those that appear in nature. If we analyze motivational systems that have evolved to solve a certain class of problems, then the parameters that that system works with have to be those that prevailed while the system was evolving. And if the parameters of this system violate the assumptions derived from other systems, that is just too bad; different systems have to serve different functions. That is the way the functionalist thinks of it. And that is quite different from the way the mechanist, over on the blue side of the spectrum, thinks of it.

The idea of separate motivational systems alerting the animal to certain classes of stimuli, priming certain classes of responses, and generally being designed to solve certain specific survival problems is very appealing to me. It is consistent with recent work from our laboratory that attempted to distinguish between a pain system and a fear system.[4] Mowrer[13] had said that fear is the conditioned form of the pain response, that the two were intimately related in that way. But what Fanselow and I concluded from our recent analysis is that they are separate systems that compete. Defensive behavior is motivated by fear, competes with recuperative behavior, which is motivated by pain. That is the way it has to be, if you think about it functionally, if you ask why animals defend themselves and why they recuperate. It appears that a functional analysis has forced us to set aside what had been the traditional associationist account of the matter.

Spear has found that the special problems that confront the neonatal rat lead us once again to set aside the general principles of association because empirically they do not seem to work. We are left with a functionalistic approach that stems from the fact that the young pup's life is dominated by its mother and its nest site. These special stimuli are so important, so overwhelmingly important for its welfare, that their presence can block conditioned taste aversion learning at a critical point in the pup's life. A few days later, as the young rat's lifestyle begins to change, then taste aversions can be conditioned just as they are in the adult.

In Booth's paper various kinds of nutritional challenges that he imposes on his subjects are described. His animals may be hungry, have an unbalanced diet, or they may be satiated. What he finds is that a variety of conditioning mechanisms come into play to connect the different body states with specific flavors and other oral stimuli. In consequence of this learning, one food may make the animal feel satiated, another may make it feel hungry, and so on. What I see reflected in Booth's work is the development of a number of feeding strategies that an omnivore like the rat can adopt. Thus, for example, I would anticipate that the very hungry rat that is in body weight deficit would, when given a choice, seek out foods it knew to be satiating. That is, of course, precisely what Booth found, and that is what we have found in our own lab.[5] Notice that these effects are not just associative. We cannot give a purely associative account of this learning in part because we do not know what the CS is or what US is, so we are not sure what the learning consists of or what brings this kind of learning about. And these effects are not just regulatory. As a matter of fact, the idea of a regulation mechanism—and certainly the idea of regulation about a set point—is beginning to collapse conceptually because, while it is attractive from a mechanistic point of view, it makes no sense at all functionally.[2] If we think of the ingestion of a balanced diet and the attainment of sufficient calories in functionalistic terms, if we think of it first as a practical problem that the animal has to solve, then we may have some hope of ultimately finding what the mechanisms are. Historically, the mechanists have always made the strategic error of believing they knew what the mechanism had to be; then they became perplexed when they could not find it. As Collier will make clear in his discussion, mechanisms are likely to be very complicated even when the problem seems quite simple from a functionalistic point of view.

In Domjan's paper there is explicit consideration of the fact that the associative principles that appear to apply to conditioned taste aversions really do appear to be somewhat distinct from those that apply to other kinds of associative learning. There is first the problem of stimulus specificity, or relevance. A sick animal learns nothing about bright, noisy water, as we learned long ago, because bright noisy water is, functionally speaking, irrelevant to its illness. Second, the long interstimulus interval over which conditioning is possible also makes sense functionally because illnesses generally do not come immediately but only some time after eating the wrong thing. Domjan points out that we have gradually come to take all of this for granted to such a great extent that we really do not know what the mechanisms are that make it possible. But no one except an associationist, a true blue associationist, would be seriously concerned about knowing why this particular system, the food system, is set aside from other kinds of associative learning or why it follows somewhat different principles. Functionalistically it has to follow different principles. I do not think Domjan is too worried about it, and that is to his credit. Let the associationists and the mechanists worry about how it is possible. After all it is really their problem. We functionalists can simply celebrate the fact that conditioned taste aversion should be different and is different from other kinds of conditioning.

One of the nice things about a functionalistic approach is that it forces us to look at behavior. It is, after all, behavior that interfaces the animal with reality on the output side; it is behavior that produces consequences. There is reality on the input side, too. But let us not worry about that at the moment. The important thing is that if we are going to call ourselves behaviorists we should focus on behavior. One of the things that has happened to associationism in recent years is that the nature of the association and the process of association formation has so obsessed some of our leading scholars, that they have forgotten why we have associations in the first place, which is to organize behavior adaptively. One of our leading scholars, Dickinson[8] tells us that his book is not going to focus on behavior; he is not really interested in what the animal does, but with how the animal learns that this event is linked to that event. He is interested in the animal's perception of causation. In another recent monograph we discover that the primary reason for studying second order conditioning is that it enables us to examine the associative process more or less directly without interference from the animal's behavior.[14] I'm happy to let them have associative processes; I will take the behavior.

One thing that pleased me about this first set of papers is the diversity of responses that are considered. We not only have consumption measures on the substance to be avoided, we also have frequent references to locomotion as the animal approaches or withdraws from the food source. We also have frequent references to the emotional expression about particular foods. What an exciting thing it is that thanks to the work of Grill and his colleagues we can get what is, in effect, a direct statement from the rat about whether it likes or dislikes a particular substance. And another thing that we see in the diversity of response, thanks largely to Booth's contribution, is conditioned preferences to supplement conditioned aversions. Thus, the data base has gotten much broader, guaranteeing generality and pretty much guaranteeing prosperity to all workers in this area. We also have a broadening of the data base in terms of Spear's work on infant animals, and the physiological work now coming out of Garcia's lab and Booth's efforts to build a broader base in terms of the animal's total nutritional problems, rather than restricting study just to the avoidance of toxins. I find all of these diversifying factors very exciting.

I want to focus briefly on two small points that emerged in these papers. My interest in these phenomena is, as you might expect, that they are related to my own research. Booth makes the distinction between oral and post-ingestive consequences of ingestion, and he observes that both kinds of event can serve as USs to reinforce taste preferences. I like that because it is very similar to what I have been saying recently. Booth finds that post-ingestive consequences can be either negative, such as toxicosis, or positive, such as caloric repletion. Conditioning occurs either way. We have found that if you put orange flavoring in 5% ethanol and expose rats to this concoction for 24 hours, they develop a preference for orange. They are tested with orange-flavored water against plain water, and they like it more than do appropriate control animals. It is interesting that our animals are still not too keen on ethanol at 5%, but they do like the orange. We find that this preference is probably due to the caloric benefit of the alcohol, because the preference is only revealed in our animals when they are tested hungry. If they are satiated at the time of testing, then they do not like the ethanol, and they are indifferent toward orange-flavored water. Sometimes we let our imagination run wild and think of conditioning as an attribution kind of process.[1] When the US comes along, the animal looks back and says, in effect, "What caused this US? Why do I feel good? It could not have been that terrible tasting ethanol; it must have been that orange stuff that makes me feel good when I am hungry." So, when it is hungry, it likes orange. We have also worked with the other part of Booth's distinction, his emphasis on the importance of purely oral stimuli. If you put orange flavoring in a saccharin solution, you find that the animal will begin to prefer orange-flavored water—that it will come to prefer the orange flavoring in water to plain water. So caloric repletion is not the only reinforcer. Purely hedonic stimuli, such as saccharin can also serve as reinforcers for establishing food preferences.[3]

The second small point I want to make has to do with the hedonic shift that surely occurs in conditioned taste aversions and maybe also occurs with conditioned preferences. Garcia has always stressed that when conditioning occurs in the gut-defense system, it produces a change in the incentive value of some taste; there is a hedonic shift in the flavor. This outcome can be contrasted with what happens if a taste cue is used to control instrumental behavior. The signal value of that particular taste turns out to be situation specific. Thus, animals that could avoid an electric shock whenever they tasted salt learned to run away from saline solutions. But they continued to drink salt solutions in their home cage.[11] The taste of salt could be used as a predictive cue without changing hedonic value, but when illness is the consequence, then hedonic value changes. So we began to suspect that perhaps change in hedonic value is a peculiar and unique property of what the conditioning consists of in the conditioned taste aversion situation.

Other kinds of evidence provide some support for this idea. Even conditioned preferences may be different. Recall that I just reported that the pairing of a taste like orange with sweetness only produced a preference for orange when the animal was hungry. And this, paradoxically, is true even though sweets are preferred by both hungry and sated animals. Some years ago when Perry Duncan was working in my lab, he paired a white noise with shock in a conditioning chamber. The animals were then taken back to the Skinner box where they had been bar pressing for food, and the white noise, or one much like it, was introduced as a probe on the bar-press baseline. He found essentially no suppression. We did not understand at the time how that was possible, because we had assumed that emotional responses get conditioned to CSs, and if a noise is paired with shock then we ought to get fear conditioned to that noise. Why did we find no fear? We now know that probably there was little fear because the contexts of conditioning and testing were so different, but it was a great mystery at the time. Apparently the skin defense system produces emotional responses (along with changes in motor behavior) that are highly specific to the conditioning context. It is as if the CS has signal value that might be compromised or augmented, by a particular test context, but the value of the CS itself, i.e., its intrinsic worth, is not changed. I do not think I can really defend the argument that there is no change in the CS's intrinsic value, but let me suggest that it does not change very much in comparison with the enormous change that occurs in its signal value when it is set up to predict shock. And the signaling of caloric benefit seems to be much the same, in that it is at least not primarily a matter of hedonic change.

Now, I have to admit that I am not entirely sure how one distinguishes a change in intrinsic or hedonic value of a CS and a change in its signal value that occurs as a result of conditioning, but I do think that these are very real alternatives. What sorts them out is probably the motivational system in which they are operative. One way to sort them out experimentally has already been suggested, and that is their generality over contexts. A loss of potential signal value occurs when the animal has no reason to expect a US in a new context. If a tone predicts shock in one situation, it does not necessarily implicate shock in a different situation. On the other hand, if you have an aversion to sauce Bernaise that was eaten in a particular restaurant, that aversion is usually going to appear whether you eat in that restaurant, a different restaurant, at home, or a friend's house. It is universal across contexts.

Another handle on the distinction may be obtained by varying motivation. A tone that signals shock brings its motivation, fear, with it. But fear is also controlled by contextual stimuli. On the other hand, if you have a flavor, such as vanilla, which signals a caloric load, that will be true whether the animal is hungry or satiated. Accordingly, one might anticipate a preference for vanilla when the animal is hungry and an aversion to it (see Booth) when the animal is satiated. But, on the other hand, there is the dessert phenomena. We know that having satiated itself on Purina, the rat will continue to ingest sugar. Unfortunately, we do not know whether the sugar taste signals something calorically rich or whether sugar is just hedonically good. Perhaps we could sort these things out by pairing an arbitrary taste such as vanilla with calories, on the one hand, and with a sweet taste, on the other, and then test animals hungry or satiated. We have not yet done that experiment properly.

We have taken a third approach to the question, however, which is to look at second-order conditioning. I mentioned this because I want to make clear to everyone that I came to this conference with some relevant new data. Its relevance is insured by my preceding remarks, which make it relevant, and its newness is attested by the fact it was produced specifically for this occasion. What we did was expose animals for a few days to sugar solutions that had, say, orange flavoring (actual flavors were counterbalanced). Then there were a few days in which orange flavoring was associated with vanilla in non-caloric fluids. The animals were then made hungry and given a two-bottle test between vanilla and plain water. They showed no preference at all for the second-order CS, vanilla. We ran large groups of animals; we obtained substantial levels of first-order conditioning; in short, we did everything that had to be done to obtain second-order conditioning, and it just was not there. So the conditioning of positive taste preferences seems to be much like conditioned taste aversions, in that second-order conditioning is very difficult to demonstrate. It can be done (e.g., Bond & Di Guisto[6]), but it is evidently problematic and tricky. Perhaps hedonic change per se is not subject to second-order conditioning. It may be recalled that reports of appetitive second-order conditioning only appear every fifty years or so in the literature,[9,12] and perhaps the thing is mainly limited to those situations in which it is the predictive-cue value of the CS that is critical, as in fear-conditioning.

In summary, I want to make three points. One is that all of the papers in this session reveal, to me at least, a movement away from purely associationistic and mechanistic explanation of behavior toward more functionalist accounts. Increasingly we seem to be more interested in why certain learning occurs and asking questions like if this kind of learning occurs, then what kinds of properties ought it to have? I view that as a very good sign. Second, there has been a diversity of response systems that have been linked to conditioned taste aversions, so that we have a much richer data base. And I think that is a very healthy development. Finally, these papers reveal that there is a growing effort to incorporate conditioned taste aversions and the learning mechanisms that have been revealed in that system within the broader context of food preferences, diet selection, nutritional balance, and caloric regulation. So conditioned taste aversions is not just an isolated phenomenon. It is becoming integrated with, and it is helping to integrate, the entire food intake literature, and I see that as a good thing, too.

REFERENCES

1. Bolles, R. C. 1976. Some relationships between learning and memory. *In* Processes of Animal Memory. D. L. Medin, W. A. Roberts & R. T. Davis, Eds. Hillsdale, NJ.
2. Bolles, R. C. 1980. Some functionalistic thoughts about regulation. *In* Analysis of Motivational Processes. F. M. Toates & T. R. Halliday, Eds. Academic Press. London.
3. Bolles, R.C. 1983. A mixed model of taste preferences in the rat. *In* Cognition and Animal Behavior. R. Mellgren, Ed. University of Oklahoma Press. Norman, OK.
4. Bolles, R. C. & M. S. Fanselow. 1980. A percetual-defensive-recuperative model of fear and pain. Behav. Brain Sci. **3**: 291–323.
5. Bolles, R. C., L. Hayward & C. Crandall. 1981. Conditioned taste preferences based on caloric density. J. Exp. Psychol. Anim. Behav. Proc. **7**: 59–69.
6. Bond, N. W. & E. L. DiGuisto. 1976. One-trial higher-order conditioning of a taste aversion. Austr. J. Psychol. **28**: 53–55.
7. Capretta, P. J. 1961. An experimental modification of food preferences in chickens. J. Comp. Physiol. Psychol. **54**: 238–242.

8. DICKINSON, A. 1980. Contemporary Animal Learning Theory. Cambridge University Press. London.
9. FROLOV, Y. (Cited by Pavlov, I. P., Conditioned reflexes. London: Oxford University Press, 1927).
10. GARCIA, J. & R. KOELLING. 1966. Relation of cue to consequence in avoidance learning. Psychon. Sci. **4**: 123–124.
11. GARCIA, J., R. KOVNER & K. GREEN. 1970. Cue properties vs palatability of flavors in flavor learning. Psychon. Sci. **20**: 313–314.
12. HOLLAND, P. C. & R. RESCORLA. 1975. Second-order conditioning with food unconditioned stimuli. J. Comp. Physiol. Psychol. **88**: 459–467.
13. MOWRER, O.H. 1947. On the dual nature of learning—a reinterpretation of "conditioning" and "problem solving." Harvard Ed. Rev. **17**: 102–148.
14. RESCORLA, R. A. 1980. Pavlovian second-order conditioning. Erlbaum Associates. Hillsdale, NJ.

A General Theory of Aversion Learning[a]

JOHN GARCIA,[b] PHILLIP S. LASITER,
FEDERICO BERMUDEZ-RATTONI, AND DANIEL A. DEEMS

Department of Psychology
Mental Retardation Research Center
University of California
Los Angeles, California 90024

> Infinitely various are the modifications of light and sound, whence they are each capable of supplying an endless variety of signs, and, accordingly, have been each employed to form languages; the one by the arbitrary appointment of mankind, the other by that of God himself. A connection established by the Author of Nature, in the ordinary course of things, may surely be called natural; as that made by men will be called artificial.
>
> GEORGE BERKELEY, *1733*

Not all associations are formed by the action of external events impinging upon the mind in concert. Strong associations exist without benefit of empirical cohesion owing to coexistence, causality, or similitude. Anticipating Darwin, Bishop Berkeley[6] said that these were natural connections instituted by the "Author of Nature." The same dichotomy is apparent in associative learning theory today. In contrast to Berkeley, who discussed natural connections as well as empirical associations, modern learning theorists attempt to base their explanatory constructs solely upon the stimuli presented in the laboratory, often ignoring the neural pathways along which the stimuli must travel.

Take, for example, Rescorla's[64] "Pavlovian Conditioning and its Proper Control Procedures." The initials CS and US, representing conditioned and unconditioned stimuli, respectively, coexist in his article about 130 times. The letter S, for subject, appears much less, about 30 times. The abbreviation CR, representing conditioned response, appears perhaps ten times, but we did not notice a single UR, which would imply a natural US-UR connection within S. On the ninth page of Rescorla's ten-page paper he finally reveals that S is a dog, CS is a tone, US is an electric shock, and that "fear" is conditioned. The use of abstract letters implies great generality for Rescorla's proposals, however, the limitation of his proposals are immediately apparent when concrete facts are substituted for abstract initials.

Rescorla proposes a "truly random control procedure," in which the CS and the US are presented without any contingency whatsoever between them. Rescorla admits, "What is explicitly unpaired for E, may not be explicitly unpaired for S." Then, he puts these doubts behind him and says, "A solution to this problem requires an ability, which we do not yet have, to identify psychological processes; until we do, *there is little choice but to associate psychological processes in Pavlovian conditioning with experimental operations*" (our italics). This is what we dare not do, for the psycho-

[a] Supported by National Institutes of Health Research Grant NS 11618 and Program Project Grant HD 05958.

[b] Address correspondence to: Dr. John Garcia, Neuropsychiatric Institute, Room 58-228, 760 Westwood Plaza, Los Angeles, California 90024.

logical processes within the subject are precisely what we perceive to be our subject matter.

Contrary to Rescorla's disavowal, a good deal is known about canine psychology. Dogs are orderly social animals. Their wild progenitors live in hierarchical packs communicating vocally, hunting cooperatively, and sharing food socially. The pack leaders enforce their authority with vocal threats (CS) followed by painful bites upon the skin (US); the subordinate members offer fearful ritualistic submission. Evolution, the Author of Nature, prepared the dog for domestication by human masters and for submissive performance in the shock-avoidance laboratory under an authoritative experimenter.

Methods, procedures, and controls are not Platonic universals, they are derived from particular theories and objectives. Since our aims differ from Rescorla's,[64] our procedures also will differ. For example, we never use the CS-US chaotic control procedure,[64] as suggested by Rescorla. Quite the contrary, we usually present the animal with various CS-US contingencies, some natural and others artificial, and then we observe what the animal learns best. But first, we heed the ethologist and learn all we can about our animal in its natural niche. After evaluating learning ability with natural stimuli we heed the haruspex and sacrifice the animal to seek explanations for behavior in its entrails and its neural matter. This is the neuroethological approach to learning.

GENERALIZING WITHIN SYSTEMS ACROSS SUBJECTS

Conditioned taste aversion research[27] has established two general principles, namely, cue-consequence specificity and long-delay learning. These principles specify that if other sensory inputs are substituted for Rescorla's tone and shock, his procedural propositions can be violated with impunity. For example, captive coyotes were given fresh ground beef (CS) and subsequently poisoned with lithium chloride in a single trial.[33] In about a half-hour or more, they became ill (US) and vomited (UR). Several days later they were presented with fresh, untainted ground beef. They sniffed, retched, and refused to eat. They displayed canine "disgust" reactions, urinating on the ground beef and rolling over it as dogs do when they encounter putrid matter. The signals, the procedures, and the conditioning parameters, drawn from Rescorla's analysis of noise-pain-fear training, have little validity for taste-toxin-disgust training, even within the same subject. This does not mean that there are no general laws of learning, quite the contrary, if we confine our analysis to an integrated sensory-motive-reaction system, be it noise-pain-fear or taste-toxin-disgust, we can generalize across a whole host of vertebrate subjects who share a common evolutionary history.

There are remarkable parallels in taste-toxin-disgust learning even between vertebrate and invertebrate species. When aposematically colored insects, such as milkweed bugs (*Lygacidae*) and monarch butterflies (*Danaidae*), feed on toxic milkweed, they incorporate the emetic cardenolide poison and thus become toxic themselves.[5] When they feed on other plants, they look the same but they are not toxic. When the eastern bluejay eats a toxic monarch butterfly, it becomes ill and vomits. Thereafter, the bird learns to distinguish toxic and safe butterflies by taste when seizing its prey in its beak, and it also learns to avoid capturing both toxic and safe monarch butterflies using only visual cues.[13,14] When the poisonous milkweed bug is captured by a predatory mantis a similar sequence is observed.[5] The mantis seizes the bug and takes a few voracious bites. After ingesting part of the bug, the mantis actively discards the remainder and then regurgitates copiously. After a few taste-illness trials, mantises learn to reject toxic milkweed bugs on sight. Subsequently, mantises will reject nontoxic milkweed bugs on the basis of visual cues, yet they will seize and eat other insects.

The natural history of the garden slug (*Limax*) indicates that it also must be an expert at toxic food learning. Conditioning experiments using vegetable flavors (odors and tastes) and poisons prove this is the case.[72] Furthermore, the association of food and toxin has been demonstrated *in vitro* using only a preparation of the slug's lips, cerebral ganglia, and buccal ganglia.[31,62] This is an elegant example of the neuroethological approach to learning.

Procedural learning propositions cannot distinguish between divergent and convergent evolution. The vertebrate feeders (coyote, bluejay) and the invertebrate feeders (mantis, slug) all learn about toxic food and behave in similar ways, despite the fact that their ancestral lines diverged prior to the Cambrian Period, some 500 million years ago. It is possible, then, that vertebrates and invertebrates share some common neural mechanisms because the gut is an ancient system. The common ancestor may have been a tube-like creature lined with internal chemical sensors of a primitive sort that later evolved into the oral receptors of food taste and the visceral monitors of food effect. On the other hand, it is more likely that vertebrate and invertebrate feeders independently evolved toxiphobic mechanisms as they faced the similar toxic defenses evolved by plants under pressure from generalized herbivores, perhaps during the Carboniferous Period about 300 million years ago. These speculative notions have one great heuristic advantage over bodiless learning theories; the implications can be tested by neuroethological, neuroanatomical, and neurophysiological research upon today's organisms.

SKIN-DEFENSE AND GUT-DEFENSE IN VERTEBRATES

In 1961, Garcia, Kimeldorf, and Hunt[28] set the stage for cue-consequence specificity by discussing the differential effects of X-ray exposure on taste aversion and place-avoidance learning in the rat. In 1968, Garcia and Ervin[25] presented a neural convergence hypothesis to explain cue-consequence phenomena in a paper entitled "Gustatory-Visceral and Telereceptor-Cutaneous Conditioning: Adaptation in the Internal and External Milieus." Since that time, neuroethological and psychobiological research has made much progress in modifying and extending the neural convergence hypothesis. Accordingly, we were surprised by Domjan's[20] contention that food aversion research has ignored the cue-consequence and long-delay characteristics of taste aversion learning in recent years. Domjan confined his discussion to purely associationistic theories, rejecting them all, but he did not consider neural convergence as an alternate theory. Therefore, we wish to summarize the evidence indicating that the convergence hypothesis is heuristically alive and well to this day.

The organization of the vertebrate brain reveals two specialized defensive systems that have evolved in response to selection pressures inherent in the food chain. To protect its skin from predatory attack, the vertebrate selectively associates exteroceptive stimuli with peripheral insults. To protect its gut from toxic foods, the animal selectively associates taste with delayed illness. The tiger salamander, a representative vertebrate feeder, has a modest central nervous system, yet somatosensory and auditory information converge at a common portion of the brain (FIGURE 1).[37] Such convergence provides a neural substrate for skin defense. Gustatory and visceral (gastrointestinal) information converge at common central neural pathways that are distinct from exteroceptive integrative systems (FIGURE 1). Convergence between gustatory and visceral pathways provides a substrate for gut defense. Olfactory pathways (and also the visual pathways) belong to neither system but have access to both skin defense and gut defense (FIGURE 1). Thus, evolution has arranged the central nervous system in a manner that affords relatively direct and independent integration of skin-defense and gut-defense processes.

FIGURE 2 is a block diagram incorporating much of the behavioral evidence for the dual-defense system.[27] Across the top, reflecting its dorsal position in body and brain, is the skin-defense system. The most effective way to challenge this system is to pair an externally referred CS (e.g., a noise) with immediate insult to the skin (e.g., an electric shock US). Subsequently, on hearing the noise CS, the vertebrate modifies its behavior to defend against shock: The noise is useful and the shock is fearful, as before conditioning, but a new coping behavior has been learned. Across the bottom of FIGURE 2, reflecting its ventral position in body and brain, is the gut-defense system. The most effective way to challenge this system is to pair a taste CS with an emetic toxic US. The emetic US may be applied an hour later, as indicated by the lateral extension of the time scale shown across the base of FIGURE 2. Vertebrates acquire a hedonically shifted response to a previously palatable taste CS following toxiphobic conditioning; the taste becomes aversive even in cases where the vertebrate has no "memory" of a CS-US association. Whether or not a human is aware of the "true cause" of its illness has little effect upon the learning of a taste aversion. Therefore, we have labeled this outcome as an "incentive modification."[29]

An inhibitory mechanism separates the two systems in FIGURE 2, simply illustrating the common observations that excitation of the external coping mechanisms is accompanied by inhibition of the internal digestive processes. For example, fear or apprehension abolishes feeding, appetite, and gastric motility. Reciprocally, activation of the ventral gut system has an inhibitory effect upon the dorsal coping mechanism. For example, a heavy meal often is followed by drowsiness and muscular relaxation.

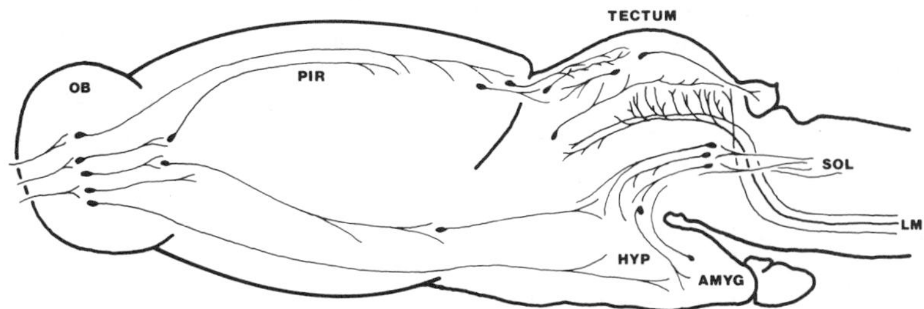

FIGURE 1. Organization of "external" and "internal" systems in the tiger salamander, redrawn from Herrick.[37] Somatosensory and auditory pathways converge at dorsal portions of the brain, particularly within the tectum. Gustatory and visceral projection pathways converge at ventral portions of the brain, particularly in the postero-ventral thalamic region, hypothalamus, and amygdala. Note that olfactory projections terminate both in dorsal and in ventral portions of the brain, providing a substrate for the putative gating mechanism for external and internal systems. Abbreviations are: AMYG, amygdala; HYP, hypothalamus; LM, lemniscal tracts, including somatosensory and auditory projections; OB, olfactory bulbs; PIR, piriform cortex; SOL, solitary nucleus. Optic radiations to the tectum are not shown for ease of visual presentation (cf. Fig. 11 in Herrick.[37])

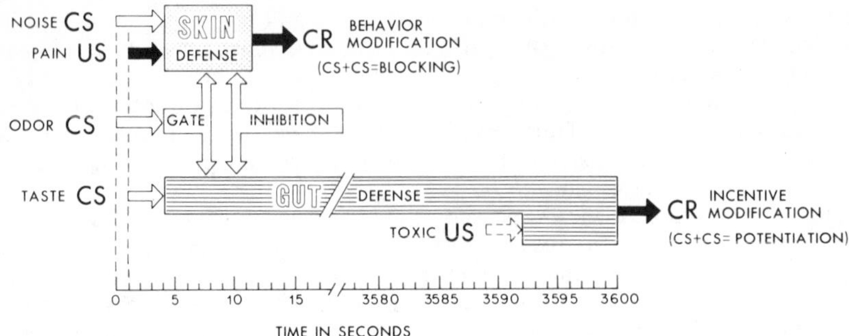

FIGURE 2. Block diagram of external (skin) defense and internal (gut) defense illustrating selective association of cue to consequence and differential CS-US delays within the two systems. Note that odor can be gated into either skin defense where it takes on the functional properties of a noise CS, or gut defense where it takes on the characteristics of a taste CS. In skin defense, behavior is modified as signals are used to defend against pain; and compound conditioning produces blocking. In gut defense the incentive value of taste is modified and compound conditioning produces potentiation.

THE ELUSIVE US IN TASTE AVERSION EXPERIMENTS

No single word can describe the US in taste aversion learning. Thus, the use of words such as "toxin," "nausea," and "emesis" are often challenged on semantic grounds. For example, Riley[66] semantically criticized the use of the word "toxin" by pointing out that cyanide will not induce a taste aversion. However, it is well known that cyanide produces its deadly effects through anoxia, without apparent emesis. Perhaps cyanide in nonlethal doses will induce place-avoidance learning. Gamzu[24] semantically criticized the use of the word "nausea," saying that the rat does not vomit. Notwithstanding, all behavioral indices of emesis can be observed in a poisoned rat. The abdomen retches, the back arches, the head lowers, the mouth gapes, and the tongue protrudes. The ingesta are not expelled because of anatomical and physiological limitations in the rat's upper gastric system. This fact is well known by those poisoning wild rats as pests. They take advantage of this peculiarity to produce rat-specific poisons; strong emetic agents that are easily vomited by children and pets are lethal for the rat, often rupturing the gastric system.

Vomiting, *per se*, is not a requisite defense against poison. The rat has other defenses. As Mitchell[54] points out, the rat is neophobic. On encountering a new food, or a familiar food in a new place, the rat examines the situation extensively, neck stretched, head extended, and vibrissae twitching as it sniffs. But neophobia cannot explain food aversions. Taste aversions and neophobia are distinguished by their unique expressions in behavior.[26] Characteristic behavioral signs of food aversions are retching, gaping, tongue protrusion, and chin rubbing.[32] Another defensive behavior is seen in the poisoned rat; it will ingest soil and dirt, which probably serve to chelate and/or absorb the ingested toxin. Dogs and other carnivores will ingest plants during toxicosis, perhaps for similar purposes.

The US in taste aversion learning is a complex homeostatic process that is impossible to describe in a single word or phrase. However, it can be concluded that internal malaise sets the occasion for food aversion learning. Lett[49] recently presented a crucial series of experiments that clarify the semantic issues raised regarding "internal," "external," "nausea," and "emesis." Each rat in the Lett study was given a distinctive taste and a distinctive place associated with poison. Another taste and another place was safe for each rat. Three kinds of toxic drugs were tested: (a) gallamine, producing neuromuscular blockade, (b) naloxone, blocking the action of endogenous opiates on pain, and (c) lithium chloride, inducing an emetic reaction. Gallamine and naloxone each produced strong place avoidances and weak taste aversions. Conversely, lithium chloride produced strong taste aversions and weak place avoidances.

Significantly, Lett[49] produced cue-consequence effects using only "toxic" injections. When she poisoned the skin-defense system with gallamine or naloxone, the behavioral effects were similar to those obtained with "external" pain consequences (e.g., shock). When she poisoned the emetic mechanisms of the gut-defense system with lithium chloride, she obtained the effects of "internal" nausea. But her injected drugs do not provide the "event-covariance" information required by Testa[75] for selective learning; rather, it was the biological site of drug action within the rat that produced differential cue-consequence associations.

Semantic confusion also arises because drugs rarely produce binary pharmacological actions, and hence, singular psychological and/or behavioral effects. For example, morphine has an emetic effect, an analgesic effect, a euphoric effect, and a stupefacient effect, all of which are dose dependent. Gallamine[49,50] produces muscular paralysis and strong place avoidance, yet it also produces weak taste aversions, indicating that it also has an emetic action. Other drugs have contradictory behavioral effects. Amphetamine[38] produces a taste aversion and a place preference, probably by producing an emetic effect on the ventral gut system and a euphoric effect upon the dorsal coping system. Thus, a particular drug may produce various behavioral effects, depending upon dose and biological locus of action.

It can be argued that even the use of the term "unconditioned stimulus" is inappropriate in taste-aversion learning because food aversions can be induced with low-dose gamma radiation treatments or emetic treatments that evoke no obvious behavioral signs of illness.[15,28,68] Flavor (odor and taste) aversions are the most sensitive behavioral index of prior emetic toxicosis in an ascending series of psychological reactions including anorexia, nausea, vertigo, and finally emesis. Therefore, a food aversion is often manifested in the absence of any other behavioral corroboration. Aversions can be induced by any agent that, at a higher dose, will produce emetic malaise. Thus, aversions are also produced by vestibular stimulation, by intense pain and emotion, or by verbal suggestion in humans. Consequently, aversions may be manifested in the absence of any "memory" of the US event, because the critical psychological process is a hedonic shift in the palatability of a taste and/or odor CS, not a CS-US association.[26,27,29] The CS has become "disgusting."

THE GATE: POTENTIATION OF LEARNING TO EXTEROCEPTIVE CUES

A sensory gate is illustrated between the skin and gut-defense systems in FIGURE 2. The gating action was demonstrated by Rusiniak and his associates,[70] using an array of acquisition conditions whereby odor was combined with taste concentrations ranging from low to high. A compound odor-taste stimulus was presented to thirsty rats followed either by immediate foot-shock or by delayed poison. Subsequently, odor alone was tested in extinction. The opposing effects observed in extinction covaried as a function of reinforcement condition and taste concentration. In the poisoned rats, taste potentiated odor-illness aversions. In the shocked rats, taste blocked odor-pain associations. However, the blocking effect was the opposite to that described by Kamin[39] because a weak taste component blocked associations with a strong odor component.[35,36] Furthermore, since the shock US and the toxin US produced opposing effects, an explanation based solely on CS interactions is inadequate.[21]

Normally, the gate is open to the skin-defense system so that odor is utilized as a external signal for painful peripheral insults such as foot-shock (FIGURE 2). Once odor is sequestered in the skin-defense system it cannot be utilized by the gut-defense system, at least not in one-trial conditioning procedures. The gate is closed to skin defense and opened to gut defense by the presence of taste and other feeding cues. Thus, odor attended by taste is sequestered in the gut-defense system where it is unavailable for association with shock and where it takes on the parametric properties of a taste.[60,69] The gating schema also is applicable to the potentiation of visual cues in rats[23] and in birds.[12,17,50] The blocking and potentiating implications indicated in the outputs of the skin-defense and gut-defense systems would be similar for visual cues. However, to date, most of the behavioral and neurological gating functions have been tested with odor.

GUSTATORY-VISCERAL CONVERGENCE AS A SUBSTRATE FOR TASTE-ILLNESS LEARNING

The idea that learned associations are mediated by convergence between central neural pathways can be traced to Ramon y Cajal.[63] It was Cajal's contention that higher-order "mental" functions depended upon the development or elimination of functional connections between convergent neural pathways. Presumably, increased activity in convergent pathways facilitates subsequent neural transmission along a common "output" channel, whereas decreased activity in convergent pathways diminishes such transmission. Kandel and Schwartz[40] have recently summarized observations that show that neural convergence mediates skin-defense learning in the invertebrate *Aplysia*. Prior and Gelperin[62] also have shown that neural convergence mediates gut-defense learning in the garden slug *Limax*. Cajal's so-called use-disuse hypothesis[71] suggests that convergence between gustatory, olfactory, and visceral projection pathways sets the occasion for aversion learning in mammals.

At the central level, aversion learning occurs when projection pathways associated with gustatory, olfactory, and visceral systems are activated in a specific temporal sequence. If illness information, conveyed by visceral projections, is relayed to projection pathways that have been recently activated by a gustatory and/or olfactory CS, taste-illness and/or flavor-illness connections may be established. On subsequent occasions "disgust" responses characteristic of emetic malaise may be manifested in response to the taste and/or odor CS.

As shown in FIGURE 1, gustatory and visceral projections converge in the neuraxis of the amphibian. In point of fact, convergence between gustatory and visceral projection pathways occurs in most vertebrate forms.[79] In mammals, gustatory-visceral convergence is established at first-order relays in the afferent gustatory and visceral pathways. Peripheral gustatory afferents of nerves VII, IX, and X synapse in the rostral two-thirds of the solitary nucleus.[1,2,77] Afferent fibers arising from the vagus nerve, which innervate the gastrointestinal tract, synapse in the caudal one-third of the solitary nucleus.[1] Gustatory and visceral areas of the solitary nucleus are connected by an abundant number of reciprocal connections.[52] It was this close anatomical relationship between gustatory and visceral projection systems within the solitary nucleus that led Garcia and Ervin[25] to suggest gustatory-visceral convergence as a mechanism for cue-consequence specificity.

Since then, the contribution of the vagus nerve and area postrema to learned aversions has been evaluated by vagotomy techniques and manipulations that challenge projection systems associated with the solitary nucleus. For instance, vagotomy will abolish vomiting in dogs.[10] Vagotomy will also attenuate taste aversion learning in rats,[42] whether induced by lithium chloride or by local irritation of the gastrointestinal tract with cupric sulfate. However, vagotomized dogs vomit in response to bloodborne toxins or to toxins that cross the blood-brain barrier. Area postrema, the so-called emetic center located at the obex of the medulla in the floor of the fourth ventricle, appears implicated in emetic responses to circulating toxins. Lesions of area postrema attenuate taste aversions induced by gamma radiation,[59] which are produced by histamine-like compounds present in the serum of irradiated rats.[51]

Area postrema lesions will not attenuate aversions induced by stimulation of the vestibular system. Internal malaise induced by rotational stimulation can establish taste aversions[45] and lesions in area postrema actually enhance rotation-induced aversions.[58] Apparently, the "emetic center" is normally inhibitory with regard to vestibular stimulation in the intact rat. Interestingly, the caudal solitary nucleus contains histamine receptors and most motion-sickness remedies contain antihistamine agents. Since projections of both the area postrema and the vestibular apparatus discharge to the caudal solitary nucleus[18,55] and alterations of input to the caudal solitary nucleus either facilitate or impair aversion learning, it is apparent that the caudal solitary nucleus is a primary relay station for aversion learning.

Gustatory and visceral projections of the solitary nucleus co-terminate within the second-order "gustatory" relay. Axons originating from neurons both in rostral and in caudal divisions of the solitary nucleus synapse at the parabrachial complex within regions described as the pontine taste area.[57,65] Rogers and associates[67] recently demonstrated that most, if not all, gustatory-response neurons in the parabrachial complex respond to electrical and chemical stimulation of the hepatic branch of the vagus nerve. DiLorenzo and Garcia[19] demonstrated that responses of parabrachial neurons to "palatable" tastes are altered as a function of taste-illness conditioning. Initial excitatory responses of parabrachial neurons to saccharin are greatly attenuated following toxiphobic conditioning and the altered responses resemble normal neural responses to "unpalatable" tastes such as quinine hydrochloride. Thus, the hedonic-shift hypothesis based upon behavioral observations has been supported by electrophysiological studies of parabrachial neurons. Such alterations in taste coding may be the basis for behavioral expressions of "disgust."

Gustatory-responsive neurons of the parabrachial complex project axons to the posterior ventromedial thalamic nuclei (FIGURE 3). Ventromedial thalamus receives projections from "visceroceptive" regions of the solitary nucleus,[3,22] and neurons in ventromedial thalamus respond both to sapid stimuli and to electrical and chemical stimulation of the hepatic branch of the vagus nerve.[67] Therefore, anatomical and physiological observations confirm that the thalamic "gustatory" relay receives convergent input from gustatory and visceral sources. Destruction of ventromedial thalamus severely impairs taste-illness learning in the rat,[44,53] yet destruction of ventromedial thalamus does not prevent odor-illness learning.[44] That observation implies that the gustatory thalamic relay is critical for taste-illness learning, but not for odor-illness learning. Taste-aversion learning impairments, observed following ventromedial thalamic damage, cannot be attributed strictly to attenuations in gustatory sensibility because rats lacking forebrain taste pathways respond to the hedonic characteristics of gustatory stimuli.[32] Thus, the damage induced "gustatory" thalamic relay mainly impairs taste-illness learning.

As illustrated in FIGURE 3, gustatory thalamocortical projections synapse both in

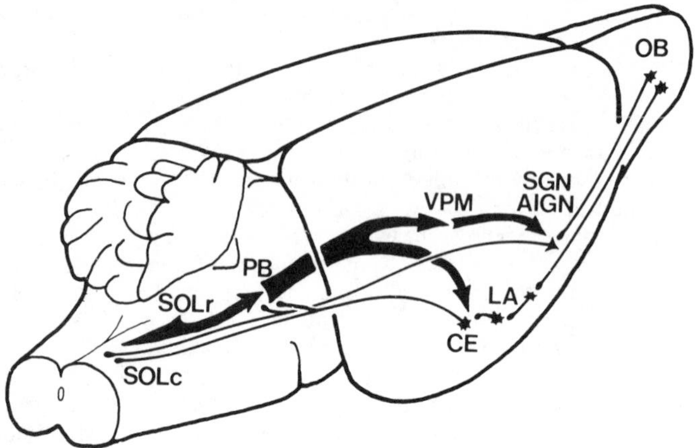

FIGURE 3. Convergent projection pathways implicated in aversion learning. Destruction of the somatic gustatory neocortex will disrupt taste aversions, but not taste-potentiated odor aversions. Lesion placement in the insular gustatory neocortex will disrupt taste aversions and taste-potentiated odor aversions. Lesion placements or pharmacological manipulations directed at the amygdala will disrupt odor-toxin associations, but not taste-toxin or odor-shock associations. Abbreviations are: AIGN, anterior insular gustatory neocortex; CE, central nucleus of amygdala; LA, lateral nucleus of amygdala; OB, olfactory bulbs; PB, parabrachial complex; SGN "somatic" gustatory neocortex; SOLc and SOLr, caudal and rostral solitary nuclei, respectively; VPM, posterior ventromedial thalamic nuclei.

the ventral somatosensory (gustatory) neocortex and in the anterior insular (gustatory) neocortex.[4,11] Destruction of gustatory thalamocortical projections attenuates taste-illness learning.[44,48] Lesion placements centered either in the somatic gustatory neocortex or in the insular gustatory neocortex disrupt taste aversion acquisition, and the retention of preoperatively established taste avoidance responses.[11,41,44,46,48] Aversion learning deficits observed following destruction of the gustatory thalamocortical relay are similar to those observed following elimination of ventromedial thalamus: Animals lacking the gustatory thalamocortical relay respond to the hedonic characteristics of each basic taste and show behavioral signs of illness, yet those animals exhibit impaired taste aversion learning.[11,46] Thus, gustatory thalamocortical projections, and the neocortical projection field of gustatory thalamocortical projections, contribute to taste-illness learning. It is apparent that gustatory pathways in the thalamus and neocortex play an integral role in taste aversion learning.

OLFACTORY-GUSTATORY-VISCERAL CONVERGENCE AS A SUBSTRATE OF FLAVOR-ILLNESS LEARNING

Olfactory and gustatory information has relatively direct access to the insular gustatory neocortex (FIGURE 3). Direct electrical stimulation of the lateral olfactory tract produces slow-wave potentials in the insular gustatory neocortex.[34] The insular gustatory neocortex also receives direct projections from the olfactory bulbs and intracortical projections from anterior and posterior divisions of the piriform cortex.[30,34] Norgren and Grill,[56] and more recently Saper[73] and Shipley,[74] have shown that neurons in the insular gustatory neocortex project axons to the parabrachial complex and to the caudal solitary nucleus. Therefore, "output" circuits of the insula can directly modulate the activity of neurons in lower-order relays of the gustatory and/or visceral projection pathways.

The nature of convergence between olfactory, gustatory, and visceral projections within the somatic and insular gustatory neocortices must ultimately dictate the differential effects observed following destruction of those neocortical regions. The somatic and insular gustatory neocortices can be distinguished anatomically with regard to gustatory-visceral convergence and olfactory-gustatory-visçeral convergence, respectively. Accordingly, Kiefer and associates[41] have shown that aspirations of the somatic gustatory neocortex disrupt taste aversion learning, but not taste-potentiated odor aversion learning. On the other hand, electrolytic lesion placements centered in the insular gustatory neocortex impair both taste aversion learning and taste-potentiated odor aversion learning.[47]

The behavioral results obtained following destruction of either the somatic gustatory neocortex or the insular gustatory neocortex reflect the intrinsic connectivity of those neocortical regions. The somatic and insular gustatory neocortices each receive gustatory thalamocortical projections, but only the insular gustatory neocortex receives direct olfactory input. Neurons in the somatic gustatory neocortex project axons to insular neurons. In turn, axons of insular neurons discharge to the parabrachial complex and solitary nuclei. Thus, intracortical projections from the somatic gustatory neocortex to the insula normally establish one source of gustatory-visceral convergence. Damage induced to the somatic gustatory region will eliminate gustatory-visceral convergence, disrupting taste-illness learning. Conversely, olfactory-gustatory-visceral convergence is normally established at the insula, and destruction of the insula impairs both taste-illness learning and flavor-illness learning.

The amygdaloid complex is recognized as a telencephalic structure that participates in olfactory-guided behaviors. A prominent and well-recognized source of olfactory input to the amygdala arises via axons from the accessory olfactory bulbar formation and projections from that region synapse at the cortico-medial amygdaloid nuclei.[18] "Gustatory" regions of the amygdala (central nucleus[11]) also receive projections from the olfactory cortex.[77] Finally, neurons within the central amygdaloid nuclei project axons to the parabrachial complex and caudal solitary nucleus, similar to that described for the insular gustatory neocortex.[43,61] Thus, the insular gustatory neocortex and the central nucleus of amygdala each shares direct reciprocal connectivity with lower-order relays in the gustatory and/or visceral projection pathways.

Application of novocaine to the dorsolateral amygdaloid region preferentially degrades taste-potentiated odor aversion learning as opposed to taste aversion learning.[8] Amygdaloid anesthesia does not disrupt simple odor-shock or taste-illness learning. In fact, novocaine injections tend to enhance odor-shock avoidance and taste-illness aversions. Therefore, the amygdaloid complex mainly appears to mediate flavor-illness learning. Lesions restricted to the lateral amygdaloid nuclei also produce impairments in potentiated odor aversion learning.[7] Again, it is noteworthy that olfactory-gustatory-visceral convergence is established at the central and lateral amygdaloid nuclei, and that invasive manipulations directed at the amygdala primarily affect flavor-illness learning.

Applications of cholinergic agonists and antagonists to the amygdala produce weak disruptions and enhancements of odor aversions, respectively, but taste aversion learning remains unaffected.[7] Much stronger effects are found when those drugs are infused in the dorsal hippocampus, but not when they are infused in the overlying parietal neocortex.[7] Such effects indicate that cholinergic agonists disrupt flavor-illness learning and that cholinergic antagonists enhance flavor-illness learning. Those results suggest that cholinergic systems of the hippocampus normally inhibit the amygdala with regard to flavor-illness learning.

The foregoing neurobehavioral observations illustrate that convergence between gustatory, olfactory, and visceral pathways is a requisite condition for normal taste-illness learning, odor-illness learning, and flavor-illness learning. Invasive manipulations that affect portions of the brain where gustatory-visceral convergence occurs alter taste-illness learning; manipulations that affect olfactory-gustatory-visceral convergence alter flavor-illness learning.

TWO KINDS OF LEARNING

As Bolles[9] commented, there must be many sensory-motive-reaction systems within any complex animal. We have discussed only two such systems in vertebrates, but we consider each to be a subsystem representative of two more general systems. The skin-defense subsystem is part of the external coping mechanisms by which the vertebrate makes contact with its goals in time and space. The instrumental approach to food, guided by vision and olfaction, is part of the external coping system, so is the approach to a receptive mate or to a warm shelter.

The gut-defense subsystem is part of the internal homeostatic system, where the hedonic value of goal objects are set according to their usefulness in the internal economy.[16] Accordingly, if a particular food satisfies metabolic needs, it will be more palatable the next time it is encountered. If a particular mate leads to sexual satisfaction, then that mate becomes more desirable. When the core temperature is cold, a warm shelter is pleasant. In each case, the peripheral receptors that contact the goal object during consummation play a pivotal role; on the one hand, by receiving the internal feedback that adjusts the hedonic value of the goal object, and on the other hand, by potentiating the distal stimuli that lead to successful consummation.

In a paper entitled "There is more than one kind of learning," Edward C. Tolman[76] discussed two kinds of learning that resemble the conditioning we have described herein: A field expectancy is acquired as the animal is repeatedly presented with an environmental situation to which it is sensitive, and through which it moves. As a result, the animal appreciates not only the immediate stimulation, but it learns to expect subsequent stimulation. That animal also learns to take appropriate shortcuts and roundabout routes through the field. Cathexes are formed when, under a given drive, the animal performs a consummatory reaction upon a specific type of goal; if the drive is satisfied, that specific goal is positively cathected. Thus, we acquire ". . . cathexes for new foods, drinks, sex objects, etc., by trying out the corresponding consummatory responses on such objects and finding that they work."[76]

Tolman suggested that ". . . if we can agree that there are really a number of different kinds of learning . . . then it may turn out that the theory and laws appropriate to one kind may well be different from those appropriate to other kinds." That is exactly what the cue-consequence and long-delay characteristics of conditioned food aversions have demonstrated.

REFERENCES

1. Allen, W. F. 1923. Origin and distribution of the tractus solitarius in the guinea pig. J. Comp. Neurol. **35**: 171–204.
2. Åstrom, K. E. 1953. On the central course of afferent fibers in the trigeminal, facial, glossopharyngeal, and vagal nerves and their nuclei in the mouse. Acta Physiol. Scand. (suppl. 106) **29**: 209–320.
3. Beckstead, R. M. & R. Norgren. 1979. An autoradiographic examination of the central

distribution of the trigeminal, facial, glossopharyngeal, and vagal nerves in the monkey. J. Comp. Neurol. **184**: 455–472.
4. Benjamin, R. M. & H. Burton. 1968. Projection of taste nerve afferents to anterior opercular-insular cortex in squirrel monkey (*Saimiri sciureus*). Brain Res. **7**: 221–231.
5. Berenbaum, M. R. & E. Miliczy. 1983. Mantids and milkweed bugs: Efficacy of aposematic coloration against invertebrate predators. Amer. Mid. Natural. **111**: 64–68.
6. Berkeley, G. 1733. The Theory of Vision, or Visual Language, Shewing the Immediate Presence and Providence of a Deity, Vindicated and Explained (London, 1733) sect. 39–43. *In* History of Psychology. W. S. Sahakian. F. E. Peacock. Itasca, IL.
7. Bermudez-Rattoni, F. 1984. Flavor-illness aversions: Potentiation of taste is regulated by the limbic system. Unpublished doctoral dissertation. University of California. Los Angeles.
8. Bermudez-Rattoni, F., K. W. Rusiniak & J. Garcia. 1983. Flavor-illness aversions: Potentiation of odor by taste is disrupted by application of Novocaine into amygdala. Behav. Neural Biol. **37**: 61–75.
9. Bolles, R. 1985. Associative processes in the formation of conditioned food aversions. Ann. N.Y. Acad. Sci. This volume.
10. Borison, H. L. & S. C. Wang. 1953. Physiology and pharmacology of vomiting. Pharm. Rev. **5**: 193–230.
11. Braun, J. J., P. S. Lasiter & S. W. Kiefer. 1982. The gustatory neocortex of the rat. Physiol. Psychol. **10**: 13–45.
12. Brett, L. P., W. G. Hankins & J. Garcia. 1976. Prey-lithium aversions. III. Buteo hawks. Behav. Biol. **17**: 87–98.
13. Brower, L. P. & J. V. Z. Brower. 1964. Birds, butterflies and plant poisons: A study in ecological chemistry. Zoologica **49**: 137–159.
14. Brower, L. P. & J. V. Z. Brower. 1974. Palatability dynamics of cardenolides in the monarch butterfly. Nature **249**: 280–283.
15. Buchwald, N. A., J. Garcia, B. H. Feder & Y. Bach-y-Rita. 1964. Ionizing radiation as a perceptual and aversive stimulus II. Electrophysiological studies. *In* The Responses of the Nervous System to Ionizing Radiation. T. J. Haley & R. S. Snyder, Eds.: 687–721. Little Brown Co. Boston, MA.
16. Cabanac, M. 1979. Sensory pleasure. Quart. Rev. Bio. **54**: 1–29.
17. Clarke, J. C., R. F. Westbrook & J. Irwin. 1979. Potentiation instead of overshadowing in the pigeon. Behav. Neural. Biol. **25**: 18–29.
18. Crosby, E. C., T. Humphrey & E. W. Lauer. 1962. Correlative Anatomy of the Nervous System. Macmillan Co. New York.
19. DiLorenzo, P. M. & J. Garcia. 1983. Taste responses of parabrachial units to NaCl and saccharin in rats that were pretrained to avoid Na saccharin. Soc. Neurosci. Abst. **9**: 1023.
20. Domjan, M. 1985. Long-delay learning revisited. Ann. N.Y. Acad. Sci. This volume.
21. Durlach, P. J. & R. A. Rescorla. 1980. Potentiation rather than overshadowing in odor-aversion learning: An analysis in terms of within compound associations. J. Exp. Psychol. **6**: 175–187.
22. Fukushima, T. & W. L. Kerr. 1979. Organization of trigeminothalamic tracts and other thalamic afferent systems of the brainstem in the rat: Presence of Gelatinosa neurons with thalamic connections. J. Comp. Neurol. **183**: 169–184.
23. Galef, B. G. 1985. Social transmission of food preferences in rats. Ann. N.Y. Acad. Sci. This volume.
24. Gamzu, E. 1985. A pharmacological perspective of drug used in establishing conditioned food aversions. Ann. N.Y. Acad. Sci. This volume.
25. Garcia, J. & F. R. Ervin. 1968. Gustatory-visceral and telereceptor-cutaneous conditioning. Adaptation in the internal and external milieus. Comm. Behav. Biol. **1**: 389–415.
26. Garcia, J., D. Forthman-Quick & D. White. Conditioned disgust and fear from mollusk to monkey. *In* Primary Neural Substrates of Learning and Behavioral Change. D. L. Alkon & J. Farley, Eds.: 47–61. Harvard University Press. Cambridge, MA.
27. Garcia, J., W. G. Hankins & K. W. Rusiniak. 1974. Behavioral regulation of the milieu interne in man and rat. Science **184**: 824–831.
28. Garcia, J., D. J. Kimeldorf & E. L. Hunt. 1961. The use of ionizing radiation as a motivating stimulus. Psychol. Rev. **68**: 383–395.
29. Garcia y Robertson, R. & J. Garcia. 1984. X-rays and learned taste aversions: Historical and psychological ramifications. *In* Nutrition and Eating Behavior: A Biobehavioral Per-

spective. T. G. Burish, S. M. Levy & B. E. Meyerowitz, Eds. Lawrence Erlbaum. New York. (In press.)

30. Geinisman, Y., M. T. Shipley & J. F. Disterhoft. 1982. Anatomical evidence for a convergence of olfactory and gustatory-visceral afferent pathways in mouse cerebral cortex. Soc. Neurosci. Abst. **8**: 9.
31. Gelperin, A., J. J. Chang & S. C. Reingold. 1978. Feeding motor program in Limax. I. Neuromuscular correlates and control by chemosensory input. J. Neurobiol. **9**: 285–300.
32. Grill, H. & R. Norgren. 1978. The taste reactivity test. II. Mimetic responses to gustatory stimuli in chronic thalamic and chronic decerebrate rats. Brain Res. **143**: 281–297.
33. Gustavson, C. R., J. Garcia, W. G. Hankins & K. W. Rusiniak. 1974. Coyote predation control by aversive conditioning. Science **184**: 581–583.
34. Haberly, L. B. & J. L. Price. 1978. Association and commissural fiber systems of the olfactory cortex of the rat: I. Systems originating in the piriform cortex and adjacent areas. J. Comp. Neurol. **178**: 711–740.
35. Hankins, W. G., J. Garcia & K. W. Rusiniak. 1973. Dissociation of odor and taste in baitshyness. Behav. Biol. **8**: 407–419.
36. Hankins, W. G., K. W. Rusiniak & J. Garcia. 1976. Dissociation of odor and taste in shock-avoidance learning. Behav. Biol. **18**:345–358.
37. Herrick, C. J. 1948. The Brain of the Tiger Salamander. pp. 329–331. University of Chicago Press. Chicago, IL.
38. Holman, E. W. 1975. Immediate and delayed reinforcers for flavor preferences in rats. Learn. Motiv. **6**: 91–100.
39. Kamin, L. J. 1969. Predictability, surprise, attention and conditioning. *In* Punishment and Aversive Behavior. B. A. Campbell & R. M. Church, Eds.: 279–296. Appleton-Century-Crofts. New York.
40. Kandel, E. R. & J. H. Schwartz. 1982. Molecular biology of Learning: Modulation of transmitter release. Science **218**: 433–443.
41. Kiefer, S. W., K. W. Rusiniak & J. Garcia. 1982. Flavor-illness aversions: Potentiation of odor by taste in rats with gustatory neocortical ablations. J. Comp. Physiol. Psychol. **96**: 540–548.
42. Kiefer, S. W., K. W. Rusiniak, J. Garcia & J. D. Coil. 1981. Vagotomy facilitates extinction of conditioned taste aversions in rats. J. Comp. Physiol. Psychol. **95**: 114–122.
43. Krettek, J. E. & J. L. Price. 1978. A description of the amygdaloid complex in the rat and cat with observations on intra-amygdaloid axonal connections. J. Comp. Neurol. **178**: 255–280.
44. Lasiter, P. S. 1983. On the contribution of forebrain gustatory centres to the learning of taste aversions. I. The pigmented rat (Rattus norvegicus). Doctoral Dissertation. Arizona State University, 1982. Diss. Abs. Intl. **43**: 3400B (University Microfilms No. DA 8305858).
45. Lasiter, P. S. & J. J. Braun. 1981. Shock facilitation of taste aversion learning. Behav. Neural Biol. **32**: 277–281.
46. Lasiter, P. S. & D. L. Glanzman. 1982. Cortical substrates of taste aversion learning: Dorsal prepiriform (Insular) lesions disrupt taste aversion learning. J. Comp. Physiol. Psychol. **96**: 376–392.
47. Lasiter, P. S., D. A. Deems & J. Garcia. 1985. Involvement of the anterior insular gustatory neocortex in taste-potentiated odor aversion learning. Physiol. Behav. (In press.)
48. Lasiter, P. S., D. A. Deems & D. L. Glanzman. 1985. Thalamocortical relations in taste aversion learning. I. Involvement of gustatory thalamocortical projections in taste aversion acquisition. Behav. Neurosci. (In press.)
49. Lett, B. T. 1984. The painlike effect of gallamine and naloxone differs from sickness induced by lithium. Behav. Neurosci. (In press.)
50. Lett, B. T. 1984. Taste potentiation in poison avoidance learning. *In* Quantitative Analyses of Behavior: Vol. 3, Acquisition. M. L. Commons, R. J. Hernstein & A. R. Wagner, Eds. Ballinger. Cambridge, MA. (In press.)
51. Levy, C. K., F. R. Ervin & J. Garcia. 1970. Effect of serum from irradiated rats on gastrointestinal function. Nature **225**: 463–464.

52. Loewy, A. D., & H. Burton. 1978. Nuclei of the solitary tract: Efferent projections to the lower brain stem and spinal cord of the cat. J. Comp. Neurol. **1981**: 421–450.
53. Loullis, C. C., M. J. Wayner & F. B. Jolicoeur. 1978. Thalamic taste nuclei lesions and taste aversion learning. Physiol. Behav. **20**: 653–655.
54. Mitchell, D. 1985. Phobic responses to novelty. Ann. N.Y. Acad. Sci. This volume.
55. Morest, D. K. 1967. Experimental study of the projections of the nucleus of the tractus solitarius and the area postrema in the cat. J. Comp. Neurol. **130**: 277–300.
56. Norgren, R. & H. Grill. 1976. Efferent distribution from the cortical gustatory area in rats. Soc. Neurosci. Abst. **2**: 124.
57. Norgren, R. & C. Pfaffmann. 1975. The pontine taste area in rat. Brain Res. **91**: 99–117.
58. Ossenkopp, K. P. 1983. Area postrema lesions in rats enhance the magnitude of body rotation-induced conditioned taste aversions. Behav. Neural Biol. **38**: 82–96.
59. Ossenkopp, K. P. 1983. Taste aversions conditioned with gamma radiation: attenuation by area postrema lesions in rats. Behav. Brain. Res. **7**: 297–305.
60. Palmerino, C. C., K. W. Rusiniak & J. Garcia. 1980. Flavor-illness aversions: The peculiar roles of odor and taste in memory for poison. Science **208**: 753–755.
61. Price J. L. & D. G. Amaral. 1981. An autoradiographic study of the projections of the central nucleus of the monkey amygdala. J. Neurosci. **1**: 1242–1259.
62. Prior, D. & A. Gelperin. 1977. Autoactive molluscan neuron: Reflex function and synaptic modulation during feeding in the terrestrial slug Limax maxiums. J. Comp. Physiol. **114**: 217–232.
63. Ramon y Cajal, S. 1911. Histologie du Systeme Nerveux de L'Homme et des Vertebres. **2**: 887–890. Maloine. Paris.
64. Rescorla, R. A. 1967. Pavlovian conditioning and its proper control procedures. Psych. Rev. **74**: 71–80.
65. Ricardo, J. A. & E. T. Koh. 1978. Anatomical evidence of direct projections from the nucleus of the solitary tract to the hypothalamus amygdala, and other forebrain structures in the rat. Brain Res. **153**: 1–26.
66. Riley, A. L. 1985. Conditioned taste aversions: A behavioral index of drug toxicity. Ann. N.Y. Acad. Sci. This volume.
67. Rogers, R. C., D. Novin & L. L. Butcher. 1979. Hepatic sodium and osmoreceptors activate neurons in the ventrobasal thalamus. Brain Res. **168**: 398–403.
68. Rusiniak, K. W., W. G. Hankins & J. Garcia. 1976. Bait-shyness: Avoidance of the taste without escape from the illness. J. Comp. Physiol. Psychol. **90**: 460–467.
69. Rusiniak, K. W., W. G. Hankins, J. Garcia & L. P. Brett. 1979. Flavor-illness aversions: Potentiation of odor by taste in rats. Behav. Neural. Biol. **25**: 1–17.
70. Rusiniak, K. W., C. C. Palmerino, A. G. Rice, D. L. Forthman & J. Garcia. 1982. Flavor-illness aversions: Potentiation of odor by taste with toxin but not shock in rats. J. Comp. Physiol. Psychol. **96**: 527–539.
71. Rutledge, L. T. 1976. Synaptogenesis: Effects of synaptic use. *In* Neural Mechanisms of Learning and Memory. M. R. Rosenzweig & E. L. Bennett, Eds.: 329–339.
72. Sahley, C. L., A Gelperin & J. Rudy. 1981. One-trial associative learning modifies food odor preferences of a terrestrial mollusc. Proc. Natl. Acad. Sci. USA **78**: 640–642.
73. Saper, C. B. 1982. Reciprocal parabrachial-cortical connections in the rat. Brain Res. **242**: 33–40.
74. Shipley, M. T. 1982. Insular cortex projection to the nucleus of the solitary tract and brainstem visceromotor regions in the mouse. Brain Res. Bull. **8**: 138–148.
75. Testa, T. J. 1974. Causal relationships and the acquisition of avoidance responses. Psych. Rev. **81**: 491–505.
76. Tolman, E. C. 1949. There is more than one kind of learning. Psych. Rev. **55**: 189–208.
77. Torvik, A. 1956. Afferent connections to the sensory trigeminal nucleus of the solitary tract and adjacent structures. An experimental study in the rat. J. Comp. Neurol. **106**: 51–141.
78. Veening, J. G. 1978. Subcortical afferents of the amygdaloid complex in the rat: An HRP study. Neurosci. Lett. **8**: 197–202.
79. Watterman, A. J. 1971. Chordate Structure and Function. Macmillan. New York.

Food-conditioned Eating Preferences and Aversions with Interoceptive Elements: Conditioned Appetites and Satieties

D. A. BOOTH[a]

Department of Psychology
University of Birmingham
Birmingham B15 2TT, England

The adaptive importance of acquired feeding habits has long been acknowledged in research on obesity[1] and animal foraging[2] for example. Yet so few experiments have measured learning under physiologically and ecologically normal conditions that there is insufficient information for effective applications in the clinic and everyday life,[3] the foods[4] or pharmaceuticals[5] industries, or animal husbandry.[6]

Nevertheless, it has been established that normal feeding in the laboratory rat is associatively conditioned by nutritional consequences.[7-11] Occasionally, aversions are conditioned. However, what is usually learned is facilitation of feeding (TABLE 1), which accounts for much of the incentive to forage and the palatability of foods and drinks.[13]

CONDITIONING IN NUTRIENT SELF-SELECTION

Allowance for aversion/preference conditioning is crucial in research on dietary selection.

Behavioral Compensation for Deficiency

Davies[22] reported that human infants showed considerable "nutritional wisdom" when fed what they appeared to want from among an array of "natural" foodstuffs. The infants stayed healthy; some symptoms of nutritional deficiency even remitted.

Experiments in rats suffering from serious nutritional deficiencies (or from dietarily ameliorable hormonal disorders) demonstrated corrective selection among diets concentrated in different nutrients.[23] This indicated a considerable range of "nutritional wisdom" in the organization of the behavior of omnivores other than humans as well.

Such results have often been subsumed under "homeostatic regulation." This is either a non-explanatory classification of the observations or the invocation of a misleading and dubiously complex model. There is no evidence that ingestive behavior, or indeed any other behavioral or physiological activity, is controlled by a predetermined and measured "set point" of some physiological characteristic, such as

[a] Address correspondence to: Dr. D. A. Booth, Department of Psychology, University of Birmingham, P. O. Box 363, Birmingham B15 2TT, England.

TABLE 1. First Observations of Ingestion/Egestion or Foraging/Rejection Conditioned by Postingestional Effects of Normal Nutrients in Rats

Unconditioned Stimulus	Conditioned Stimulus	Reference
	Conditioned aversion and deappetizing/satiation	
Concentrated glucose[b]	Odor or taste	14
Continued thiamin deficiency[b]	Diet	15
Concentrated starch on near repletion	Repletion plus odor[c]	10
Undigested fat[b]	Odor/taste	16
	Conditioned preference and appetite/desatiation	
Whole diet on high deprivation	Place	17
Whole diet (on self-deprivation?)	(Taste)	18
Water on water deprivation	Taste/odor	19
Balanced amino acids on deprivation	Odor or taste	8
Concentrated or dilute starch ad lib	Taste[a]	9
Dilute starch on part repletion	Repletion (? gastric) plus odor, taste, or texture	10 11
Part withdrawal of whole diet	(Repletion plus taste)	12
(Delayed oral) glucose[b] on low deprivation	Odor	20
Partly digested fat on low deprivation	Odor/taste	16
(Intravenous) glucose on part repletion	Odor	21

[a] An absolute preference CR, and to an odor CS, demonstrated subsequently (TABLE 2).
[b] Arguably not part of a natural nutritional occurrence.
[c] Can include an absolute aversion CR to an odor CS during repletion (TABLE 3).

blood glucose concentration or uptake rate, body fat mass or cell size, body water or sodium content, body temperature, or the like.[3,6,24,25] The approximation to constancy of the internal milieu that in fact occurs is quite limited and is modulated by internal cycles[26] and by variations amongst habitats.[7]

Furthermore, healthy dietary selection is not necessarily evidence for fine control of behavior by nutritional requirements. An individual's physiology can adapt to remarkable departures from the normal average intakes of energy-rich substances, nitrogen, various minerals, and vitamins. Such buffering contributes to the limited constancy observed in the internal milieu. Only relatively coarse tuning need be invoked from dietary selection behavior. There is no indication of fine control, when one considers the pathological extremes often involved in dietary selection experiments and the wide variability in response amongst individuals.

Thus, homeostatic regulation needs only some increasing tendency, as a deficit (or excess) increases, to emit behavior suited to the habitat's capacity to help correct that error. In other words, extreme states generate an innate or learned search for remedial diets or avoidance of diets that might be deleterious. Thus, nutritional wisdom could consist merely of these simple, graded negative-feedback effects of extreme states.

For example, so-called regulation of protein intake in the rat[27] appears to be the effect of individual, highly variable encounters with extremes of amino acid metabolism. While a rat's liver has not yet adapted to high-protein diet, ammonia toxicity will limit intake or condition aversion. Any continuing risk of amino acid imbalance can be avoided by the conditioning of preferences for diets that supply limiting amino acids and aversions for diets that fail to rectify the deficiencies.[5,8]

The only behaviorally effective deficits on human beings might be water and energy. It would have had selective value to respond to deficits (or deleterious excesses) of other nutrients if energy had not carried with it in past human diets sufficient of some other nutrient for an adapted metabolism. Solid evidence for instinctive nutrient selection in people is lacking.

An organism's knowledge of the ecophysiological contingencies might be inherited or acquired.

Innate Nutrient-specific Hungers

The only well-established innate hunger is sodium appetite. During sodium deficiency, rats innately recognize the relevance of ingesting very salty tasting materials, which are normally aversive. Rats even forage for the source of such a taste remembered from the past when there was no deficiency.[28] Need-specific facilitation of salty taste preference may be inherited in other species too, including our own.[29]

A smell, taste, or texture, or even some distinctive gastrointestinal or systemic stimulation during the feeding bout, might be an ecologically valid cue that the diet contains a particular nutrient. The organism might then have inherited a preference for that cue or even a hunger or appetite[a] – i.e., a strengthening of that sensory preference during deficiency of the cued nutrient. Such an innate mechanism has been proposed for some nutrients, e.g., sugars[30] and amino acids.[31]

Stupid Rats or Impossible Diets?

The early studies of dietary selection were open to the criticism that the nutrient composition of the test diets was not fully controlled. So, experimenters began to use chemically purified nutrients such as sucrose, corn oil, and casein. In these later experiments, the rats quite often died of malnutrition. However, it is a non sequitur to conclude that the rat lacks any "nutritional wisdom." Strong sensory stimulation of ingestive or egestive reactions could in principle bias or even override inherited or acquired behavioral influences from any information contained in subtler sensory discriminations.

For example, if an eater hates the gluey oral sensation of casein, protein appetite cannot be expressed when casein is the sole protein available. Conversely, the rat's sweet tooth[32] or gluttony for grease[33] (unless moderated by dumping-conditioned aversion[34,35]) will overwhelm its intake with "empty calories" if sucrose or corn oil is provided and lethal deficiencies in amino acids, minerals, and vitamins can develop – much as the "empty calories" from chronic excess consumption of ethanol can create nutritional deficiency in human beings. The "natural foods" philosophy underpinning the studies on human infants[22] probably pre-empted such an overwhelming of

[a] The disposition to eat food or some specified type of food is called either "appetite" or "hunger" in common parlance. Both dietary and somatic influences may generate that same behavioral disposition. Furthermore, as we shall see, sometimes the external sources of feeding motivation do not simply add to the internal sources, but they are intimately combined: craving and drive may be indistinguishable in the behavior they produce. Therefore the frequent attempts to prescribe redefinitions of these terms so that they apply to different categories of cause of ingestive behavior, instead of merely classifying the behavior itself, are ultimately unworkable and should be avoided.

behavioral counterinfluences to nutritional deficiency; unlearned sweetness preference caused no serious problem because sugar was not provided.

Demonstration of Genuine Nutrient Selection

Inattention to learned sensory control of eating behavior has also undermined recent work on dietary selection, inspired by demonstrations of effects of dietary composition on neurotransmitter activity.[36] Experimenters have designed diets that confound nutrient differences and sensory differences and then fallaciously interpreted the dietary choices as "nutrient selection." An attempt has been made recently to equate the basic palatability (or its balance with satiating power) of diets varying in nutrient composition.[37] This effort to minimize differences in diet palatability still leaves unmeasured the rat's use of remaining perceptible characteristics of the diets. Known sensory cues for innate hungers have to be eliminated. During adaptation to diets, when the rat could be learning, sensory differences between nutrients have to be completely masked or matched and the experimenter has to provide arbitrary learnable cues predictive of any postingestional effects of the nutrient in question (not dependent on its physical form): the only valid measure of nutrient selection is the rat's reactions to those arbitrary cues when tested later in the absence of nutrient differences.

None of the work published on the effects of neurotransmitter-modulating drugs (or indeed hormones) on dietary selection has used a minimally controlled learning design, although the likely importance of learning in nutrient selection[5] is now beginning to be acknowledged in this literature.[38]

Nevertheless, there are longstanding experiments, albeit limited in number, that have been both behaviorally analytic and nutritionally controlled. These have conclusively demonstrated that the rat has the capacity for a limited degree of nutritional wisdom, based on associative conditioning of aversions and preferences by nutritional effects. Wisdom might also be acquired from experience of conspecifics' foraging and feeding and (in our species) linguistic communication of behavior-controlling genuine information about the nutritional benefits of eating certain foods in certain circumstances. Such social transmission of eating habits may still rest on nutritional conditioning at base.[4,13]

AVERSIONS CONDITIONED BY NUTRIENTS

Although innate sodium hunger is accepted as a genuine preference, acquired hungers are widely regarded as mere artifacts of conditioned aversions to the available deficient diets. This paradoxical view ignores limitations of traditional experimental procedures, involving grossly pathological states induced by nutrient-depletion or by administration of unnatural forms of nutrients, poisons, and pharmaceuticals.

Aversive Pathological States

The first fully controlled experiment on the acquisition of a nutrient-specific hunger appears to be that published by Harris and colleagues in 1933.[39] After eating a thiamin-containing diet and a thiamin-free diet differing only in flavor, rats came to select the thiamin-containing diet. This was proved to be an acquired thiamin-specific hunger mediated by a conditioned relative preference for the arbitrary flavor paired with the effects of ingesting thiamin: experienced rats chose the hitherto thiamin-paired flavor even when the diet having that flavor no longer contained thiamin.

Intensive study of this behavior was taken up by Rozin and colleagues in the late 1960s. To eliminate the possibility that the rat sensed the thiamin in the diet, the conditioning effects of thiamin were generated by injecting the vitamin intraperitoneally into the thiamin-depleted rat after presenting a distinctive diet. The results of this excellent series of experimental analyses were most simply interpreted as evidence that absence of relief of the thiamin deficiency conditioned an aversion to the distinctive sensory characteristics of a diet, rather than thiamin conditioning an actual preference for the predictive dietary characteristics.[40] Thiamin deficiency also appeared to reduce the rat's normal neophobia—at least to the extent of producing substantial sampling of a new diet followed by abstinence from eating for a period that would allow postingestional effects of the eaten sample to be detected. If no aversion was conditioned by lack of thiamin, the usual habituation and safety-learning processes encouraged a subsequent increase in consumption of the beneficial diet.

This line of interpretation of the mechanism for a learned nutrient appetite had the merit of consistency with the facts of a phenomenon that was then coming to the attention of American psychologists and is the central focus of this volume. Toxic effects of eating can condition aversion to the diet, even when there is delay between onset of oronasal cues and onset of visceral or systemic consequences, as first demonstrated in learned "poison-bait shyness" by Rzoska in 1953.[41] Then in 1955, Garcia and colleagues[42] reported that gamma irradiation conditioned an aversion to fluid drunk in its presence, either when flavored with saccharin or when presented again in the presence of gamma rays (which presumably generated an olfactory stimulus such as from ozone). Eventually, from 1965, Garcia and subsequently many others were able to publish evidence that drinking of saccharin-flavored water in 24-hour water-deprived rats was suppressed relative to unflavored water (after the decline of illness that would disrupt any drinking), if the first drink of saccharin had been followed (even by some hours) by the effects of cytotoxic agents or, as subsequently materialized, some apparently non-toxic or even addictive drugs.

Thus, the work on learned components of thiamin appetite (and other vitamin and mineral hungers) showed the importance of aversive conditioning by chronic extreme nutritional deficiency, as by toxic and drugged states. Such learning is presumably crucial for omnivores in order to colonize new habitats and survive discovery of deficient and poisonous vegetation and prey.

The ease of such aversion conditioning contrasted with the difficulty of conditioning preferences by varying the technique so that a distinctive drink or food was paired with recovery from the vitamin deficiency[43] or the toxic state.[44] Work on such abnormal nutrition has left a persisting impression that aversions are easier to condition than preferences[45] and even that genuine absolute preferences cannot be generated by associative conditioning. Such a view can only be sustained by ignoring both how ill the rats are in these experiments and the results of many other experiments using milder conditioning states that are more common in nature. Chronic depletion of thiamin makes a very sick animal. Gross deficiency of a vitamin or mineral, or the administration of a toxin, creates a complex pathological state that will at best be only partly normalized after administration of the deficient nutrient or cessation of toxin administration. Even though overt behavioral symptoms may have subsided, it is surprising that partial "recovery" conditions the slightest preference at all. That it sometimes does may indeed be evidence for a relative theory of reinforcement—improvement from very bad to bad is sufficient to condition preference (or to reward discriminatively).

Aversive Abnormal Nutrients

Any conditioning involved in the routine control of nutrient intake must be based on the acute effects of ordinary foodstuffs on relatively mild deprivation; not on the effects of non-nutritive drinks and drugs on extreme hunger or thirst. Yet, just like the avoidance of pathology, both food selection and meal sizes have to anticipate nutritional consequences that arise with delays of probably at least a minute or two. Nevertheless, the earliest work on learned food selection provided clear evidence of conditioning by delayed consequences.[39,41] From 1955 onwards, Le Magnen repeatedly observed conditioning over an oral-visceral delay before the toxin-conditioned taste aversion paradigm had developed, in experiments examining learned control of selection and amounts eaten by manipulation of the rat's acute nutritional status.[14,46–48] Unfortunately these findings were not effectively absorbed into either physiological psychology or animal learning, even though presented in 1967 in an American handbook on the physiology of ingestion[49] and at a 1969 conference of the New York Academy of Sciences.[50]

However, the usual experimental manipulations of hunger and satiety at that time were not physiologically or ecologically normal and have all since proved to be aversive. Caloric dilution of the diet with dry bulk such as cellulose, kaolin, or chalk has sensory effects that condition aversion,[51] which has again recently been misinterpreted as energy-conditioned preferences.[52] The drug amphetamine[53] and hormone insulin[54] that Le Magnen used condition aversion also (even though rats self-administer them). Oral, intragastric,[9,34] or intraperitoneal[55] administration of hypertonic glucose has aversive[9] osmotic effects that do not arise from carbohydrate in its usual macromolecular dietary form[9,11] or from intermittent delivery of glucose into the bloodstream at normal absorption rates.[21] Deutsch and colleagues failed to condition preference with hypertonic glucose[16] but have subsequently confirmed[56] the preference-conditioning effects of starch,[9,11] which does not stress the gut osmotically.

NUTRITIONAL PREFERENCE CONDITIONING

Although very few laboratories have used them, ordinary foodstuffs have been known for decades to have postingestional effects that reward foraging and condition ingestion (TABLE 1). The effects of various amounts of starch and protein on mild depletion must be experienced at most meals throughout life.[13] Yet a single pairing of a beneficial nutritional consequence with either a taste or an odor is sufficient to condition a substantial increase in relative preference for that flavor. Furthermore, the preference conditioned to an odor by pairing it with the effects of dilute starch in the mildly hungry rat is a genuine absolute preference (TABLE 2). It is not a choice of an aversive conditioned odor relative to some even more aversive flavor.

Strength of Preference Conditioning

It is not obvious how to make a legitimate comparison of the strengths of the two directions of conditioning.[58] In the nature of the case, the conditioning consequence in preference conditioning must have an optimum strength beyond which the organism is receiving "too much of a good thing." Sufficient excess of even an essential nutrient can be toxic.

TABLE 2. Intake in Absence of Starch after Exposure to Odorized Water or Saccharin Solution with or without 10% Starch Added

	Water Intake (ml)			
	Starch-conditioned Group		No Starch Group	
Test Day and Condition	M	SD	M	SD
Saccharin-varied Unyoked Training (three days)				
First test (odor alone)	5.4	3.3[a]	0.9	1.5
Second test (saccharin alone)	5.1	4.4	5.3	4.9
Saccharin-constant Yoked Training (one day)				
First test (odor alone)	4.4	1.8[b]	1.7	1.9
Second test (saccharin alone)	6.5	2.2	6.2	2.0

[b] $p < 0.01$, [a] $p < 0.05$ by t test. M = mean, SD = standard deviation.

In contrast, the conditioning consequence in aversion conditioning has no upper limit, except that the organism recover sufficiently to be testable for learning later. So, any attempts to compare the strengths of conditioned preferences and conditioned aversions must be founded on demonstrable equality of the strengths of the two sorts of conditioning consequence. It is not easy to formulate a sound behavioral criterion for equating strengths of different types of US, especially as it is their associative strengths that have to be equated, without circularity. If physical dose is any criterion (which I doubt), it should be noted that virtually identical doses of appetitively and aversively conditioning amino acid mixtures conditioned somewhat stronger preferences than aversions,[8] relative to various arguably neutral consequences in hungry rats.

Odor Conditioning

Although the view cannot be reconciled with the palatability of food aromas (and appearances), the conditioned aversion literature has been strongly influenced by the idea that tastes can be conditioned by internal events and that odors and the appearance of a food in a visual species like ours cannot. Yet food odor conditioning was evidenced by Le Magnen many times.[47] Our early proof that pairing with a toxic drug would condition odors[59] was criticized for leaving open the possibility that the rat tasted the odorant. This objection was an instance of logic overwhelming empirical good sense. Our experiments were two-odor discriminative designs, using odorants that are insoluble in water (unlike flavors), that created similar and very slight sensations when applied to the human tongue in raw fluid form, and that were used in minute concentrations in complex fluid or solid diets. It has since been demonstrated that conditioned preferences and aversions for such insoluble odorants presented at these low concentrations within the test diet are eliminated when temporary anosmia is created by placing tubes in the nares.

Potentiation and Overshadowing

It should be emphasized that our earlier experiments on odor conditioning involved some taste that was the same in each of two diets given different odors. This non-discriminative taste may have been potentiating odor conditioning.[60] However, potentiation of odor conditioning by increasing levels of non-discriminative saccharin in the odorized fluid was not seen in the starch-conditioned preference experiment of TABLE 2, unlike the saccharin-potentiated odor-aversion conditioning seen with similar procedures in Garcia's and others' laboratories. That may be because the starch-fed hungry rats were given much longer periods of access to the odorized fluid than were the lithium-injected thirsty rats: brief exposure to the odor may be critical to generate potentiation rather than overshadowing.[61]

Acting on the mild depletion that recurs during free feeding, the satiating effects of eating ordinary foods may condition incentive to even exteroceptive cues.[62] Earlier failures to condition hunger[63] are probably attributable to experimental designs based on a stimulus-substitution model of conditioning, using levels of food deprivation that disrupt the postintestinal satiety that conditions preference,[21,55] leaving only sensory conditioning.[20,52]

DEPLETION-DEPENDENT PREFERENCES IN FOOD-HUNGER AND THIRST

If much palatability is based on conditioned preferences, then hunger (or thirst) might be based on conditioning of preferences specifically elicited by deficiencies in gastric fill and energy supply (or water deficit).

Sweet Preference

Sweet preference is increased during food deprivation.[64] There is no evidence that this arises specifically from carbohydrate deficiency, rather than from a more general energy depletion. Furthermore, it is not clear how much of this potentiation of sweetness preference by hunger results from merely an energizing effect that any deprivation might have on any movement in response to any stimulus (i.e. general drive or arousal),[65–67] with a disproportionately large effect on a strong incentive.

Insulin-induced hypoglycemia does not facilitate saccharin preference in sugar-naive rats.[68] Insulin-induced sugar intake in the rat[70] and the sweet craving reported in human hypoglycemia[71] may therefore be learned.[69]

Acquired Carbohydrate Hunger

The rat's saccharin preference can be increased still further by prior drinking of carbohydrate-containing sweet solutions, such as glucose solution[46] or saccharin-flavored starch solutions.[9] Evidence that administration of insulin increases starch intake (i.e. a carbohydrate appetite independent of sweet taste) has been obtained only in experiments with designs that did not exclude transfer from prior learning of the ameliorative efforts of that starchy diet on ordinary self-imposed food deprivation.[72]

If carbohydrate hunger is entirely learned and unlearned sweet preference may not be specific to carbohydrate need, the question arises whether ordinary hunger for food during general depletion is in fact inherited, as widely assumed in physiology and pharmacology. It may be all an acquired preference or appetite for carbohydrate (or for any source of energy),[9,13] or at least some combination of learned and unlearned processes.

Water Hunger

The same question arises for the ordinary appetite for water. Thirst (the disposition to drink watery fluids) includes a specific hunger for water during water deficit. Repair of water deficit conditions flavor preferences,[19] and so the liking for watery fluids might be at least partly acquired. In that case a compound stimulus of watery cues and water deficit might be an acquired part of the specific hunger. Despite great interest in the physiology of drinking, no fully controlled experiments appear to have been published to distinguish inherited and acquired behavioral mechanisms in normal repair of water deficit.

Thirst also often occurs in the absence of measurable systemic deficit. It has been claimed that need-free drinking functions to anticipate need, i.e. to avoid water deficit (such as might be generated systemically by digestive secretions after a meal). We await clear demonstration of a discriminative avoidance of water deficit or a conditioned preference for characteristics of fluids that repair incipient water deficits.[73]

SATIATION AS STATE-DEPENDENT AVERSION

Satiety is a term for an impermanent behavioral state in which appetite is absent. During the normal satiation process, the hungry state is removed by the ingestion of food; the term anorexia is usually reserved for an absence of hunger induced by other means, e.g. administration of an anorexigenic drug. Because many of us are conscious of sensations of abdominal fullness, the lack of a diposition to eat food (satiety itself) has been confused with visceral sensations arising from visceral stimulation, or with the activation of physiological signals or even visceral responses to ingest food. However, a behavioral state is not the same thing as its behavioral or physiological causes and concomitants.

The satiated lack of interest in, or even positive aversion to, eating food can be viewed as a reduction in facilitation of the ingestion of foods. That is, satiety is a reduction in preference for food stimuli. However, it is not a permanent reduction of ingestion in all circumstances: by definition, the reduction must depend on the normal effects of ingesting foodstuffs. The evidence is that this transient reduction in ingestive preferences can arise from the preceding sensory stimulation by food, from strong internal stimulation from accumulated food and water, or from some learned combination of current external and internal stimuli.

HABITUATION-BASED SATIATION

The satiation that arises from immediately prior stimulation from the process of eating is a dispositional change that is selective to foods that are perceived as similar to those just eaten.[25,57,74] It appears that the starting preference undergoes a non-associative habituation process.

Intake can be stimulated by variety of odorants in a rat's diet or by other purely sensory variety in the human diet. If eating produces food-specific habituation, then the variety effect may be attributable to dishabituation of ingestive reactions by the next food available. It has been suggested that long-term facilitation of habituation by prior exposure to the food to be varied is a precondition of sufficiently strong dishabituation of intake incentive,[25] but there is recent evidence to the contrary.[76]

Le Magnen initially interpreted the variety effect as evidence for conditioned satiation.[75] Recent workers have also posed a conflation of the two.[76] However, the two effects are operationally quite distinct. Immediately prior stimulus presentation is necessary to habituate and so provide a base for dishabituation of ingestion. In contrast, long-past presentation of the conditioned stimulus, along with the conditioning consequence, is sufficient to inhibit eating by conditioned satiation. No immediately preceding presentation is necessary. Indeed, any prior satiation conditioning of the dis-habituating (second) stimulus would eliminate or reduce the variety effect. That is, so far from being related, habituation satiation and conditioned satiation can be antagonistic.

CONDITIONED SATIATION

Definition of Satiation Conditioning

Since satiety is not a permanent relative aversion or loss of palatability but a relative aversion temporarily induced by food, conditioned satiation has to be defined as a conditioned aversion distinguished by its dependence on the effects of ingested food.[10]

Le Magnen was interested in learned control of amounts eaten (meal sizes and satiation), not just in learned dietary selection. He demonstrated that anorexigenic manipulations differentially conditioned the relative amounts eaten of two cued diets when each was presented alone (one-stimulus tests).[14,47,48] However, as we have already seen, the relative amounts chosen of the two diets when experimental and control cues were presented together for the first time (two-stimuli tests) were also conditioned. That is, by the usual operational definition there was evidence, from both the usual types of test, for aversion for the conditioned cue, even when the test was started during hunger. Hence, the small meal might not reflect satiation conditioning but merely the conditioning of an aversion that was independent of effects of food ingested during the test meal. This interpretation was supported by inspection of average cumulative intakes in conditioned and control meals:[48] the ratio of initial intake rates was identical to the ratio of meal sizes. This suggested an operational criterion for genuine satiation conditioning: it should yield small meals that could not be attributed to low preference or intake rate from the start of the meal.[10] Later, the converse of this criterion was also applied: learned satiation would be demonstrated by the conditioning of a relative aversion with some specificity to the later part of meals.[57] In other words, by definition, the partly or completely replete state is also an element, as well as the food element(s), in an acquired stimulus complex eliciting conditioned satiation.[10,57,58]

Demonstration of Satiation Conditioning

These criteria of true conditioning of satiation were met when rats[7,10,11,57] (and, later, people[77–79]) were given the experience of the effects of disguised variations of dietary composition in the normal range, namely concentrated and dilute solid and liquid starch diets. Initially, the criterion of satiation conditioning was a dissociation of the acquired meal-size differences from the acquired intake-rate and choice-preference differences at the start of the test meal while hungry.[10,11] The mechanism by which the preferred dietary stimulus at the start of the conditioned meal came to elicit the smaller meal was postulated to be that the conditioned flavor became suffi-

TABLE 3. Depletion- and Repletion-dependent Relative Preferences and Aversions to Odor Conditioned by Effects of Starch Concentration on Depleted or Repleted State

Starch (%) Previously Paired with Odor	Preference Ratio for Conditioned Odor Relative to Control Odor in Test Meal			
	First 2 min of Test Meal		Last 10 min of Test Meal	
	M	SD	M	SD
10	0.77[a]	0.23	0.56	0.38
40	0.84[a]	0.21	0.29[a]	0.38

[a] $p < 0.05$ for difference from 0.5, i.e. indifference relative to control odor. M = mean, SD = standard deviation.

ciently little preferred towards the end of the meal that it did not sustain ingestion.[7,57] The effect could not be attributed to habituation because less and more preferred stimuli were often eaten in similar amounts early in meals.[10,11,57] When conditioned rats were required to make new flavor choices repeatedly during a test meal (TABLE 3), their selective intakes confirmed that smaller meals involved relative aversion specific to the near-replete state of the second half of the meal.[7,57]

Thus, by definition and by demonstration, satiation conditioning results in a conditioned response that is elicited by a combination of a dietary stimulus and a repletion state—in other words, a compound conditioned stimulus. The learned behavior depends quite as much on the concurrent internal effects of food as it depends on the external flavor elements. Yet learned satiation has been dismissed as a mere effect of flavor,[80] even when the complementary part of the analysis of satiated behavior as relative aversion has been invoked,[81] the original dissociation of preference conditioning and meal size conditioning has been reproduced in review,[82] and the reviewers' laboratory had demonstrated the claimed interdependence of oral and gastric stimuli.[83,84] Indeed, failure to allow for the fact that foods have postingestional effects that may differ with nutrient composition (differences that are acknowledged to cause the differentiation of meal size in the first place) has resulted in illegitimate comparisons that confound conditioned and innate effects.[82] When the differentially conditioned flavors are compared in diets having the same nutrient composition (thus generating comparable internal states towards the end of the meal) then the flavor-specific differentiation of meal size is incontrovertibly evident.[7,10,11,57] Equally clearly, the preference difference early in a choice between nutritionally identical conditioned flavors is opposite in direction from the flavor-specific meal size difference.[7,10,11,57] That is, the relative aversion for flavor also involves specifically the partly replete state later in the meal. The satiety signals involved, such as gastric distension presumably, are therefore themselves learned to that extent. It should be noted that the satiety effect of cholecystokinin may result from augmentation of gastric distension[85] and that cholecystokinin satiety may extinguish[86] as the new gastric-postgastric contingency is learned.

Strength of Conditioned Satiation

The speed and strength of satiation conditioning has been compared unfavorably with aversion conditioning.[63] This involves a misinterpretation of the original data and is directly refuted by later results. In the original experiments on conditioned satiety, there was a highly variable but sometimes lengthy "incubation" period before responses differentiated.[10] Follow-up work[7,57] has indicated that this lag is attributable to procedural incidentals such as aversive tastes, disruptive diet-presentation procedures, and interactions between training trials when more than one was given during a day. Even in the original experiments, the data published clearly show that when an individual rat's differentiation of meal sizes began, it developed very rapidly; sometimes reaching asymptote in one or two training trials.[10] In later experiments,[7] most of the differentiation has been seen by the second training trial (i.e., learning could not be faster).

Furthermore, the original reports[10,11] showed that relearning, by elimination of the differential contingencies between cues and consequences, also occurred after a single trial. Based on the correct conception of the associative strengths of conditioning consequences, this is evidence of rapid and therefore strong conditioning, not of weak conditioning.

The importance of conditioned satiation in meal size control has also been miscalculated.[82] Fractional decrease in meal size is not a valid measure of any satiety effect. The total amount eaten at a meal is a result of many interacting processes, such as the initial emptiness of the gut and the food's basic palatability, not just satieties. The tradition of regarding meal sizes (and intermeal intervals) as outputs of the system, rather than epiphenomenal measurements, suffers from the fallacy of misplaced concreteness. (The common use of single-bottle tests for conditioned aversion runs similar risks of confusing conditioned satiation, sickness,[59] or lack of thirst[53] with aversion: indeed, some conditioned satiation has been detected in just such a conditioned aversion drink[87]). Therefore, the measure of the strength of a satiating influence must be the fraction it accounts for of the variability that is evident in meal sizes when factors other than satiating influences have been controlled. The published data clearly show that conditioning accounts for at least half, and sometimes virtually all, of the difference in meal size between dilute and concentrated carbohydrate diets after that difference has been fully elaborated by training.[10,11]

Direction of Satiation Conditioning

Other experiments, using the techniques of gastric loading and withdrawal, show that the size of a meal taken in familiar circumstances can change immediately without new learning.[12,56] It has yet to be determined whether this satiation mechanism is unlearned or is a process of generalization from schedule adaptation and a lifetime of learning.

With repeated sessions of gastric withdrawal, however, there is a large further increase in meal size.[12,88] This increase in meal size is specific to the dietary cues associated with withdrawal.[12] As in the gastric withdrawal experiments, most or all of the meal-size differentiation in starch-conditioned satiety experiments[10] is attributable to increases in size of meals on dilute diet, with little or no decrease in meal size on even the most highly concentrated diet. That is, to be strict, desatiation (preference) conditioning is more evident than satiation (aversion) conditioning. This may be because, with voluntarily ingested natural nutrients, preference-conditioning consequences are much more likely than aversively conditioning consequences.

The Conditioned Internal Elements

The conditioning of flavors in combination with postingestional signals is in fact the learning of postingestional signals of satiety and hunger (specific to the relevant flavor). Therefore, nearly all the usual experimental designs on the physiology of satiety are liable to have been misleading because they do not measure the effects of learning and relearning on the suppression of food intake that gastric distension or other signals may produce.

Some recent experiments that have measured learning have demonstrated once again that, as a result of conditioning experience, the effects of gastric distension are contingent on test-diet flavor.[56] These results were interpreted as evidence for inheritance of complex attentional mechanisms deciding intake control between mouth and stomach. Also, the original satiation conditioning experiments were misdescribed as diet-dilution procedures to accommodate this "two memories" hypothesis. Both these recent results[56] and the original conditioned differences in reaction to two flavors,[7,10,11] when the stomach was partly filled and the flavors were presented at the same intermediate dietary concentration, are more simply explained in terms of conditioned combinations of flavor cue elements and gastric cue elements.

MECHANISMS OF THE CONDITIONING OF SATIETIES AND APPETITES

The basic phenomenon of (de)satiation conditioning can be demonstrated as a switch from relative preference to relative aversion on passing from depletion to repletion, when the flavor(s) presented in those states have previously been paired with the effects of concentrated starch (which differ between depletion and repletion)[7,55,57] (TABLE 3). Thus, the relative preference for an odor paired with 10% starch persists from early to late in the meal, whereas 40% starch conditions a relative aversion specifically to the latter part of the meal (TABLE 3). This is as clear a demonstration of external-internal compound stimulus conditioning as can be expected from a within-subjects design.

Facilitatory Conditioned Responses and Their Repletion-Specific Absence

My working hypothesis is that replacement of slowed absorption by the normal postintestinal satiety signals is the major source of learned palatabilities, appetites, and desatiations. This is consistent even with data that have been interpreted to the contrary.[56,89]

When the consequence of eating a starchy food is no rectification of energy deficit because rapid prandial or postprandial absorption has already begun, then desatiation (repletion-dependent preference) will not be conditioned to that food. Therefore, carbohydrate eaten late in a meal will fail to condition desatiation if concentrated starch has been eaten early in the meal. This appears to be the major learning mechanism limiting meal sizes.

Preference conditioning of both depleted and replete states in compound with flavor has been demonstrated now in women with a between-subjects design. Each woman was trained only in one state, either before or after lunch. A preference for dilute-paired flavor conditioned and tested during satiety did indeed not generalize to hunger (TABLE 4). Furthermore, in other women, a preference for concentrated-paired flavor conditioned and tested during hunger did not generalize to satiety (TABLE 4).

TABLE 4. Differentially Conditioned Stimulus Control by Flavor and by Internal State, Following Pairing Each of Two Flavors Once with a Different Starch Concentration during One of Two Internal States (Before/After Lunch)

Category of Woman	*N*	Flavor Stimulus Control[a] M	Flavor Stimulus Control[a] SE	Internal Stimulus Control[b] M	Internal Stimulus Control[b] SE
Non-dieters	28	7.0[d]	3.3	8.3[e]	5.0
Unsuccessful dieters	16	3.8	5.7	−2.2	4.7
Successful dieters	20	16.7[c]	5.1	15.3[d]	5.5

[c] $p < 0.01$, [d] $p < 0.02$, [e] $p < 0.05$, by one-tailed t test against zero or unsuccessful dieters.

[a] Difference between flavors, tested during the trained internal state, in the change in pleasantness that had been conditioned by pairing with different starch concentrations in one internal state (whether hungry or satiated).

[b] Difference between trained and untrained internal states in the difference in conditioned change in flavor pleasantness.

(Unpublished data, A-M. Toase & D.A. Booth.[79])

Repletion-Specific Conditioned Aversion

However, even a normal food may occasionally be eaten to excess, perhaps creating unpleasant bloating effects that would counterbalance the appetitive conditioning effects that the food creates following absorption. A genuine absolute aversion can indeed be acquired from the effects of voluntarily ingested starch. When the rat is "tricked" into ingesting a large volume of odorized concentrated starch (by prior desatiation conditioning, to instill a habit of taking large meals), then it shows an aversion to the conditioned odor, relative even to a novel odor (TABLE 4) that from past work would be expected to be mildly aversive itself. The aversively conditioning effect may arise from gastrointestinal distension, sedation, or discomfort: some rats are briefly prostrated after drinking over 10 ml of 60% starch, whereas rapid intravenous glucose infusion conditions only preference.[21] We are currently testing whether this absolute aversion is specific to the repletion state as is the relative aversion conditioned by concentrated starch (TABLE 3).[7] Failure of the aversion to generalize to hunger would be proof of compound external-internal conditioning.

This basic theory of conditioning of compounds of incentive and drive stimuli was first applied to ingestion by Revusky[90] who also influenced me to opt for this working hypothesis among the several interpretations admitted in the original satiation conditioning papers.[10,11] Early evidence for acquired control of respondents or operants by drive cues has been difficult to interpret conclusively.[91] However, abundant evidence has recently been accumulated in diverse paradigms, from drive-dependent maze learning[92,93] to the many operant drug discrimination studies. Drug states are harder to condition aversively than strong tastes[94] and extreme hunger and thirst may be impossible to discriminate.[95] Mood-dependent recall, currently under study as a mechanism of depression, can also be interpreted as compound stimulus conditioning.[96]

The consequences that condition facilitation (desatiation or appetite) and inhibition (satiation or de-appetizing) to compound oral-visceral stimuli will presumably include mild versions of those that condition simple state-independent flavor preferences and aversions respectively (TABLES 1, 2, and 5).

TABLE 5. Odor Aversion in Second Half of Test Meal, Previously Conditioned by Pairing the Odor and Repletion with Effects of Concentrated Starch

	Odor Intakes (ml)				Preferences for Conditioned Odor (%)	
	Conditioned Odor		Novel Odor			
Test Period	M	SD	M	SD	M	SD
Odor throughout test meal (N = 12)						
First half of meal	1.0	0.9	1.5	1.2	41	29
Second half of meal	1.2	0.9[a]	2.1	1.3	37	26
No odors during first 6 min of test meal (N = 12)						
6–10 min	0.1	0.1	0.6	0.2	30	17[b]
10–16 min	0.1	0.1	0.2	0.3	27	24[c]
16–25 min	0.2	0.2	0.2	0.1	40	22

[c] $p < 0.005$, [b] $p < 0.01$, [a] $p < 0.05$, less than novel intake or 50%.

This test for true aversion was suggested by E.W. Holman, in collaboration with whom the experiment with odor throughout the meal was performed (1980). Second experiment: E.L. Gibson & D.A. Booth (1983).

Deutsch has emphasized that flavor preference conditioning is better than intake suppression as evidence of the return of a true satiety signal because direct suppression of feeding may result from adverse effects, not from normal satiation. Only energy-providing nutrients have met this criterion to date (TABLES 1 and 2).

However, still stronger evidence than this apparently state-independent preference conditioning would be depletion-dependent preference (appetite) conditioning by moderate doses of the putative satiety agent and repletion-dependent aversion (satiation) conditioning by the highest normal doses of the agent. Again, only the actions of food starch have met these criteria so far (TABLES 2–5).

Recent discussions[56,97] have been confused by failures to recognize that voluntary satiety can be sufficiently extreme to condition an aversion, but an aversion that is limited to near-replete states (TABLES 3–5). Aversion conditioning has been taken as proof that an agent such as cholecystokinin is not inducing satiety, and satiation conditioning has been dismissed as a counter-example.[9] Aversive conditioning undoubtedly raises questions about the mechanism of an intake suppression produced by the same procedure, and cannot be itself dismissed because non-toxic drugs condition aversively.[98] Yet it is not a knock-down disproof of the claim that an agent genuinely satiates. Any procedure at high enough intensity is liable to produce adverse physical effects that may or may not suppress food or water intake and may and may not condition aversion. When some cholecystokinin preparations do not condition aversion at doses sufficient to suppress intake, it is circular to argue that intake is more sensitive than aversion conditioning; indeed, even though certain tests of lithium chloride can be so interpreted, it is not even true for irradiation.[42] When cholecystokinin has met the preference and state-dependent conditioning criteria that food starch has, it will merit attention as a neuropeptide acting outside the brain to satiate or to amplify a major satiating influence.[85]

PRACTICAL IMPLICATIONS

Implications for current research experimentation have been drawn throughout this review. For application in conservation and animal husbandry, one might conclude that omnivores can be left to select an adequate diet so long as excessively high or low palatability and perceived availability (e.g. predation risk) are avoided for sole sources of essential nutrients. The implications for the human home, commerce, and clinics are virtually analogous: a balanced variety of types of foodstuffs, each near complete in nutrient content, would permit automatic tuning of the amount of energy intake towards need by the appetite and satiety conditioning mechanisms described here. Other nutritional requirements should then also be met (excepting special conditions and of course acute disease) even if human beings have no other specific hungers besides those for energy and water.

These implications for human behavior are far from laissez-faire. The interactions of customer demand, technological invention, and commercial financing have generated a food market in which it can be very hard for some people to express their nutritional wisdom. Also, domestic eating practices, even without market pressures, may be best adapted to the needs of only the average individual in the culture in question. So, for example, someone with efficient metabolism may have his appetites conditioned and elicited by attractive nutritious foods, and his conditioned and even inherited satieties overwhelmed by over-frequent eating times or over-large "proper" meals.[3]

Even though some conditioned satiations may be true aversions, they are state-dependent and are conditioned by everyday consequences of the food stimuli in question. Therefore, the present analysis implies that artificial and state-independent aversive conditioning of food stimuli or eating places will be quite ineffective at inhibiting eating. Aversion conditioning has been proved a failure at supporting efforts to reduce weight.[99] To date, when the concept of satiation conditioning has been invoked in weight reduction studies, the procedures sufficient to condition human satiation have not been used and evidence of satiation conditioning has not been provided. So the usefulness of satiation conditioning remains to be tested.

However, in our recent study (TABLE 4), the successful dieters acquired better stimulus control than the unsuccessful dieters, by both the food stimulus elements and the internal stimulus elements. Maybe it was good conditionability of eating that helped them lose weight and keep it off. If so, then the less fortunate might benefit from organized naturalistic state-dependent conditioning experiences and supportive autosuggestive focusing on the everyday contingencies.[3] Alternatively or as well, this experimental result may mean that dieting makes one's appetites and satiations more readily conditionable. If so, we have more evidence of the pervasiveness of nutritional external-internal conditioning. Also, if dieting succeeds by inducing better conditionability, this implies that weight reduction strategies would be more effective if they were structured to exploit these nutritional conditioning mechanisms, whatever social, pharmaceutical, or cognitive supports are also recruited. Nevertheless, it must be remembered that the conditioning effects of ingestion are merely one set of negative feedbacks in a much more complex system from which the problem of overweight arises.[3]

ACKNOWLEDGMENT

This paper is dedicated to the memory of George Wolf, whose incomparable contributions to the scientific understanding of sodium appetite were complemented by a generosity with intellectual insights and personal friendship that is sadly missed.

REFERENCES

1. Bruch, H. 1969. Hunger and instinct. J. Nerv. Ment. Dis. **149**: 91–114.
2. McFarland, D. J., Ed. 1982. Functional Ontogeny. Pitmans. London.
3. Booth, D. A. 1980. Acquired behavior controlling energy intake and expenditure. *In* Obesity. A. J. Stunkard, Ed.: 101–143. W. B. Saunders, Philadelphia, PA.
4. Booth, D. A. 1981. Momentary acceptance of particular foods and processes that change it. *In* Criteria of Food Selection. J. Solms & R. L. Hall, Eds.: 49–68. Forster. Zurich.
5. Booth, D. A. & D. Stribling. 1979. Neurochemistry of appetite mechanisms. Proc. Nutr. Soc. **37**: 181–191.
6. Booth, D. A. 1979. Feeding control systems within animals. *In* Food Intake Regulation in Poultry. K. M. Boorman & B. M. Freeman, Eds.: 13–62. British Poultry Science, Ltd. Edinburgh.
7. Booth, D. A. 1980. Conditioned reactions in motivation. *In* Analysis of Motivational Processes. F. M. Toates & T. R. Halliday, Eds.: 77–102. Academic Press. London.
8. Booth, D. A. & P. C. Simson. 1971. Food preferences acquired by association with variations in amino acid nutrition. Q. J. Exp. Psychol. **23**: 135–145.
9. Booth, D. A., D. Lovett & G. M. McSherry. 1972. Postingestive modulation of the sweetness preference gradient in the rat. J. Comp. Physiol. Psychol. **78**: 485–512.
10. Booth, D. A. 1972. Conditioned satiety in the rat. J. Comp. Physiol. Psychol. **81**: 457–471.
11. Booth, D. A. & J. D. Davis. 1973. Gastrointestinal factors in the acquisition of oral sensory control of satiation. Physiol. Behav. **11**: 23–29.
12. Davis, J. D. & C. S. Campbell. 1973. Peripheral control of meal size in the rat: effect of sham feeding on meal size and drinking rate. J. Comp. Physiol. Psychol. **83**: 379–387.
13. Booth, D. A., R. Stoloff & J. Nicholls. 1974. Dietary flavor acceptance in infant rats is established by association with effects of nutrient composition. Physiol. Psychol. **2**: 313–319.
14. Le Magnen, J. 1959. Effets des administrations post-prandiales de glucose sur l'établissement des appétits. C. R. Soc. Biol., Paris **153**: 212–215.
15. Rozin, P. 1967. Specific aversions as a component of specific hungers. J. Comp. Physiol. Psychol. **64**: 237–242.
16. Puerto, A., J. A. Deutsch, F. Molina & P. L. Roll. 1976. Rapid discrimination of rewarding nutrient by the upper gastrointestinal tract. Science **192**: 485–487.
17. Miller, N. E. & M. L. Kessen. 1952. Reward effects of food via stomach fistula compared with those of food via mouth. J. Comp. Physiol. Psychol. **45**: 555–564.
18. Holman, G. 1968. Intragastric reinforcement effect. J. Comp. Physiol. Psychol. **69**: 432–441.
19. Revusky, S. H. 1968. Effects of thirst level during consumption of flavored water on subsequent preferences. J. Comp. Physiol. Psychol. **66**: 777–779.
20. Holman, E. W. 1975. Immediate and delayed reinforcers for flavor preferences in rats. Learn. Motiv. **6**: 91–100.
21. Mather, P., S. Nicolaidis & D. A. Booth. 1978. Compensatory and conditioned feeding responses to scheduled glucose infusions in the rat. Nature **273**: 461–463.
22. Davis, C. M. 1928. Self selection of diet by newly weaned infants. Am. J. Dis. Child. **36**: 651–679.
23. Richter, C. P. 1943. Total self-regulatory functions in animals and human beings. Harvey Lecture Series **38**: 63–103.
24. Booth, D. A., F. M. Toates & S. V. Platt. 1976. Control system for hunger and its implications in animals and man. *In* Hunger. D. Novin, W. Wyrwicka & G. A. Bray, Eds.: 127–142. Raven Press. New York.
25. Booth, D. A. 1976. Approaches to feeding control. *In* Appetite and Food Intake. T. Silverstone, Ed.: 417–478. Abakon & Dahlem Konferenzen. West Berlin.
26. Newman, J. C. & D. A. Booth. 1981. Gastrointestinal and metabolic consequences of a rat's meal on maintenance diet ad libitum. Physiol. Behav. **27**: 929–939.
27. Booth, D. A. 1974. Food intake compensation for increase and decrease in the protein content of the diet. Behav. Biol. **12**: 31–40.
28. Krieckhaus, E. E. & G. Wolf. 1968. Acquisition of sodium by rats: interaction of innate mechanisms and latent learning. J. Comp. Physiol. Psychol. **65**: 197–201.

29. DENTON, D. A. 1982. The Hunger for Salt. Springer. Berlin.
30. CABANAC, M. 1971. The physiological role of pleasure. Science **173**: 1103–1107.
31. AMOORE, J. 1975. Four primary odor modalities of man: experimental evidence and possible significance. *In* Olfaction and Taste V. D. A. Denton & J. P. Coghlan, Eds.: 283–289. Academic Press, Inc. New York.
32. JACOBS, H. L. 1964. Observations on the ontogeny of saccharin preference in the neonate rat. Psychon. Sci. **1**: 105–106.
33. HAMILTON, C. F. 1964. Rat's preference for high fat diets. J. Comp. Physiol. Psychol. **58**: 459–460.
34. HARPER A. E. & H. E. SPIVEY. 1958. Relationship between food intake and osmotic effect of dietary carbohydrate. Am. J. Physiol. **193**: 483–487.
35. DEUTSCH, J. A., A. PUERTO & M.-L. WANG. 1977. The pyloric sphincter and differential food preference. Behav. Biol. **19**: 543–547.
36. WURTMAN, R. J. & J. D. FERNSTROM. 1975. Control of brain monoamine synthesis by diet and plasma amino acids. Am. J. Clin. Nutr. **28**: 638–647.
37. MARKS-KAUFMAN, R. & R. KANAREK. 1980. Morphine selectively influences macronutrient intake in the rat. Pharmacol. Biochem. Behav. **12**: 42–430.
38. LEATHWOOD, P. D. & D. V. M. ASHLEY. 1984. Behavioural strategies in the regulation of food choice. Experientia **44** Suppl.: 171–196.
39. HARRIS L. J., J. CLAY, F. J. HARGREAVES & A. WARD. 1933. Appetite and choice of diet. The ability of the vitamin B deficient rat to discriminate between diets containing and lacking the vitamin. Proc. R. Soc. Lond. Ser. B **113**: 161–190.
40. ROZIN, P. & J. W. KALAT. 1971. Specific hungers and poison avoidance as adaptive specializations of learning. Psychol. Rev. **78**: 459–486.
41. RZOSKA, J. 1953. Bait shyness: a study in rat behaviour. Br. J. Anim. Behav. **1**: 128–135.
42. GARCIA, J., D. J. KIMELDORF & R. A. KOELLING. 1955. Conditioned aversion to saccharin resulting from exposure to gamma radiation. Science **122**: 157–158.
43. GARCIA, J., F. R. ERVIN, C. YORKE & R. A. KOELLING. 1967. Conditioning with delayed vitamin injections. Science **155**: 716–718.
44. GREEN, K. F. & J. GARCIA. 1971. Recuperation from illness: flavor enhancement for rats. Science **173**: 749–751.
45. ZAHORIK, D. M. 1979. Learned changes in preferences for chemical stimuli: asymmetrical effects of positive and negative consequences and species differences in learning. *In* Preference Behaviour and Chemoreception. J. H. A. Kroeze, Ed.: 233–243. Information Retrieval Ltd. London.
46. LE MAGNEN, J. 1954. Le processus de discrimination par le rat blanc des stimuli sucres alimentaires et non alimentaires. J. Physiol., Paris **46**: 414–418.
47. LE MAGNEN, J. 1956. Effets sur la prise alimentaire du rat blanc des administrations postprandiales d'insuline et le mécanisme des appetits. J. Physiol., Paris **48**: 789–802.
48. LE MAGNEN, J. 1963. La facilitation differentielle des reflexes d'ingestion par l'odour alimentaire. C. R. Soc. Biol. **157**: 1165–1170.
49. LE MAGNEN, J. 1967. Food habits. *In* Handbook of Physiology. Alimentary Canal, Vol. 1: 11–30. American Physiological Society. Washington, D.C.
50. LE MAGNEN, J. 1969. Peripheral and systemic actions of food in the caloric regulation of intake. Ann. N.Y. Acad. Sci. **147**: 1126–1157.
51. BOOTH, D. A. 1972. Caloric compensation in rats with continuous or intermittent access to food. Physiol. Behav. **8**: 891–899.
52. BOLLES, R. C., L. HAYWARD & C. CRANDALL. 1981. Conditioned taste preferences based on caloric density. J. Exp. Psychol.: Anim. Behav. Proc. **7**: 59–69.
53. BOOTH, D. A., C. W. T. PILCHER, G. D. D'MELLO & I. P. STOLERMAN. Comparative potencies of amphetamine, fenfluramine and related compounds in taste aversion experiments in rats. Br. J. Pharmacol. **61**: 669–677.
54. LOVETT, D. & D. A. BOOTH. 1970. Four effects of exogenous insulin on food intake. Q. J. Exp. Psychol. **22**: 406–419.
55. BOOTH, D. A. 1979. Metabolism and the control of feeding in man and animals. *In* Chemical Influences on Behaviour. K. Brown & S. J. Cooper, Eds.: 79–134. Academic Press. London.

56. Deutsch, J. A. 1983. Dietary control and the stomach. Prog. Neurobiol. **20**: 313–332.
57. Booth, D. A. 1977. Appetite and satiety as metabolic expectancies. *In* Food Intake and Chemical Senses. Y. Katsuki, M. Sato, S. F. Takagi & Y. Oomura, Eds.: 317–330. University of Tokyo Press. Tokyo.
58. Booth, D. A. 1982. Normal control of omnivore intake by taste and smell. *In* Determination of Behaviour by Chemical Stimuli. J. E. Steiner, Ed.: 233–243. Information Retrieval Ltd. London.
59. Pain, J. & D. A. Booth. 1968. Toxiphobia to odors. Psychon. Sci. **10**: 363–364.
60. Rusiniak, K. W., W. G. Hankins, J. Garcia & L. P. Brett. 1979. Flavor-illness aversions: potentiation of odor by taste in rats. Behav. Neural Bio. **25**: 1–17.
61. Westbrook, R. F., J. Homewood, K. Horn & J. C. Clarke. 1983. Flavour-odour compound conditioning: odour-potentiation and flavour-attenuation Q. J. Exp. Psychol. 35B: 13–33.
62. Weingarten, H. P. 1984. Meal initiation controlled by learned cues: basic behavioral properties. Appetite **5**: 147–158.
63. Mineka, S. 1975. Some new perspectives on conditioned hunger. J. Exp. Psychol: Anim. Behav. Proc. **1**: 134–148.
64. Valenstein, E. S. 1967. Selection of nutritive and non-nutritive solutions under different conditions of need. J. Comp. Physiol. Psychol. **63**: 429–433.
65. Booth, D. A. 1972. Taste reactivity in satiated, ready to eat and starved rats. Physiol. Behav. **8**: 901–908.
66. Booth, D. A. 1979. Preference as a motive. *In* Preference Behaviour and Chemoreception. J. H. A. Kroeze, Ed.: 317–334. Information Retrieval Ltd. London.
67. Coons, E. E. & H. A. White. 1978. CNS weighting of external and internal factors governing reward. Ann. N.Y. Acad. Sci.
68. Booth, D. A. & T. Brookover. 1968. Hunger elicited in the rat by a single injection of crystalline bovine insulin. Physiol. Behav. **3**: 439–446.
69. Siegel, S. & N. Nettleton. 1972. Conditioning of insulin-induced hyperphagia. J. Comp. Physiol. Psychol. **70**: 390–398.
70. Richter, C. P. 1942. Increased dextrose appetite of normal rats treated with insulin. Am. J. Physiol. **135**: 781–787.
71. Mayer-Gross, W. & J. Walker. 1946. Taste and selection of food in hypoglycaemia. Br. J. Exp. Pathol. **27**: 297–305.
72. Kanarek, R. B., R. Marks-Kaufman & B. J. Lipeles. 1980. Increased carbohydrate intake as a function of insulin administration in rats. Physiol. Behav. **25**: 779–782.
73. Booth, D. A. 1979. Is thirst largely an acquired specific appetite? Behav. Brain. Sci. **2**: 103–104.
74. Rolls, B. J., E. A. Rowe & E. T. Rolls. 1982. How sensory properties of foods affect human feeding behavior. Physiol. Behav. **29**: 409–417.
75. Le Magnen, J. 1956. Hyperphagie provoquée chez le rat blanc par alteration du mécanisme de satiété peripherique. C. R. Soc. Biol., Paris **150**: 31–32
76. Treit, D., M. L. Spetch & J. A. Deutsch. 1983. Variety in the flavor of food enhances eating in the rat: a controlled demonstration. Physiol. Behav. **30**: 207–211.
77. Booth, D. A., M. Lee & C. McAleavey. 1976. Acquired sensory control of satiation in man. Br. J. Psychol. **67**: 137–147.
78. Booth, D. A., P. Mather & J. Fuller. 1982. Starch content of ordinary foods associatively conditions human appetite and satiation. Appetite **3**: 163–184.
79. Booth, D. A. & A. M. Toase. 1983. Conditioning of hunger/satiety signals as well as flavour cues in dieters. Appetite **4**: 235–236.
80. Smith, G. P. 1983. The peripheral control of appetite. Lancet **ii**: 88–90.
81. Smith, G. P. 1982. Satiety and the problem of motivation. *In* The Physiological Mechanisms of Motivation. D. W. Pfaff, Ed.: 133–143. Springer Verlag. New York.
82. Smith, G. P. & J. Gibbs. 1979. Postprandial satiety. Prog. Psychobiol. Physiol. Psychol. **10**: 179–242.
83. Kraly, F. R., W. J. Carty & G. P. Smith. 1978. Effect of pregastric food stimuli on meal size and intermeal interval in the rat. Physiol. Behav. **20**: 779–784.

84. Kraly, F. S. & G. P. Smith. 1978. Combined pregastric and gastric stimulation is sufficient for normal meal size. Physiol. Behav. **21**: 405–408.
85. Moran, T. H. & P. R. McHugh. 1982. Cholecystokinin suppresses food intake by inhibiting gastric emptying. Am. J. Physiol. **242**: R491–R497.
86. Crawley, J. N. & M. C. Beinfeld. 1983. Rapid development of tolerance to the behavioural actions of cholecystokinin. Nature **302**: 703–706.
87. Davies, J. D., B. J. Collins & M. W. Levine. 1978. The interaction between gustatory stimulation and gut feedback in the control of ingestion of liquid diets. *In* Hunger Models. D. A. Booth, Ed.: 109–142. Academic Press. London.
88. Mook, D. G., R. Culberson, R. J. Gelbart & K. McDonald. 1983. Oropharyngeal control of ingestion in rat: acquisition of sham drinking patterns. Behav. Neurosci. **97**: 574–584.
89. Van Vort, W. & G. P. Smith. 1983. The relationships between the positive reinforcing and satiating effects of a meal in the rat. Physiol. Behav. **30**: 279–284.
90. Revusky, S. H. 1967. Hunger level during food consumption: effects on subsequent preference. Psychnom. Sci. **4**: 109–110.
91. Beck. R. C. 1978. Motivation: Theories and Principles. Prentice-Hall. Englewood Cliffs, NJ.
92. Capaldi, E. D. & F. Friedman. 1976. Deprivation and reward as compound stimuli. Learn. Motiv. **7**: 17–30
93. Capaldi, E. D. & T. L. Davidson. 1979. Control of instrumental behavior by deprivation stimuli. J. Exp. Psychol.: Anim. Behav. Proc. **5**: 355–367.
94. Revusky, S. H., S. Coombes & R. W. Pohl. 1982. Drug states as discriminative stimuli in a flavor-aversion learning experiment. J. Comp. Physiol. Psychol. **96**: 200–201.
95. Revusky, S. H., R. W. Pohl & S. Coombes. 1980. Flavor aversions and deprivation state. Anim. Learn. Behav. **8**: 543–549.
96. Bower, G. H., S. G. Gilligan & K. P. Monteiro. 1981. Selectivity of learning caused by affective states. J. Exp. Psychol.: Gen. **110**: 451–473.
97. Deutsch, J. A. 1980. Bombesin—satiety or malaise? Nature **285**: 592.
98. Gibbs, J. & G. P. Smith. 1980. Bombesin—satiety or malaise? Reply. Nature **285**: 592.
99. Cole, A. D. & N. W. Bond. 1983. Olfactory aversion conditioning and overeating: a review and some data. Percept. Mot. Skills **57**: 667–678.

Contextual Influences on Conditioned Taste Aversions in the Developing Rat

NORMAN E. SPEAR, DAVID KUCHARSKI, AND HEATHER HOFFMANN

Department of Psychology
State University of New York
Binghamton, New York 13901

For about 15 years we have been studying infantile amnesia, why we don't remember what happened to us before the age of three or so. Our tests have addressed this effect with the rat. Animals show something akin to infantile amnesia—it is practically impossible to study it experimentally with humans—and the rat model has well-known advantages. In this case a major advantage is that the rat is altricial like the human but develops more quickly. For instance, two weeks postnatal the preweanling rat has only 10–20% of the neocortical synapses it will have as an adult and yet achieves adult-like levels of synapses by four weeks postnatal.

Our story begins eight or nine years ago, when we set out to test infantile amnesia for conditioned taste aversion. We eventually found that infantile amnesia does occur in this situation, pretty much as in any other. But first we had to solve a sticky problem of experimental design.

Basically, we needed to compare the long-term forgetting of taste aversion conditioning in preweanlings and adults. This provided a circumstance in which the contexts of training and later testing might be drastically different for the younger animals, which could inflate our estimates of how much the long retention interval actually contributed to their forgetting. One solution might be to condition the preweanlings in their home nest, continue to house them in a maternity cage, and test them there later as adults. But there are great changes that take place in the developing rat's response to home, changes that serve to promote the weaning process. The mothers and siblings change in appearance and how they respond to one another, odors change, and visual and structural characteristics of the nest change, so that psychologically and biologically, the rats' preweaning residence can never be maintained in exactly the same form when the rat reaches adulthood. Like the human the adult rat cannot go home again, and cannot even stay at home without changing it, and so this solution did not work.

Another solution might be to train the preweanling in an adult-like environment and then test them as adults in the same environment. But here, too, there is potentially a contextual change between conditioning and testing, at least in effect. The conditioning environment would be totally unfamiliar and uncomfortable to the preweanling rat, but familiar and reasonably comfortable when that rat becomes an adult. An experimental solution was called for—a direct test of the effects of contextual change on the preweanling's retention of conditioned taste aversion.

The results of this experiment were quite unexpected. It did not matter whether the contexts of conditioning and testing for the preweanlings were the same or different. But in a long series of more than 10 extensive experiments, what did matter was where the animals were conditioned. Conditioning preweanlings in the home led to a weaker taste aversion than conditioning in a novel location.[3]

As our experimental analysis evolved it became clear that the basic effect was straightforward and really quite easily described. When the conditioning solution was consumed at home followed shortly by an illness, percentage preference for that solution was two or three times greater than if that same solution had been consumed away from the home (percentage preference following consumption at home versus elsewhere did not differ for control subjects not given the taste-illness pairing). It did not matter where the animal was made ill, where it became ill, where it was tested, or where it spent the interval between conditioning and testing. The effect occurred even if the preweanling previously was given several hours of experience with the novel location in which they consumed the conditioning solution. Yet the effect was sharply dependent on age. The conditioning of adults did not differ if conditioned at home or in a novel location, even when their home was made similar structurally to that of the preweanling. And, although the impairment of conditioned taste aversion inevitably occurred in animals conditioned when 18 days of age, it was not present in animals 21 days of age. This latter difference was particularly puzzling initially but now seems understandable. The characteristics of this general effect, retarded conditioning of taste aversion in preweanlings conditioned at home, are summarized in TABLE 1.

We were surprised by the nature of this effect of home on conditioned taste aversion. We had reason to expect some differences in conditioning at home compared to a novel place, but not the particular difference we found. Before our tests of conditioned taste aversion we had been investigating how isolating the preweanling from its home might affect other kinds of learning. This requires some appreciation of the preweanling rats' ecological plight when conventional tests of learning are administered in the laboratory. Nearly all of these tests have required that the preweanling be plucked from a home of warmth, tactual comfort, and familiar tastes, odors, sounds, and movements, and taken to an experimental apparatus that is quite different in most of these respects. When isolated from their home in this way, striking changes occur in the preweanling rat, quite independent of the experimental test.[18] For instance, within a minute or so the infant rat's general activity triples; its vocalizations increase more

TABLE 1. Characteristics of the Effect of Home Stimuli on Conditioned Taste Aversions[3]

Preweanling rats (18 days postnatal) given a single pairing of 15% sucrose solution and 0.15 M (or 0.3 M) LiCl develop relatively weak sucrose aversions if the conditioning takes place in the pup's home.

This effect seems to depend primarily on where the taste is experienced.

It occurs regardless of:

- whether the pups are exposed to the toxicosis at home or in a novel location.
- whether the pups spend the interval between conditioning and testing at home or in a novel location.
- whether or not the pups are given several hours of prior familiarization with the novel location, even when the prior familiarization includes ingestion of fluids (infusion of plain water or almond-flavored water).

Conditioning at home does not attenuate aversions for adults or slightly older (21 days) preweanlings.

than sixfold over five minutes, and over the same five-minute period, heart rate increases 25% or so, from about 400 beats per minute to nearly 500.

What triggers this array of immediate responses to isolation from the nest? We guessed that the absence of nest odors is a particularly salient signal in view of the dominant role of olfaction in the developing rat.[8] To make the context of testing more "home-like," Gregory Smith and I simply placed the materials from the preweanling's own home nest under and around the experimental apparatus. This crude manipulation made some striking differences in learning. We found that the presence of home nest materials increased the rate at which these young rats could learn passive avoidance, essentially doubled the probability of spontaneous alteration to the level of adults, and facilitated acquisition of a discriminated escape task.[9,10] Rats a week older (23 days) were unaffected by the home odors.

The presence of home-nest odors has not facilitated all types of learning tested with preweanlings. In unpublished studies we have found no influence of these odors on learning one-way active avoidance or on classical conditioning of aversion to an odor paired with footshock. In several experiments, however, presence of these materials has facilitated conditioning of an aversion to a particular location-brightness combination. By way of analysis of these effects, the home-nest facilitation of discriminated escape learning seemed to be a matter of the mere familiarity of the home odors, because a similar effect occurred when non-rat odors were made familiar and placed near the training apparatus.[17] Also, this effect was observed at the beginning of the second postnatal week as well as the beginning of the third postnatal week[10] even though the "meaning" of home odors during conditioning seemed different for animals of these two ages.[1] These effects of home odors on aversive conditioning, excluding conditioned taste aversions, are summarized in TABLE 2. The effects of home odors on these kinds of learning are of particular interest here because they are so different from their impact on conditioned taste aversion.

At about the same time that we were examining conditioned taste aversion in preweanlings, a particularly elegant study was published by Martin and Alberts.[6] They discovered that the 15-day-old rat could acquire no aversion whatsoever to a taste consumed while it was on the nipple of its mother, although when in the same context, but off the nipple, a conditioned taste aversion was acquired. We will discuss later more recent work from this laboratory. At this point, however, we will examine basic issues in order to integrate three of the facts just illustrated: (1) the conditioning of a taste aversion is impaired in the home for 18-day-olds, but not for 21-day-olds nor

TABLE 2. Effects of Home Odors on Learning in Preweanling Rats[a]

Enhances acquisition of passive avoidance for 16-day-olds but not for 23-day-olds

Enhances acquisition of discriminated escape
  for 9-, 11-, or 16-day-old rats but not for 28-day-old rats
  Similar enhancement occurs for 16-day-olds, but not for 28-day-olds, in the presence of familiar odors

Increases spontaneous alternation
  for 16-day-olds but not for 23-day-olds

Enhances classical conditioning of a location/brightness aversion
  for 16-day-olds but not for weaned 23–30-day-olds

No effect on one-way active avoidance or on classical conditioning of aversion to novel odor (paired with footshock)

[a] Excludes conditioned taste aversions; from a variety of studies with Smith, Wigal, and Richter.

for adults; (2) the presence of home-nest odors can facilitate test performance of rats during their second and third postnatal weeks in a variety of learning tasks, although this same facilitation does not occur after weaning at the beginning of the fourth postnatal week; and (3) the conditioning of a taste aversion is quite drastically impaired or impossible for 15-day-old rats conditioned when suckling.

EXPERIMENTAL TESTS OF THE ISSUES

We designed several experiments in order to help answer three questions about "home" effects: (1) Is the odor of home-nesting materials sufficient to retard the conditioning of a sucrose aversion? (2) Is the drastic impairment in conditioning of a flavor aversion during suckling a simple extension of the lesser impairment observed in the home environment in the absence of suckling? (3) Is learning about tastes in general retarded for preweanlings when they are in their home, or is retardation of the association between taste and illness a relatively special case? The results of these particular experiments are easy to describe and have been confirmed by data from other experiments in our laboratory.

Are Home Odors Sufficient to Retard Conditioning of a Sucrose Aversion in Preweanling Rats?

The core design of this experiment was simple, essentially four conditions with general procedures like those of Infurna, Steinert, and Spear.[3] Briefly, 18-day-old preweanling rat pups were injected with LiCl immediately after one hour of access to a tube delivering 15% sucrose solution. Half the animals consumed the sucrose solution from tubes placed directly into their maternity cage and half did so from the same type of tubes presented in a typical hanging metal cage that was novel to the preweanling rats. Individual compartments inserted into the maternity cage separated one animal from another during ingestion, and a similar compartment of exactly the same dimensions was inserted into the hanging metal cages in order to equate area of the range permitted during access to the sucrose solution. For half the animals in the maternity cages, nesting material had not been changed for seven days; for the other half, nesting material was changed just prior to presentation of the sucrose solution. In both cases, the preweanling's mother and father were removed from the maternity cages and held in another cage elsewhere until after the animal consumed sucrose solution and was injected with LiCl. Of the preweanlings that ingested sucrose solution in the metal cages, half had seven-day-old nesting materials on the floor and half did not. Immediately after access to the sucrose solution, each animal was injected with LiCl (0.15 M) administered in a dose of 20 ml solution per kg of body weight. All animals remained in their conditioning environment for one hour, then spent the five days prior to testing in their home with parents and littermates.

The results replicated the usual effect (FIGURE 1). For animals conditioned in the home (with soiled nest shavings) the conditioned aversion was clearly weaker than for animals conditioned in a novel location. Animals conditioned in a maternity cage but with clean nesting materials showed aversions intermediate between these two. But it is the fourth group that is most pertinent here—those animals conditioned in the novel location but in the presence of odors and tactual characteristics of the nesting materials from the home. Their conditioning was significantly stronger than that of the animals similarly conditioned in the presence of nesting materials and in the fa-

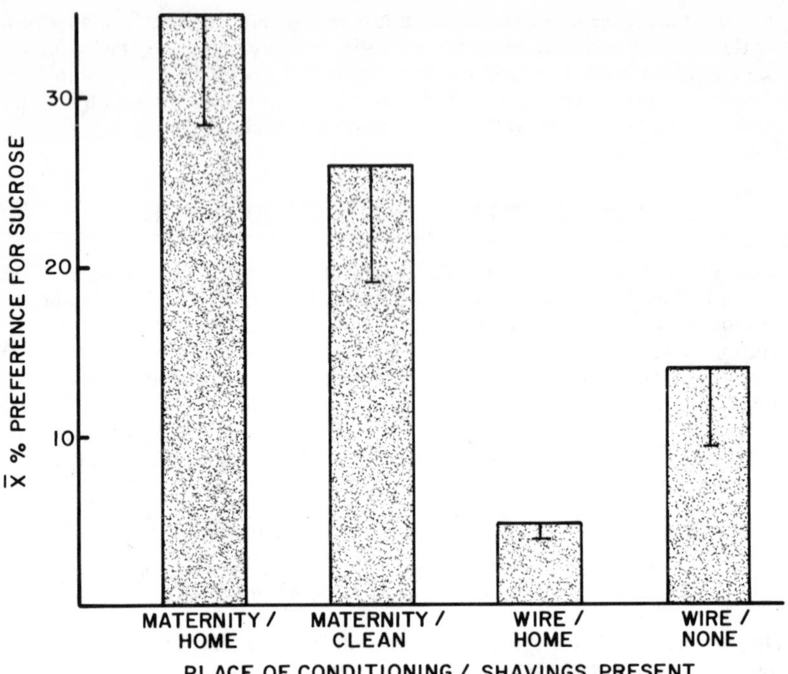

FIGURE 1. Mean percent preference for sucrose during test [sucrose intake/(sucrose intake + water intake)] as a function of conditioning group. For the maternity/home group, animals were conditioned and tested in a maternity cage with litter shavings from the animals' own home present. For the maternity/clean group, animals were conditioned and tested in a maternity cage with clean shavings present. For the wire/home group, animals were conditioned and tested in a wire cage with litter shavings from the animals' own home present. For the wire/none group, the animals were conditioned and tested in a wire cage with no litter shavings present.

miliar maternity cage. Conditioning in the novel cage with nest materials on the floor was in fact no weaker (in this case it was significantly stronger) than conditioning in the novel environment without nesting materials. This indicates that even when combined with the tactual aspects of home, odors from the home are not sufficient for the retardation of a conditioned aversion to sucrose. We have replicated this general result in other experiments. In two of these, delays of 10 or 15 minutes were introduced between the sucrose solution and LiCl in order to combat anticipated measurement problems; the third experiment was like the present one in having no CS-US delay but it included a different dose of LiCl in order to examine the generality of this effect over different intensities of US. In each of these experiments, as in the present one, the preweanlings conditioned in a novel environment with home odors and tactual stimuli tended to show stronger conditioned aversions than those in the novel environment without these home stimuli.

The lesson of this experiment is that the odors of the home are not sufficient to retard conditioning of an aversion to sucrose solution, even when combined with the tactile stimulation from home-nest materials. It would appear that visual aspects of the maternity cage contribute to this effect, to the extent that the concept of "home" can be so divided for the preweanling in terms of sensory dimensions.

Is the Retardation of Conditioning During Suckling Simply an Extension of the Lesser Retardation in the Home Without Suckling?

The conditioned stimulus in the Martin and Alberts experiment[6] was not sucrose solution but geraniol mixed in warm milk. Geraniol has a distinctive odor as well as a distinctive flavor. Also, Martin and Alberts conditioned preweanlings at 15 days of age whereas we conditioned 18-day-old preweanlings; and, their test for aversion was different, measuring intake of differently flavored foods in separate locations, which may allow more influence from aversion to a particular compartment on the basis of its odor rather than the taste of the food there. It was therefore unclear whether 18-day-olds with a sucrose CS would show severely retarded conditioning when suckling, and it is equally uncertain whether 15-day-old rat pups given geraniol-flavored milk as their CS would show retarded conditioning in their home. Our initial study used cannulated 15-day-old rat pups as in the Martin and Alberts study, but with sucrose solution as the CS and a two-bottle drinking test to assess conditioning. We chose this particular approach because we have a great deal of data using the sucrose CS. Also, sucrose solution has less of a distinctive odor than geraniol and we wished to maximize the taste and minimize the olfactory consequences of conditioning.

The initial experiment was to assess the idea of a continuum that defines similarity to home from completely novel locations at one extreme to suckling-in-nest at the other. One might expect from this continuum that the strongest conditioned aversions would be acquired in a novel location, somewhat weaker aversions acquired when in the home but not actually suckling, and the weakest aversion, perhaps no aversion at all, in the home nest while suckling.

This experiment included six groups of 15-day-old rat pups, all of which were cannulated in order to have sucrose solution infused into their mouths (rats of this age are of course too young to drink from tubes). For the three circumstances of conditioning, the "suckling" group had their sucrose infused for one minute while they were actually suckling on their anesthetized mother's nipple. The "home" group had their sucrose solution infused for one minute while they were in the nest near the mother, but for these pups the mother's nipples were inaccessible (the dam was placed lying on her ventrum). The third group had their sucrose solution infused for one minute while in a Plexiglas® cage with a wire mesh floor that was completely novel to them. For half the subjects in each of these conditions, LiCl was injected immediately after infusion of the sucrose solution; for the other half, the explicitly unpaired control animals, LiCl was not injected until 24 hours after infusion of the sucrose solution. All animals were tested for sucrose preference five days after sucrose infusion. During this test access was permitted to two tubes, one containing 15% sucrose solution and one water.

The results basically replicated those of Martin and Alberts (FIGURE 2). There was no conditioning of an aversion to sucrose for animals that consumed it while suckling on the nipple. The conditioned animals in this case showed nearly 100% sucrose preference and tended to consume more sucrose than did the unpaired controls. The other two groups apparently developed some conditioned aversion to the sucrose solution, clearly more aversion than was seen for animals conditioned on the nipple but really quite weak conditioning in both condtions. There was some tendency for

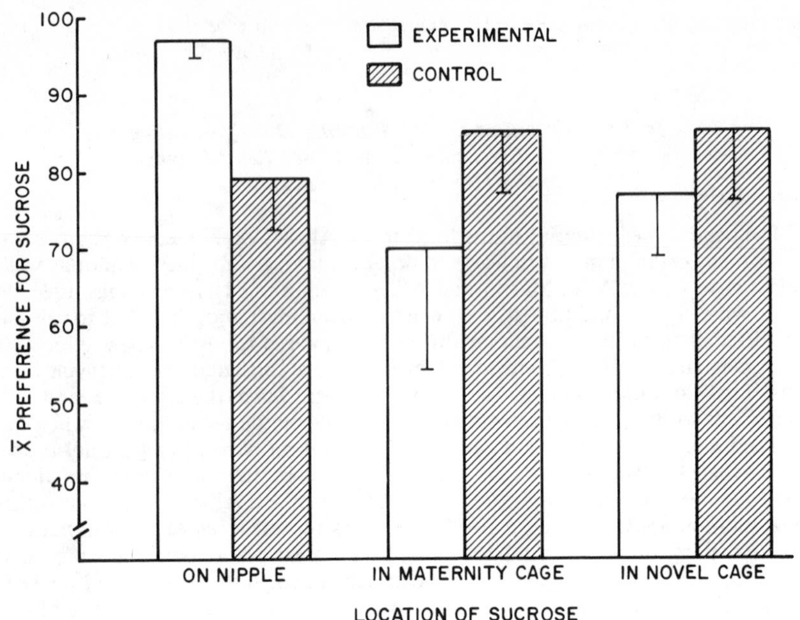

100
90
80
70
60
50
40
X̄ PREFERENCE FOR SUCROSE
EXPERIMENTAL
CONTROL
ON NIPPLE
IN MATERNITY CAGE
IN NOVEL CAGE
LOCATION OF SUCROSE

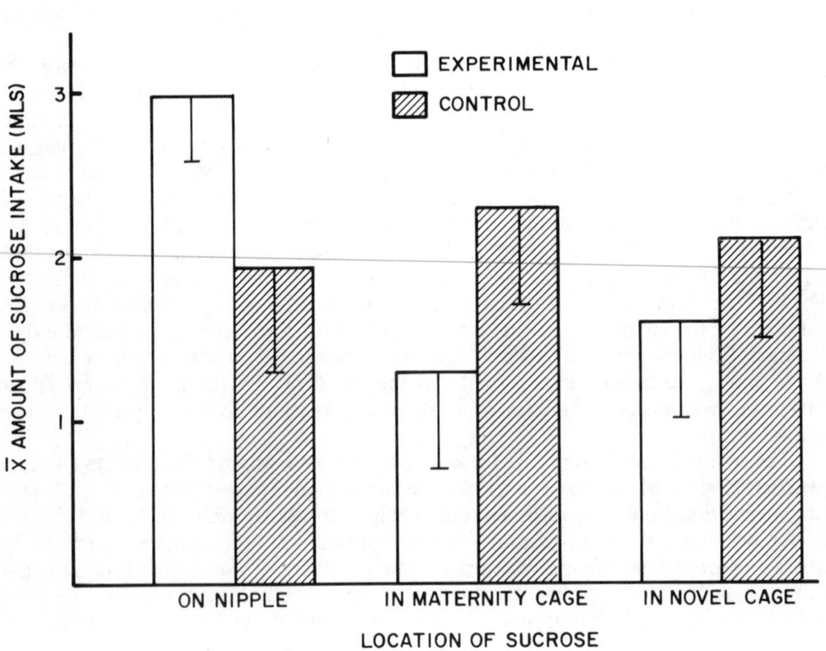

3
2
1
X̄ AMOUNT OF SUCROSE INTAKE (MLS)
EXPERIMENTAL
CONTROL
ON NIPPLE
IN MATERNITY CAGE
IN NOVEL CAGE
LOCATION OF SUCROSE

less sucrose preference among animals conditioned in the novel environment than for those conditioned at home off the nipple, but this difference did not approach statistical significance. Although somewhat aside from our main point, the LiCl-linked increase in sucrose preference and intake for pups conditioned on the nipple is notable; Martin and Alberts[6] also reported such an effect in some of their experiments.

This experiment extends the Martin-Alberts effect of suckling-related impairment to conditioning with sucrose solution as the CS. There was no indication, however, that at this age (15 days) conditioning of an aversion to a taste is weaker in the home without suckling than in a novel location. Perhaps this is to be expected if visual characteristics of the home are important for this effect (as our previous experiment implied), to the extent that the recent eye-opening of 15-day-olds leaves them less adept visually than 18-day-olds. However, we do not want to make much of this lack of difference. With further tests and procedures to promote stronger conditioning, the effects of the home environment without suckling might emerge in animals of this age as well.

Is Learning About Novel Tastes Uniformly Suppressed in the Home Environment of the Preweanling?

At first glance this seems a ridiculous question. There is no doubt that what the preweanling consumes at home must have been novel at some point and that its early consumption can influence markedly what it eats later in life, probably due to associative mechanisms. The issue here, however, is not whether anything can be learned about novel tastes but whether less is learned about them in the home than elsewhere.

This experiment, conducted in collaboration with Tim Wigal, was to test the effects of the home environment on learning the relationship between two tastes, sucrose and coffee (sweet and bitter). We wanted to assess in a single situation the learning of the relationship between two tastes and that between the tastes and induced illness. The idea was to determine whether the context of home affects all types of learning equally or whether there is a singular effect on conditioning an aversion to a particular taste. Common sense favors the latter. It would be an unfortunate rat pup that became ill following ingestion of mother's milk and then developed an aversion to it. As the pup's only food source during the first two weeks postnatal and major food source for the next week or so, mother's milk must be consumed by the rat pup if it is to survive. But in spite of this ostensible advantage in having the home context retard conditioned taste aversion, there would seem little advantage to having all classes of learning about tastes retarded when at home. The present study was to test this version of common sense.

There were two separate experiments in this study. The first tested learning of an association between two tastes, sucrose and coffee mixed in a common solution. We

---

FIGURE 2. (*Top*) Mean percent preference for sucrose during test as a function of experimental manipulation (experimental or control) and where the sucrose was ingested during conditioning [on nipple (the animals consumed the solution in a maternity cage while attached to a nipple), in maternity cage (the animals consumed the solution while in a maternity cage), or in novel cage (the animals consumed the solution while in a novel wire cage)]. (*Bottom*) Mean amount of sucrose ingested during test as a function of experimental manipulation (experimental or control) and where the solution was ingested during conditioning (on nipple, in maternity cage, in novel cage).

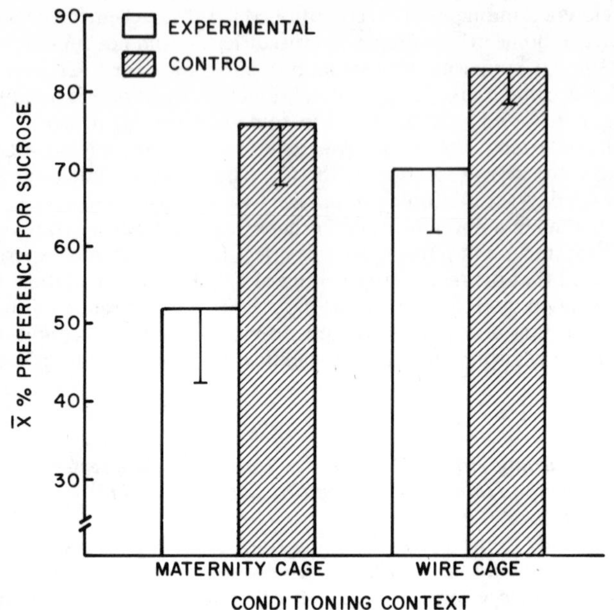

EXPERIMENTAL
CONTROL
X̄ % PREFERENCE FOR SUCROSE
90
80
70
60
50
40
30
MATERNITY CAGE
WIRE CAGE
CONDITIONING CONTEXT

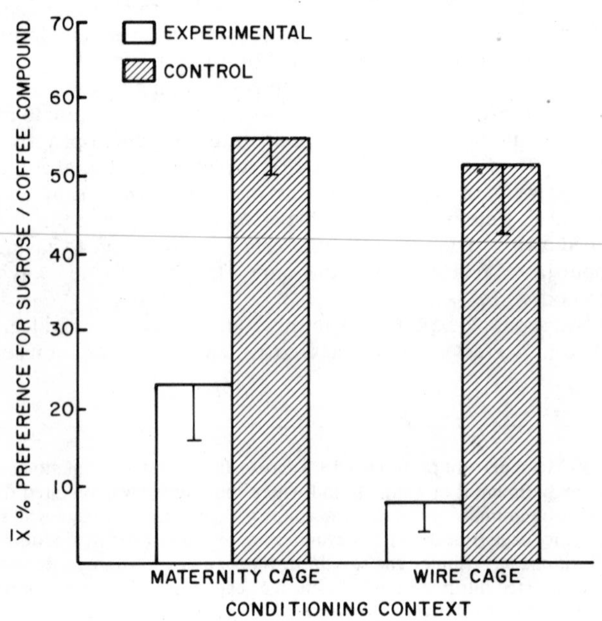

EXPERIMENTAL
CONTROL
X̄ % PREFERENCE FOR SUCROSE / COFFEE COMPOUND
70
60
50
40
30
20
10
MATERNITY CAGE
WIRE CAGE
CONDITIONING CONTEXT

chose this particular combination of tastes because several of our experiments had indicated that preweanling rats do learn the relationship between them.[5,14] The concentrations of each (15% sucrose solution, 1.25% decaffeinated coffee) were such that when paired separately with LiCl, equivalent aversions are acquired. The procedure applied the sensory preconditioning paradigm, involving two steps. First, the preweanlings consumed the sucrose-coffee compound either at home or in a novel metal cage. Next, the "value" of one taste was decreased by pairing it with LiCl. To the extent that this caused a decrease in the ingestion of the other taste (sucrose), we may infer an association between sucrose and coffee. To summarize, preweanlings consumed a compound of sucrose and coffee either at home or in a novel location. Then, later, half the animals consumed coffee followed immediately by injections of LiCl. The other half, the controls, consumed coffee but received no LiCl injection until 24 hours later. Several days later all animals were tested for sucrose preference. The results are shown in FIGURE 3 (top). Quite unlike the learning of the relationship between sucrose solution and LiCl discussed earlier, there was no indication that learning the association between sucrose and coffee was poorer at home than elsewhere. The results were in fact quite the opposite. The differences, albeit statistically weak, suggested stronger conditioning of the sucrose-coffee relationship when those elements occurred at home than when they occurred in a novel location.

Was learning of the association between the coffee-sucrose compound and LiCl impaired at home? It was possible that the addition of the bitter coffee component to our CS might alter the influence of home on conditioning an aversion to that compound. For instance we once entertained the possibility that for preweanlings, home has special effects on conditioning to sucrose solution because it is sweet.[15] The sweetness of mother's milk might lead to a context-specific latent inhibition so that home might impair conditioning to only sweet tastes. The results indicated otherwise (FIGURE 3, bottom). As with our previous experiments using sucrose solution as the CS, conditioning of the aversion to the sucrose-coffee compound was weaker in the home than in the novel location. There was no difference between the unpaired control conditions. So, learning about novel tastes is not inevitably retarded in the home. Quite the opposite, learning the relationship between two such tastes tends to be facilitated there. There seems little doubt, however, that for the preweanling 18-day-old rat learning of the relationship between taste and illness is retarded in the home.

Finally, we feel that in this case, sensory preconditioning might not be associative and could be qualitatively different from taste-toxicosis learning. We have found that preweanlings are especially likely to form a configured representation of a compound taste, more so than adults.[14] Rescorla[7] has suggested that such configuration enhances sensory preconditioning. It is possible that when in their home, preweanlings are more likely to use the "infantile" strategy of configuring the taste stimuli than when in the novel wire cage. In other words, we do not know at this point whether preweanlings condition differently in the home because they are more likely to associate two tastes

---

FIGURE 3. (*Top*) Mean percent preference for sucrose as a function of experimental manipulation (experimental or control) and the conditioning context (animals were either conditioned and tested in a maternity cage with litter shavings from the animals' own home present or in a novel wire cage). (*Bottom*) Mean percent preference for the sucrose-coffee compound solution [sucrose-coffee compound solution intake/(sucrose-coffee compound solution intake + water intake)] as a function of experimental manipulation (experimental or control) and the conditioning context (maternity cage or wire cage).

together, or because they are more likely to form a configured representation of a compound stimulus. In any case, the result suggests stronger or equal sensory preconditioning in the home cage than elsewhere.

DISCUSSION AND CONCLUSIONS

Taken as a whole these studies support two generalizations. First, the context of home can have special impact on what is learned by the developing rat pup and how strong that learning will be. These are explicitly developmental effects—learning by older, weaned rats is relatively unaffected whether it takes place in the home or elsewhere. Second, conditioned taste aversion is affected differently by the home than are other kinds of learning. Whereas the presence of home nest stimuli facilitates learning in many other instances, the conditioning of an aversion to a taste is impaired in the home for preweanlings. The locus of this impairment is not only home odors, which might conceivably interact with taste perception on a relatively peripheral level, but other sensory modalities, such as vision, may also be implicated.

It is still unclear whether the impairment of conditioned taste aversion by mere presence in the home is related to that observed during suckling. Like Martin and Alberts,[6] we found no indication that conditioned taste aversion could be acquired by the 15-day-old rat while engaged in suckling. But when our 15-day-olds were not suckling, there seemed little difference between the sucrose preference or intake of pups conditioned in the home and those conditioned elsewhere.

Other data also suggest that the impairment of conditioning by suckling may have a different basis than that by home stimuli alone. Gubernick and Alberts[2] have evidence to indicate that the suckling-related impairment is fundamentally a failure in expressing an acquired taste aversion. This failure was observed throughout the first four postnatal weeks, so long as the rat pups were not weaned or otherwise exposed to an alternative food source. As soon as an acceptible food alternative to mother's milk was experienced, the aversion previously acquired while on the nipple was expressed. These pups also readily acquired aversions to new substances presented while on the nipple. Our effect of home-stimuli impairment of conditioned taste aversion does not seem to be a matter of expression, however. There is little doubt that all of our pups conditioned at 18 days of age consume an alternative food source before they are tested at 22–24 days of age. The arrangement of our maternity cages is such that during the latter part of the third postnatal week, preweanling rats can reach the same hard food source as the mother, and they do so. We do not know how prevalent this is before 18 days of age, but it seems common to all pups by the age of 21 days. Perhaps it is the increasing familiarity with this hard food source that leads to the disappearance of the home-stimuli impairment in our studies by the time the preweanlings are 21 days old. Yet, our animals conditioned at 18 days of age show the home-stimuli impairment even though they are not tested until 22–24 days of age, by which time they have had ample experience with the hard food alternative to mother's milk.

Finally, that home stimuli influence the conditioning of a taste aversion differently than other cases of conditioning and learning is worthy of emphasis. This could be taken as confirmation that conditioned taste aversion has its own set of governing rules. We look at it as one more piece of evidence against the hypothesis that memory is a unitary system. Evidence is rapidly mounting against this hypothesis from a variety of sources, such as studies of dysfunction in human memory, but ontogenetic evidence like that described here has seemed equally pertinent.[11–13,16]

REFERENCES

1. CORBY, J., P. A. CAZA & N. E. SPEAR. 1982. Ontogenetic changes in the effectiveness of home nest odor as a conditioned stimulus. Behav. Neural Biol. **35**: 354–367.
2. GUBERNICK, L. T. & J. R. ALBERTS. 1985. A specialization of taste aversion learning during suckling and its weaning-associated transformation. Dev. Psychobiol. (In press.)
3. INFURNA, R. N., P. A. STEINERT & N. E. SPEAR. 1979. Ontogenetic changes in the modulation of taste aversion learning by home environmental cues. J. Comp. Physiol. Psychol. **93**: 1097–1108.
4. KUCHARSKI, D. & N. E. SPEAR. 1985. Potentiation of a conditioned taste aversion in preweanling and adult rats. Behav. Neural Biol. (In press.)
5. KUCHARSKI, D. & N. E. SPEAR. 1985. Potentiation and overshadowing in preweanling and adult rats. J. Exp. Psychol. Anim. Behav. Proc. (In press.)
6. MARTIN, L. T. & J. R. ALBERTS. 1979. Taste aversions to mother's milk: The age-related role of nursing in acquistion and expression of a learned association. J. Comp. Physiol. Psychol. **93**: 430–455.
7. RESCORALA, R. A. Simultaneous associations. 1982. *In* Predictability, Correlation Contiguity. P. Harzem & M. D. Zeiler, Eds. John Wiley & Sons. New York.
8. ROSENBLATT, J. S. 1983. Olfaction mediates developmental transition in the altricial newborn of selected species of mammals. Dev. Psychobiol. **16**: 347–375.
9. SMITH, G. J. & N. E. SPEAR. 1978. Home environmental effects on witholding behaviors in infant and neonatal rats. Science **202**: 327–329.
10. SMITH, G. J. & N. E. SPEAR. 1980. Facilitation of odor-aversion conditioning by the presence of conspecifics. Behav. Neurobehav. Biol. **28**: 491–495.
11. SPEAR, N. E. 1984. The future study of learning and memory from a psychobiological perspective. *In* Perspective in Psychological Experimentation. V. Sarris & A. Parducci, Eds.: 87–103. Lawrence Erlbaum Associates. Hillsdale, NJ.
12. SPEAR, N. E. 1985. Psychobiological and cognitive studies relevant to the issue of a unitary memory system. *In* New Directions in Cognitive Sciences. T. M. Schlecter & M. P. Toglia, Eds. Ablex Publishing Co. Norwood, NJ.
13. SPEAR, N. E. & R. L. ISAACSON. 1982. The problem of expression. *In* The Expression of Knowledge. R. L. Isaacson & N. E. Spear, Eds. Plenum Press. New York.
14. SPEAR, N. E. & D. KUCHARSKI. 1984. The ontogeny of stimulus selection: Developmental differences in what is learned. *In* Memory Development: Comparative Perspectives. R. Kail & N. E. Spear, Eds.: 227–252. Lawrence Erlbaum Associates. Hillsdale, NJ.
15. STEINERT, P. A., R. N. INFURNA, M. F. JARDULA & N. E. SPEAR. 1979. Effects of CS concentration on long-delay taste aversion learning in preweanling and adult rats. Behav. Neural Biol. **27**: 487–502.
16. TULVING, E. 1983. Elements of Episodic Memory. Oxford University Press. Oxford.
17. WIGAL, T., D. KUCHARSKI & N. E. SPEAR. 1985. Familiar contextual odors promote discrimination learning in preweanlings but not older rats. Dev. Psychobiol. (In press.)

Cue-consequence Specificity and Long-delay Learning Revisited[a]

MICHAEL DOMJAN

Department of Psychology
University of Texas at Austin
Austin, Texas 78712

The present volume and the proceedings of the conference held at Baylor University eight years ago[1] attest to the great importance and popularity of the food-aversion learning paradigm in a variety of psychobiological investigations. Much of this popularity was stimulated by two characteristics of food-aversion learning, cue-consequence specificity and long-delay learning.

At the time of their discovery, cue-consequence specificity and long-delay learning were contrary to prevailing ideas about the mechanisms of association formation.[2] This made food-aversion learning of great interest to investigators of learning processes. Cue-consequence specificity and long-delay learning also contributed to the use of food-aversion learning as an investigative technique in other areas of research. Cue-consequence specificity makes the conditioning of aversions to nongustatory cues unlikely. This liberates investigators from the usual burdens of conducting learning studies in experimental chambers specially designed to limit exposure to disruptive exteroceptive stimuli. Many aversion-conditioning experiments can be conducted in the home cages of animals in a colony room. The characteristic of long-delay learning has served to increase the range of chemicals that can be employed as aversion-inducing agents in food-aversion experiments. Because of long-delay learning, the delayed onset of many drugs does not preclude their use in the food-aversion paradigm.

Even though cue-consequence specificity and long-delay learning have been critical in stimulating use of the food-aversion learning paradigm, much of the resulting research, particularly in recent years, has not focused on these phenomena. This shift away from interest in cue-consequence specificity and long-delay learning is evident, for example, in the contents of the present volume in comparison to the Baylor volume published eight years ago. Whereas in the latter volume 8 of 22 papers were concerned primarily with some aspect of cue-consequence specificity or long-delay learning, in the present volume only 2 of 24 contributions have those two phenomena as their focus. The decline in interest in cue-consequence specificity and long-delay learning may reflect the resolution of outstanding research questions or simply abandonment of these questions. The purpose of the present paper is to consider, through a review of recent work, which of these alternatives seems to be the case.

[a] Preparation of the manuscript was supported by Grant MH 38529-01 from the Public Health Service.

CUE-CONSEQUENCE SPECIFICITY

Cue-consequence specificity refers to the fact that when rats are made ill following exposure to novel audiovisual and taste cues, they evidence much stronger aversions to the taste than to the audiovisual stimuli. In contrast, if they receive brief foot-shock following the same cues, they evidence much stronger aversions to the audiovisual than to the taste cues.[3] These findings are of particular interest because they show that aversion performance is not determined primarily by the nature of either conditioned or unconditioned stimuli but their combinations. Particular combinations of conditioned and unconditioned stimuli (taste and illness, for example) may condition aversions because of genetic predispositions to associate these stimuli selectively with one another. Alternatively, the cue-consequence specificity effect may reflect processes that do not involve experience-independent associative predispositions.[4] Much of the research on the cue-consequence specificity effect has focused on ruling out such alternative explanations.

Alternatives to Experience-Independent Associative Predispositions

Problems with Conditioned and Unconditioned Stimuli

Early research on the cue-consequence specificity effect was concerned with the possibility that the phenomenon reflected aspects of the ways in which the conditioned stimuli were presented during conditioning trials. Animals typically receive access to taste stimuli contingent on ingesting a food or drink. In contrast, audiovisual cues may be experienced independent of particular responses. Garcia and Koelling[3] addressed this issue by presenting both taste and audiovisual cues contingent on licking a drinking tube. In a later study, both taste and auditory exteroceptive cues were presented independent of behavior.[5] Strong evidence of cue-consequence specificity was obtained in both studies, suggesting that the method of presentation of taste and exteroceptive cues is not responsible for the phenomenon.

A second early concern focused on the possibility that the cue-consequence specificity effect reflected some type of competition between taste and audiovisual cues during conditioning trials. In their landmark experiment, Garcia and Koelling[3] presented taste and audiovisual cues simultaneously during the conditioning trials. However, subsequent work has involved comparing independent groups that received exposure to only a taste or only an audiovisual conditioned stimulus during training.[5–7] Evidence obtained in these studies suggests that stimulus competition during training is not responsible for the cue-consequence specificity effect.

Other attempts to explain cue-consequence specificity without invoking selective associations have focused on the unconditioned stimuli used. Rescorla and Holland[8] suggested that shock and illness induce differential orientations to taste and audiovisual cues, and these differential orientations may be responsible for cue-consequence specificity. Van Miller and I have taken two approaches to evaluating this possibility. First, we attempted to document the nature of differential orientations to shock and lithium-induced illness in rats.[9] We found that foot-shock sensitized rats to novel auditory or visual cues but not to novel taste stimuli. In contrast, lithium-induced illness sensitized rats to novel taste stimuli but not to novel auditory or visual cues. However, these proactive selective sensitization effects decayed in minutes (in the case of shock) or hours (in the case of lithium). Therefore, they could not explain the selective aversion performance that is typically observed one day or more following conditioning trials in cue-consequence specificity experiments.

In a second series of studies,[7] we attempted to rule out selective sensitization effects in cue-consequence specificity by exposing all subjects to both foot-shock and lithium-induced illness. Independent groups had the shock or lithium paired with a visual or taste conditioned stimulus. Even though all subjects received exposure to both unconditioned stimuli, they evidenced aversions to visual cues only if the visual cues had been paired with shock, and they evidenced aversions to taste only if the taste had been paired with lithium. Differential orientations induced by the unconditioned stimuli could not have led to these results.

Problems with Response Measures

Another possibility is that cue-consequence specificity reflects differential sensitivity of the responses used to measure aversion conditioning.[10] In most experiments, suppression of ingestion is used as an index of aversion. Perhaps suppression of ingestion is sensitive to taste-illness and audiovisual-shock associations but is not sensitive to taste-shock and audiovisual-illness associations. Van Miller has taken several approaches to investigating this issue.[11] In one experiment, he devised a locomotor measure of taste- and visual-aversion conditioning. The study was conducted in an experimental chamber that measured 60 × 20 × 20 cm. Two lines were drawn on the floor of the chamber, dividing it into three 20 × 20 cm areas. A stainless steel drinking spout and a 15-watt light bulb were positioned at one end of the chamber (the "front"). After habituation to drinking in the chamber, subjects received one of two conditioned stimuli contingent on licking the spout (.15% saccharin or the 15-watt light), paired with one of three consequences (foot-shock, lithium injection, or saline injection). On the two days that followed the single conditioning trial, subjects received whichever unconditioned stimulus (or stimuli in the case of saline-injected subjects) they were not exposed to during the conditioning trial. Three water-drinking sessions were then conducted to extinguish any aversions that might have been conditioned to background cues of the experimental chamber. Each subject was then tested with its conditioned stimulus. During this test session, saccharin-conditioned rats received a drinking spout containing saccharin and light-conditioned rats received a drinking spout containing water; licks at the water spout activated the light. One minute after the first lick, the drinking spouts were removed and the position of each subject was monitored continuously for the next 10 min.

The amount of time each group spent in the front of the experimental chamber, where conditioned stimuli had been presented, is shown in FIGURE 1. Among groups conditioned and tested with saccharin, subjects that received lithium during the conditioning trial (Group S-Li) spent significantly less time at the front of the chamber than either the control group (S-C) or subjects conditioned with shock (S-Sh). Among groups conditioned and tested with the light, subjects that received shock during the conditioning trial (Group L-Sh) spent significantly less time near the front than control subjects (Group L-C) or subjects conditioned with lithium (Group L-Li). In addition, there was no evidence that shock conditioned an aversion to saccharin or that lithium conditioned an aversion to the light. These results indicate that cue-consequence specificity in aversion learning can be demonstrated with a locomotor as well as an ingestive measure of aversion performance.

In a subsequent experiment, Miller[11] obtained continuous recordings of various

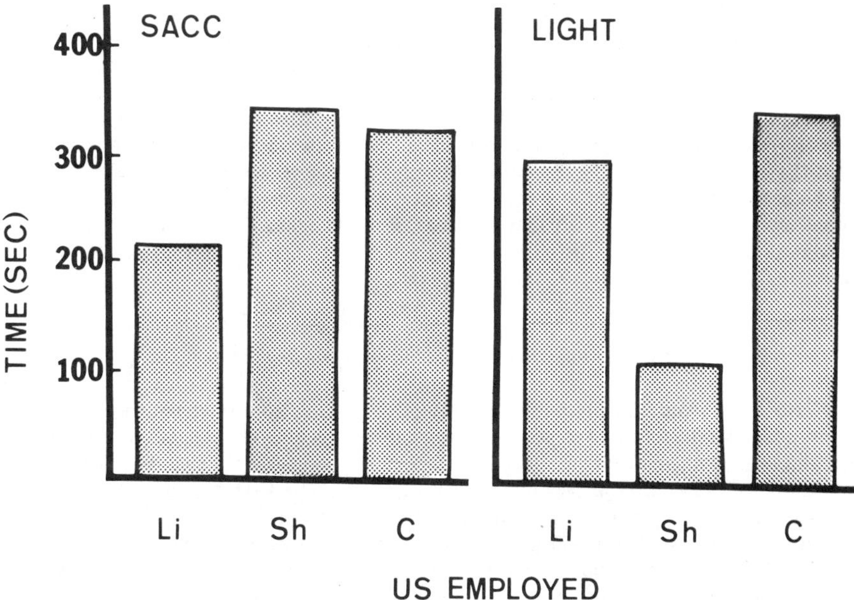

FIGURE 1. Amount of time subjects spent in the front of the experimental chamber where they were exposed to saccharin (sacc) or a cue light following conditioning with lithium (Li), foot-shock (Sh), or control injection of physiological saline (c). (After Miller.[11])

action patterns of rats before, during, and after presentation of a conditioned taste or white noise stimulus. Both types of conditioned stimuli were presented in a response-independent manner, the saccharin being infused through an oral cannula. Test sessions were recorded on video tape for later analysis, and behavior was coded in terms of the following categories: freezing, rearing, grooming, chin-wiping, head shaking, gaping, drinking, and "other" (see Miller[11] for definitions of the response classes). Following conditioning with shock, the noise CS elicited increased freezing and decreased rearing and grooming. Following conditioning with lithium, the taste of saccharin elicited increased chin wiping, head shaking, gaping, and decreased drinking. No evidence of conditioning was observed in any response measure to the noise stimulus paired with lithium or to the saccharin flavor paired with shock (see also Pelchat, Grill, Rozin, and Jacobs,[12] and Parker[13]). These results indicate that the cue-consequence specificity effect can be observed with multiple noningestive measures of behavior. Therefore, the phenomenon is not likely to result from the use of particular inappropriate response measures of aversion.

Problems with Learning History

Another alternative to the idea that cue-consequence specificity reflects a genetic predisposition for selective associations focuses on the learning history of animals. According to this interpretation, by the time animals reach adulthood and participate in a cue-consequence specificity experiment, they have experienced a history in which orosensory stimuli (taste, for example) are highly correlated with consequent interoceptive effects (malaise or nutritional repletion) and exteroceptive cues (sounds and sights), are correlated with consequent exteroceptive effects (cutaneous pain). These experiences are assumed to result in acquisition of a learning set that subsequently facilitates the association of taste with illness and audiovisual cues with foot-shock.[14] One way to test this idea is to investigate cue-consequence specificity at an early age, before subjects have had opportunity to acquire the presumed learning sets. Gail Gemberling and I recently investigated cue-consequence specificity in rats conditioned one day after birth and obtained results that were analogous to findings with adult rats.[15] These results suggest that acquisition of learning sets is not necessary for cue-consequence specificity.

Explanations of Selective Associations

Efforts to find alternatives to a selective association interpretation of cue-consequence specificity have not met with much success. This leads us to consider possible mechanisms that might lead to selective associations. Two not necessarily mutually exclusive alternatives have been proposed. The first of these assumes that the similarity of the temporal-intensity patterns of conditioned and unconditioned stimuli facilitates their association.[16,17] Such a mechanism leads to selective associations when conditioned and unconditioned stimuli of similar and dissimilar temporal-intensity patterns are employed. The cue-consequence specificity effect in aversion learning is explained by assuming that tastes and drug-induced malaise are similar in both having slow onset and slow offset characteristics. In contrast, audiovisual cues and foot-shock are assumed to be similar in being punctate, with rapid onset and offset features. Presumably tastes are not easily associated with subsequent foot-shock and audiovisual cues are not easily associated with illness because of the contrasting temporal-intensity patterns of these cues. (For a related hypothesis, see Krane and Wagner.[18])

Although several efforts have been made to manipulate the time course of drug-induced illness and shock,[19-21] these have not provided strong evidence for or against the stimulus-similarity hypothesis. The fundamental difficulty has been that we do not have precise knowledge about the time course of drug or shock-induced physiological changes that are relevant to aversion conditioning. In fact, the relevant physiological changes themselves are often difficult to identify. We also do not have precise information about the time course of taste sensations. In the absence of such knowledge, effects of variations in US temporal-intensity patterns are difficult to interpret.

The technical difficulties in evaluating the stimulus-similarity hypothesis in aversion learning have led investigators to employ other conditioning preparations and response systems (see Domjan,[22] for a recent review). Generally, these efforts have yielded evidence supportive of the stimulus-similarity hypothesis. This evidence suggests that stimulus similarity contributes to cue-consequence specificity in aversion learning. However, the extent of this contribution is unknown and may not be substantial. Evidence of one-trial long-delay visual aversion learning is particularly difficult to explain in terms of the stimulus-similarity hypothesis. Visual aversions have been conditioned in one trial with toxicosis delayed 30 min or more in chicks,[23,24] Japanese quail,[25] guinea pigs,[26] and monkeys.[27] Furthermore, these aversions are not likely to have been mediated by novel tastes.[28] The stimulus similarity hypothesis is assumed to apply to all species capable of acquiring aversions based on illness. If one assumes that the punctuate nature of visual cues interferes with the association of visual cues with illness in rats, such interference should also be observed in other species.

A second effort to explain selective associations has focused on differences in the neurophysiological processing of various types of conditioned and unconditioned stimuli.[29] According to this hypothesis the neurophysiological convergence of sensory systems involved in processing taste and gastrointestinal stimuli and audiovisual and cutaneous cues is assumed to facilitate their association. The neurophysiology of aversion learning is discussed in detail by other participants in this volume. Therefore, I will not comment on it, except to note that as evidence concerning the neurophysiology of aversion learning accumulates, the adequacy of the neurophysiological convergence hypothesis will have to be evaluated in mammalian as well as in avian species.

LONG-DELAY LEARNING

Most of the research on long-delay learning has been conducted with mammals exposed to a novel flavor followed minutes or hours later by illness induced by a drug or radiation exposure. The typical finding has been that subjects learn an aversion to the flavor despite the long delay between exposure to the flavor and subsequent poisoning.[30] Early considerations of this phenomenon sought explanations that avoided acknowledging that the aversion performance reflected association of the novel flavor with illness over a long delay. One approach emphasized the role of aftertastes. According to this hypothesis, aversion learning occurs with delayed toxicosis because aftertastes of the earlier flavor exposure are present at the time of the induced illness, thus permitting association of the aftertaste and toxicosis by temporal contiguity. Aversions thus acquired were assumed to generalize to the original flavored solution. Several lines of evidence argue against the aftertaste interpretation.[31,32] However, because the nature and duration of aftertastes are difficult to specify and manipulate experimentally, proponents of the aftertaste hypothesis can always resurrect it in some *ad hoc* fashion. The most convincing evidence against aftertaste as a general explanation of long-delay learning is provided by demonstrations of long-delay aversion learning to visual cues.[23-27] A second early approach attributed acquisition of flavor aversions in delayed toxicosis situations to nonassociative effects of the aversion-inducing agent. This account is also not convincing (see Domjan,[33] for a detailed discussion).

Much of recent research on long-delay learning has ignored aftertaste and nonassociative interpretations and has focused on various other behavioral mechanisms that are expected to lead to long-delay learning. Initially, these experiments were conducted using the taste-aversion conditioning paradigm. More recently, the critical experiments have been performed in other types of learning situations. This raises the question of whether the findings are applicable to taste-aversion learning.

Flavor-aversion Experiments

Traditionally, instances of delayed conditioning have been explained as special cases of association by contiguity by assuming that the conditioned stimulus has a gradually decaying neural trace that persists until the unconditioned stimulus is presented. The trace is assumed to become associated with the unconditioned stimulus by temporal contiguity, and the conditioned response to the stimulus trace is assumed to generalize to the CS. Difficulties in measuring and experimentally manipulating neural traces make this trace-decay hypothesis as difficult to test as the aftertaste hypothesis, if not more so. Therefore, early efforts to explain long-delay learning sought alternatives to trace decay. One of these, the learned safety or learned noncorrelation hypothesis,[34,35] did not succeed because critical experimental evidence was subject to alternative interpretations.[36] A more promising alternative was provided by the concurrent interference theory, according to which associations are formed between two events over a long delay provided that other stimuli do not occur in the delay interval that become associated with either of the target stimuli.[37,38] In the typical long-delay learning procedure, rats are exposed to a novel taste, followed some time later by toxicosis. The concurrent interference theory predicts that learning will occur with this procedure because subjects are likely to experience only nongustatory cues during the delay interval, and such stimuli are not likely to become associated with toxicosis because of the cue-consequence specificity effect. Thus, the concurrent interference theory predicts long-delay learning on the basis of cue-consequence specificity.

The concurrent interference theory is supported by a variety of evidence. For example, as predicted by the theory, long-delay learning is disrupted by nontarget flavor stimuli presented during the delay interval, and the degree of this disruption is related to the extent that these interposed stimuli become associated with the consequent toxicosis.[37] These results suggest that limiting concurrent interference is necessary for long-delay learning. However, it may not be sufficient. One-day-old rats, for example, display cue-consequence specificity, which should limit concurrent interference in a long-delay experiment, as it is presumed to do in adult rats. However, one-day-old rats do not display long-delay aversion learning.[15] Evidently, infant rats lack other memorial mechanisms that are also important in long-delay learning. Without further elaboration, the concurrent interference theory also has difficulties explaining instances of long-delay aversion learning to tactile cues in rats and monkeys,[39,40] and visual cues in birds, monkeys, and guinea pigs.[24-27] Subjects in these experiments no doubt experienced numerous tactile and visual stimuli during the delay interval that should have interfered with long-delay learning. Long-delay aversion learning may have occurred in these studies because the tactile and visual stimuli were encountered during the course of ingestion. The ingestive context may serve to direct tactile and visual information to a special ingestion-related memory register in which the information is protected against interference from other sources of exteroceptive stimulation.[33,39]

Long-delay Experiments in Other Stimulus-response Systems

Some of the interesting ideas about long-delay learning have been tested in experiments that did not involve flavor stimuli and toxicosis. I will consider three of these, the marking hypothesis, affective response conditioning, and interrelations of cue, response, and consequence (for a more complete discussion, see Domjan[22]).

The marking hypothesis was formulated during efforts to evaluate procedures for long-delay learning of spatial and visual discriminations in a T-maze developed from concurrent interference theory.[41-43] The concurrent interference theory was extended to maze learning situations by postulating a principle of situational relevance, according to which animals only learn associations between events that occur in the same situation. With this principle, the concurrent interference theory predicts that animals will associate a response with delayed reward in a T-maze provided they are removed from the maze during the delay interval. Lett obtained results consistent with this prediction.[41-43] However, subsequent research indicated that the critical aspect of her procedure probably was not removal of the subjects from the maze during the delay interval but handling of the subjects after each choice response. Lieberman, McIntosh, and Thomas[44] found that rats learned a spatial discrimination with reward delayed one minute provided that they were handled briefly after choice responses. Whether or not they were placed back into the maze for the delay interval was unimportant. Based on these results, they suggested that handling serves to mark the preceding choice response and thereby makes the response memorable. Subsequent research showed that marking can be also accomplished by a brief burst of noise or light.[44] The marking stimulus only has to be presented in conjunction with the instrumental response (not the reinforcer) and is equally effective in facilitating learning whether it is presented just before or immediately after the instrumental response.[45]

The above findings clearly indicate that marking an instrumental response can greatly facilitate long-delay learning of spatial discriminations. The implications of this for understanding long-delay poison-avoidance learning are less clear. The marking hypothesis does not specify what stimuli act as good markers other than to assume that such stimuli must be salient and possibly surprising. What might serve to mark the to-be-conditioned stimulus in poison-avoidance experiments? One possibility involves orosensory stimuli experienced during the course of ingestion of a novel-flavored food or drink. Consistent with this suggestion, long-delay taste-aversion learning is attenuated by presenting flavored solutions through an oral fistula in the absence of ingestive responses.[46]

D'Amato and his associates[47] have suggested that one of the critical aspects of flavor-aversion learning that permits conditioning over long delays is that it involves the conditioning of an affective rather than an instrumental response. Consistent with this suggestion, they have shown that conditioning of affective responses can occur with much longer delays of reinforcement than conditioning of instrumental behavior.[48] They have also devised procedures for appetitive conditioning of spatial preference behavior in one trial with long delays of reinforcement. In one of the studies,[49] cebus monkeys were conditioned in one trial with a 30-minute delay of reinforcement to increase their preference for the previously nonpreferred arm of a T-maze. One day after a pre-test for side preference, experimental subjects were placed in the nonpreferred arm of the T-maze for one minute. They were then placed in a holding cage in the test room for the 30-minute delay interval, after which they were returned to the start box of the maze to receive 10 raisins. Control groups received only either exposure to the CS or the US. Subsequent tests of side preference indicated that experimental subjects increased their preference for the previously nonpreferred arm significantly more than the control groups. An analogous study with rat subjects provided evidence of one-trial spatial-preference learning with reward delayed 30 and 120 minutes in experimental as compared to control subjects.[50] However, in this case the critical group differences arose from decreases in CS preference evidenced by the control groups rather than increases in preference evidenced by experimental subjects.

Another interesting proposal concerning long-delay learning was made by Testa and Ternes,[17] who suggested that a critical feature of flavor-aversion procedures is that they involve a special relation among cue, response, and consequence. When animals ingest a poisonous food, the extent of exposure to the food's flavor as well as the amount of poison that is received depend on ingestive behavior, which is then used to provide evidence of the aversion learning that results. If this interdependence of cue, reponse, and consequence is critical for long-delay learning, then long-delay learning should be evident wherever cues, responses, and consequences are highly correlated. In an interesting test of this idea, Sullivan[51] first allowed rats to touch small objects and then presented periodic shocks 35 minutes later that were correlated with the extent of prior touching. This procedure resulted in a significant suppression of contact with the shock-paired objects. Evidence in support of the Testa-Ternes hypothesis has also been provided by studies of poison-avoidance learning to visual cues in rats and pigeons that demonstrated that aversion learning is facilitated by making the visual cue a part of the ingested food or liquid.[52,53]

The above studies have identified factors important for long-delay learning. They have led to demonstrations of long-delay learning outside the taste-toxicosis situation and therefore provide evidence critical to evaluating the generality of long-delay learning.[22] However, these studies provide insights into long-delay taste-aversion learning only by implication. The experiments were conducted with nongustatory cues and also often involved unconditioned stimuli other than toxicosis. Therefore, the importance for taste-aversion learning of marking, affective conditioning, and interdependence of cue, response, and consequence has yet to be experimentally demonstrated. We also do not know what is the relative importance of each of these factors in long-delay taste-aversion learning. Some of the mechanisms may turn out to be less important in taste-aversion learning than they are in other stimulus-response systems. For example, in the typical taste-aversion experiment, administration of the illness-inducing agent is independent of how much of a flavored solution subjects drink because the toxin is not contained in the ingested fluid. Thus, cue, response, and consequence are not as interdependent as they are when subjects ingest a poisonous food. This lack of correlation between response and consequence does not preclude long-delay learning of strong taste aversions in the laboratory.

The Delay Gradient: A Remaining Problem

Long-delay learning may be considered from two perspectives. One perspective focuses on the occurrence of learning despite a long interval between conditioned and unconditioned stimuli (or between response and reinforcer). Much of the research on long-delay learning to date has been conducted from this perspective. Long-delay learning also may be investigated by focusing on the gradient of learning that occurs as a function of the delay interval. This second perspective on the problem has received far less attention than the first. The fact that learning can occur with delays of 30 minutes or more is so impressive that it has overshadowed the fact that learning declines with increasing delay intervals.

Most of the proposed mechanisms of long-delay learning have little to say about the delay gradient. Nothing about the proposition that affective conditioning is less easily disrupted by delays than instrumental conditioning implies that learning will be inversely related to the delay interval. This proposition is a statement about the relative slopes of the delay gradient in affective and instrumental conditioning and does not specify the absolute characteristics of the delay gradient in either case. The marking hypothesis and the proposition that close relations among cue, response, and consequence are important for long-delay learning similarly do not explain why learning is inversely related to the delay interval.

As was noted earlier, investigators have tried to avoid the concept of trace decay in explaining long-delay learning. The only nontrace mechanism of long-delay learning that may be used to deduce a delay gradient is the concurrent-interference theory. This theory predicts a delay gradient by assuming that the longer the interval is between two events that are to be associated, the more likely subjects are to experience stimuli during the delay interval that can provide concurrent interference. What these intervening stimuli are in the typical long-delay taste aversion experiment is a matter of speculation. This makes the concurrent-interference explanation of the delay gradient *post hoc* in most cases and not much of an improvement on a poorly specified trace-decay theory.

The gradient of learning that occurs as a function of the delay interval in taste-aversion learning may be considered a result of memory failure, retrieval failure, or both. The traditional trace-decay hypothesis views the delay gradient as an instance of memory failure—memory of the taste exposure is assumed to be lost gradually and in a passive manner as a function of time. Some of the manipulations suggested by new ideas about long-delay learning may be incorporated into the trace-decay hypothesis as variables that control the magnitude of the stimulus trace. For example, introducing a marker may be viewed as increasing the initial strength of a stimulus trace without changing its decay parameter. Although strengthened by marking, the stimulus trace is still assumed to decay with time, leading to a delay gradient in learning.

Although the trace-decay hypothesis can be supplemented by other concepts to explain certain new phenomena such as the marking effect, the trace-decay hypothesis is inconsistent with variations in taste memory in different situations. In sensory preconditioning involving the association of one flavor with another, delays of more than a few seconds between the two flavors seem to preclude their association.[54] In contrast, delays of several hours are possible in taste-aversion conditioning with lithium-induced malaise.[31] Even longer delays (one week or more) are possible when the retention test involves presentation of the original flavor a second time in a test of the attenuation of neophobia.[35] This diversity in the duration of taste memory probably reflects differences in the effectiveness of various events as retrieval cues for an earlier flavor experience. Presentation of a new flavor (as in the sensory preconditioning procedure) is evidently less effective as a retrieval cue than presentation of toxicosis (in aversion conditioning), and toxicosis is less effective as a retrieval cue than a second presentation of the original flavor (in tests of neophobia attenuation).

Covariation of cue, response, and consequence[17] may facilitate long-delay learning by enhancing the effectiveness of the unconditioned stimulus in retrieving memory of the conditioned stimulus. Stimulus similiarity is an important determinant of the effectiveness of retrieval cues. The greater the correlation of cue and consequence, the greater their similarity, and this should increase the effectiveness of the consequence as a retrieval stimulus for the cue.[22]

Postulating that various events are differentially effective as retrieval cues for flavor experiences helps explain differences in taste memory observed in diverse situations. However, such assumptions do not help explain why a given event (lithium-induced malaise, for example) is less effective in association with a taste memory as a function of time since the taste presentation. Nothing obvious about lithium-induced malaise changes as a function of time after a flavor presentation. Therefore, there is no reason to suspect that lithium-induced malaise becomes less effective as a retrieval cue for the prior flavor presentation. This makes retrieval failure difficult to invoke as an explanation of the delay gradient in flavor-aversion conditioning.

The above considerations suggest that some form of the concept of trace may be inescapable in attempts to explain the delay gradient. A flavor presentation may be assumed to result in a gradually decaying neural trace. Other events (toxicosis, for example) may act as retrieval cues for the flavor memory. The extent to which memory of the original flavor is retrieved may be jointly determined by the strength of the stimulus trace at the time of the retrieval event and the effectiveness of the event as a retrieval cue for flavor stimuli. Thus, a particularly effective retrieval cue (such as re-presentation of the original flavor) may fully reinstate the memory of the original flavor even if the stimulus trace of the flavor was weak. In contrast, less effective retrieval cues (such as presentation of a different flavor) may reinstate memory of the original flavor only if the stimulus trace of the original flavor is still strong.

CONCLUDING COMMENTS

Nearly 20 years have passed since John Garcia and his colleagues published their findings of cue-consequence specificity and long-delay learning in aversion conditioning. We have obtained a great deal of information about the two phenomena during those years. However, some of the questions that were with us then are still with us today. Research on the cue-consequence specificity effect has told us much about mechanisms that are not responsible for the phenomenon. We know that the cue-consequence specificity effect is not caused by various nonassociative processes related to the conditioned or unconditioned stimuli involved. We also know that the phenomenon is not likely to be the result of inappropriate response measures and that historical factors are not necessary for its expression. The most viable behavioral explanation of the phenomenon is that it reflects the power of stimulus similarity in the formation of associations. But that mechanism is difficult to reconcile with rapid long-delay learning of aversions to visual cues. Research on long-delay learning has told us much about mechanisms that can lead to long-delay learning outside the taste-aversion system and as such has provided important information about the generality of long-delay learning. However, we do not know what the relative importance of these mechanisms is for taste-aversion learning. We also have not been able to abandon entirely the traditional trace-decay interpretation of long-delay learning, although we may have more ideas about processes controlling stimulus traces and have had to supplement the trace-decay hypothesis with retrieval mechanisms.

REFERENCES

1. Barker, L. M., M. R. Best & Domjan, Eds. 1977. Learning mechanisms in food selection. Baylor University Press. Waco, TX.
2. Seligman, M. E. P. 1970. On the generality of the laws of learning. Psychol. Rev. **77**: 406–418.
3. Garcia, J. & R. A. Koelling. 1966. Relation of cue to consequence in avoidance learning. Psychon. Sci. **4**: 123–124.
4. LoLordo, V. M. 1979. Selective associations. *In* Mechanisms of Learning and Motivation. A. Dickinson & R. A. Boakes, Eds.: 367–398. Erlbaum. Hillsdale, NJ.
5. Domjan, M. & N. E. Wilson. 1972. Specificity of cue to consequence in aversion learning in the rat. Psychon. Sci. **26**: 143–145.
6. Garcia, J., B. K. McGowan, F. R. Ervin & R. A. Koelling. 1968. Cues: Their relative effectiveness as a function of the reinforcer. Science **160**: 794–795.
7. Miller, V. & M. Domjan. 1981. Specificity of cue to consequence in aversion learning in the rat: Control for US-induced differential orientations. Anim. Learn. Behav. **9**: 339–345.
8. Rescorla, R. A. & P. C. Holland. 1976. Some behavioral approaches to the study of learning. *In* Neural Mechanisms of Learning and Memory. M. R. Rosenzweig & E. L. Bennett, Eds.: 165–192. MIT Press. Cambridge, MA.
9. Miller, V. & M. Domjan. 1981. Selective sensitization induced by lithium malaise and footshock in rats. Behav. Neur. Bio. **31**: 42–55.
10. Parker, H. B. & R. F. Smith. 1981. Flavor- vs. tone-cued shock avoidance. Anim. Learn. Behav. **9**: 335–338.
11. Miller, V. 1984. Selective association learning in the rat: Generality of response system. Learn. Motiv. **15**: 58–84.
12. Pelchat, M. L., H. J. Grill, P. Rozin & J. Jacobs. 1983. Quality of acquired responses

to taste by *Rattus norvegicus* depends on type of associated discomfort. J. Comp. Psychol. **97**: 140–153.
13. PARKER, L. A. 1982. Nonconsummatory and consummatory CRs elictied by lithium- and amphetamine-paired flavors. Learn. Motiv. **13**: 281–303.
14. MACKINTOSH, N. J. 1974. The Psychology of Animal Learning. Academic Press. London.
15. GEMBERLING, G. A. & M. DOMJAN. 1982. Selective associations in one-day-old rats: Taste-toxicosis and texture-shock aversion learning. J. Comp. Physiol. Psychol. **96**: 105–113.
16. TESTA, T. J. 1974. Causal relationships and the acquisitions of avoidance responses. Psychol. Rev. **81**: 491–505.
17. TESTA, T. J. & J. W. TERNES. 1977. Specificity of conditioning mechanisms in the modification of food preferences. *In* Learning Mechanisms in Food Selection. L. M. Barker, M. R. Best & M. Domjan, Eds.: 229–253. Baylor University Press. Waco, TX.
18. KRANE, R. V. & A. R. WAGNER. 1975. Taste-aversion learning with a delayed shock US: Implications for the "generality of the laws of learning." J. Comp. Physiol. Psychol. **88**: 882–889.
19. DOMJAN, M., K. FOSTER & D. G. GILLAN. 1979. Effects of distribution of the drug unconditioned stimulus on taste-aversion learning. Physiol. Behav. **23**: 931–938.
20. GOUDIE, A. J. & D. W. DICKINS. 1978. Nitrous oxide-induced conditioned taste aversion in rats: The role of duration of drug exposure and its relation to the taste aversion-self-administration "paradox". Pharm. Biochem. Behav. **9**: 587–592.
21. GREEN, L., A. BOUZAS & H. RACHLIN. 1972. Test of an electric-shock analog to illness-induced aversion. Behav. Bio. **7**: 513–518.
22. DOMJAN, M. 1983. Biological constraints on instrumental and classical conditioning: Implications for general process theory. *In* The Psychology of Learning and Motivation. G. H. Bower, Ed. **17**: 215–277. Academic Press. New York.
23. GENOVESE, R. F. & M. P. BROWN. 1978. Sickness-induced learning in chicks. Behav. Bio. **24**: 68–76.
24. MARTIN, G. M. & W. P. BELLINGHAM. 1979. Learning of visual food aversions by chickens (Gallus gallus) over long delays. Behav. Neur. Biol. **25**: 58–68.
25. CZAPLICKI, J. A., D. E. BORREBACH & H. C. WILCOXON. 1976. Stimulus generalization of an illness-induced aversion to different intensities of colored water in Japanese quail. Anim. Learn. Behav. **4**: 45–48.
26. BRAVEMAN, N. S. 1974. Poison-based avoidance learning with flavored or colored water in guinea pigs. Learn. Motiv. **5**: 182–194.
27. JOHNSON, C., R. BEATON & K. HALL. 1975. Poison-based avoidance learning in nonhuman primates: Use of visual cues. Physiol. Behav. **14**: 403–407.
28. LETT, B. T. 1980. Taste potentiates color-sickness associations in pigeons and quail. Anim. Learn. Behav. **8**: 193–198.
29. GARCIA, J., W. G. HANKINS & K. W. RUSINIAK. 1974. Behavioral regulation of the milieu interne in man and rat. Science **185**: 824–831.
30. GARCIA, J., F. R. ERVIN & R. A. KOELLING. 1966. Learning with prolonged delay of reinforcement. Psychon. Sci. **5**: 121–122.
31. REVUSKY, S. H. & J. GARCIA. 1970. Learned associations over long delays. *In* The Psychology of Learning and Motivation. G. H. Bower, Ed. **4**: 1–84. Academic Press. New York.
32. ROZIN, P. & J. W. KALAT. 1971. Specific hungers and poison avoidance as adaptive specializations of learning. Psychol. Rev. **78**: 459–486.
33. DOMJAN, M. 1980. Ingestional aversion learning: Unique and general processes. *In* Advances in the Study of Behavior. **11**: 275–336. Academic Press. New York
34. KALAT, J. W. 1977. Status of "learned safety" or "learned non-correlation" as a mechanism in taste aversion learning. *In* Learning Mechanisms in Food Selection. L. M. Barker, M. R. Best & M. Domjan, Eds.: 273–293. Baylor University Press. Waco, TX.
35. KALAT, J. W. & P. ROZIN. 1973. "Learned Safety" as a mechanism in long-delay taste-aversion learning in rats. J. Comp. Physiol. Psychol. **83**: 198–207.
36. BEST, M. R. & L. M. BARKER. 1977. The nature of "learned safety" and its role in the delay of reinforcement gradient. *In* Learning Mechanisms in Food Selection. L. M. Barker, M. R. Best & M. Domjan, Eds.: 295–317. Baylor University Press. Waco, TX.
37. REVUSKY, S. 1971. The role of interference in association over a delay. *In* Animal Memory. W. K. Honig & P. H. R. James, Eds.: 155–213. Academic Press, New York.

38. Revusky, S. 1977. The concurrent interference approach to delay learning. *In* Learning Mechanisms in Food Selection. L. M. Barker, M. R. Best & M. Domjan, Eds.: 319–366. Baylor University Press. Waco, TX.
39. Domjan, M. & M. J. Hanlon. 1982. Poison-avoidance learning to food-related tactile stimuli: Avoidance of texture cues by rats. Anim. Learn. Behav. **10**: 293–300.
40. Domjan, M., V. Miller & G. A. Gemberling. 1982. Note on aversion learning to the shape of food by monkeys. J. Exp. Anal. Behav. **38**: 87–91.
41. Lett, B. T. 1973. Delayed reward learning: Disproof of the traditional theory. Learn. Motiv. **4**: 237–246.
42. Lett, B. T. 1974. Visual discrimination learning with a 1-min delay of reward. Learn. Motiv. **5**: 174–181.
43. Lett, B. T. 1975. Long delay learning in the T-maze. Learn. Motiv. **6**: 80–90.
44. Lieberman, D. A., D. C. McIntosh & G. V. Thomas. 1979. Learning when reward is delayed: A marking hypothesis. J Exp. Psychol.: Anim. Behav. Proc. **5**: 224–242.
45. Thomas, G. V., D. A. Lieberman, D. C. McIntosh & P. Ronaldson. 1983. The role of marking when reward is delayed. J. Exp. Psychol.: Anim. Behav. Proc. **9**: 401–411.
46. Domjan, M. & N. E. Wilson. 1972. Contribution of ingestive behaviors to taste-aversion learning in the rat. J. Comp. Physiol. Psychol. **80**: 403–412.
47. D'Amato, M. R., W. R. Safarjan & D. Salmon. 1981. Long-delay conditioning and instrumental learning: Some new findings. *In* Information Processing in Animals. N. E. Spear & R. R. Miller, Eds.: 113–142. Erlbaum. Hillsdale, NJ.
48. D'Amato, M. R. & W. R. Safarjan. 1981. Differential effects of reinforcement on acquisition of affective and instrumental responses. Anim. Learn. Behav. **9**: 209–215.
49. D'Amato, M. R. & J. Buckiewicz. 1980. Long-delay one-trial conditioned preference and retention in monkeys (Cebus apella). Anim. Learn. Behav. **8**: 359–362.
50. Safarjan, W. R. & M. R. D'Amato. 1981. One-trial, long-delay, conditioned preference in rats. Psychol. Rec. **31**: 413–426.
51. Sullivan, L. 1979. Long-delay learning with exteroceptive cues and exteroceptive reinforcement in rats. Australian J. Psychol. **31**: 21–32.
52. Galef, G. B. Jr. & A. J. Dalrymple. 1981. Toxicosis based aversions to visual cues in rats: A test of the Testa and Ternes hypothesis. Anim. Learn. Behav. **9**: 332–334.
53. Logue, A. W. 1980. Visual cues for illness-induced aversions in the pigeon. Behav. Neur. Biol. **28**: 372–377.
54. Lavin, M. 1976. The establishment of flavor-flavor associations using a sensory preconditioning training procedure. Learn. Motiv. **7**: 173–183.

PART II. PHYSIOLOGICAL SUBSTRATES OF CONDITIONED FOOD AVERSIONS

Introduction: Physiological Mechanisms in Conditioned Taste Aversions[a]

HARVEY J. GRILL

Graduate Groups of Psychology and Neuroscience
University of Pennsylvania
Philadelphia, Pennsylvania 19104

The behavioral effects of associating a taste with visceral malaise are rapid and dramatic. Following this association, animals avoid consuming a taste which they had once readily consumed. In conceptualizing the physiological mechanisms responsible for the production of this conditioned taste aversion (CTA) we should consider how the central nervous system (CNS) integrates taste and visceral stimuli and within which of its structures this integration takes place. This integration(s) changes the animal's response to the paired taste stimulus and to other tastes that are processed similarly by its nervous system. The physical properties of the taste stimulus have not changed, yet due to the association, the neural coding of the taste has been altered to yield an opposite response. The factors integrated by the CNS derive from the peripheral and central gustatory system, peripheral and central afferent systems sensitive to emetic stimuli, and hormones and neurotransmitters that modulate the excitability of both central synapses and even perhaps the taste receptors themselves, if there are ancillary aspects to this neural integration. The five papers in the physiological section of this book focus on separate aspects of this central integration problem, though none has focused on the sites of action of, and neural channels mediating, the variety of agents that can function as USs in CTAs. I will discuss some issues raised by these papers, as well as material of my own, in a topic format.

THE TASTE FACTOR: INPUT AND ITS CENTRAL INTEGRATION

Behavioral Measures of the Effects of the Taste-Visceral Association: The Use of Intake and Taste Reactivity Measures of Palatability

Responses to taste stimuli have traditionally been measured by comparing the intake of the taste stimulus in question with that of its solvent, distilled water. FIGURE 1 displays the relative intake results from two-bottle preference tests for a concentration series of a particular taste solution, e.g. sodium chloride (NaCl), and is referred to as a "preference-aversion curve." Relative intake has also provided the principle measure of the effect of taste-visceral associations. Despite the use of the word aver-

[a] Supported by National Institute of Health grant AM-21397.

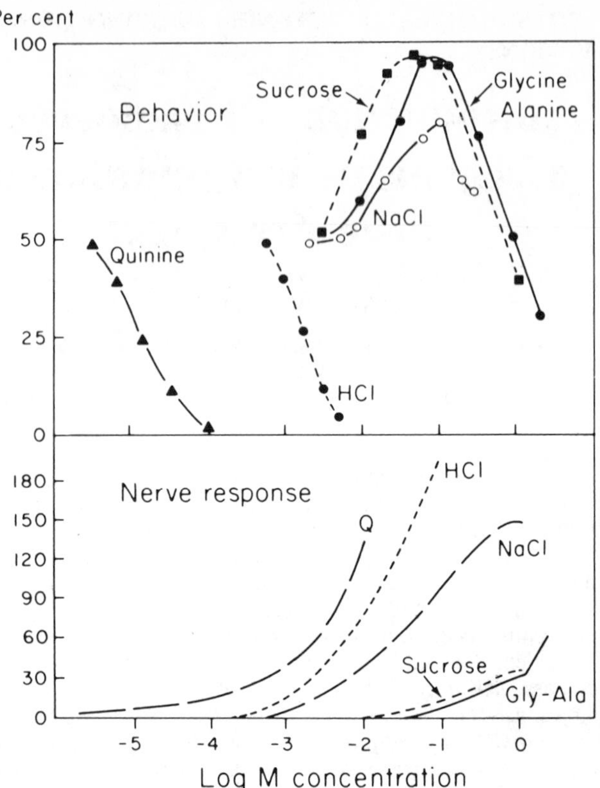

FIGURE 1. Correlation of intake measure of palatability with composite electrophysiological responses of chorda tympani and glossopharyngeal nerve to indicated solutions of taste stimuli. The upper panel shows intake of indicated taste solution as a percentage of total fluid intake (solution + H_2O) in a 24 hr two-bottle preference test. The lower panel shows neural responses to the same stimuli relative to the 0.1 M NaCl response.

sion in both the preference-aversion curve and conditioned taste aversion contexts, the alteration of relative preference by a reduction in the intake of the paired solution is a measure of avoidance and should not be viewed as a measure of aversion (note: White and Boudreau[37] use the term preference-avoidance curves to describe these data). In fact, the interpretation of reductions in intake poses a serious problem. Are we to assume that a reduction in intake must always mean that the taste stimulus has been evaluated as unpalatable by the animal's nervous system?

My colleague Kent Berridge and I[18] have taken the position that all tests that measure palatability, measure the behavioral output of a CNS integration of gustatory afferent, internal state, and associative neural signals. The fact that a measure like intake can reflect this integration should not imply that palatability is the only thing it measures. Other central states might also be expected to affect this measure. For example, fear might stop a rat from drinking sucrose, but does fear alter sucrose palatability?

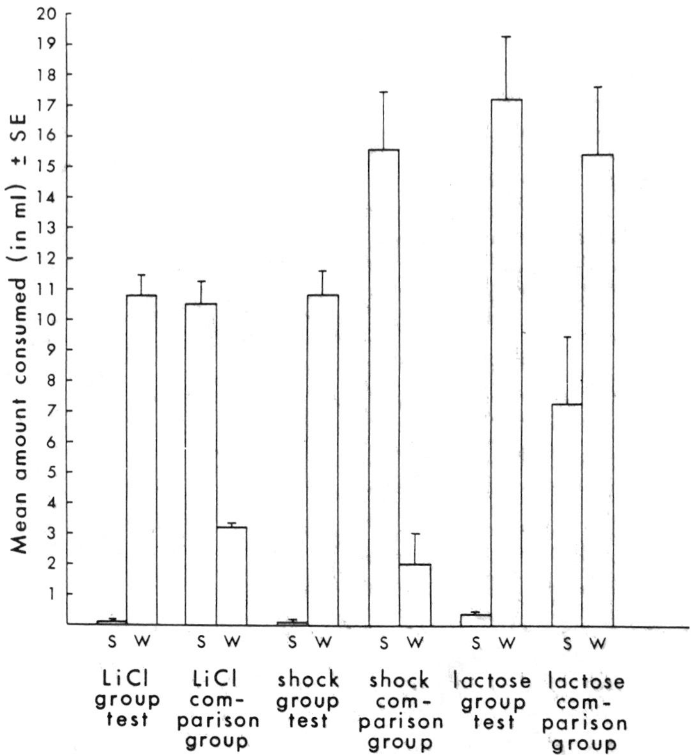

FIGURE 2. Mean intake (±SE) for sugar (s) and water (w) for rats that had associated sugar with LiCl, shock, or lactose.

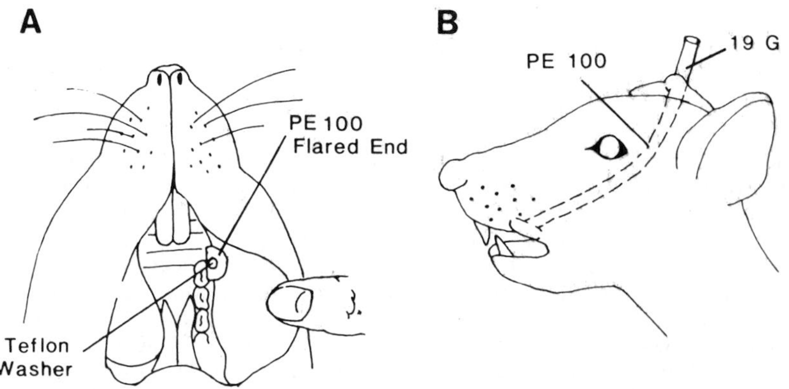

FIGURE 3. Diagram of the intraoral catheter. The intraoral end is placed just rostral to the first maxillary molar. The tubing is led out subcutaneously to the skull and secured to a short piece of 19-gauge (19 G) stainless steel tubing with dental acrylic. (A) Ventral view. (B) Lateral view.

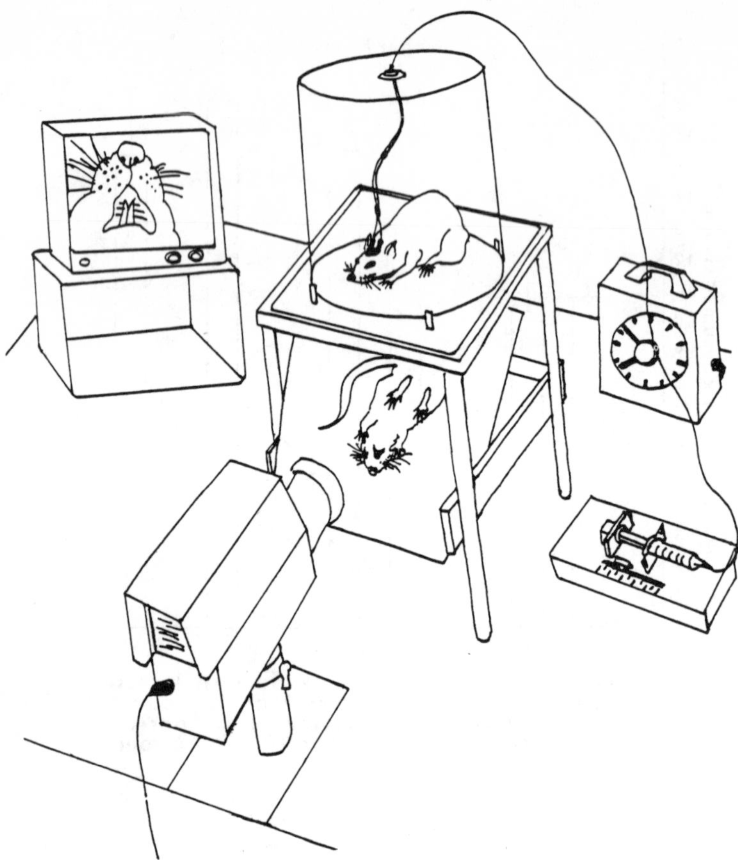

FIGURE 4. Apparatus for videotaping taste reactivity responses to taste stimuli injected into the mouth via chronic intraoral catheters. Videotaping is done via a mirror located beneath the plexiglass floor.

My colleagues Marci Pelchat, Paul Rozin, Joel Jacobs and I[32] have found that pairing a taste with the consequences of either footshock, lithium chloride (LiCl) injection, or lactose intolerance can produce an equivalent reduction of taste intake as seen in FIGURE 2. Using intake as the only measure of palatability would lead to the conclusion that all three types of pairings result in a similar decrease in sucrose palatability. This conclusion, however, would be incorrect. There may be a degree of overlap in the constellation of effects produced by two functional variables such as fear and palatability; however this overlap is not complete for all measures of any one of these variables. When another measure of palabatility, taste reactivity, was used to compare the effects of these three taste-US associations, the results were different.

Let me first describe the taste reactivity method. The activity of lingual, masticatory and facial muscles is videotaped during oral contact with taste stimuli. Contact with taste stimuli can be achieved by either normal drinking, or by the direct oral application of taste solutions via indwelling catheters like those pictured in FIGURE

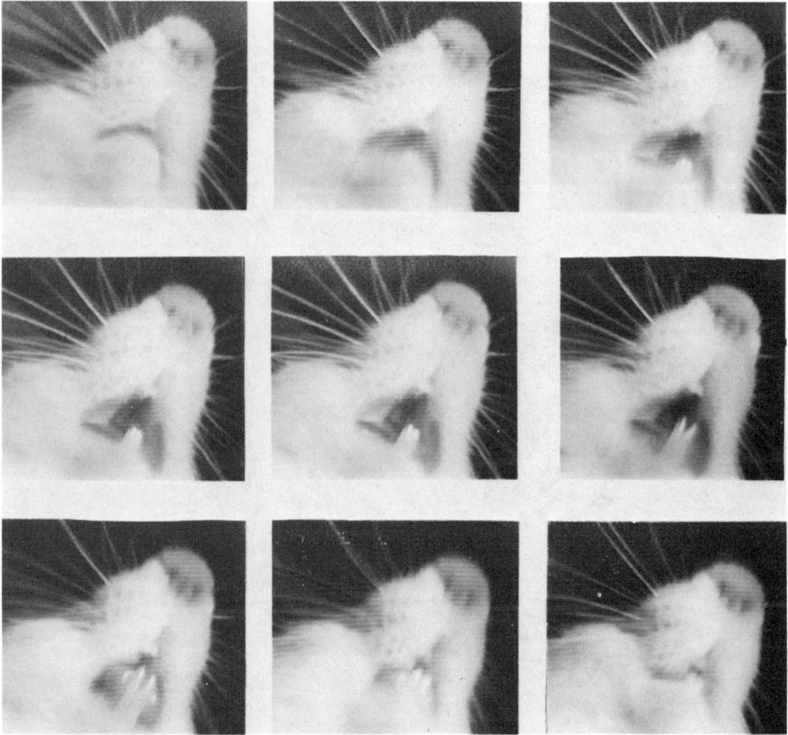

FIGURE 5. Consecutive videofields (16.6 msec separating each frame) of an individual gape response elicited by a 3×10^{-4} M QHCl stimulus. The response begins in the upper left proceeding vertically from left to right. The corners of the mouth retract to a maximal mouth opening. The lower lip retracts to reveal the incisors. The tongue is initially retracted from its extended resting position and then extends at jaw closure.

3. An apparatus suited for the macrophotography of oral behavior, like the one shown in FIGURE 4, is used in either free drinking or direct oral application paradigms. Taste stimuli evoke eight separate responses involving primarily the muscles just specified. These taste reactivity responses (e.g. the sequence and number of these responses) are analyzed using a single frame analysis of videotape (60 fields/sec; 2 fields/frame). An example of consecutive single fields of videotape for one of these responses, the gape response, is shown in FIGURE 5. The eight stereotyped taste reactivity responses tend to cluster into two response patterns depicted in FIGURE 6. In sated intact rats, novel taste stimuli like sucrose elicit an ingestive pattern displayed in conjunction with swallowing, while others like quinine evoke an aversive response pattern and rejection of the tastant.

Unlike intake tests, the taste reactivity test does measure aversion by quantifying the occurrences of aversive responses. The responses in the aversive pattern are called aversive because they meet the criteria established by the ethologist Wallace Craig[9] for aversive behavior; that is, the production of each response facilitates the removal of the taste stimulus from the oral cavity.

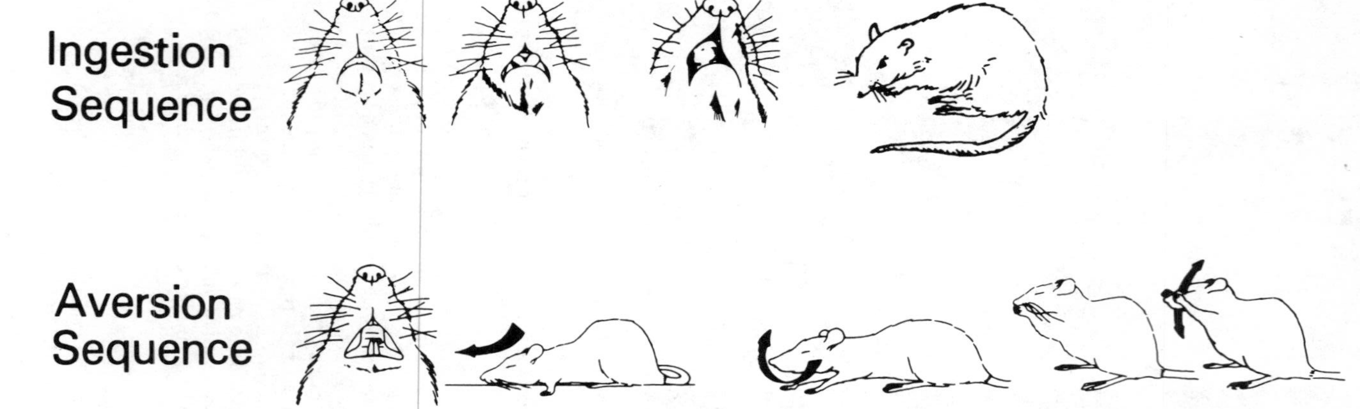

FIGURE 6. Taste-elicited fixed action patterns. Ingestive responses (top) are elicited by oral infusions of glucose, sucrose, isotonic sodium chloride, and include rhythmic mouth movements, tongue protrusions, lateral tongue protrusions and paw licking. Aversive responses (bottom) are elicited by infusions of quinine, caffeine, and morphine solutions and include gapes, chin rubs, head shakes, paw wipes, forelimb flailing, and locomotion (not shown).

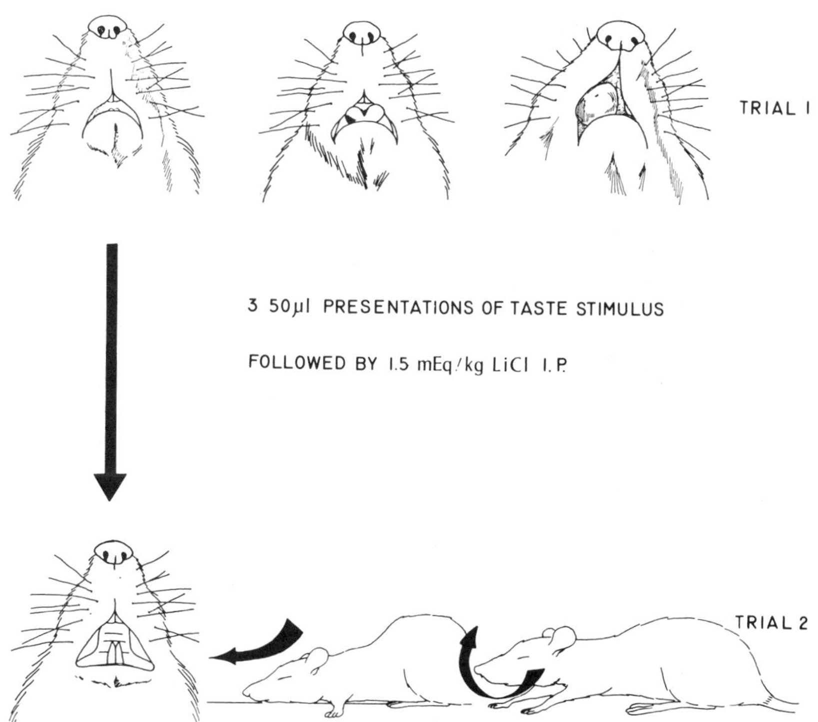

FIGURE 7. Taste reactivity for unpaired and paired stimuli. Sucrose, NaCl, and HCl stimuli when presented intraorally in 50 µl presentations elicit an ingestion sequence composed of rhythmical movements of mandible and tongue and lateral tongue extensions (trial 1). After a single pairing of the taste stimulus with LiCl injection, the taste elicits a replica of the rejection response to quinine. This rejection response is composed of gaping, chin rubbing, and head shaking (trial 2).

Following taste-LiCl association there is a dramatic shift in the pattern of taste reactivity responses elicited by the paired taste stimulus. FIGURE 7 reveals that the very same sucrose stimulus that had elicited an ingestive response pattern before LiCl association evokes a quinine-like aversive pattern after LiCl pairing.[2,17] Recall that intake test results did not discriminate between the effects of pairing sucrose with LiCl, shock, or lactose intolerance, leading one to the conclusion that sucrose palatability was altered in each type of association (FIGURE 2). Taste reactivity results enabled us to reject this conclusion. As seen in FIGURES 8, 9, and 10, sucrose continued to elicit an ingestive taste reactivity pattern following either shock or lactose pairing, but not after LiCl pairing. These data suggest that the taste reactivity technique can be used to distinguish between the effects of separate psychological variables, like palatability and fear, that are not distinguished by more traditional measures of palatability, like intake. While the taste reactivity test is new and has not yet been extensively used, its obvious utility in this and other contexts is evidenced in recent applications by Parker,[31] Garcia, Forthman-Quick and White,[13] and Domjan (this volume).

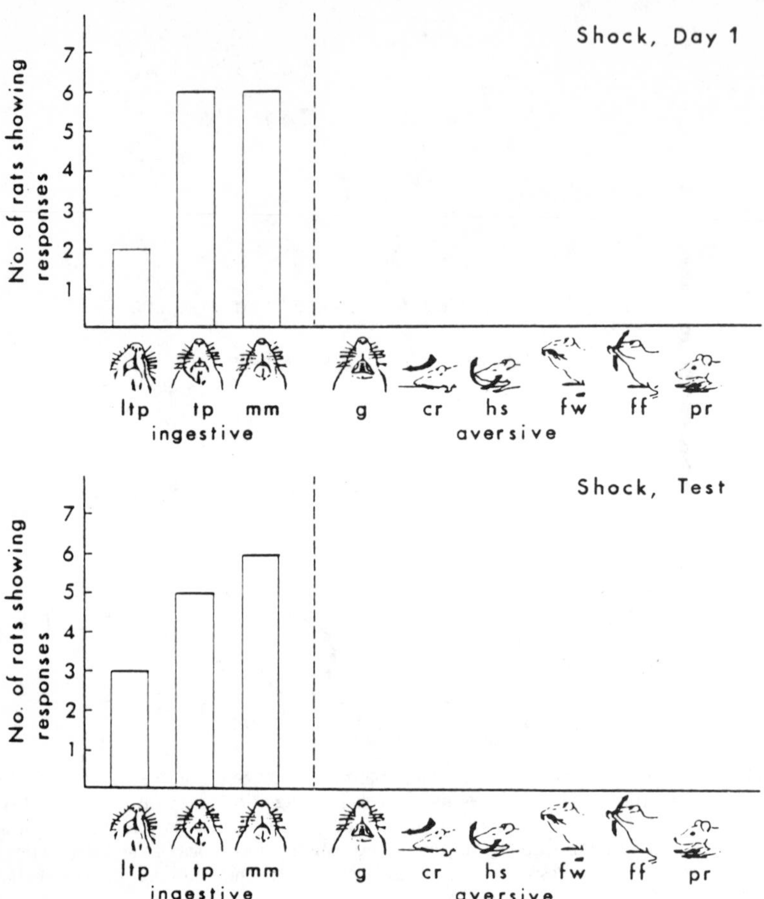

FIGURE 8. Taste reactivity responses of rats trained to associate sucrose with foot shock. (Top) Taste reactivity responses to sucrose on first day of training. (Bottom) Taste reactivity responses to sucrose during intake test following training. Ingestive taste reactivity responses noted on the abcissa are lateral tongue protrusions (ltp), tongue protrusions (tp), head shaking (hs), face washing (fw), forelimb flailing (ff), and paw rubbing (pr).

The Nature of the Effective Gustatory Stimulus for a CTA

It is useful to note that while previous exposure to a taste inhibits the rate of CTA acquisition, all taste stimuli are not equal in this regard. FIGURE 11 compares the shift in the taste reactivity response pattern following the association of novel (left panel) and familiar tastes (right panel) with LiCl injection. Familiarity with salt and acid tastes reduced the rate of shifting the taste reactivity pattern from ingestive to aversive. In contrast, prior exposure to a sucrose taste seemed to totally block the shift to an aversive pattern (compare novel sucrose to familiar sucrose results).

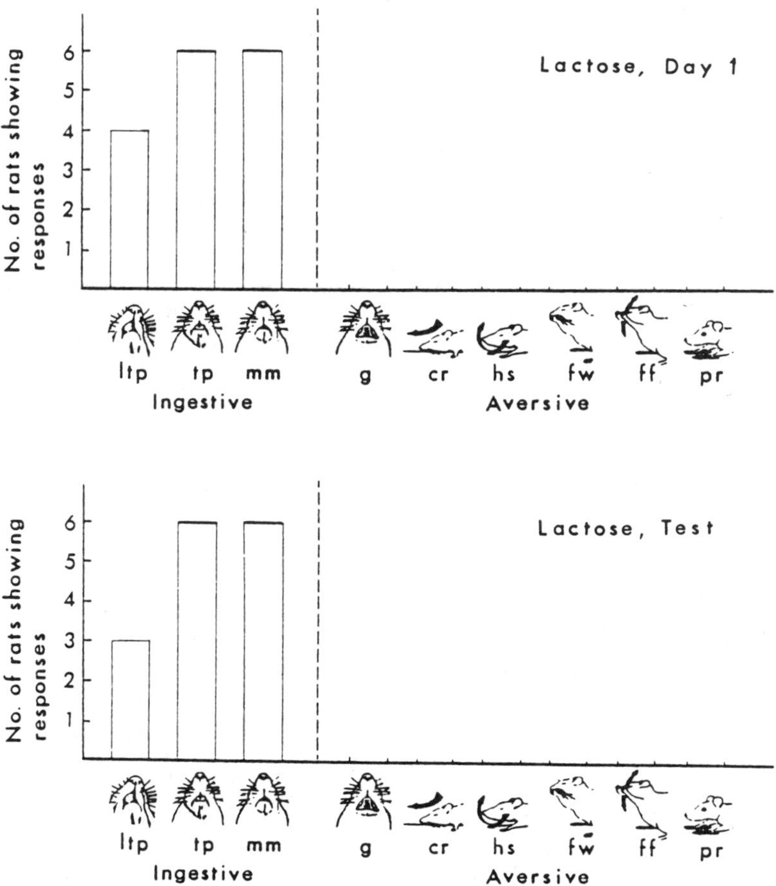

FIGURE 9. Taste reactivity responses of rats trained to associate lactose with its intestinal malabsorptive effects. (Top) Taste reactivity responses of rats to lactose prior to the postingestive effects of lactose. (Bottom) Taste reactivity responses of rats to lactose following several exposures to the taste of lactose followed by the effects of its malabsorption.

The CTA Paradigm as a Method of Determining Similarities between Taste Stimuli for Nonverbal Species

The physiological analysis of the gustatory system requires the use of animal models. In selecting these models it is important to determine, rather than assume, that the animals chosen respond to categories of taste stimuli in ways similar to our own with respect to both neurophysiological coding and behavioral responses. The use of the CTA paradigm to test for similarities between taste stimuli and their classification into categories in nonverbal animals by Frank and her colleagues Nowlis and Pfaffmann[12] has been an important development in gustatory research (see Frank,

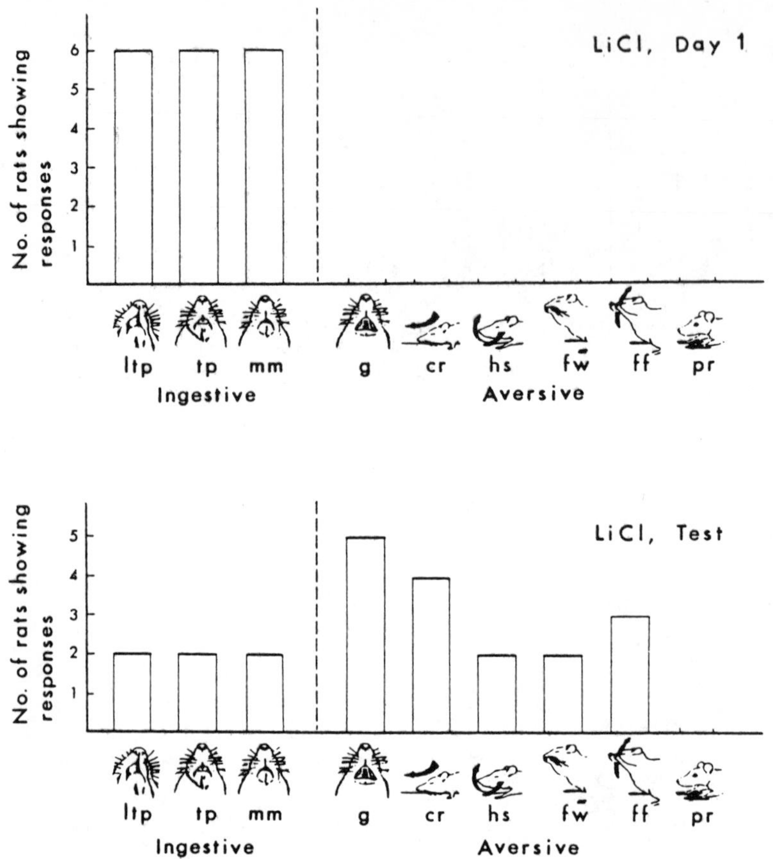

FIGURE 10. Taste reactivity responses of rats trained to associate sucrose with LiCl. (Top) Taste reactivity responses to sucrose prior to pairing with LiCl (first training day). (Bottom) Taste reactivity responses to sucrose after two pairings with LiCl (during intake test).

this volume). The utility of this method is evidenced by its recent application by others, e.g. Pritchard and Scott[34] to determine categorization of amino acid taste stimuli by rats and Jakinovich[21] for similar questions for nonnutritive sweeteners in gerbils.

For the results of this approach to be generalizable, however, it is imperative for the field to develop a valid methodology for equating the intensity of the taste stimuli to be examined. Differences in taste stimulus intensity can markedly alter human psychophysical taste judgments. For example, for humans the bitter quality of sodium saccharin and the sour quality of urea increase with increasing stimulus concentrations. No single method of equating taste intensity will be perfect, but some methods have more apparent pitfalls than others. Using human judgements of taste intensity to select taste intensities for animal experiments seems particularly suspect. For reasons noted earlier, equating intake volume is also a dubious method, as this measure can

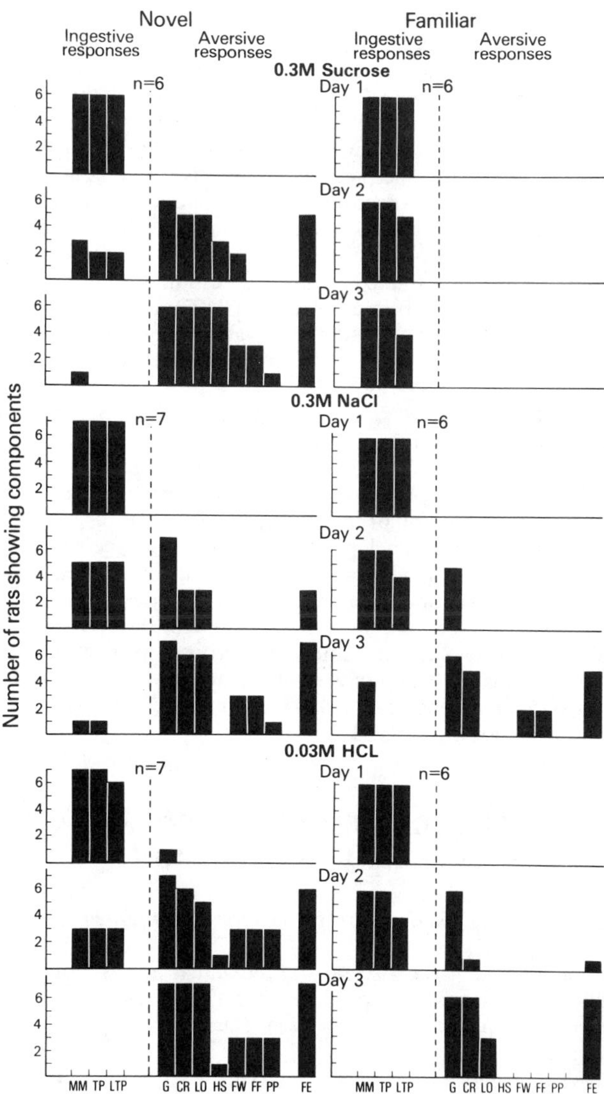

FIGURE 11. Growth of aversive responses as a function of taste quality and its novelty. Behavioral response to oral infusions of novel or familiar sucrose (top), salt (middle), and acid (bottom) in naive rats (day 1) and in the same rats after one (day 2) or two pairings (day 3) of these tastes with lithium chloride injection. The number of animals displaying a particular response component is represented in the height of each histogram. The response components elicited by 50 μl presentations of sucrose, salt, and acid stimuli are rhythmic mouth movements (MM), rhythmic tongue protrusions (TP), lateral tongue protrusions LTP), gapes (G), chin rubs (CR), locomotion (LO), head shakings (HS), face washing (FW), forelimb shakes (FF), paw pushes (PP), and ejection of fluid from the mouth (FE).

be affected by too large a variety of irrelevant factors. Selecting the concentration equivalent to the half-maximal response of one peripheral nerve is of limited utility. The wisest course is to examine a range of CS+ and CS− concentrations.

The usefulness of the CTA generalization paradigm is seen in the following example. Ammonium chloride (NH_4Cl) as well as other non-sodium salts like potassium chloride (KCl) and calcium chloride (CaCl) have traditionally been viewed as categorically similar to NaCl and assumed to act through the same "salt" receptor system. Recently, Boudreau *et al.*[3] have demonstrated that these non-sodium salts act via a different peripheral channel than do sodium salts. This channel is pH sensitive and is therefore responsive to acids. It is interesting that in the presentation by Frank it has been shown that hamsters trained on a NH_4Cl stimulus in a CTA paradigm generalize to hydrochloric acid (HCl) and not to NaCl. These data reveal an interesting parallel between peripheral nerve electrophysiological and behavioral responses within the gustatory system and are useful in developing models of quality coding in this sensory modality.

Frank's use of taste mixtures as paired stimuli in the CTA paradigm demonstrates that the component tastes of a mixture are discernible to the animal based on their CTA response generalization to these individual component tastes as well as to the taste mixture itself. For example, when an acid-sugar mixture was used as the CS+ in a CTA paradigm consumption of the mixture as well as of the sugar and acid component stimuli themselves were each reduced. These data suggest that taste can function as an analytic sense for animals as it can for humans.[11] For example, we can discern the sweet and sour components of lemonade. Lemonade is not a synthetic or an emergent property of the mixture of sugar and acid tastes as the color brown is for our visual system. Brown is the synthetic property of the mixture of red and green; the components of a mixture that produced brown are not decipherable. It is our ability for deciphering or analyzing complex tastes into simpler component tastes that guides the cook in the preparation of food.

THE VISCERAL FACTOR: INPUT AND ITS CENTRAL INTEGRATION

The Nature of the Effective Visceral US for Conditioned Taste Aversion

What are the qualities that the visceral stimulus must possess following its pairing with a novel taste in order for it to produce a CTA? The relevant effects of USs, like LiCl, irradiation, and apomorphine, have been referred to as toxicosis. This term refers to the pathological effects of poisons. However, Nachman and Hartley[28] have demonstrated that several widely used rodenticides, while clearly toxic, are not effective as USs in CTAs. These data argue against the use of the toxicosis concept in CTA. A proviso to reducing the importance of the toxicosis concept for CTAs is seen in a suggestion made in Riley's paper that an adequate dose range of these exceptional toxins has not yet been examined.

Getting beyond the broadly defined toxicosis concept, investigators have attempted to factor out the visceral site of effective US action (e.g. mouth, stomach, small intestine, large intestine), as well as attempting to assign a qualitative descriptor to this sensation (e.g. nausea, cramps, gas). The component symptoms of emesis including nausea and vomiting appear to be the most widely accepted symptoms that predict the formation of CTAs. A variety of data support this notion. Antiemetic drugs block the expression of previously acquired CTAs; dose levels were critical for the effect and correspond well with levels prescribed for antiemetic activity in dogs.[7] LiCl, the most widely used US agent in CTA experiments, is known to produce nausea and vomiting in humans.[1] Even more compelling are the recent findings of Pelchat and Rozin.[33] Humans who experienced a non-gastrointestinal symptom (e.g. hives or mouth sores) showed little or no mean decrease in their hedonic rating of the food that preceded the symptom, whereas other subjects experiencing gastrointestinal malaise (e.g. nausea, diarrhea, gas) showed a decreased hedonic rating of the associated food item. Only those experiencing nausea or vomiting after eating a particular food shifted their palatability evaluation from positive to negative, that is they developed a net dislike for the paired food. These data argue for a special role for nausea in altering human responses to taste stimuli. It should be noted, however, that while nausea (i.e., the visceral manifestation of a particular agent) may be sufficient for the formation of a CTA it is not necessary. Eliminating the visceral effects of toxins by vagal section neither eliminates their action upon central sites in and around the area postrema nor their effectiveness as USs in CTAs.[8]

LiCl is the most widely used US agent in CTA studies. The dosage of LiCl used, however, varies widely. Nachman and Ashe[27] examined a wide range of isotonic LiCl doses and three sites of application, intraperitoneal, intragastric, and intravenous. A direct relationship of LiCl dose (in mEq/l) was found for intake suppression irrespective of site of application. However, some investigators have used hypertonic LiCl doses, which result in pain[16] in addition to other visceral symptoms. Greater efforts to use isotonic solutions of LiCl, as well as expanding the use of other US agents like apomorphine and copper sulfate ($CuSO_4$), will lead to greater interlaboratory reliability and greater generalization of CTA effects.

Satiety Versus the Effects of US Agents in CTA

The association of a food's taste with either an aversive visceral experience (CTA) or the visceral events that accompany the digestion of this food (satiety) can produce the same effect (i.e., reduction of intake of that food). This result has led some to the question: Are the behavioral effects of the internal state changes following consumption of a meal (satiety) similar to those of the nausea or visceral malaise in CTA? To further focus the question it can be asked whether both treatments produce a similar shift in palatability. While both treatments may reduce food intake,[36] we should be prepared to reject equating the effects of satiety and gastrointestinal malaise based on similarities in intake suppression alone. Other measures of palatability would, therefore, be useful. Cabanac[6] notes that human palatability judgements of glucose shift from highly palatable to aversive following the consumption of concentrated glucose solutions. Cabanac's data argue for a reversal in palatability rather than a reduction in palatability. This distinction is critical because, as we know, taste reactivity testing reveals that the association of a taste with the symptoms produced by LiCl injection reverses the palatability response from ingestion to aversion. In contrast, the majority of other data on satiety and palatability have argued for a reduction in the palatability evaluation of a particular food following the consumption of that food rather than reversing the evaluation to aversion (see Booth, present volume).[35] It is possible that the volume and concentration of glucose consumed by subjects in Cabanac's experiment produced gastrointestinal symptoms more similar to LiCl than to the normal satiety state that he was attempting to produce (see Deutsch *et al.*[10] on use of glucose in CTA).

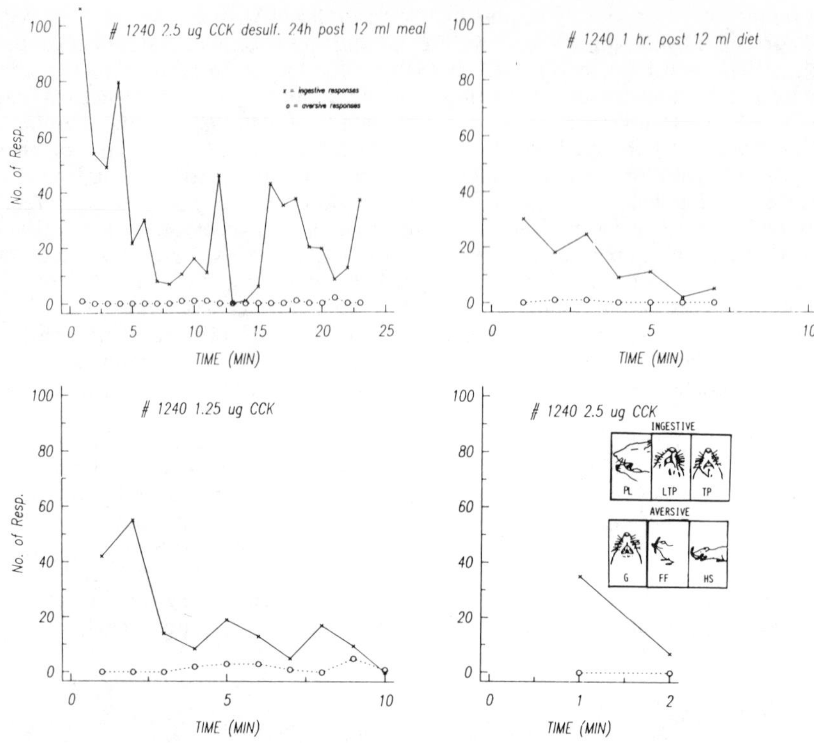

FIGURE 12. The sum of the ingestive (x) and aversive (o) taste reactivity responses occurring during each minute of an intraoral intake test to a 0.1 M sucrose stimulus. The four testing conditions of the same rat are indicated. The amount consumed in each condition equals the duration of the test in minutes times the rate of infusion, which was 1.1 ml/min.

Putting aside the issue of the extremes of satiety in which pronounced gastric distension, osmotic stress, or rapid intestinal absorption are factors, can we compare the effects of normal meal termination with the associative aversive consequences of taste-gastrointestinal malaise? This question has been quite difficult to resolve. It is clear from the presentation by Kulkovsky that he and his colleagues Smith and Gibbs have made some progress on the issue. These investigators compared the effects of LiCl and putative satiety agents like cholecystokinin (CCK) and bombesin (BBS) as US agents in a CTA after first matching the effective dose of these agents on the reduction of intake. Doses of CCK and BBS that reduced food intake to the same degree as a given dose of LiCl did not function as effective US agents in a CTA test.[36] This experiment circumvents a problem that previous attempts to unravel the action of CCK from aversive learning had failed to do, namely how one compares the effects of LiCl and CCK without anchoring dosage selection in some way.

As these authors note, despite this evidence it is still possible to argue that CCK and BBS are more aversive when administered before a feeding test in food- or water-deprived rats than they are in a CTA paradigm, which measures the effect of an injection of these putative satiety agents after the ingestion of flavored water. These paradigmatic differences are critical, e.g. before versus after. Kulkovsky[25] has examined this possibility by administering vehicle control, CCK, or LiCl doses to separate groups prior to the presentation of flavored water to thirsty rats in the presence of food. CCK and LiCl decreased food intake to the same extent but did not act in similar ways on drinking. LiCl suppressed drinking, but CCK did not. When the three groups of rats were subsequently tested on a two-bottle preference test for flavored versus plain water, the LiCl group demonstrated a CTA by suppressing their flavored water intake while the vehicle and CCK groups did not.

Some preliminary data from my laboratory support the similarity between the effects of meal-induced satiety and CCK treatment on palatability. In FIGURE 12, note that the total number of ingestive taste reactivity responses elicited at the beginning of an intraoral infusion of 0.1 M sucrose was dramatically greater in the food-deprived condition (upper left) than in either meal-fed (upper right) or CCK conditions (remaining panels). Following an intragastric meal (meal-induced satiety) the termination of intraoral sucrose intake was not reliable associated with aversive taste reactivity responses. In the same paradigm, when two different doses of CCK were administered to food-deprived rats, sucrose intake termination was similarly not accompanied by aversive taste reactivity components. The decline in the number of ingestive taste reactivity responses emitted per minute rather than the appearance of aversive taste reactivity responses predicted meal termination in both intragastric meal and CCK injection conditions, as well as in the food deprivation condition.

SITES OF TASTE-VISCERAL INTEGRATION WITHIN THE CNS

In making the transition to considering sites of central integration, I would like to stress the fact that the taste reactivity method has another advantage over measures of palatability, like intake, which require spontaneous intake or appetitive behavior. A variety of neural lesions and ablations produce animals that do not seek out food. An animal that does not seek out food may nevertheless be able to evaluate a taste

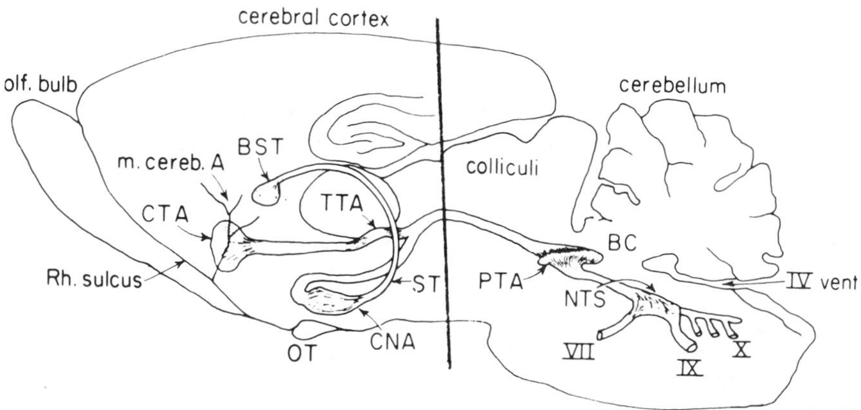

FIGURE 13. Cartoon schematization of the central gustatory system of the rat.

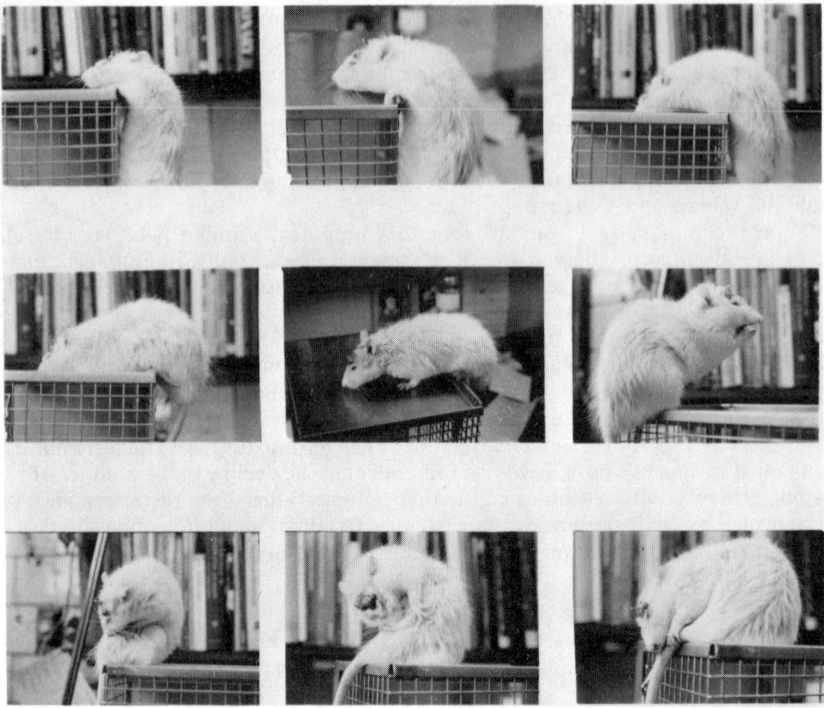

FIGURE 14. Decerebrate rats exhibit no spontaneous activity other than grooming but often overreact with well-coordinated movements to seemingly inappropriate stimuli. Tail pinch facilitates a brisk, well-coordinated cage climb. Decerebrate rats maintain their fur: face washing, grooming of the flanks, anal, and genital grooming involve complicated postures that are executed in a coordinated fashion by decerebrate rats.

that is placed directly onto the gustatory receptors; appetitive and evaluative capacities should not be confused.

Are Taste and Visceral Afferent Information Integrated within the Nucleus of the Solitary Tract and If So Is This Integration Sufficient To Produce CTAs?

Taste and visceral afferent neurons make their first central synapse within adjacent areas of the same nucleus within the caudal brainstem, the nucleus of the solitary tract (NTS). Their juxtaposition within NTS, however, should not imply that a behaviorally relevant convergence or integration occurs at this level of the neuraxis since these two types of afferent signals are also closely associated at more rostral levels of the brain. Recent examinations of primary afferent distributions within the NTS have extended the gustatory nerve terminations caudally and the vagal field rostrally, raising the possibility of some convergence within the NTS.[29] However, the subdiaphragmatic vagus, which carries most of the vagal afferent information implicated in ingestive control,[29] terminates caudomedially in the NTS adjacent to the area pos-

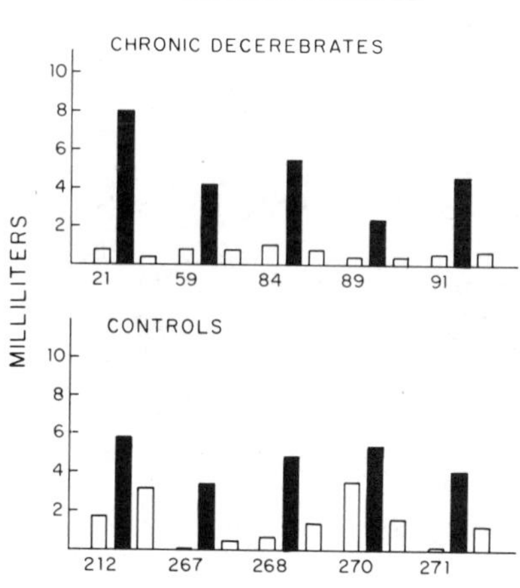

FIGURE 15. Intraoral intake of 0.03 M sucrose in chronic decerebrate and control rats. The open histograms represent the amount of sucrose consumed in the meal fed condition (1 hr post intragastric feeding) and the filled histogram the amount of the same sucrose stimulus consumed following food deprivation (24 hr of food deprivation, but 1 hr after intragastric intubation of water).

trema and thus contributes little, if anything, to the more rostrolateral area of taste and visceral afferent overlap.[22,29]

The results of an integration between taste and visceral information within the caudal brainstem could be directly examined behaviorally. Norgren and I[19] used the taste reactivity method to examine whether the chronic decerebrate rat or caudal brain-

TABLE 1.

Treatment	Decerebrate	Control
Sucrose		
Saline	3.2 + 1.0	8.1 + 1.1
Insulin (5 U/kg)	6.7 + 1.4	11.3 + 1.2
Change	3.5 + 0.9[a]	3.2 + 0.8[b]
Water		
Saline	2.5 + 1.2	4.7 + 1.0
Insulin (5 U/kg)	1.7 + 0.7	5.8 + 1.0
Change	−0.9 + 0.9	0.7 + 1.2
Sucrose		
Saline	2.2 + 0.5	11.6 + 2.9
Insulin (10 U/kg)	5.5 + 0.7	15.8 + 2.2
Change	3.3 + 0.7[b]	3.8 + 2.1[a]
Water		
Saline	1.1 + 0.2	8.9 + 1.7
Insulin (10 U/kg)	1.0 + 0.2	6.3 + 2.5
Change	−0.2 + 0.1	−2.6 + 0.9

[a] $p < 0.05$ [b] $p < 0.01$; paired t-test comparisons, significantly different from saline of that group. Sucrose = 0.03 M. Intake values are in milliliters.

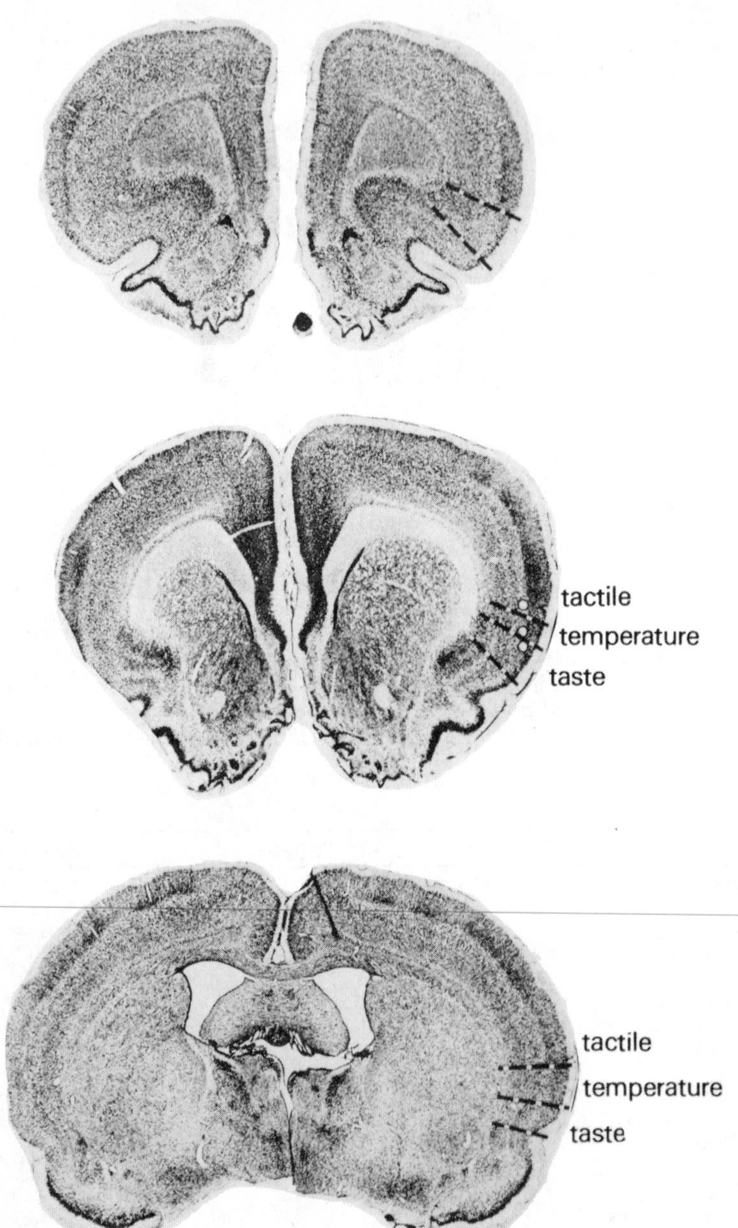
tactile
temperature
taste
tactile
temperature
taste

stem preparation could acquire a CTA. The level of the transection with respect to the central gustatory system is shown in FIGURE 13. The chronic decerebrate rat is a viable neurological preparation; these rats maintain a righted posture and spontaneously groom as shown in FIGURE 14. While this preparation never produces spontaneous ingestion food or water, the lack of appetitive behavor can be circumvented by direct oral application of taste stimuli using intraoral catheters. Intraoral taste stimulation of chronic decerebrate rats elicits the same patterns of taste reactivity responses at the same concentrations as it does from intact rats.[20] Furthermore, the chronic decerebrate rat can behaviorally demonstrate its integration of taste and caloric state signals by altering its taste reactivity to, and intake of, sucrose when challenged with food deprivation (FIGURE 15) or insulin-induced hypoglycemia (TABLE 1). In contrast, despite 12 times as many taste-LiCl pairings as were necessary to shift the taste reactivity pattern of intact rats, the decerebrate rats continued to display ingestive taste reactivity whether they were retested 1 or 24 hrs after taste-LiCl pairings. Therefore, in spite of repeated assertions[13-15] that the NTS constitutes the neural basis of taste-illness association, there is currently no behavioral data to support an integration of taste and visceral afferent signals that is sufficient to produce behavioral aspects of CTAs within the NTS.

Are Taste and Visceral Afferent Signals Relevant to the Acquisition of CTAs Integrated within the Cortical Gustatory Relay?

While there is some disagreement on the effect of gustatory cortical ablation on the rat's ability to acquire and retain a CTA, this may be explained by a lack, until recently, of an adequate anatomical description of this region. Kosar *et al.*[30] have recently defined the cytoarchitectural boundaries of the cortical gustatory area of the rat. Using electrophysiological recording within cortex, autoradiographic analysis of thalamocortical projections derived from electrophysiologically guided VPMpc injections and cortical cytoarchitecture, these authors defined the gustatory cortical representation as agranular insular cortex (FIGURE 16). This definition contrasts with previous assertions that the cortical gustatory representation was more dorsal in granular insular cortex.[23] The work of Kiefer (this volume) and his colleague Braun, as well as Yamamoto, Matsuo, and Kawamura[39] have demonstrated that cortical ablations that include the cytoarchitectural region defined by Kosar *et al.* blocks the retention of a prelesion CTA. This retention deficit has been interpreted by Braun and colleagues[4,5] to mean that the cortical gustatory representation is functionally integral in the learning and memory of taste stimuli. This same neural lesion how-

FIGURE 16. (Top) Cresyl violet stained, coronal section of a normal rat brain showing cytoarchitectural boundaries of gustatory neocortex as defined by the autoradiographic tracing of afferent projections from the gustatory relay nucleus in the thalamus. (Middle) Coronal sections showing lesions placed at electrophysiologically determined functional transitions within anterolateral cortex. The most dorsal lesion is placed within a region responding to tactile stimulation of the mouth and is marked by a well-developed layer IV. The middle lesion is situated in an oral temperature responsive region at a point where layer IV is thinning. The most ventral lesion is placed in agranular gustatory cortex. (Bottom) Cytoarchitectural boundaries of oral tactile, temperature, and gustatory cortical regions. The regions are derived from studies involving the physiological placement of tritiated amino acid injections within portions of the ventrobasal nucleus of the thalamus.

TABLE 2.

Decorticate			Control		
Rat	H_2O	NaCl	Rat	H_2O	NaCl
177	0	336	5		584
014	4	238	2		260
119	0	98	3		217
176	0	78	6		180
046	0	69	4		115
043		60	1		75
107		54	7	28	
120	13	36	8	18	
013	0	36			

Rank-ordered bar-press values during a one-hour extinction period for individual sodium-depleted decorticate and control rats as a function of 4–6 hours of previous taste experience with distilled water or 0.15 M sodium chloride.

ever, does not appear to eliminate the rats capacity to acquire a postlesion taste-LiCl association or to retain this association.[4,26] As a proviso to conclusions derived from these data, it should be noted that only the intake suppression measure and not taste reactivity responses have thus far been measured. Since intake responses do not distinguish between taste avoidance and taste aversion, as noted above, it will be important to reexamine these experiments using the taste reactivity measure of palatability.

The use of paradigms other than CTA reveals that completely decorticate rats learn taste associations. Wirsig and Grill[38] examined completely decorticate rats for their ability to latently learn the taste of NaCl. Using the paradigm of Krieckhaus and Wolf,[24] water-deprived rats were trained to perform a bar pressing task to obtain either water (one group) or isotonic NaCl (another group). After approximately four daily, one-hr sessions, bar pressing rates stabilized. The following sequence of events then occurred: rats were allowed *ad libitum* access to water (water deprivation ameliorated), next they were treated with a diuretic to promote urine sodium loss (salt appetite facilitated), and were then returned to the operant situation, but now the bar presses did not yield fluid reward (extinction). As seen in TABLE 2, decorticate rats that had been trained to receive NaCl when thirsty resisted extinction when tested sodium deprived, whereas water-trained decorticates rapidly extinguished. In other experiments, intact rats were trained on this paradigm, then decorticated, and finally tested on the extinction condition. Retention of the preablation salt taste experience was evidenced in this group by their resistance to extinction. The rat's neocortex is, therefore, not necessary for the retention or acquisition of at least some types of complex taste associations.

ACKNOWLEDGMENTS

The author wishes to acknowledge the collaboration of Ralph Norgren and Kent Berridge. Eva Kosar and Gary Schwartz's critical readings of earlier drafts improved the quality of this manuscript.

REFERENCES

1. Baldessarini, R. J. 1980. Drugs and the treatment of psychiatric disorders. *In* The Pharmacological Basis of Therapeutics. A. G. Gilman, L. S. Goodman & A. Gilman, Eds. 6th edit. Macmillan. New York.
2. Berridge, K., H. J. Grill & R. Norgren. 1981. Relation of consummatory responses and preabsorptive insulin release to palatability and learned taste aversions. J. Comp. Physiol. Psychol. **95**: 363–382.
3. Boudreau, J. C., N. K. Hoang, J. Oravec & L. T. Do. 1983. Rat neurophysiological taste responses to salt solutions. Chem. Senses **8**: 131–150.
4. Braun, J. J., S. W. Kiefer & J. V. Ouellet. 1981. Psychic ageusia in rats lacking gustatory neocortex. Exp. Neurol. **72**: 711–715.
5. Braun J. J., P. S. Lasiter & S. W. Kiefer. 1982. The gustatory neocortex of the rat. Physiol. Psychol. **10**: 13–45.
6. Cabanac, M. 1971. Physiological role of pleasure. Science **173**: 1103–1107.
7. Coil, J. D., W. G. Hankins, D. J. Jenden & J. Garcia. 1978. The attenuation of a specific cue-to-consequence association by anti-emetic agents. Psychopharmacology **56**: 21–25.
8. Coil, J. D., R. C. Rogers, J. Garcia & D. Novin. 1978. Conditioned taste aversions vagal and circulatory mediation of the toxic US. Behav. Biol. **24**: 509–519.
9. Craig, W. 1918. Appetites and aversions as constituents of instincts. Biol. Bull. **34**: 91–107.
10. Deutsch, J. A., F. Molina & A. Puerto. 1976. Conditioned taste aversion caused by palatable nontoxic nutrients. Behav. Biol. **16**: 161–174.
11. Erickson, R. P. 1977. The role of primaries in taste research. *In* Proceedings of the Sixth International Symposium on Olfaction and Taste. J. Le Magnen & P. MacLeod, Eds. Information Retrieval Ltd. London.
12. Frank, M. E., G. H. Nowlis & C. Pfaffmann. 1980. Specificity of acquired aversions to taste qualities in hamsters and rats. J. Comp. Physiol. Psychol. **94**: 932–942.
13. Garcia, J., D. Forthman-Quick & B. White. 1984. Conditioned disgust and fear from mollusk to monkey. *In* Primary Neural Substrates of Learning and Behavioral Change. D. L. Alkon & J. Farley, Eds. Cambridge University Press. New York.
14. Garcia, J., W. G. Hankins & K. W. Rusiniak. 1974. Behavioral regulation of the milieu interne in man and rat. Science **185**: 824–831.
15. Garcia, J., K. W. Rusiniak, S. W. Kiefer & F. Bermudez-Rattoni. 1982. The neural integration of feeding and drinking habits. *In* Conditioning: Representation of Involved Neural Functions. C. D. Woody, Ed.: 567–579. Plenum Press, New York.
16. Giesler, G. J., Jr. & J. C. Liebeskind. 1976. Inhibition of visceral pain by electrical stimulation of the periaqueductal gray matter. Pain **2**: 43–48.
17. Grill, H. J. 1975. Sucrose as an aversive stimulus. Neurosci. Abstr. **1**: 525.
18. Grill, H. J. & K. Berridge. 1985. Taste reactivity as a measure of the neural control of palatability. Progr. Psychobiol. Physiol. Psychol.
19. Grill, H. J. & R. Norgren. 1978. The taste reactivity test. I. Mimetic responses to gustatory stimuli in neurologically normal rats. Brain Res. **143**: 263–279.
20. Grill, H. J. & R. Norgren. 1978. The taste reactivity test. II. Mimetic responses to gustatory stimuli in chronic thalamic and chronic decerebrate rats. Brain Res. **143**: 281–297.
21. Jakinovich, W. 1981. Stimulation of the gerbil's gustatory receptors by artificial sweeteners. Brain Res. **210**: 69–81.
22. Hamilton, R. B. & R. Norgren. 1984. Central projections of gustatory nerves in the rat. J. Comp. Neurol. **222**: 560–577.
23. Krettek, J. E. & J. L. Price. 1977. The cortical projection of the medio-dorsal nucleus and adjacent thalamic nuclei in the rat. J. Comp. Neurol. **171**: 157–192.
24. Krieckhaus, E. E. & G. Wolf. 1968. Acquisition of sodium by rats: Interaction of innate mechanisms and latent learning. J. Comp. Physiol. Psychol. **65**: 197–201.
25. Kulkovsky, P. J. 1980. Reduction of drinking-associated feeding by c-terminal octapeptide of cholecystokinin-pancreozymin. Behav. Neural Biol. **29**: 111–116.
26. Lasiter, P. S. & D. L. Glanzman. 1982. Cortical substrates of taste aversion learning: dorsal

prepiriform (insular) lesions disrupt taste aversion learning. J. Comp. Physiol. Psychol. **96**: 376–392.

27. Nachman, M. & J. H. Ashe. 1973. Learned taste aversions in rats as a function of dosage, concentration, and route of administation of LiCl. Physiol. Behav. **10**: 73–78.
28. Nachman, M. & P. L. Hartley. 1975. Role of illness in producing learned taste aversions in rats: a comparison of several rodenticides. J. Comp. Physiol. Psychol. **89**: 1010–1018.
29. Norgren, R. 1983. Afferent interactions of cranial nerves involved in ingestion. J. Autonomic Nerv. System **9**: 67–77.
30. Norgren, R., E. Kosar & H. J. Grill. 1982. Gustatory cortex in the rat delimited by thalamocortical projections, physiological properties, and cytoarchitecture. Neurosci. Abst. **8**: 201.
31. Parker, L. A. 1982. Nonconsummatory and consummatory behavioral CRs elicited by lithium- and amphetamine-paired flavors. Learning Motiv. **13**: 281–303.
32. Pelchat, M. L., H. J. Grill, P. Rozin & J. Jacobs. 1983. Quality of acquired responses to tastes by Rattus norvericus depends on type of associated discomvort. J. Comp. Psychol. **97**: 140–153.
33. Pelchat, M. L. & P. Rozin. 1982. The special role of nausea in the aquisition of food dislikes by humans. Appetite **3**: 341–351.
34. Pritchard, T. C. & T. R. Scott. 1982. Amino acids as taste stimuli. II. Quality coding. Brain Res. **253**: 93–104.
35. Rolls, B. J., E. T. Rolls, E. A. Rowe & K. Sweeney. 1981. Sensory specific satiety in man. Physiol. Behav. **27**: 137–142.
36. Smith, G. P., J. Gibbs & P. J. Kulkovsky. 1982. Relationships between brain-gut peptides and neurons in the control of food intake. *In* The Neural Basis of Feeding and Reward. B. G. Hoebel & D. Novin, Eds.:149–165. Haer Institute. Brunswick, ME.
37. White, T. D. & J. C. Boudreau. 1975. Taste preferences of the cat for neurophysiologically active compounds. Physiol. Psychol. **3**: 405–410.
38. Wirsig, C. R. & H. J. Grill. 1982. Contribution of the rat's neocortex to ingestive control: I. Latent learning for the taste of sodium chloride. J. Comp. Physiol. Psychol. **96**: 615–627.
39. Yamamoto, T., R. Matsuo & Y. Kawamura. 1980. Localization of cortical gustatory area in rats and its role in taste discrimination. J. Neurophysiol. **44**: 440–455.

Sensory Physiology of Taste and Smell Discriminations Using Conditioned Food Aversion Methodology[a]

MARION E. FRANK

School of Dental Medicine
University of Connecticut Health Center
Farmington, Connecticut 06032

INTRODUCTION

Physiological studies of taste quality discriminations in animals have been designed and interpreted in light of human taste quality experience as studied psychophysically. The three sensory systems that contribute to flavor in humans: taste, olfaction, and the common chemical sense are distinct; chemoreceptors activated in oral and nasal cavities are located either in taste buds, olfactory mucosa, or are endings of general sensory nerve fibers. But, unlike other senses such as hearing or vision, the separate stimulation of the chemical senses is not easily accomplished. Psychophysical experiments on taste use chemical solutions that may not exclusively stimulate the taste system; in fact, some, such as acids, may stimulate all three chemosensory systems involved in flavor.[1,2] Study of the physiological processes in animals allowing the discrimination of taste quality has strongly reflected conclusions about human sensory experience gleaned from psychophysical studies carried out during the past century. A mammal such as the hamster possesses three additional separate chemoreceptive systems that may contribute to reactions to chemical solutions: vomeronasal, *nervous terminalis*, and septal organs within the nasal cavity; capacities for taste discrimination and taste physiology should be studied in the same species.

A common practice is to divide human taste quality experience into four categories described by the adjectives sweet, salty, sour, and bitter, although it may merely be a convenience.[3,4] The speculation that all taste experience can be accounted for by four categories is supported by the presence of four adjectives in many human languages that abstractly describe taste quality similarly. But some languages[5,6] contain words for special flavors; for example, *umami* for the flavor of monosodium glutamate in Japanese.[7] However, such words may identify flavors of familiar food additives that stimulate several of the oral-nasal chemosensory systems. Because humans can reliably divide the experience of taste quality elicited by single chemicals or mixtures into components that they comfortably describe as sweet, salty, sour, and bitter[8,9] has been taken to suggest taste is an analytic sense in which the qualities are separately processed and therefore separately available to experience. Many solutions of pure

[a] Supported by a grant from the National Science Foundation (BNS-81-12180).

chemicals are described by several quality adjectives,[10] implying individual molecules, or individual ions in salt and acid solutions, can interact with several physiological taste systems. In a representative psychophysical experiment, McBurney and Shick[10] asked subjects to estimate the magnitude of sweetness, saltiness, sourness, and bitterness of many solutions matched in overall intensity. Results suggested sucrose (or fructose or saccharin) and quinine (or caffeine) are excellent prototypal sweet and bitter stimuli, respectively; one and the same taste quality was attributed to these solutions by most people. Salt and acid solutions, characteristic stimuli for the salty and sour tastes, were often described by more than one taste quality adjective; salts were described as salty, sour, and bitter, and acids as sour and bitter by the majority of people. HCl and NaCl are reasonable prototypes of the sour and salty tastes although a minority of people ascribed considerable saltiness to HCl and sourness to NaCl. Of sodium salts, NaCl has been shown to be the purest salty stimulus;[11] in contrast, $NaNO_3$ and Na_2SO_4 are described as salty-sour-bitter, for example. Nonsodium-lithium salts are often described as predominantly bitter (e.g. $MgSO_4$) or equally bitter and salty (e.g., KCl and NH_4Cl).[10] Many of the acids, besides having a sour taste, are also irritants and have odors (e.g., the "vinegar" odor of acetic acid).

Cells in the gustatory peripheral[12-15] and central[13,16,17] nervous system of animals such as rats and hamsters have been most frequently characterized for sensibilities to lingual application of chemical solutions prototypal for human taste qualities. It has been generally assumed that animals discriminate a few classes of taste stimuli and place chemicals into similar classes as do humans. Preference-aversion[18-22] and learned response generalization[23-26] data have generally shown that other species behave toward solutions of gustatory stimuli in a way predictable from the human's reaction. For example, the sweet quality of sucrose, fructose, and sodium saccharin is associated with preference in many but not all animal species; but, other sweet solutions are not. NaCl, which has a salty taste, is also preferred by some species although its taste quality is easily discriminated from sucrose by humans; preference-aversion data cannot give precise information about taste quality discrimination in animals. Generalization of learned responses are better suited for this purpose. Such data also suggest there are species similarities and differences; the similar salty-bitter profile of NH_4Cl and KCl is associated with strong cross-generalization of responses trained to the two salts in rats, but responses to neither of these salts generalize to the salty NaCl; it is possible these nonsodium salts do not have the same taste quality to rats as to humans, or, the limited taste vocabulary available to humans does not allow a distinction between two "salties." Data on the cross-adaptation between salts[27,28] argue for the species difference. Neural responses to human taste quality prototypes recorded from single peripheral taste neurons of a number of species have suggested to sensory physiologists the form in which information about taste quality may be transmitted to the central nervous system.[12,23,29-33] Of primary concern is whether there are discrete types of peripheral neurons that differ essentially from one another in a given species; the most complete set of data available on this issue is from the rat[13-15,34] and most of these data describe response spectra for neurons to stimuli of known taste to humans. Peripheral taste neurons that are highly and selectively sensitive to bitter quinine,[35] salty sodium and lithium salts,[15,34] sweet sucrose, saccharin, and D-phenylalanine,[36,37] or highly, although less selectively, sensitive to sour acids[15,34] have been described for the rat and the latter three for the hamster whose chorda tympani contains many sweetener-sensitive fibers.[30,37] But these direct comparisons of human sensations with animal neural responses will ultimately fail unless the animal's sensory abilities are identical to the human's, which is unlikely.[18,22]

TASTE QUALITY IN ANIMALS

Taste quality discrimination in animals can be efficiently determined by establishing a conditioned food aversion[38] to flavored drinking water and examining generalization of the aversion to other taste solutions.[26,39–42] Quality profiles for taste solutions of humans who are asked to partition their sensations into amounts of sweetness, saltiness, sourness, and bitterness can be approximated by profiles of generalization of aversions learned by animals to the taste solutions across the four prototypes of human taste quality.[40] Such generalization profiles for hamsters for some solutions resemble taste quality profiles based on human magnitude estimates of four taste qualities.[32,33,40] Aversions to sucrose, sodium-saccharin, or D-phenylalanine generalize strongly only to the sweet prototype; an aversion to NaCl generalizes only to the salty prototype; and aversions to mixtures generalize to stimuli that are quality prototypes of the ingredients indicating the animals can identify mixture components as can humans. On the other hand, generalization profiles for some taste solutions suggest there is no precise congruity of human and hamster taste discrimination. A $NaNO_3$ aversion generalizes only to the salty prototype but is as bitter-sour as salty to humans,[10] HCl and NH_4Cl aversions generalize to the sour and bitter prototypes whereas to humans these stimuli do not taste similar;[10] and aversions to a mixture of sucrose and HCl do not show lesser generalization of the aversion to the sweet prototype than does the mixture of sucrose and NaCl[33] as would be expected by the greater reduction in sweetness produced by adding acid than by adding salt to sucrose in humans.[43,44] For that matter, generalizations of aversions do not reflect reductions in peripheral neural responses to sweeteners demonstrated in the hamster chorda tympani.[37] It is possible stimulus intensity[45] is not as salient a cue as stimulus quality for the establishment of conditioned taste aversions.

As the psychophysical experiments are restricted by the four adjectives in our language for taste quality, conditioned taste aversions tested for generalization to four prototypal taste stimuli[40] characteristic for those adjectives to humans may impose our language limitations upon the animals. This is not necessary since each stimulus in an array can be a conditional as well as generalization test stimulus if the food aversion is periodically reestablished.[32] Generalization patterns for aversions established to many solutions that primarily activate the gustatory system and are known to be attributed sweet, salty, sour and/or bitter qualities by humans can correspondingly be accounted for by postulating four sensory processes or elementary "sensations" in hamsters.[32] Aversions to some taste stimuli yielded nearly identical patterns of generalization across thirteen test stimuli; pairs of such stimuli are sucrose and fructose, NaCl and $NaNO_3$, citric acid and acetic acid, and quinine and KCl. FIGURE 1 shows the pattern of generalization for two of these pairs: the sugars and the sodium salts; striped bars indicate drinking of a test solution was suppressed (+) by a significant ($p \leqslant 0.05$) percentage. Aversions to other pairs of stimuli yielded similar, but less redundant patterns of generalization. Examples of such pairs are HCl and acetic acid, and sucrose and saccharin; an aversion to HCl generalized more strongly to non-sodium salts and quinine than did an aversion to acetic acid; and, as seen in FIGURE 1, an aversion to saccharin generalized significantly to test stimuli besides the three sweeteners. "Off-tastes" of saccharin are described by humans and can be clearly demonstrated in hamsters if aversions to saccharin are established in animals familiarized with sucrose by its presence in their daily drinking water.[40] An aversion to one stimulus, urea, which is described as predominantly bitter by humans, yields a com-

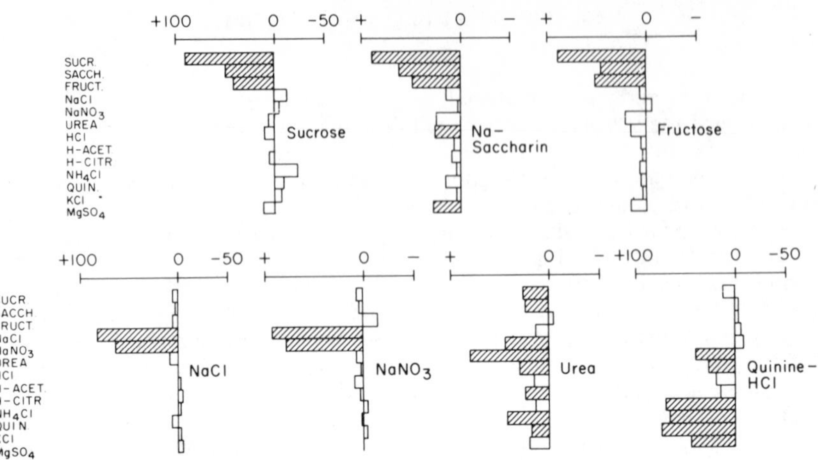

FIGURE 1. Generalization patterns of learned aversions to .1 M sucrose, .001 M Na-saccharin, .3 M fructose, .1 M NaCl, .1 M $NaNO_3$, 3.0 M urea, and .001 M quinine hydrochloride in hamsters. Test stimuli included the conditional stimuli (1.0 M urea was substituted for 3.0 M) and .01 M HCl, .01 M acetic acid, .003 M citric acid, .3 M NH_4Cl, .3 M KCl, and .1 M $MgSO_4$. Groups of twelve hamsters were used, one for each conditional stimulus; animals were conditioned, tested with four stimuli (one on each day), then reconditioned before a second four-day cycle of testing with four other stimuli; cycles were continued until all stimuli were tested. Conditioning was effected by injection of the emetic agent apomorphine.[32] Percent suppression of drinking of the 13 test stimuli is shown for each of the conditional stimuli. + 100% suppression would indicate the animals drank none of the test solution in the hour-long test session; 50% suppression would indicate they drank half as much as did a control group conditioned to water; negative suppressions indicate the animals drank more of the test solution than did the control group of animals.

plex generalization pattern (FIGURE 1). After conditioning an aversion to 3 M urea, small but significant suppression of drinking of most of the taste solutions resulted. Of these effects, only that to 1 M urea was strong (81% suppression) and only that to quinine was reciprocated; when the conditional stimulus was quinine, test 1 M urea drinking was suppressed; but when the conditional stimulus was sucrose, $NaNO_3$, or saccharin, for examples, no suppression of 1 M urea drinking was observed. Either a conditioned flavor aversion to a strong unpalatable stimulus has general effects on drinking taste solutions, or, looking at it from the other perspective, when the conditional stimulus was $NaNO_3$ for example, a strong NaCl-like taste quality dominated in the learning, as demonstrated for a strong sucrose-like taste of saccharin.

Relationships between tastes of stimuli, judged by cross-generalizations of aversions between pairs of stimuli, can be displayed simultaneously in a spatial arrangement with distance between points directly related to taste dissimilarity (multidimensional scaling: KYST II, Bell Laboratories). A three-dimensional solution ("stress" or "badness of fit" mimimized) was obtained that described data on cross-generalizations between taste solutions with points falling in a roughly tetrahedral pattern (FIGURE 2), suggesting four elemental taste processes contribute to their discrimination.[32,46] Sucrose-fructose, NaCl-$NaNO_3$, acetic-citric acid, and KCl-quinine are positioned near the corners of the tetrahedron suggesting they are reasonably pure examples of stimuli activating one process. Other stimuli such as saccharin, urea, HCl, and NH_4Cl fall

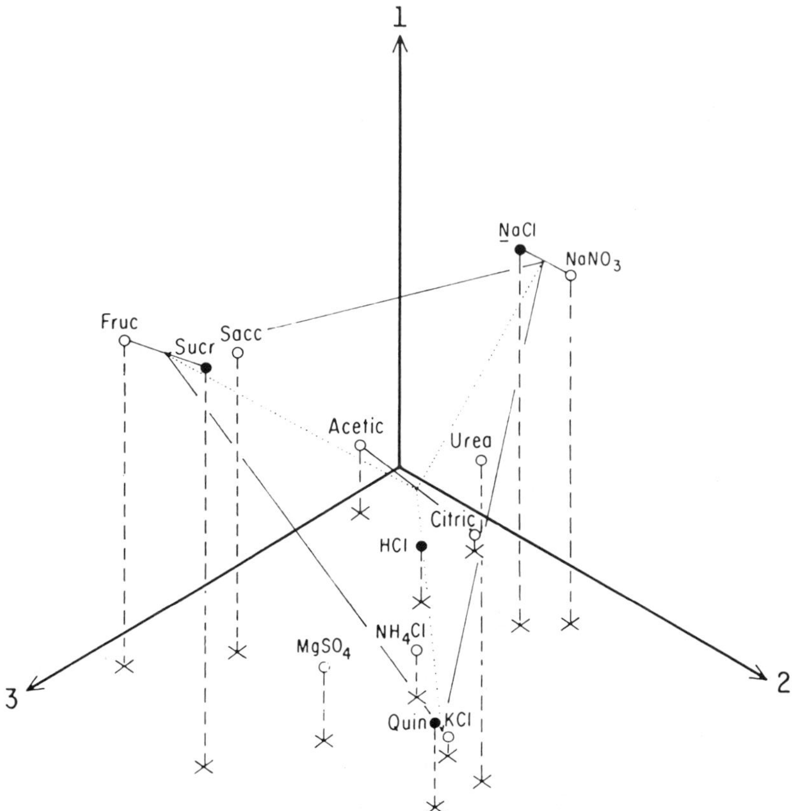

FIGURE 2. A three-dimensional space depicting discriminations among thirteen taste stimuli by hamsters. Stimuli were at the same concentrations as indicated for FIGURE 1. The multidimensional scaling program KYST II of Bell Laboratories[58] was used to generate the space in which distance represents dissimilarity; "stress" of the solution was minimized in three dimensions.[32] Data similar to those presented in FIGURE 1 were used; groups consisted of six animals, however.

at points within the tetrahedron indicating their activation of several of the processes. The relationship between the tastes of stimuli to hamsters suggests there are profound similarities among gustatory systems of mammalian species as diverse as humans and hamsters. Stimuli that are described as comprising four qualities by humans are discriminated on the basis of four factors by hamsters. On the other hand, many individual solutions are not identically perceived by the two species as indicated by positions of $NaNO_3$, KCl, NH_4Cl, HCl, and urea in the space representing taste discrimination in hamsters; this conclusion could not have been drawn from preference studies. KCl provides an excellent example of a species difference; this salt, used as a salt-taste substitute for people on low-sodium diets, does not appear to taste at all like NaCl to hamsters but to taste exactly like quinine, the prototypal bitter.

Binary mixtures of prototypal stimuli for human taste qualities, which are reasonably pure representatives of four gustatory processes identified for hamsters, have qualitative sensory characteristics in common with the components of the mix-

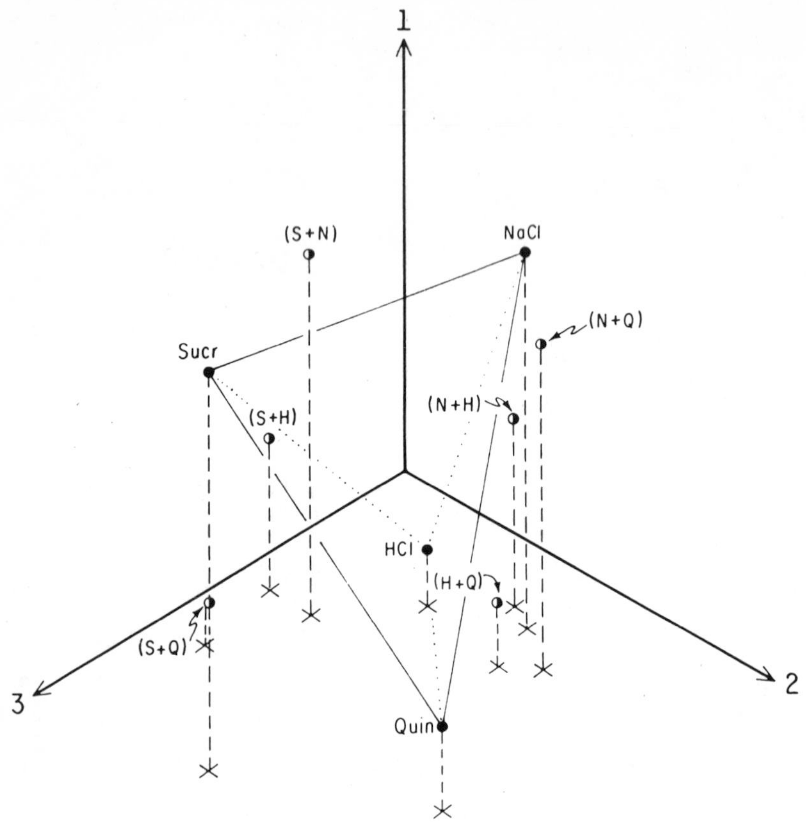

FIGURE 3. A three-dimensional space depicting discriminations among four prototypal taste stimuli and their six binary mixtures by hamsters. Technical details about stimuli and the generation of the space are given in the legend for FIGURE 2.

ture.[32,46] In a three-dimensional space depicting discriminability among prototypal taste stimuli and their binary mixtures (FIGURE 3), points for mixtures generally fall between points for components, indicating mixtures taste similar to both components. The pattern of generalization for one mixture, NaCl-quinine, was not discriminable from the pattern for one of its components; the animals behaved as if the quinine were not present in the mixture. A comparable reduction of the bitter taste of quinine by NaCl has been reported for humans.[47] Aversions to mixtures of prototypal stimuli typically result in a strong suppression of drinking of both component stimuli, which is about 85% of that observed to a component after an aversion is established to the component; a slight (about 10%) enhancement of drinking of prototypes not contained in the mixture is also seen. These characteristics of generalization of food aversions result in points for mixtures outside a tetrahedron defined for the prototypes by multidimensional scaling. The extent of generalization of food aversions may not be quantitatively equivalent to similarity between conditional and test stimuli; the method may be better suited to identify qualities taste stimuli elicit in common than to quantify their relative similarities.

TASTE: ANALYTIC OR SYNTHETIC SENSE?

Sensory systems have been considered analytic to the extent sensations elicited by two stimuli presented simultaneously could be individually identified (as in adding notes in a chord) and synthetic to the extent a new experience is generated by the mixture that is not seen in the components (as in adding colors). Analytic systems suggest different forms of sensory processing than synthetic systems. Psychophysical studies of human sensations suggest the gustatory system can operate analytically;[9,48] generalizations of conditioned taste aversions in hamsters suggest the same. Aversions established to a binary taste mixture generalize to the mixture (a mean 79% suppression of drinking) and to the components of the mixture (71%); aversions established to a component generalize to the component (82%) and taste mixtures containing the component (54%) and, to a lesser extent, aversions established to a taste mixture generalize to mixtures of stimuli of which one of the components but not the other was a component of the conditional stimulus (34%). These results are consistent with discriminations based on an analytic sensory system although addition of a new taste component tends to disrupt generalization more than subtraction of a mixture component.

Aversions conditioned to mixtures of stimuli prototypal for the taste processes identified for the hamster (e.g., NaCl and sucrose or acetic acid and quinine) after animals are accustomed to the presence of one component in their drinking water are learned to the unfamiliar component of the conditional stimulus.[49] The familiar component is ineffective for learning[50] and drinking of the unfamiliar component and mixture are equally suppressed, suggesting there is no new quality synthesized from the mixture.[32] Since it is likely the animals can taste the familiar component, these result demonstrate their ability to extract one part from a mixture stimulus, which is consistent with discriminations based on an analytic sensory system.

QUALITIES OF FLAVOR

The sensory qualities that make up flavor are usually considered to include those mediated by the gustatory, olfactory, and general sensory systems that are associated with food. Study of generalizations of conditioned food aversions should be as useful in determining characteristics of general sensory[51] and olfactory[52,53] discriminations of animals as it has been for taste.

Conditioned aversions to stimuli that may have either taste, olfactory, or general sensory, or combined taste, olfactory, and general sensory components to humans generalize to simple and compound stimuli in characteristic ways to suggest the sensory modalities involved.[54] For example, aversions to stimuli that have sulfurous, sulfurous plus sour, or sour flavors to humans cross-generalize in hamsters in a manner to suggest two sensory processes are involved in their discrimination (FIGURE 4); Cleland's reagent has a sulfurous, cysteine-HCl a sulfurous-sour, and malic acid a sour flavor to humans. Experiments are required to identify the sensory systems involved perhaps utilizing a reversible lesion of the olfactory receptors with zinc sulfate[55] since sulfurous may describe an olfactory sensation[2] enhanced by retrograde stimula-

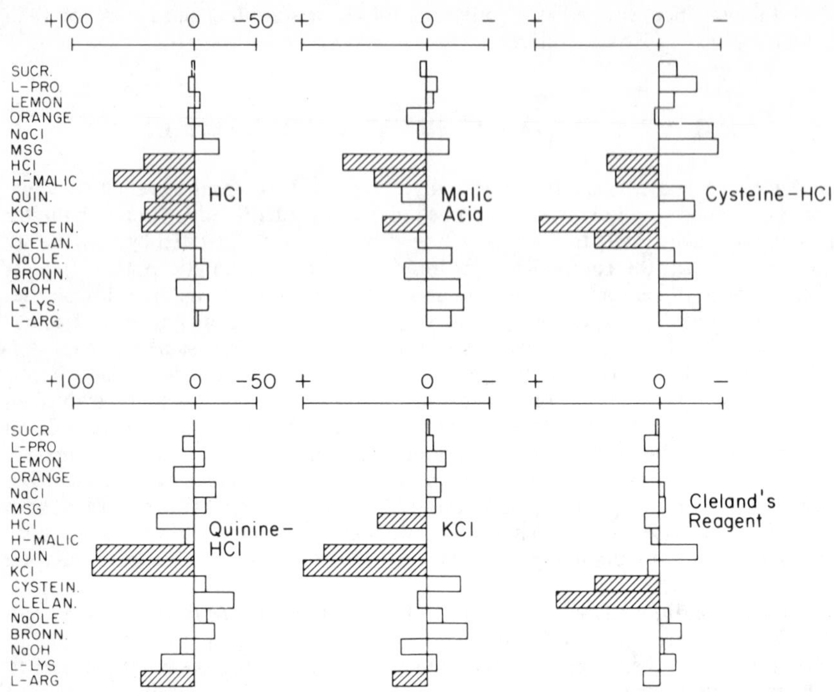

FIGURE 4. Cross-generalization patterns for learned aversions to .01 M HCl, .01 M malic acid (H-MALIC), .003 M cysteine hydrochloride, (CYSTEIN.), .001 M quinine hydrochloride (QUIN.), .3 M KCl, and .0001 M dithiotheitol (Cleland's reagent: CLELAN.) in hamsters. Test stimuli included conditional stimuli and .3 M L-proline (L-PRO.), lemonade (LEMON), orange juice (ORANGE), .1 M NaCl, .1 M monosodium glutamate (MSG), .01 M Na-oleate (NaOLE.), Dr. Bronner's Almond Soap (BRONN.), .03 M NaOH, 0.1 M L-lysine (L-LYS.), and 0.1 M L-arginine (L-ARG.) Data are presented as they are in FIGURE 1. Six animals were in each group, however, and suppressions indicated for a pair of stimuli is an average of the reciprocal results for a stimulus pair; e.g., for KCl-quinine, the median percent suppression when KCl was the conditional and quinine the test stimulus, and the suppression when quinine was the conditional and KCl the test stimulus were averaged. Striped bars indicate a median suppression outside the semi-interquartile range for each reciprocal result.

tion, or with the establishment of the effects of pure sulfurous stimuli on peripheral gustatory nerves. In another example, aversions to stimuli that evoke a soapy (Bronner's soap), soapy plus salty (Na-oleate), or salty (NaCl, monosodium glutamate) flavor cross-generalize in a way to suggest two sensory processes are involved. Experiments are required to identify the sensory system mediating the specific soapy flavor that does not cross-generalize with bitter (quinine, KCl) or other prototypal taste stimuli; perhaps a general sensory component is discriminated.

Identification of a specific sensory component of a stimulus involved in discrimination requires careful study with appropriate test stimuli for generalization of learned aversions and use of the familiarization of animals with components of a compound qualitative sensation. Without appropriate test stimuli to establish a generalization pattern, potential qualitative components of flavor would not be identified; for example, if Cleland's reagent had not been a test stimulus, cysteine-HCl could not be easily distinguished from other acids; its greater generalization to itself than to other chemicals could be due to a stronger intensity, affecting the strength of conditioned response and the learning.[45] Sweetened lemonade and orange juice were not distinguished from sucrose despite their more complex sensory properties, at least to humans, because of such a limitation. The cross-generalization of binary taste mixtures containing only one component in common is not strong: potential stimulus aspects used in discrimination may be obscured unless familiarization is judiciously used to uncover them. For example, the qualitative characteristics of a stimulus such as hydrochloric acid may be clarified if conditioned food aversions were established after malic acid (a potential pure sour taste stimulus) or KCl (a potential pure bitter stimulus) were familiar to an animal because of its presence in daily drinking water. Learning would be effective only for the non-sour or the non-bitter aspects of HCl, respectively.

CONCLUSIONS

The characteristics of food aversion learning made study of its generalization efficient for establishing discriminative capacities of chemosenses in animals and holds advantage over human psychophysics with its reliance on language. The olfactory system, which is capable of a multitude of qualitative discriminations and may be a synthetic sensory system[56,57] could hold advantage over the other chemosenses in providing a specific cue for flavor aversion; the gustatory and general sensory systems may be capable of but a few, discrete qualitative discriminations; a response learned to such cues would generalize to a good proportion of all flavor stimuli. Identification of the chemosensory system involved in a discrimination and the system's methods of processing neural information require parallel physiological experimentation.

ACKNOWLEDGMENTS

The inspiration and assistance of C. Pfaffmann and G. H. Nowlis were significant.

REFERENCES

1. SILVER, W. L. & J. A. MARUNIAK. 1981. Trigeminal chemoreception in the nasal and oral cavities. Chemical Senses **6**: 295–305.
2. ROZIN, P. 1982. "Taste-smell confusions" and the duality of the olfactory sense. Percept. Psychophys. **31**: 397–401.
3. ERICKSON, R. P. 1977. Role of primaries in taste research. Olfaction Taste Proc. Int. Symp. **6**: 369–376.
4. SCHIFFMAN, S. S. & R. P. ERICKSON. 1980. The issue of primary tastes versus a taste continuum. Neurosci. Biobehav. Rev. **4**: 109–117.
5. O'MAHONY, M. & M. D. MANZARRO ALBA. 1980. Taste descriptions in Spanish and English. Chemical Senses **5**: 47–62.
6. O'MAHONY, M. & T. TSANG. 1980. A preliminary comparison of Cantonese and American-English as taste languages. Brit. J. Psychol. **71**: 221–226.
7. YAMAGUCHI, S. 1977. Taste of monosodium L-glutamate and its psychophysical properties. Olfaction Taste Proc. Int. Sym. **6**: 493.
8. BARTOSHUK, L. M. 1978. History of research on taste. *In* Handbook of Perception. E. C. Carterette & M. P. Friedman, Eds. **VIA**: 3–18. Academic Press. New York.
9. MCBURNEY, D. H. 1978. Psychological dimensions and perceptual analysis of taste. *In*

Handbook of Perception. E. C. Carterette & M. P. Friedman. Eds. **VIA**: 125–155. Academic Press. New York.
10. McBurney, D. H. & T. R. Schick. 1971. Taste and water taste of 26 compounds for man. Percept. Psychophys. **10**: 228–232.
11. Murphy, C., A. V. Cardello & J. G. Brand. 1981. Tastes of fifteen halide salts following water and NaCl: anion and cation effects. Physiol. Behav. **26**: 1083–1095.
12. Sato, M. 1971. Neural coding in taste as seen from recordings from peripheral receptors and nerves. *In* Handbook of Sensory Physiology. L. Beidler, Ed. **IV**(part 2): 116–147. Springer-Verlag KG. Berlin.
13. Pfaffmann, C., M. Frank & R. Norgren. 1979. Neural mechanisms and behavioral aspects of taste. Ann. Rev. Psychol. **30**: 283–325.
14. Erickson, R. P., E. Covey & G. S. Doetsch. 1980. Neuron and stimulus typologies in the rat gustatory system. Brain Res. **196**: 513–519.
15. Frank, M. E., R. J. Contreras & T. P. Hettinger. 1983. Nerve fibers sensitive to ionic taste stimuli in chorda tympani of the rat. J. Neurophysiol. **50**: 941–960.
16. Travers, J. B. & D. V. Smith. 1979. Gustatory sensitivities in neurons of the hamster *nucleus tractus solitarius*. Sensory Processes **3**: 1–26.
17. Van Buskirk, R. L. & D. V. Smith. 1981. Taste sensitivity of hamster parabrachial pontine neurons. J. Neurophysiol. **45**: 144–171.
18. Carpenter, J. A. 1956. Species differences in taste preferences. J. Comp. Physiol. Psychol. **49**: 139–144.
19. Pfaffmann, C. 1957. Taste mechanisms in preference behavior. Am. J. Clin. Nutr. **5**: 142–147.
20. Morrison, G. R. 1972. Detectability and preference for sodium chloride and sodium carbonate. Physiol. Behav. **8**: 25–28.
21. White, T. D. & J. C. Boudreau. 1975. Taste preferences of the cat for neurophysiologically active compounds. Physiol. Psychol. **3**: 405–410.
22. Hellekant, G. & T. W. Roberts. 1983. Study of the effect of gymnemic acid on taste in hamster. Chem. Senses **8**: 195–202.
23. Erickson, R. P. 1963. Sensory neural patterns and gustation. Olfaction Taste Proc. Int. Symp. **1**: 205–213.
24. Nachman, M. 1963. Learned aversion to the taste of lithium chloride and generalization to other salts. J. Comp. Physiol. Psychol. **56**: 343–349.
25. Morrison, G. R. 1967. Behavioral response patterns to salt stimuli in the rat. Can. J. Psychol. **21**: 141–152.
26. Tapper, D. N. & B. P. Halpern. 1968. Taste stimuli: a behavioral categorization. Science **161**: 708–709.
27. Smith, D. V., & D. H. McBurney. 1969. Gustatory cross-adaptation: Does a single mechanism code the salty taste? J. Exp. Psychol. **80**: 101–105.
28. Smith, D. V. & M. Frank. 1972. Cross adaptation between salts in the chorda tympani nerve of the rat. Physiol. Behav. **8**: 213–220.
29. Pfaffmann, C. 1955. Gustatory nerve impulses in rat, cat and rabbit. J. Neurophysiol. **18**: 429–440.
30. Fishman, I. Y. 1957. Single fiber gustatory impulses in rat and hamster. J. Cell. Comp. Physiol. **49**: 139–144.
31. Nagai, T. & K. Ueda. 1981. Stochastic properties of gustatory impulse discharges in rat chorda tympani. J. Neurophysiol. **45**: 574–592.
32. Nowlis, G. H. & M. E. Frank. 1981. Quality coding in gustatory systems of rats and hamsters. In Perception of Behavioral Chemicals, D. M. Norris, Ed.: 59–80. Elsevier/No. Holland. Amsterdam.
33. Frank, M. E. 1985. On the neural code for sweet and salty taste. *In* Olfactory and Gustatory Influences on the Central Nervous System. D. W. Pfaff, Ed. The Rockefeller University Press. New York.
34. Boudreau, J. C., N. K. Hoang, J. Oravec & L. T. Do. 1983. Rat neurophysiological taste responses to salt solutions. Chemical Senses **8**: 131–150.
35. Frank M. 1975. Response patterns of rat glossopharyngeal taste neurons. Olfaction Taste Proc. Int. Symp. **5**: 59–64.

36. Ogawa, H., M. Sato & S. Yamashita. 1969. Gustatory impulse discharges in response to saccharin in rats and hamsters. J. Physiol. (Lond). **204**: 311–329.
37. Hyman, A. M. & M. E. Frank. 1980. Sensitivities of single nerve fibers in the hamster chorda tympani to mixtures of taste stimuli. J. Gen. Physiol. **76**: 143–173.
38. Garcia, J. & F. R. Ervin. 1968. Appetites, aversion, and addiction: A model for visceral memory. Rec. Adv. Biol. Psychiatry **10**: 284–293.
39. Smith, D. V., J. B. Travers & R. L. Van Buskirk. 1979. Brainstem correlates of gustatory similarity in the hamster. Brain Res. Bull. **4**: 359–372.
40. Nowlis, G. H., M. E. Frank & C. Pfaffmann. 1980. Specificity of acquired aversions to taste qualities in hamsters and rats. J. Comp. Physiol. Psychol. **94**: 932–942.
41. Jakinovich, W., Jr. 1982. Taste aversion to sugars by the gerbil. Physiol. Behav. **28**: 1065–1071.
42. Pritchard, T. C. & T. R. Scott. 1982. Amino acids as taste stimuli. II. Quality coding. Brain Res. **253**: 93–104.
43. Pangborn, R. M. 1961. Taste interrelationships. II. Suprathreshold solutions of sucrose and citric acids. J. Food Sci. **26**: 648–655.
44. Pangborn, R. M. 1962. Taste interrelationships. III. Suprathreshold solutions of sucrose and sodium chloride. J. Food Sci. **27**: 495–500.
45. Nowlis, G. H. 1974. Conditioned stimulus intensity and acquired alimentary aversions in the rat. J. Comp. Physiol. Psychol. **86**: 1173–1184.
46. Nowlis, G. H. & M. E. Frank. 1977. Qualities in hamster taste: Behavioral and neural evidence. Olfaction Taste Proc. Int. Symp. **6**: 241–248.
47. Bartoshuk, L. M. 1979. Taste interactions in mixtures of sucrose with NaCl and sucrose with QHCl. Soc. Neurosci. Abstr. **5**: 125.
48. Bartoshuk, L. M. 1975. Taste mixtures: Is mixture suppression related to compression? Psychol Behav. **14**: 643–649.
49. Nowlis, G. H. & M. E. Frank. 1981. On the hamster's response to mixtures. AChemS III. Abstract.
50. Franchina, J. J., S. Selber & M. Brian. 1981. Novelty and temporal continguity in taste aversion learning: Within subjects conditioning effects. Bull. Psychonom. Soc. **18**: 99–102.
51. Mason, J. R. & W. L. Silver. 1983. Trigeminally mediated odor aversions in starlings. Brain Res. **269**: 196–199.
52. Palmerino, C. C. & J. Garcia. 1980. Flavor-illness aversions: the peculiar roles of odor and taste in memory for poison. Science **208**: 753–755.
53. Panhuber, H. 1982. Effect of odor quality and intensity on conditioned odor aversion learning in the rat. Physiol. Behav. **28**: 149–154.
54. Frank, M. E., G. H. Nowlis & C. Pfaffmann. Cross-generalizations of flavor aversions to taste, odor and general sensory stimuli in hamsters. (Unpublished observations.)
55. Slotnick, B. M. & L. A. Gutman. 1977. Evaluation of intranasal zinc sulfate treatment on olfactory discrimination in rats. J. Comp. Physiol. Psychol. **91**: 942–950.
56. Cain, W. S. 1978. History of research on smell. *In* Handbook of Perception. E. C. Carterette & M. P. Friedman, Eds. **VIA**: 197–229. Academic Press. New York.
57. Gesteland, R. C. 1978. The neural code: Integrative neural mechanisms. *In* Handbook of Perception. E. C. Carterette & M. P. Friedman, Eds. **VIA**: 259–276. Academic Press. New York.
58. Kruskal, J. B. 1964. Multidimensional scaling by optimizing goodness of fit to a non metric hypothesis. Psychometrika **29**: 1–27.

Neural Mediation of Conditioned Food Aversions[a]

STEPHEN W. KIEFER

Department of Psychology
Kansas State University
Manhattan, Kansas 66506

As with most scientific endeavors, the search for the understanding of underlying neural mechanisms in behavior necessitates the use of an appropriate experimental paradigm. Several learning procedures have already proven quite useful in providing information: maze learning in rats,[23] classical conditioning of the rabbit nictitating membrane,[34] and brightness discrimination in rats[25] to name just a few. The conditioning of a specific food aversion is yet another valuable behavioral situation from which a great deal can be learned about the neural basis of behavior.

Since the early publications of Garcia and colleagues,[11] conditioned food aversions have been used extensively in a variety of disciplines. As evidenced by the present volume, individuals such as pharmacologists, learning theorists, and clinicians have exploited conditioned aversions to provide information about their particular field. One obvious reason for the extensive use of this paradigm is the ease with which one can produce the effect. An animal is presented with a particular food which is then followed by experimentally induced illness; upon later presentation of the food, the animal typically will refuse to consume it. For the same reasons that others have used the paradigm, neuroscientists have also employed food aversion learning to provide them with information about the underlying neural mechanisms of learning and memory.

The present review will examine the neural basis of two important aspects of aversion learning: taste and illness (a summary diagram is shown in FIGURE 1). A section then will review what is known about how these two events become associated or, more specifically, what neural factors are known to be involved in the associations. Finally, a relatively new aspect of aversion learning will be discussed, one which involves the interaction of both taste and smell as cues in food aversion learning.

TASTE

The majority of information available about the anatomical and physiological basis of taste has been published in the last two or three decades. As Patton pointed out in his 1950 review on the chemical senses,[32] little information about gustatory sensibility was available relative to other senses (vision, audition) possibly because of the difficulty of studying taste and also because taste processes were not thought to be that important for the survival of an organism. Such a view, of course, is question-

[a] Supported by the Department of Psychology at Kansas State University, and the National Institute of Alcohol Abuse and Alcoholism (Grant AA05898).

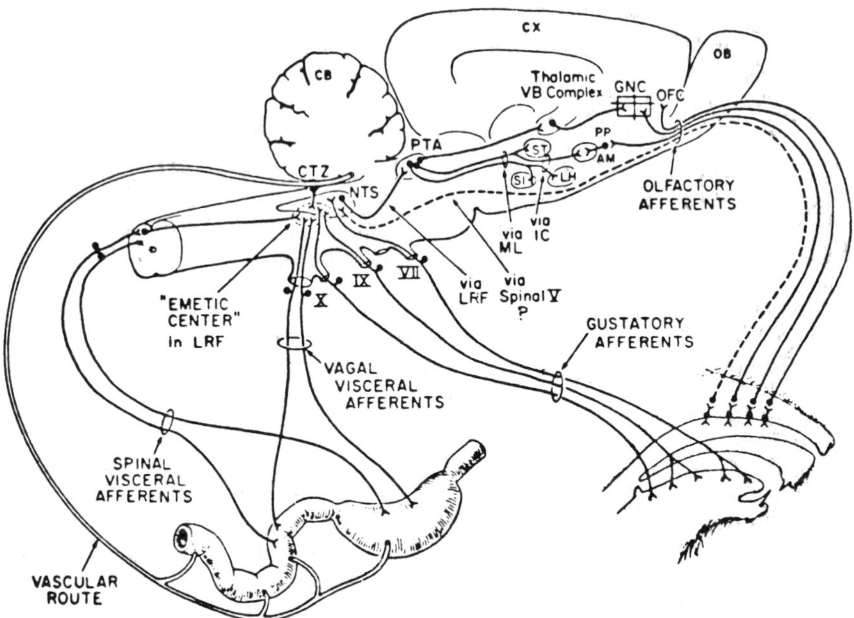

FIGURE 1. Schematic drawing outlining the gustatory and visceral pathways in the rat. Olfactory afferents are also included in an intentionally simplified manner. See text for a discussion of these systems. Abbreviations: (AM) amygdala, (CB) cerebellum, (CTZ) chemoreceptor trigger zone, (CX) cortex, (GNC) gustatory neocortex, (IC) internal capsule, (LH) lateral hypothalamus, (LRF) lateral reticular formation, (ML) medial lemniscus, (NTS) solitary nucleus, (OB) olfactory bulb, (OFC) orbitofrontal neocortex, (PP) prepyriform cortex, (PTA) pontine taste area, (SI) substantia innominata, (ST) subthalamic nucleus, (VB) ventrobasal thalamic complex. (Drawing provided through the courtesy of Kenneth Rusiniak and John Garcia, University of California Los Angeles.)

able because of the realization that food selection (consuming items that are good and avoiding items that are bad) plays such a pivotal role in survival.

Taste information is carried primarily in two cranial nerves: the facial (VII) and the glossopharyngeal (IX) with a small contribution from the vagus (X). These first-order fibers all converge in the anterior portion of the nucleus solitarius, a brainstem nucleus that also receives vagal afferents from the gastrointestinal tract. The course of secondary fibers was once thought to be included in the classic lemniscal system, which projected directly to the thalamus. However, work by Norgren and Leonard[29] demonstrated that the majority of solitary fibers from the taste region project a small distance rostrally to the parabrachial nucleus in the pons.

Pontine taste projections take one of two courses: the first major projection of pontine taste fibers passes to ventral forebrain structures such as the central nucleus of the amygdala (which also appears to receive projections from the solitary nucleus), the far lateral hypothalamus, and the substantia innominata.[27] A second projection is directed at the ventrobasal complex of the thalamus. Fibers from here then project to the gustatory neocortex (GN), which, in the rat, is located on the anterolateral aspect of the cortex. The GN of the rat is of particular interest and appears to include a portion of the facial region of the somatosensory neocortex and a more ventral portion, which includes insular cortex.

Although there is some disagreement regarding the sensory encoding of taste, behavioral responses to taste are relatively straightforward. A given taste can either be accepted or rejected, indicating that the taste is hedonically positive or hedonically negative, respectively. The hedonic property of any particular taste can be determined for an intact organism by simply seeing whether the animal accepts or rejects the substance, something revealed by measuring consumption. In animal research one typically determines a baseline level of consumption (usually water) and then compares consumption of tastes (assuming the taste is in an aqueous solution) relative to water baseline. Preference is indicated by a level of consumption that is higher than baseline and rejection is indicated by consumption that is below baseline. One can also use a similar rationale to determine absolute thresholds for taste stimuli, thereby determining empirically when the animal detects a given taste.

Behavioral acceptance or rejection of a given taste stimulus has been convincingly shown to be a brainstem reflexive behavior. To demonstrate this fact, one is presented with special problems. Preparations in which significant tissue rostral to the brainstem has been either removed or severed have meager behavioral repertoires. One of the more obvious problems is that these animals fail to exhibit consummatory behavior and must be force-fed to survive. To circumvent these difficulties, Grill and Norgren developed a taste reactivity (mimetic) test that involves video recording of mouth movements in response to the placement of taste substances directly onto the tongue of the animal.[13] At least in rats, a stereotyped set of mouth and tongue movements reflects the acceptance-rejection dichotomy. Sweet substances produce a series of tongue lapping and lateral tongue movements that eventually result in swallowing. Bitter substances, on the other hand, produce tongue protrusions and "gaping," which serve to prevent the substance from being swallowed and provide for the removal of the material from the mouth. The taste mimetic test has been used to demonstrate that brainstem mechanisms are sufficient for an animal to display normal responses to taste stimuli. Decerebrate rats display normal mouth and tongue responses to various categories of taste and they also show normal detection thresholds.

Given that hedonic responding to taste stimuli is reflexive, a further question regards taste perception or how animals categorize gustatory stimuli. To determine the properties of a stimulus, a conditioned aversion paradigm has been used. The rationale is that if an animal has an aversion for a specific substance, it will generalize the aversion to similar tasting substances: the greater the similarity, the greater the rejection. Nachman found that if rats were trained to avoid a lithium chloride (LiCl) solution, they also refused to consume an equimolar solution of sodium chloride (NaCl).[26] The conclusion that NaCl and LiCl have similar taste properties was supported by the demonstration that these two salts produce similar electrophysiological responses in the chorda tympani, solitary nucleus, and pons. Nowlis, Frank, and Pfaffmann have employed a similar approach to determine the similarity of a wide range of tastants in hamsters and rats.[30]

We have also used the generalization of a conditioned aversion to provide information about the taste of alcohol.[10] Rats were trained to avoid a mild alcohol (6%) solution and then given various taste solutions to test for aversion generalization. Interestingly, rats tended to generalize the alcohol aversion to compound tastants, specifically sucrose and quinine mixtures. Rats also showed a small amount of generalization to a sucrose-hydrochloric acid solution. These data suggested that alcohol has a sweet component to it, a conclusion supported by further electrophysiological data: the only substance with which the neural response to alcohol was correlated was sucrose, although the correlations were relatively weak.

ILLNESS

In the same manner that responses to taste stimuli can be seen as brainstem reflexes, illness or emesis also is reflexive with the neural involvement being at the brainstem level. Borison and Wang have shown that the emetic center is an area in the lateral reticular formation adjacent to the solitary nucleus.[2] In vomiting species, stimulation of this region will produce emesis, a reflex with a complex set of motor responses (intake of a deep breath, opening of the esophageal sphincter, closing of the glottis, etc.). For the present purposes, the motor outputs of the emetic center are not as important as the stimuli that engage the emetic mechanism.

As suggested by Borison and Wang, there are two major inputs to the emetic center (two ways of producing illness).[2] The first is by gastric irritation, which can be produced by particular chemicals. When a substance such as copper sulfate is introduced into the gastrointestinal tract of a dog, the dog will vomit. The information about the gastric distress is conveyed by the vagus nerve. Vagal afferents project and synapse in the caudal region of the nucleus solitarius, the same nucleus to which primary gustatory afferents project. Presumably, information from the vagus eventually reaches the emetic center and can trigger the reflex. The second route by which a stimulus can produce vomiting is blood borne. Toxins that enter the blood are detected by a chemosensitive region on the floor of the fourth ventricle, the area postrema. The area postrema is in a strategic position to monitor not only blood (the blood-brain-barrier at this point is relatively weak) but also the cerebrospinal fluid. Once the area postrema detects something toxic, it too triggers the emetic reflex.

Experimental studies of emetic mechanisms demonstrate a classic double dissociation.[33] Severing of the vagus just below the esophagus, thus denervating the gastrointestinal tract, eliminates the vomiting normally produced by intubated copper sulfate. Vagotomy does not eliminate the vomiting that results from the administration of blood-borne toxins such as apomorphine hydrochloride. Conversely, area postrema lesions disrupt illness induced by blood-borne toxins but do not affect emesis induced by gastrointestinal irritation. It might be added that copper sulfate administered intravenously in a vagotomized animal still produces emesis as one would expect because the area postrema would still be present to detect the toxin in the blood.

Coil, Rogers, Garcia, and Novin[8] have shown that the Borison and Wang model of emesis predicts quite well the results of taste aversion learning situations. Rats with subdiaphragmatic vagotomies do not acquire a saccharin aversion if the illness is induced by intubation of copper sulfate. Vagotomized rats do acquire significant taste aversions, however, if the copper sulfate is administered intravenously. More recently, Coil and Norgren have completed the double dissociation by showing that area postrema lesions disrupt aversion learning with blood-borne toxins; normal taste aversions result when illness is induced with gastric irritants.[9]

It might be added that conditioned emesis may play a role in the maintenance of a learned taste aversion. Presumably the conditioned response would be mediated predominantly by vagal efferents that could produce the gastric response. In experiments where rats were trained to avoid saccharin and vagotomized after training, it was found that the aversion in the vagotomized rats was severely attenuated and that these rats quickly extinguished the aversion relative to control rats.[22] It was hypothesized that the vagotomy eliminated the conditioned gastric response to the aversive taste and that, lacking this aspect of the conditioned aversion, it extinguished quickly. Anti-emetic drugs given to rats just prior to testing for an aversion conditioned earlier also appear to attenuate the expression of an aversion.[7]

A knowledge of emetic mechanisms allows one to deduce the mode of action of some toxin. For instance, if vagotomy disrupts the normal emetic action of a chemical, that substance probably acts as a gastric irritant. Conversely, if area postrema lesions eliminate the emesis normally induced by a drug, the mode of action of the drug is probably blood borne. In non-vomiting species (e.g. the rat), one can use conditioned aversions as a guide.

One particular chemical used frequently for conditioned aversion studies is LiCl. Exactly how LiCl produces illness is not entirely clear. Martin, Cheng, and Novin showed in a two-bottle test that vagotomized rats learned to shift fluid preference when an initially preferred solution was paired with LiCl illness.[24] We have confirmed this result using a one-bottle test by showing that vagotomized rats developed essentially normal saccharin aversions when consumption was followed immediately by intragastric intubation of LiCl. These results indicate that LiCl operates via a blood-borne route but the possibility remains that this chemical also has some gastric irritative properties.

A second substance particularly effective in producing illness and subsequent aversions is alcohol. Again, the exact mode of action of alcohol was assumed to be blood borne but the possibility remained that it might produce gastric irritation. However, vagotomized rats developed normal saccharin aversions following alcohol-induced illness, thus suggesting that alcohol is indeed a blood-borne toxin.[18]

TASTE-ILLNESS ASSOCIATIONS

Theoretically, the acquisition of a learned food aversion could be accomplished with only brainstem mechanisms. It will be recalled that both taste and gastric information converge at the solitary nucleus. In addition, the emetic center also operates at this relatively low level. In a direct test of this hypothesis, Grill and Norgren attempted to train decerebrate rats to avoid a saccharin solution by pairing its presentation with LiCl illness.[15] Normal rats trained to avoid saccharin display mouth and tongue movements (particularly the gaping response) when presented with the saccharin. These responses were typical of the response to bitter or hedonically negative substances. Using a similar measure of aversion learning, these authors failed to find evidence that brainstem animals were capable of acquiring the aversion. It is possible that more stringent procedures (e.g. increased doses of LiCl) may prove effective in producing significant taste aversions.

Although the reflexive components of taste and illness are at a brainstem level, these mechanisms do not operate in a neural vacuum. Rostral structures are capable of providing the fine-tuning of an organism's response to a particular food. As in many other learning and memory tasks, certain brain regions have been demonstrated to be involved in taste-illness associations. The general strategy has been to produce some sort of disruption of the structure's function (lesions) and then to determine if any aspect of aversion learning or retention is affected. And, as one might guess, a host of central structures appear to be involved in some aspect of aversion conditioning, structures such as the hypothalamus, hippocampus, amygdala, and neocortex. As Gaston has indicated,[12] it is difficult to synthesize all of the available data on various brain structures because such different results are obtained by different investigators. Further, the exact nature of the deficit in aversion learning is sometimes not evident. Many of the differences might be due to the method of testing, variables such as one or two-bottle tests, deprivation conditions, and illness agent. Each of these factors may interact with the effects of brain damage in ways that are difficult to quantify. A good example of the confusion involves the ventromedial hypothalamus where investigators have found either deficits, no effect, or facilitation of aversion conditioning.

The gustatory neocortex (GN) of the rat provides a system the function of which has been discerned by exploiting some of the strategies mentioned above. This cortical region, which lies on the anterolateral aspect of the brain, presents a clear dissociation between the hedonic and associative aspects of taste responding. The hedonic response of rats lacking GN are relatively normal. These rats consume sucrose and mild concentrations of sodium chloride at above water baseline levels. GN rats also reject quinine and acid solutions normally. It was concluded by Braun, Lasiter, and Kiefer that the GN was not necessary for normal taste responsiveness,[5] a result not surprising considering Grill and Norgren's[14] demonstration that taste responsiveness was intact even in decerebrate rats.

Despite the fact the GN is not involved in hedonic responses to taste, this area is intimately involved in the association of specific tastes with illness. Following the initial report of a taste aversion learning deficit in rats lacking GN,[6] associative deficits have been shown for both preferred and nonpreferred tastes. The deficits appear to be evidenced by slower acquisition of aversions. In addition, GN rats show abnormal tendencies to generalize a learned taste aversion to other, safe taste stimuli.[17]

Experiments have also shown that the GN was critically involved in the retention of learned taste aversions.[4,20] Rats were trained to avoid specific tastes and this was followed by ablation of the GN; postoperative testing indicated that the GN rats showed no evidence of retention. The losses were complete because the trained GN rats consumed the same amount of the taste as naive GN rats. The one exception to this generalization was an aversion to a mild hydrochloric acid solution. Retention of the acid aversion was found in GN rats, as evidenced by their significantly lower consumption than naive GN rats. However, the retention was still not as complete as that found in normal rats. Correlations between acid aversion retention and amount of damage to the taste region suggested that larger lesions were more effective in disrupting the acid aversion. These correlations were computed between the amount of acid consumed on the retention test and the amount of tissue removed on the side of cortex which had the smallest lesion.

A summary of the data obtained from rats lacking GN suggested that one can dissociate hedonic responses from associative responses in the gustatory system.[5] The employment of conditioned aversion paradigms to elucidate the associative mechanisms and GN involvement obviously has been an invaluable tool for the theoretical developments.

TASTE-ODOR INTERACTIONS

A relatively recent finding in the food aversion literature is that taste and odor interact in a manner not predicted by traditional learning theories. Briefly, taste alone is a strong cue for illness whereas odor alone is a weak cue. When the weak odor cue is compounded with the strong taste cue and followed by illness, rats develop strong odor aversions.[31]

By using odor and taste as cues for aversion conditioning, one has the opportunity to determine if a particular brain area is involved in some specific aspect of conditioning. One obvious area that receives both olfactory and gustatory input is the amygdala. In an initial experiment an attempt was made to dissociate odor and taste by employing selective lesions in the amygdala.[1] It was hypothesized that discrete lesions would disrupt a specific aspect of aversion conditioning. Rats with lesions in the basal amygdala region (lateral and medial nuclei) and rats with central nucleus lesions were trained to avoid taste alone, odor alone, or the odor-taste compound using LiCl-induced illness. In general, the results failed to produce the predicted dissociation. Odor aversions, both alone and potentiated, were normal in all of the operated rats. A further experiment demonstrated that larger lesions effectively disrupted potentiation, but the lesions also affected taste and odor learning.

The GN has again been used as a model system to examine the possible neural mechanisms of potentiation. In an initial report,[21] it was shown that GN rats failed to develop normal saccharin aversions induced by LiCl. GN rats did develop normal odor aversions, however. Such a result indicates that the gustatory neocortex is involved primarily in taste associative functions. Interestingly, rats lacking GN still displayed potentiation. When given a taste-odor compound that was followed by illness, the GN rats failed to develop an aversion to the taste but did develop potentiated odor aversions (the odor aversions were stronger than those shown by rats which had odor alone training).

A further experiment in the same report examined the effect of GN ablations on flavor aversions that were acquired prior to the surgery. Normal rats were trained to avoid a saccharin-almond compound and after strong aversions were developed, half the rats were subjected to removal of GN. Retention testing involved the presentation of the saccharin taste and the almond odor on separate tests. As one would predict, the GN rats displayed no retention of the saccharin aversion. All GN rats consumed saccharin at baseline levels. In contrast, the same rats still showed normal retention of the odor aversion, refusing to consume water in the presence of the almond odor.

While testing the GN rats for aversion retention, casual observation of their behavior was made in the presence of both the saccharin and the almond odor. When presented with saccharin, the GN rats began drinking immediately for essentially the entire five-minute testing period. This was in contrast to trained normal rats that, when presented with aversive saccharin, quickly ceased licking and showed signs of agitation. The response of both normal rats and GN rats when presented with the almond odor was similar. The rats refused to approach the spout and demonstrated signs of disgust (gaping). When the extents of cortical damage were correlated with the odor test data, no significant relationships could be found.

To examine odor retention in more detail, an experiment was conducted where rats received a portion of their daily water in an olfactometer, a specialized chamber that was made of clear Plexiglas for viewing and that had an air stream flowing over the drinking spout. The air stream was arranged so that an odor could be presented by the simple switching of a solenoid. Using this chamber, a group of normal rats was trained to avoid a saccharin-almond solution by pairing its presentation with illness that was induced by apomorphine hydrochloride. Two independent observers recorded the rats' behavior during the session. Most important for the present discussion was that gaping was one of the behaviors noted, an indication that the rats found the stimuli aversive. All rats quickly acquired an aversion. On the third acquisition trial, the mean number of licks was only 13.0 (compared to 789.0 on the first acquisition trial). In addition, 18 out of 20 rats displayed gaping responses on the last trial, many as soon as they were placed in the chamber and the odor was introduced.

Surgical removal of the GN was done after training and the rats were given three weeks of postoperative recovery. The rats were reintroduced to the olfactometer and then tested with the saccharin and almond in separate tests. The results of these tests are shown in FIGURE 2 where the number of licks on each test, expressed as a percent of water baseline, is plotted for each rat. One can see that the GN rats form quite

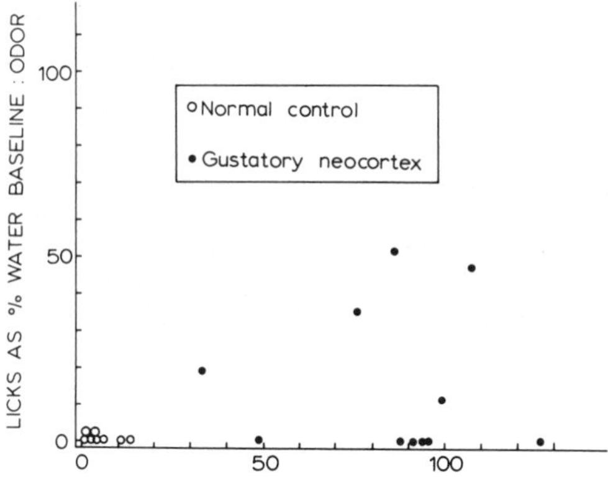

FIGURE 2. A scatterplot diagram of the lick amounts, expressed as a percent of water baseline, during the separate taste and odor tests. Each point represents the data for a single rat. Note the separate populations formed by the control rats and the rats lacking gustatory neocortex.

a different population from the control rats. As predicted, the normal rats retained the saccharin aversion whereas the GN rats showed little sign of retention, consuming the saccharin solution at water baseline levels. On the odor tests, normal rats showed complete retention, refusing to lick the spout in the presence of the odor. Also, gaping was recorded in six of the eight normal rats. Half of the GN rats also displayed excellent retention of the odor aversion. The remaining half of GN rats did lick in the presence of the odor, albeit at a much lower rate than water baseline. Four of the six GN rats that showed perfect retention and one rat that licked 112 times showed gaping type responses, indicating aversion retention.

When correlations were computed between retention of the odor aversion and amount of cortex removed, a significant relationship was found between consumption on the odor test and the size of the lesion on the smallest side ($r = .69$), a result similar to that reported for the acid aversion retention mentioned previously. Correlations between lesion size and saccharin consumption ($r = .04$) and water consumption ($r = .01$) were nonsignificant. The issue of whether amount of cortex removed is related to odor retention deficits needs further work. In two reports, positive relationships have been found, but in a third[21] no relationship could be discerned.

The demonstration that GN rats still respond to olfactory cues may account for the acid aversion retention cited earlier. Conceivably, rats trained to avoid an acid solution acquired both a taste and odor aversion. When tested following GN ablation, the rats evidenced retention because of the olfactory cues. Similarly, it has been found recently that rats trained to avoid alcohol, a stimulus with clear gustatory and olfactory qualities, retained the aversion following GN ablation.[19] It was assumed that the olfactory nature of the alcohol was the cue that the GN rats were using to avoid the solution.

Utilization of olfactory cues by GN rats might also account for the fact that GN rats can acquire new food aversions postoperatively. These rats can relearn an aversion that had been disrupted by GN ablation,[4] an ability that may be dependent upon the rats actually learning olfactory aversions. Support for this idea was presented recently by Braun who showed that rats given combined GN ablations and olfactory bulb removals were extremely debilitated in the acquisition of a sucrose aversion.[3] This deficit was much more pronounced than the deficit seen after GN ablation alone. Olfactory bulbectomy by itself did not affect aversion acquisition.

The odor-taste interaction data briefly reviewed above should provide those interested in neural mechanisms of learning with some cautions. Although conditioned aversions are easily obtainable, some care must be exercised in the selection of the conditioned stimulus because a particular substance might have both gustatory and olfactory qualities to it. Thus two examinations of the same neural structure with an aversion paradigm might produce quite different results if one is using only a taste and the other is using a compound taste-odor stimulus.

SUMMARY

The above discussion is only a brief review of what is known about the neural mediation of conditioned food aversions. Although several other approaches were not mentioned (e.g. biochemical studies), one can still appreciate the value of the aversion paradigm for providing important information about neural mechanisms in learning and memory.

A theoretical approach that may be valuable in understanding brain function in conditioned food aversion data is Hughlings Jackson's hierarchical notions of nervous organization.[16] Hedonic responses to food stimuli appear to be brainstem reflexes. On top of these are rostral brain structures that add greater complexity to the consummatory behavior of the organism. An important aspect of this complexity is reflected in an animal's ability to form conditioned food aversions, a process undoubtedly tied intimately to particular neural mechanisms.

REFERENCES

1. Bermudez-Rattoni, F., S. W. Kiefer, C. V. Grijalva & J. Garcia. 1982. Basal and central amygdala involvement in the acquisition of taste and odor aversions. Abst. Soc. Neurosci. **8**: 310.
2. Borison, H. L. & S. C. Wang. 1953. Physiology and pharmacology of vomiting. Pharm. Rev. **5**: 193–230.
3. Braun, J. J. 1983. Foundations of residual associative taste salience in rats lacking gustatory neocortex. Bull. Psychon. Soc. **21**: 337.
4. Braun, J. J., S. W. Kiefer & J. V. Ouellet. 1981. Psychic ageusia in rats lacking gustatory neocortex. Exp. Neurol. **72**: 711–716.
5. Braun, J. J., P. S. Lasiter & S. W. Kiefer. 1982. The gustatory neocortex of the rat. Physiol. Psych. **10**: 13–45.
6. Braun, J. J., T. B. Slick & J. F. Lorden. 1972. Involvement of gustatory neocortex in the learning of taste aversions. Physiol. Behav. **9**: 637–641.
7. Coil, J. D., W. G. Hankins, D. J. Jenden & J. Garcia. 1978. The attenuation of a specific cue-to-consequence association by antiemetic agents. Psychopharm. **56**: 21–25.
8. Coil, J. D., R. C. Rogers, J. Garcia & D. Novin. 1978. Conditioned taste aversions: Vagal and circulatory mediation of the toxic US. Behav. Bio. **24**: 509–519.
9. Coil, J. D. & R. Norgren. 1981. Taste aversions conditioned with intravenous copper sulfate: Attenuation by ablation of the area postrema. Brain Res. **212**: 425–433.
10. DiLorenzo, P. D., S. W. Kiefer, A. G. Rice & J. Garcia. 1984. Taste coding of ethyl alcohol: Electrophysiological and behavioral data. (Manuscript submitted for publication.)

11. GARCIA, J. & R. A. KOELLING. 1966. Relation of cue to consequence in avoidance learning. Psychon. Soc. **4**: 123–124.
12. GASTON, K. E. 1978. Brain mechanisms of conditioned taste aversion learning: A review of the literature. Physiol. Psych. **6**: 340–353.
13. GRILL, H. J. & R. NORGREN. 1978. The taste reactivity test. I. Mimetic responses to gustatory stimuli in neurologically normal rats. Brain Res. **143**: 263–279.
14. GRILL, H. J. & R. NORGREN. 1978. The taste reactivity test. II. Mimetic responses to gustatory stimuli in chronic thalamic and chronic decerebrate rats. Brain Res. **143**: 281–297.
15. GRILL, H. J. & R. NORGREN. 1978. Chronically decerebrate rats demonstrate satiation but not bait shyness. Science **201**: 267–269.
16. JACKSON, J. H. 1958. Evolution and dissolution of the nervous system. *In* Selected Writings of John Hughlings Jackson. Vol. 2. J. Taylor, Ed. Basic Books. New York.
17. KIEFER, S. W. & J. J. BRAUN. 1979. Acquisition of taste avoidance habits in rats lacking gustatory neocortex. Physiol. Psych. **7**: 245–250.
18. KIEFER, S. W., R. J. CABRAL, K. W. RUSINIAK & J. GARCIA. 1980. Ethanol-induced flavor aversions in rats with subdiaphragmatic vagotomies. Behav. Neur. Biol. **29**: 246–254.
19. KIEFER, S. W. & G. J. LAWRENCE. 1983. Retention of learned alcohol aversions following gustatory neocortex lesions. Abst. Soc. Neurosci. **9**: 1243.
20. KIEFER, S. W., L. R. LEACH & J. J. BRAUN. 1984. Taste agnosia following gustatory neocortex ablation: Dissociation from odor and generality across taste qualities. Behav. Neurosci. **98**: 590–608.
21. KIEFER, S. W., K. W. RUSINIAK & J. GARCIA. 1982. Flavor-illness aversions: Gustatory neocortex ablations disrupt taste but not taste-potentiated odor cues. J. Comp. Physiol. Psychol. **96**: 540–548.
22. KIEFER, S. W., K. W. RUSINIAK, J. GARCIA & J. D. COIL. 1981. Vagotomy facilitates extinction of conditioned taste aversions in rats. J. Comp. Physiol. Psychol. **95**: 114–122.
23. LASHLEY, K. S. 1950. In search of the engram. Symp. Soc. Exp. Biol. **4**: 454–482.
24. MARTIN, J. R., F. Y. CHENG & D. NOVIN. 1978. Acquisition of learned taste aversion following bilateral subdiaphragmatic vagotomy in rats. Physiol. Behav. **21**: 13–17.
25. MEYER, D. R. 1972. Access to engrams. Am. Psychol. **27**: 124–133.
26. NACHMAN, M. 1963. Learned aversion to the taste of lithium chloride and generalization to other salts. J. Comp. Physiol. Psychol. **56**: 343–349.
27. NORGREN, R. 1974. Gustatory afferents to ventral forebrain. Brain Res. **81**: 285–295.
28. NORGREN, R. 1977. A synopsis of gustatory neuroanatomy. *In* Olfaction and Taste VI. J. LeMagnen & P. MacLeod, Eds. Information Retrieval. London.
29. NORGREN, R. & C. M. LEONARD. 1973. Ascending central gustatory pathways. J. Comp. Neurol. **150**: 217–238.
30. NOWLIS, G. H., M. E. FRANK & C. PFAFFMANN. 1980. Specificity of acquired aversions to taste qualities in hamsters and rats. J. Comp. Physiol. Psychol. **94**: 932–942.
31. PALMERINO, C. C., K. W. RUSINIAK & J. GARCIA. 1980. Flavor-illness aversions: The peculiar roles of odor and taste in memory for poison. Science **208**: 753–755.
32. PATTON, H. D. 1950. Physiology of smell and taste. Ann. Rev. Physiol. **12**: 469–484.
33. TEUBER, H.-L. 1955. Physiological Psychology. Ann. Rev. Psychol. **6**: 267–296.
34. THOMPSON, R. F., T. W. BERGER, C. F. CEGAVSKE, M. M. PATTERSON, R. A. ROEMER, T. J. TEYLER & R. A. YOUNG. 1976. The search for the engram. Am. Psychol. **31**: 209–227.

Sexual Dimorphisms as an Index of Hormonal Influences on Conditioned Food Aversions[a]

KATHLEEN C. CHAMBERS

Reproductive Biology and Behavior
Oregon Regional Primate Research Center
Beaverton, Oregon

Hormones are very powerful modulators of avoidance learning processes. Removal of the anterior pituitary impairs acquisition of active shock avoidance and treatment with ACTH and its fragments restores behavior in adrenalectomized and adrenal-intact rats.[1-4] Vasopressin, ACTH, and ACTH fragments prolong extinction of active and passive shock avoidance.[5-9] Corticosterone and cortisone increase the extinction rate of active shock avoidance in hypophysectomized and pituitary-intact rats and attenuate passive avoidance.[10-12]

The observation that female and male rats differ in the acquisition of avoidance behavior led to the discovery of the involvement of gonadal hormones in avoidance learning. Ultimately, any behavioral sex difference must be explained by one or a number of physiological sex differences. The most obvious explanation of the difference between females and males is in the level of gonadal hormone during the perinatal and postpubertal periods. In fact, most sex differences, if not all, are linked in some way to gonadal hormones.[13]

Sex differences have been found in several different avoidance learning tasks.[14-19] Only the sex differences in acquisition of two-way shock avoidance in rats have been studied extensively. For this behavior, the level of gonadal hormones during adulthood does not influence acquisition.[20-22] But the presence of testosterone during the perinatal period results in a slower acquisition rate in adulthood.[21]

It is not surprising, then, to find that there is a sexual dimorphism in another avoidance behavior, conditioned food aversion, or to find that this dimorphism is influenced by gonadal hormones. It has been postulated that gonadal hormones influence sexual dimorphisms by acting during the perinatal period, the postpubertal period, or during both periods.[23-25] The uniqueness of this sexual dimorphism in a conditioned food aversion lies in the fact that it is one of the few dimorphisms known to depend solely on the presence of gonadal hormones during adulthood.

A conditioned aversion to a sucrose solution is extinguished more slowly in male rats than in females (FIGURE 1).[26] Low levels of testosterone (as found in females and castrated males) are associated with a fast extinction rate, and high levels (as found in intact males and testosterone-treated females) are associated with a slow extinction rate (FIGURES 2 and 3).[27] A testosterone metabolite, dihydrotestosterone, also prolongs extinction (FIGURE 4).[28,29] I have found no influence of estrogen and progesterone on

[a] This work was supported by the National Institutes of Health Grant RR-00163. This work is described in Publication No. 1382 of the Oregon Primate Research Center.

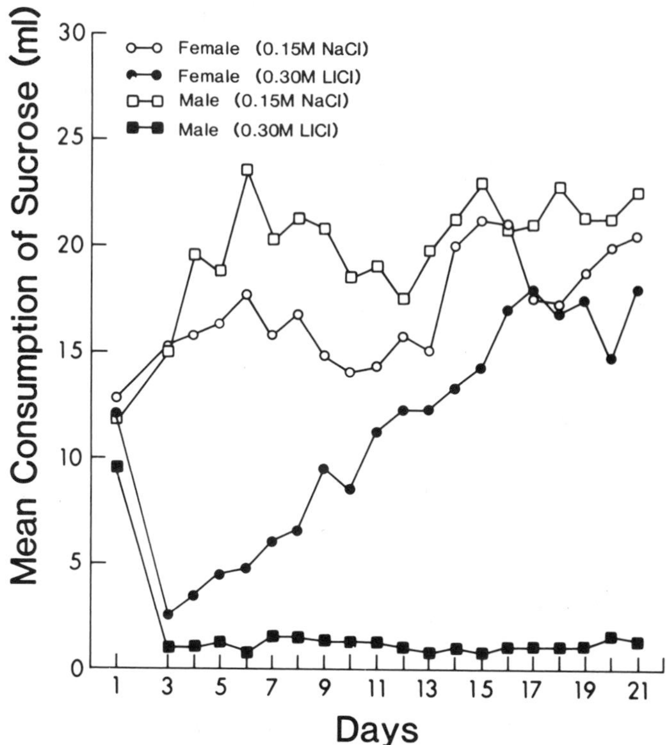

FIGURE 1. Mean sucrose consumption by female and male rats before (Day 1) and after (Day 3 through Day 21) injection of NaCl or LiCl.

extinction (FIGURE 4),[27,28] although Earley and Leonard[30] have reported that estrogen increases the extinction rate in castrated males. Except for this one discrepancy, the data clearly suggest that it is the level of testosterone, not of estrogen or progesterone, that prolongs extinction. Recently, Babine and Smotherman[31] demonstrated that the extinction rate in female rats exposed *in utero* to testosterone (from neighboring male siblings) is not different from that in unexposed females. Their data, as well as data showing that females exhibit a slow extinction when given testosterone by injection, strongly indicate that the presence of testosterone during adulthood, not the presence of this hormone during the perinatal period, is the critical factor in expression of a slow extinction rate.

Testosterone levels during the perinatal period, however, might play a role in the sexual dimorphism seen in extinction. Recent evidence suggests that female and male rats differ in their sensitivity to testosterone; the amount of testosterone required to prolong extinction is greater for females than for males (Chambers and Sengstake, unpublished data). Empty Silastic capsules or testosterone-filled capsules that were 30-, 60-, or 120-mm long were implanted in gonadectomized females and males. Sham-gonadectomized males received empty capsules. Three weeks later, all rats underwent conditioning and extinction. The extinction rates (the number of days each rat drank less than its acquisition-day volume) of gonadectomized animals were compared to

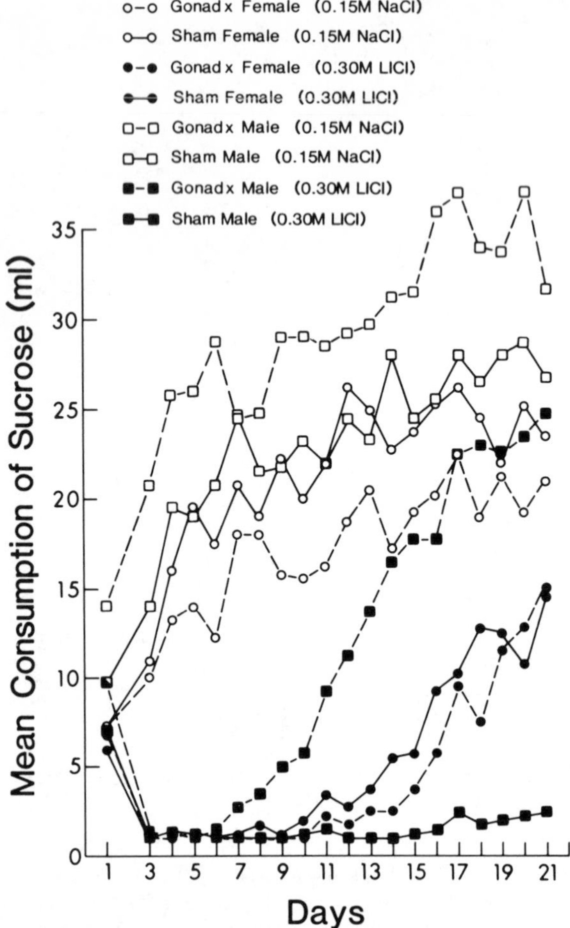

FIGURE 2. Mean sucrose consumption by gonadectomized and sham-gonadectomized female and male rats before (Day 1) and after (Day 3 through Day 21) injection of NaCl or LiCl.

those of sham-gonadectomized males. As expected, extinction was achieved more quickly in gonadectomized females and males with empty capsules than in sham-gonadectomized males (FIGURE 5). Gonadectomized females with 30-mm testosterone implants also had a faster extinction rate than sham-gonadectomized males. However, the extinction rates of gonadectomized females with 60- and 120-mm testosterone implants and gonadectomized males with 30-, 60-, and 120-mm implants were not significantly different from those of the sham-gonadectomized males. Therefore, a 30-mm implant provides enough testosterone to prolong extinction in males but not in females.

This sexual dimorphism in testosterone sensitivity cannot be attributed to differences in circulating testosterone levels. The serum levels were measured in gonadec-

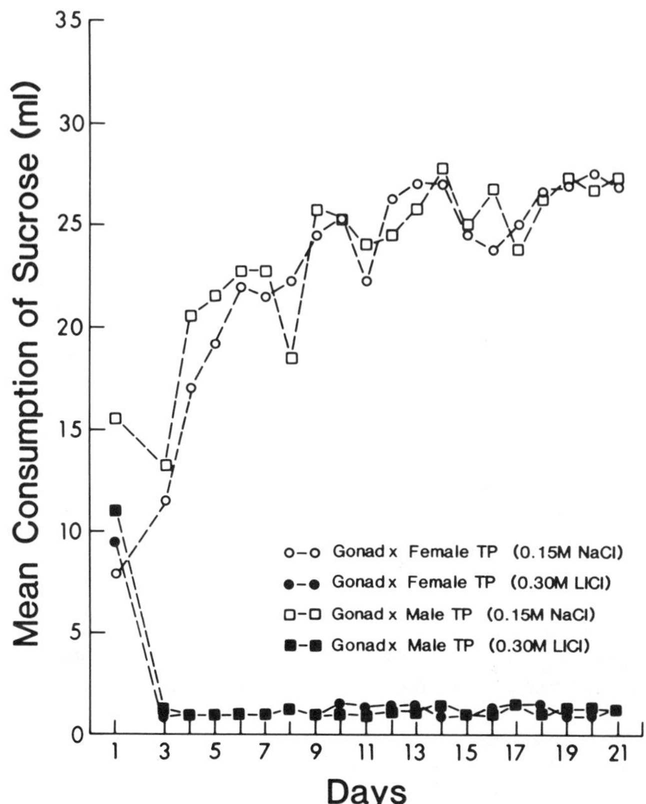

FIGURE 3. Mean sucrose consumption by testosterone-treated gonadectomized female and male rats before (Day 1) and after (Day 3 through Day 21) injection of NaCl or LiCl.

tomized females and males with 30-mm testosterone implants and in sham-gonadectomized males with empty implants (Sengstake and Chambers, unpublished data). The testosterone levels of these three groups did not differ (FIGURE 6).

I suggest that sensitivity to testosterone is established during the perinatal period. The amount of testosterone required to prolong extinction is less when testosterone is present during the perinatal period than when it is absent. In support of this hypothesis, Babine and Smotherman[31] have found that females exposed to testosterone *in utero* (from neighboring male siblings) show a prolonged extinction as adults when given low-dose injections of testosterone, whereas unexposed females do not.

The nature of the sexual dimorphism in extinction of a conditioned food aversion, therefore, is quantitative rather than qualitative. Both females and males have a testosterone-sensitive mechanism that, when activated, decreases the rate of extinction. This mechanism is activated in intact males but not females because males have higher circulating levels of testosterone.

Because of the dependence of this sexual dimorphism in extinction on the level of testosterone, any factor influencing the availability of testosterone at the site of

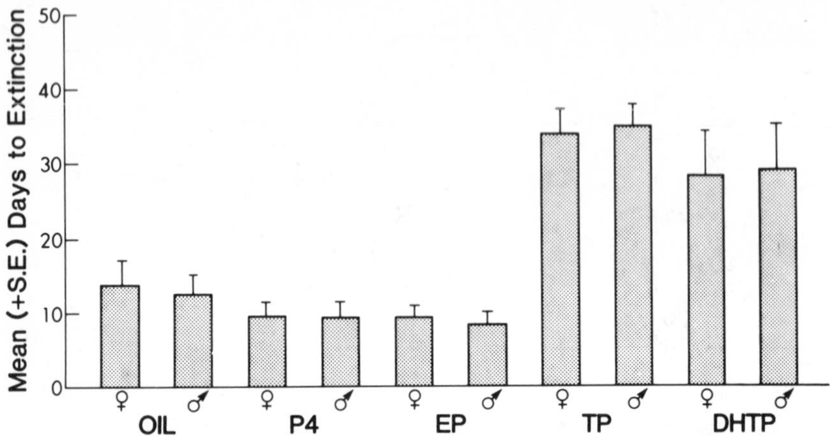

FIGURE 4. Mean number of days that gonadectomized female and male rats given injections of oil, progesterone (P4), estradiol dipropionate (EP), testosterone propionate (TP), and dihydrotestosterone propionate (DHTP) drank less than 100% of the amount consumed on acquisition day.

action in target tissues affects expression of the dimorphism. Social isolation is such a factor. It decreases the circulating levels of testosterone and abolishes the sexual dimorphism by increasing the rate of extinction in males.[32,33]

Water deprivation also eliminates the sexual dimorphism in extinction.[26,34] Males on a 22-hr water deprivation schedule reach extinction faster than males with *ad libitum* food and water and reach extinction at the same rate as females. Deprived females do not achieve extinction at a faster rate (FIGURE 7). That males and females are affected differently by water deprivation indicated to my colleague, Cord Sengstake, and me that testosterone might be involved in this abolition of sexual dimorphism.

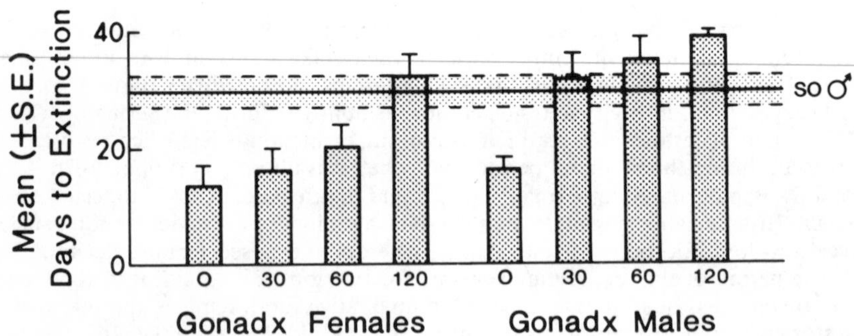

FIGURE 5. Mean number of days that sham-gonadectomized male rats with empty-capsule implants (SO) and gonadectomized females and males with empty-capsule implants (O) or testosterone-filled capsules 30-, 60, or 120-mm long drank less than 100% of the amount consumed on acquisition day.

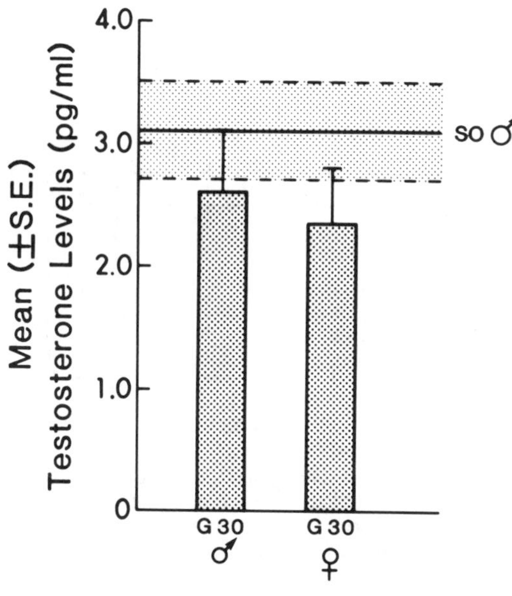

FIGURE 6. Mean serum testosterone levels of sham-gonadectomized male rats with empty capsules (SO) and gonadectomized females and males with testosterone-filled capsules 30-mm long.

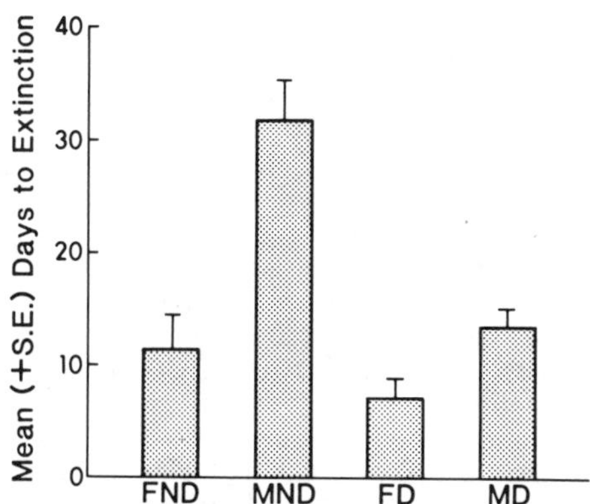

FIGURE 7. Mean number of days that nondeprived and water-deprived (22-hr water deprivation schedule) female and male rats drank less than 100% of the amount consumed on acquisition day.

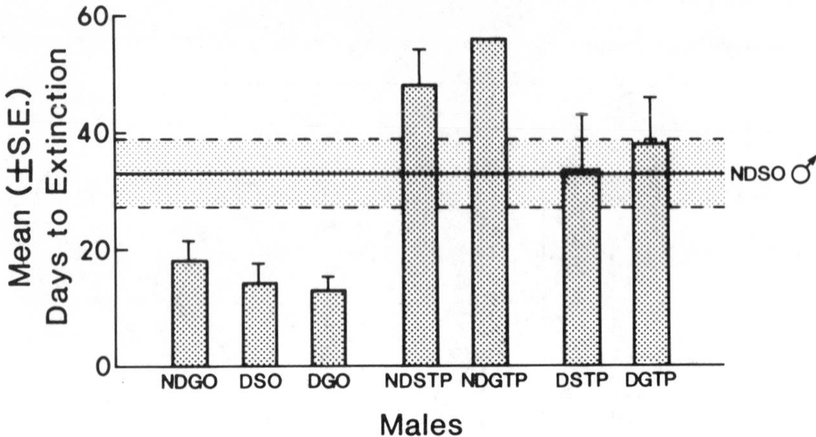

FIGURE 8. Mean number of days that sham-gonadectomized (S) or gonadectomized (G) male rats that received injections of oil (O) or testosterone propionate (TP) and that were either water-deprived (D; 22-hr water deprivation schedule) or not water-deprived (ND) drank less than 100% of the amount consumed on acquisition day.

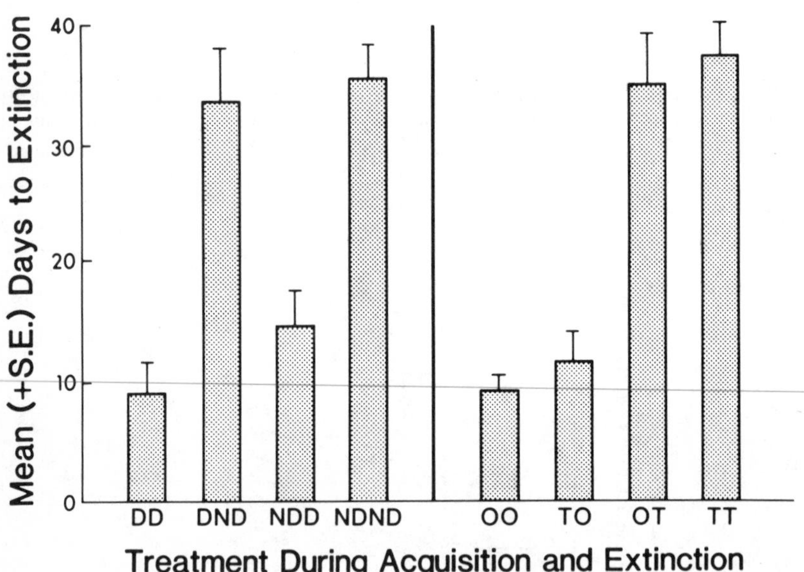

FIGURE 9. Mean number of days that male rats drank less than 100% of the amount consumed on acquisition day. The groups consisted of the following: males water-deprived during both acquisition and extinction (DD); males water-deprived during acquisition but not during extinction (DND); males not deprived during acquisition but water-deprived during extinction (NDD); males not deprived during acquisition or extinction (NDND); males receiving oil during both acquisition and extinction (OO); males receiving testosterone propionate during acquisition and oil during extinction (TO); males receiving oil during acquisition and testosterone propionate during extinction (OT); and males receiving testosterone propionate during both acquisition and extinction (TT).

The hypothesis is supported by two observations. First, increasing the level of testosterone prolongs extinction in water-deprived male rats. Injections that produce supraphysiologic levels of testosterone decrease the rate of extinction of deprived males to that of nondeprived males (FIGURE 8).[34] And ACTH, which increases testosterone levels, prolongs extinction in deprived males only if the testes are intact.[35]

Second, both testosterone and water deprivation affect extinction by acting on an extinction process not an acquisition process. The presence or absence of testosterone or water deprivation during acquisition of the aversion has no effect on the rate of its extinction (FIGURE 9).[36,37] But, the presence of testosterone during extinction decreases the rate of extinction and water deprivation during extinction increases the rate of extinction.

It was hypothesized that water deprivation either reduces the level of testosterone below threshold or increases the threshold level of testosterone required to prolong extinction to a point above normal circulating testosterone levels.[34] Three experiments were designed to test the validity of these hypotheses.

In the first experiment, testosterone levels were measured in water-deprived and nondeprived male rats (Sengstake and Chambers, unpublished data). Fifteen males were placed on a 22-hr water deprivation schedule, and an additional 15 remained on *ad libitum* food and water. All were singly housed and were given cylinders of cold water at the start of the dark cycle (12 hr long). The males were bled three times: 4, 11, and 18 days after the initiation of the deprivation schedule. Blood samples were collected prior to the daily watering at the end of the light cycle (12 hr long). The blood was analyzed for testosterone through extraction of steroids from serum by chromatography on a Sephadex column. Quantification of serum testosterone was completed by radioimmunoassay.[38,39] The testosterone levels of the water-deprived and nondeprived males did not differ and did not change differentially across the three days (FIGURE 10).

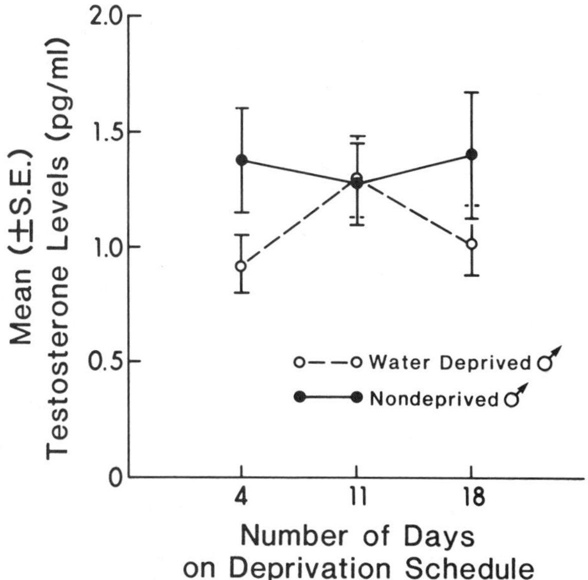

FIGURE 10. Mean serum testosterone levels of nondeprived male rats and water-deprived males 4, 11, and 18 days after the initiation of a 22-hr water deprivation schedule.

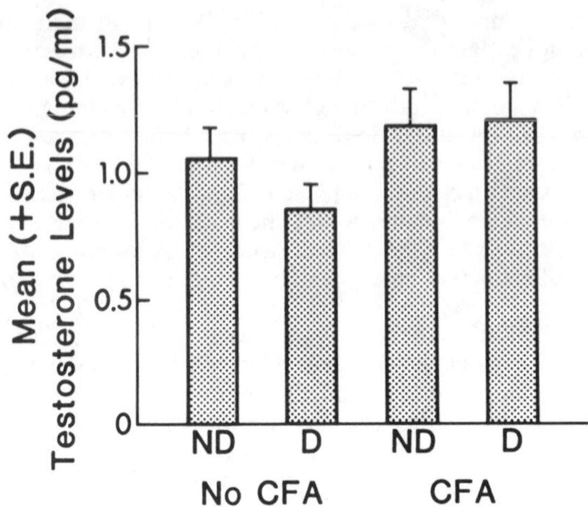

FIGURE 11. Mean serum testosterone levels of nondeprived and water-deprived male rats that had not been conditioned and those that had undergone an acquisition and extinction trial.

It is possible that water deprivation and the conditioned food aversion procedure interacted to produce lower testosterone levels. To test this possibility, the blood levels of testosterone in water-deprived and in nondeprived males that had undergone an acquisition and extinction trial were compared to those of deprived and nondeprived males that had not been conditioned (Chambers and Sengstake, unpublished data). Seventeen male rats were placed on a 22-hr water deprivation schedule, and an equal number continued to be given *ad libitum* food and water. As before, all males were singly housed and were allowed access to cold water at the start of the dark cycle (12 hr long). One week after the initiation of the deprivation schedule, eight of the deprived and eight of the nondeprived males were given access to a cylinder of sucrose solution and a cylinder of water for 2 hr. The access period was followed by LiCl injections. The rest of the males were given two cylinders of water only, and did not undergo conditioning. Two days later, the conditioned males underwent an extinction trial by giving them access to a sucrose solution and water for 2 hr. The nonconditioned males received only water. The next day, all males were bled prior to receiving any fluid. Again, the blood was analyzed for testosterone by extraction, chromatography, and radioimmunoassay techniques.[38,39]

The testosterone levels of the four male groups did not differ significantly (FIGURE 11). A 22-hr schedule of water deprivation did not reduce circulating levels of testosterone, but it might have changed the sensitivity to testosterone. To explore this possibility, the rate of extinction was measured in water-deprived and nondeprived males into which testosterone capsules of different sizes were implanted (Sengstake, unpublished data).

A blank Silastic capsule or a testosterone-filled capsule, 30-, 60-, or 120-mm long, was implanted in 48 gonadectomized males; six sham-gonadectomized males each received an empty capsule. Two weeks after implantation, all of the male rats were moved into single cages, and a 22-hr water deprivation schedule was initiated for half of the gonadectomized animals. The rest remained on *ad libitum* food and water. One week later, all of the males received LiCl by injection after access to a sucrose solution. Daily extinction trials were initiated two days after conditioning. All rats were given a cylinder of sucrose solution and a cylinder of water for 2 hr during conditioning and extinction trials.

The extinction rates for the gonadectomized rats were compared to those for the nondeprived, sham-gonadectomized males. As expected, both deprived and nondeprived gonadectomized males with empty capsules had a faster extinction rate than did sham-gonadectomized males (FIGURE 12). Nondeprived gonadectomized males with testosterone-filled implants had extinction rates that were equal to or greater than those of sham-gonadectomized males; males with 60- and 120-mm implants achieved extinction more slowly than did sham-gonadectomized males. Of the deprived males, only those with a 120-mm implant had an extinction rate as slow as that of the sham-gonadectomized males; the deprived males with 30- and 60-mm implants achieved extinction more quickly.

Water deprivation has a similar effect on females. Twelve gonadectomized females each received a 120-mm testosterone-filled capsule and 6 sham-gonadectomized males each received an empty capsule (Sengstake, unpublished data). Six of the females were placed on a 22-hr water deprivation schedule two weeks after implantation; the rest of the rats remained on *ad libitum* food and water. One week later, all of the rats underwent conditioning and extinction. The extinction rates for the gonadectomized females were compared to those for sham-gonadectomized males. Deprived gonadectomized females achieved extinction faster than sham-gonadectomized males whereas nondeprived females had the same rate as these males (FIGURE 13).

Thus, extinction is prolonged when nondeprived males have a 30-mm testosterone implant and deprived males have a 120-mm implant. Nondeprived females require a 60-mm implant to extend extinction; for deprived females, a 120-mm capsule is not sufficient. Clearly, these results indicate that water deprivation increases the amount of testosterone required to decrease the extinction rate of a conditioned food aversion in both males and females. The data are consistent with the hypothesis that water deprivation alters the extinction rate by affecting a testosterone-sensitive mechanism.

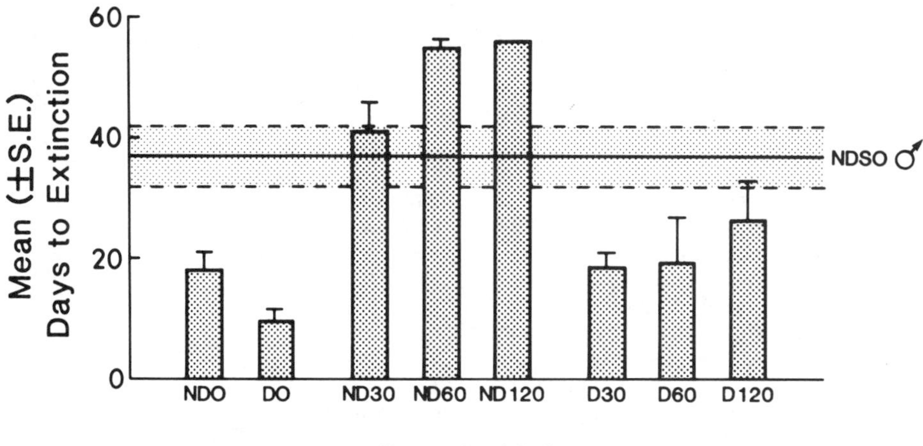

FIGURE 12. Mean number of days that nondeprived sham-gonadectomized male rats (NDSO) and nondeprived (ND) and water-deprived (D) gonadectomized males with empty-capsule implants (O) or testosterone-filled capsules 30-, 60-, or 120-mm long drank less than 100% of the amount consumed on acquisition day.

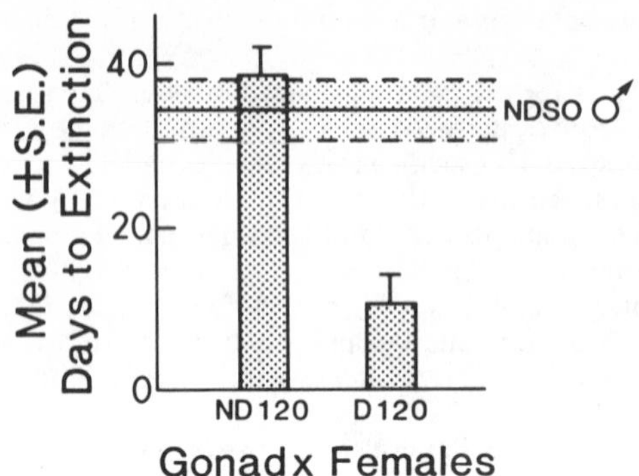

FIGURE 13. Mean number of days that nondeprived sham-gonadectomized male rats (NDSO) and nondeprived (ND) and water-deprived (D) gonadectomized females with testosterone-filled capsules 120-mm long drank less than 100% of the amount consumed on acquisition day.

Several questions regarding the testosterone-sensitive mechanism remain to be answered. For instance, what is this mechanism and where does it act? Specifically, how is it affected by water deprivation and by what means does it alter extinction? I suggest the following model as a guide to answering these questions.

Cells in the brains of male and female rats, once activated by testosterone or one of its metabolites, inhibit extinction. Receptors for testosterone and dihydrotestosterone have been found in the hypothalamus, amygdala, and cortex of both female and male rats.[40–43] In males, the preoptic area and septum also contain dihydrotestosterone receptors; investigations have not been made on females.[42] Whether any of these areas contain the testosterone-sensitive cells that extend extinction of a conditioned food aversion when activated remains to be demonstrated. It must be kept in mind that these testosterone-sensitive cells are postulated to be modulators. They only extend extinction; they are not critical for the establishment of a conditioned food aversion or for its extinction.

According to the proposed model, water deprivation blocks activation of testosterone-sensitive cells. Two major factors could account for this effect. First, less testosterone might be available to the receptors. For example, testosterone levels at the brain site might be lower, permeability of the cell membrane might be altered so that less testosterone can enter the cells, there might be an increase in the binding of testosterone so that less is available to the cells, or there might be an increase in the release of another substance that competes with testosterone for receptor sites but cannot activate the cells. Second, the receptors themselves might be affected by water deprivation; water deprivation might cause a decrease in the affinity of the receptors for testosterone or reduce receptor numbers.

When testosterone-sensitive cells are activated, extinction is prolonged. Several hypotheses have been suggested to account for the effect of testosterone on extinction: (1) testosterone facilitates the development of a stronger aversion by increasing reactivity to toxin or sensitivity to punishment, by increasing neophobia, or by facilitating the association of illness with sucrose;[26,29,36,44] (2) testosterone decreases preferences for sweet substances;[26,27,29] (3) testosterone increases persistence in behavior by increasing attention to relevant stimuli;[29,30] (4) testosterone increases fearfulness after an aversive event has occurred;[36] (5) testosterone improves performance in passive avoidance tasks by decreasing general activity levels or by enabling animals to resist making approach behaviors;[36] (6) testosterone inhibits forgetting of aversive events;[29,36] (7) testosterone inhibits relearning that the conditioned substance no longer causes illness by reducing the problem-solving ability or flexibility, or by protecting the association of sucrose-illness-avoidance from interference by an association of sucrose-preference-approach.[29,30,36]

One must take two things into consideration when identifying factors that could account for the effect of testosterone on extinction. First, testosterone affects factors that influence extinction not acquisition. When two groups of castrated male rats receive both testosterone injections and the same dose of toxin during acquisition, they presumably have acquired the same level of the aversion. But when one of these groups is given testosterone during extinction and the other is given oil, the testosterone-treated males achieve extinction slowly and the oil-treated males reach extinction rapidly (FIGURE 9).[36] If testosterone were affecting factors during acquisition, these two groups of animals would have shown the same rate of extinction since the only difference in hormonal state occurred after acquisition. When one group of castrated males is given testosterone and another is given oil during acquisition, both groups achieve extinction at the same slow rate if each is given testosterone during extinction. If testosterone were affecting factors during acquisition, these two groups of males would have shown different rates of extinction since they had different hormonal states during acquisition. Thus, testosterone-sensitive cells do not prolong extinction by facilitating the development of stronger aversions.

Second, the factor that is hypothesized to account for the effects of testosterone on extinction must itself depend on the level of testosterone.[27,36] More generally, gonadal hormones must influence this factor in the same way that they influence the extinction rate. Activity levels decrease when both female and male rats are gonadectomized.[45,46] Both estrogen and testosterone increase the activity level of castrated male rats (estrogen is more effective), whereas dihydrotestosterone has no effect.[47] Clearly, the hormonal determinants of activity are different from those of extinction of a conditioned food aversion. The same is true for sweet preferences. The expression of a strong sweet preference depends on the absence of testosterone during the prenatal period and the presence of estrogen and progesterone after this period of development.[48] Thus, testosterone-sensitive cells do not extend extinction by decreasing activity levels or preferences for sweet substances.

The remaining hypotheses that have been suggested to account for the effects of testosterone have not been adequately tested. But arguments against the persistence and fearfulness hypotheses have been made.[30,36] Although testosterone-sensitive cells might affect some aspect of the memory process, they do not decrease the rate with which the memory trace for a conditioned food aversion passively decays. Female rats normally achieve extinction in two weeks. If they do so because the memory trace decays after two weeks, they should not show an aversion if there is a delay of two weeks between acquisition and extinction. However, females still show an aversion when a delay of two and four weeks is introduced between acquisition and the initiation of extinction trials (Sengstake and Chambers, unpublished data and FIGURE 14). In addition, they achieve extinction at the same rate as females with only a two-day delay.

Extinction involves "unlearning" that consuming the conditioned stimulus has negative consequences and "relearning" that it has nonnegative consequences or it is safe.[49–51] To me, the most appealing hypothesis to explain the effect of testosterone on extinction is that testosterone-sensitive cells retard relearning.

Females appear to learn the nonnegative consequences of consuming a sweet solution more readily than males. Female and male rats given zero, two, four, or eight

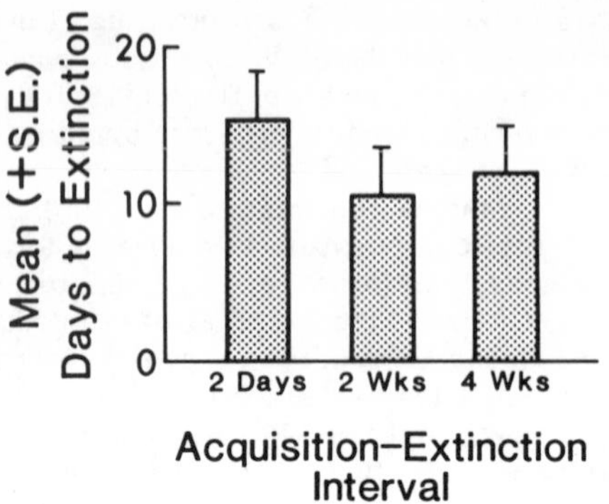

FIGURE 14. Mean number of days that female rats drank less than 100% of the amount consumed on acquisition day when extinction trials were initiated two days, two weeks, and four weeks after the acquisition trial.

preexposures to the conditioned stimulus (a sucrose solution) prior to acquisition (Chambers and Sengstake, unpublished data) do not differ in sucrose consumption on the acquisition day (FIGURE 15). During extinction, males given zero, two, and four preexposures consume less sucrose than females given zero, two, and four preexposures, respectively. Females given two, four, and eight preexposures do not differ from one

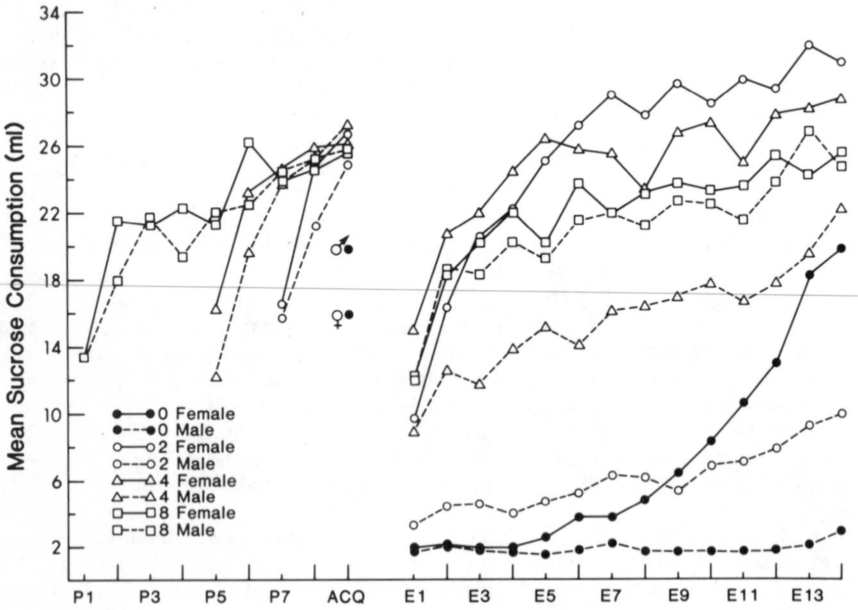

FIGURE 15. Mean sucrose consumption by female and male rats before (PI through ACQ) and after (E1 through E13) injection of LiCl when given no, two, four, or eight preexposures to sucrose.

another in the amount of sucrose consumed during extinction, but they consume significantly more during extinction than females given no preexposure. Males given zero and two preexposures do not differ from one another in the amount of sucrose consumed during extinction, but they consume significantly more than males given four and eight preexposures. Males given four and eight preexposures do not differ from one another. Thus, in males, four preexposures are equivalent to eight, but in females, as few as two preexposures are equivalent to eight.

I suggest that the following is occurring. When female and male rats are poisoned after their first exposure to a sucrose solution, they learn that consuming this solution has negative consequences, and they acquire sucrose aversions that are of equal strength. During extinction, females and males sample the substance equally, but females learn about the nonnegative consequences of consuming it more readily than males. When females and males are given more than one exposure to a sucrose solution prior to conditioning, females acquire a weaker aversion than do males because they have learned about the nonnegative consequences of consumption prior to poisoning more readily than males. Females, then achieve extinction faster when they are given preexposures to the sucrose solution because they learn about the nonnegative consequences more readily than males both before and after poisoning. Since female rats essentially are not under testosterone stimulation and males are, I hypothesize that testosterone has its effect by delaying learning about the nonnegative consequences of consuming the sucrose solution.

In summary, I think that when testosterone-sensitive cells in the brains of females and males are activated, they inhibit extinction by delaying the learning of nonnegative consequences of consumption. Environmental factors, such as social isolation and water deprivation, block the activation of cells by reducing the availability of testosterone to the receptor or by affecting the receptor itself.

ACKNOWLEDGMENTS

I thank Dr. David L. Hess, supervisor of the Oregon Regional Primate Research Center Radioimmunoassay Laboratory, in which the testosterone assays were conducted.

REFERENCES

1. Bohus, B., W. H. Gispen & D. de Wied. 1973. Effect of lysine vasopressin and $ACTH_{4-10}$ on conditioned avoidance behavior of hypophysectomized rats. Neuroendocrinology **11**: 137–143.
2. Miller, R. E. & N. Ogawa. 1962. The effect of adrenocorticotrophic hormone (ACTH) on avoidance conditioning in the adrenalectomized rat. J. Comp. Physiol. Psychol. **55**: 211–213.
3. de Wied, D. 1964. Influence of anterior pituitary on avoidance learning and escape behavior. Am. J. Physiol. **207**: 255–259.
4. de Wied, D. 1969. Effects of peptide hormones on behavior. *In* Frontiers in Neuroendocrinology. W. F. Ganong & L. Martini, Eds.: 97–140. Oxford University Press. London.
5. Ader, R., J. A. W. M. Weijnen & P. Moleman. 1972. Retention of a passive avoidance response as a function of the intensity and duration of electric shock. Psychon. Sci. **26**: 125–128.
6. Bohus, B., R. Ader & D. de Wied. 1972. Effects of vasopressin on active and passive avoidance behavior. Horm. Behav. **3**: 191–197.
7. Greven, H. M. & D. de Wied. 1973. The influence of peptides derived from corticotrophin (ACTH) on performance. Structure activity studies. *In* Progress in Brain Research.

E. Zimmermann, W. H. Gispen, B. H. Marks & D. de Wied, Eds. **39**: 429–442. Elsevier. Amsterdam.
8. LEVINE, S. & L. E. JONES. 1965. Adrenocorticotrophic hormone (ACTH) and passive avoidance learning. J. Comp. Physiol. Psychol. **59**: 357–360.
9. DE WIED, D. 1971. Long term effect of vasopressin on the maintenance of a conditioned avoidance response in rats. Nature **232**: 58–60.
10. BOHUS, B. & K. LISSAK. 1968. Adrenocortical hormones and avoidance behaviour of rats. Int. J. Neuropharmacol. **7**: 301–306.
11. DE WIED, D. 1967. Opposite effect of ACTH and glucocorticosteriods on extinction of conditioned avoidance behavior. *In* Proceedings of Second International Congress on Hormonal Steroids. (Milan, May 1966) L. Martini, F. Franschini & M. Motta, Eds.: 945–951. Excerpta Medica Foundation Amsterdam.
12. DE WIED, D. 1977. Pituitary adrenal system hormones and behaviour. Acta Endocrinol. **85** (Suppl. 214): 9–18.
13. BEATTY, W. W. 1979. Gonadal hormones and sex differences in non-reproductive behaviors in rodents: Organizational and activational influences. Horm. Behav. **12**: 112–163.
14. BARRETT, R. J. & O. S. RAY. 1970. Behavior in the open field, Lashley III maze, shuttlebox, and Sidman avoidance as a function of strain, sex and age. Develop. Psychol. **3**: 73–77.
15. BEATTY, W. W., K. C. GREGOIRE & L. L. PARMITER. 1973. Sex differences in retention of passive avoidance behavior in rats. Bull. Psychon. Soc. **2**: 99–100.
16. BENGELLOUN, W. A., D. J. NELSON, H. M. ZENT & W. W. BEATTY. 1976. Behavior of male and female rats with septal lesions: Influence of prior gonadectomy. Physiol. Behav. **16**: 317–330.
17. DENTI, A. & A. EPSTEIN. 1972. Sex differences in the acquisition of two kinds of avoidance behavior in rats. Physiol. Behav. **8**: 611–615.
18. LEVINE, S. & P. L. BROADHURST. 1963. Genetic and ontogenetic determinants of adult behavior in the rat. J. Comp. Physiol. Psychol. **56**: 423–428.
19. RAY, O. S. & R. S. BARRETT. 1975. Behavioral, pharmacological, and biochemical analysis of genetic differences in rats. Behav. Biol. **15**: 391–417.
20. BEATTY, W. W. & P. A. BEATTY. 1970. Hormonal determinants of sex differences in avoidance behavior and reactivity to electric shock in the rat. J. Comp. Physiol. Psychol. **73**: 446–455.
21. SCOUTEN, C. W., L. K. GROTELUESCHEN & W. W. BEATTY. 1975. Androgens and the organization of sex differences in active avoidance behavior in the rat. J. Comp. Physiol. Psychol. **88**: 264–270.
22. VAN WIMERSMA GREIDANUS, TJ.B. 1970. Effects of steroids on extinction of an avoidance response in rats. A structure-activity relationship study. Prog. Brain Res. **32**: 185–191.
23. GOY, R. W. & D. A. GOLDFOOT. 1973. Hormonal influences on sexually dimorphic behavior. *In* Handbook of Physiology. Sec. 7, Endocrinology. R. O. Greep & E. B. Astwood, Eds. **2** (Pt. 1): 169–186. American Physiological Society. Washington, D.C.
24. PHOENIX, C. H., R. W. GOY, A. A. GERRALL & W. C. YOUNG. 1959. Organizing action of prenatally administered testosterone propionate on the tissues mediating mating behavior in the female guinea pig. Endocrinology **65**: 269–382.
25. YOUNG, W. C. 1961. The hormones and mating behavior. *In* Sex and Internal Secretions. 3rd edit. W. C. Young, Ed. **2**: 1173–1239. Williams and Wilkins. Baltimore, MD.
26. CHAMBERS, K. C. & C. B. SENGSTAKE. 1976. Sexually dimorphic extinction of a conditioned taste aversion in rats. Anim. Learn. Behav. **4**: 181–185.
27. CHAMBERS, K. C. 1976. Hormonal influences on sexual dimorphism in the rate of extinction of a conditioned taste aversion in rats. J. Comp. Physiol. Psychol. **90**: 851–856.
28. CHAMBERS, K. C. 1980. Progesterone, estradiol, testosterone and dihydrotestosterone: Effects on rate of extinction of a conditioned taste aversion in rats. Physiol. Behav. **24**: 1061–1065.
29. EARLEY, C. J. & B. E. LEONARD. 1978. Androgenic involvement in conditioned taste aversion. Horm. Behav. **11**: 1–11.
30. EARLEY, C. J. & B. E. LEONARD. 1979. Effects of prior exposure on conditioned taste aversion in the rat: Androgen- and estrogen-dependent events. J. Comp. Physiol. Psychol. **93**: 793–805.

31. BABINE, A. M. & W. P. SMOTHERMAN. 1984. Uterine position and conditioned taste aversion. Behav. Neurosci. **98**: 461–466.
32. CHAMBERS, K. C. & C. B. SENGSTAKE. 1978. Pseudo-castration effects of social isolation on extinction of a taste aversion. Physiol. Behav. **21**: 29–32.
33. DESSI-FULGHERI, F., C. LUPO DI PRISCO & P. VERDARELLI. 1976. Effects of two kinds of social deprivation on testosterone and estradiol-17β plasma levels in the male rat. Experientia **32**: 114–115.
34. SENGSTAKE, C. B., K. C. CHAMBERS & J. H. THROWER. 1978. Interactive effects of fluid deprivation and testosterone on the expression of a sexually dimorphic conditioned taste aversion. J. Comp. Physiol. Psychol. **92**: 1150–1155.
35. CHAMBERS, K. C. 1982. Failure of ACTH to prolong extinction of a conditioned taste aversion in the absence of the testes. Physiol. Behav. **29**: 915–919.
36. CHAMBERS, K. C. & C. B. SENGSTAKE. 1979. Temporal aspects of the dependency of a dimorphic rate of extinction on testosterone. Physiol. Behav. **22**: 53–56.
37. SENSTAKE, C. B. & K. C. CHAMBERS. 1979. Differential effects of fluid deprivation on the acquisition and extinction phases of a conditioned taste aversion. Bull. Psychon. Soc. **14**: 85–87.
38. RESKO, J. A., W. E. ELLINWOOD, L. M. PASZTOR & A. E. BUHL. 1980. Sex steroids in the umbilical circulation of fetal rhesus monkeys from the time of gonadal differentiation. J. Clin. Endocrinol. Metab. **50**: 900–905.
39. RESKO, J. A., A. MALLEY, D. E. BEGLEY & D. L. HESS. 1973. Radioimmunoassay of testosterone during fetal development of the rhesus monkey. Endocrinology **93**: 156–161.
40. BAILEY, J., M. GINSBURG, B. D. GREENSTEIN, N. J. MACLUSKY & P. J. THOMAS. 1975. An androgen receptor in rat brain and pituitary. Brain Res. **100**: 383–393.
41. KATO, J. 1976. Cytosol and nuclear receptors for 5α-dihydrotestosterone and testosterone in the hypothalamus and hypophysis, and testosterone receptors isolated from neonatal female rat hypothalamus. J. Steroid Biochem. **7**: 1179–1187.
42. LIEBERBURG, I., N. J. MACLUSKY & B. S. MCEWEN. 1977. 5α-dihydrotestosterone (DHT) receptors in rat brain and pituitary cell nuclei. Endocrinology **100**: 598–607.
43. NAESS, O. 1976. Characterization of the androgen receptors in the hypothalamus, preoptic area and brain cortex of the rat. Steroids **27**: 167–185.
44. ROBBINS, R. J. 1980. Sex affects the initial strength but not the extinction of poison-based taste aversions in deer mice (*Peromyscus maniculatus bairdi*). Behav. Neural Biol. **30**: 80–89.
45. HOSKINS, R. G. 1925. Studies on vigor: II. The effects of castration on voluntary activity. Am. J. Physiol. **72**: 324–330.
46. YOUNG, W. C. & W. R. FISH. 1945. The ovarian hormones and spontaneous running activity in the female rat. Endocrinology **36**: 181–189.
47. ROY, E. J. & G. N. WADE. 1975. Role of estrogens in androgen-induced spontaneous activity in male rats. J. Comp. Physiol. Psychol. **89**: 573–579.
48. WADE, G. N. & I. ZUCKER. 1969. I. Taste preferences of female rats: Modification by neonatal hormones, food deprivation and prior experience. Physiol. Behav. **4**: 935–943.
49. KALAT, J. W. & P. ROZIN. 1971. Role of interference in taste-aversion learning. J. Comp. Physiol. Psychol. **77**: 53–58.
50. KALAT, J. W. & P. ROZIN. 1973. "Learned safety" as a mechanism in long-delay taste-aversion learning in rats. J. Comp. Physiol. Psychol. **83**:198–207.
51. ROZIN, P. & J. W. KALAT. 1971. Specific hunger and poison as adaptive specializations of learning. Psychol. Rev. **78**: 459–486.

Glucocorticoid and Other Hormonal Substrates of Conditioned Taste Aversion[a]

WILLIAM P. SMOTHERMAN

Laboratory for Psychobiological Research
Department of Psychology
Oregon State University
Corvallis, Oregon 97331

When a rat is subjected to the unpleasant effects of a drug after drinking a distinctly flavored fluid for the first time, the rat will acquire an aversion to the taste of the fluid; this is commonly referred to as a conditioned taste aversion (CTA). In the 10 years since the publication of a review article by Garcia, Hankins, and Rusiniak[1] there has been a proliferation of publications on CTA. One active area of interest has been the study of hormonal substrates of CTA, the role that hormones play in acquisition and extinction of CTA.

Investigators interested in the molecular biochemical bases of learning and memory have begun to examine the role that hormones play in modulating brain function during the learning and performance of aversively and appetitively motivated tasks. In this regard, hormones of the hypothalamic-pituitary-adrenocortical (P-A) system, namely, corticotropin releasing factor (CRF), adrenocorticotropin (ACTH), beta-endorphin, glucocorticoids, and norepinephrine (NE) have come under investigation.[2]

Hormones secreted by this system (FIGURE 1) exhibit a bidirectional response profile. Cues paired with positive reinforcement can themselves trigger a suppression of pituitary-adrenocortical activity, while cues associated with aversive stimulation can activate the P-A system and trigger conditioned increases in hormonal levels. In other words, the system can exhibit an activation or a suppression during the acquisition and performance of learned behaviors. Furthermore, manipulations of CRF, ACTH, the glucocorticoids, and NE affect the performance of rats in a variety of learning situations.

This review will focus on the brain-hypothalamic-pituitary-adrenal system and discuss the role that hormones secreted by this system play in the learning and performance of CTA. The general methods and procedures are similar in the experiments to be discussed. In all experiments, subjects were adult male Sprague-Dawley rats (300–350 g). The rats were individually housed in temperature- and humidity-controlled colony rooms on regulated 12/12-hr light/dark cycles. Subjects were trained to drink on cue in the home cage by presentation of a 20% sucrose solution. A sweetened milk

[a] W.P.S. is supported by Grant 16102 from the National Institute of Child Health and Human Development (NICHD) and an Oregon State University Research Council Biomedical Research Support Grant (RR 07079). Much of the data presented in this article was collected while W.P.S. was an NIH Postdoctoral Fellow (1F32 MH 05555-01) and supported by a grant from the C.F. Aaron Endowment Fund (Stanford Dean's Fund Postdoctoral Fellowship).

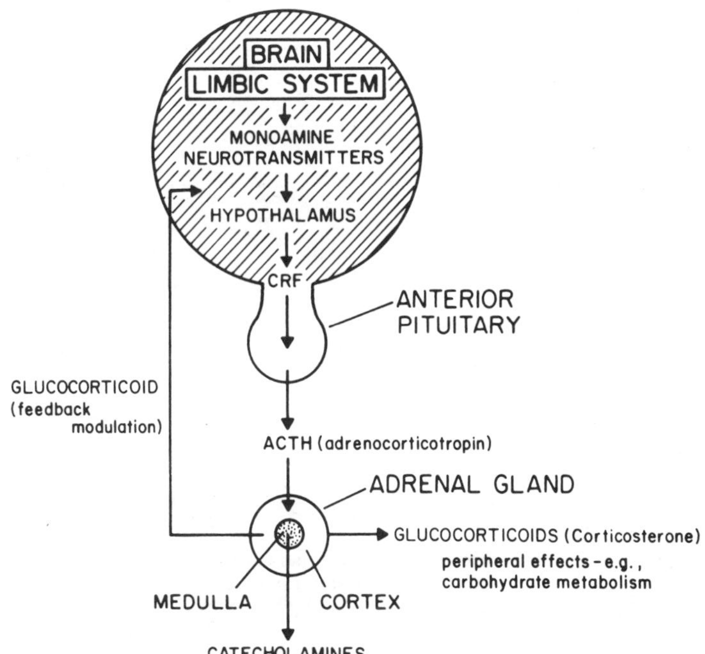

FIGURE 1. A simplified schematic representation of the neural and hormonal interrelationships of the brain-hypothalamic-pituitary-adrenal system.

solution (the CS) was then presented and, after 2 to 5 presentations, paired with an i.p. injection of LiCl (0.40 M; 7.5 ml/kg) after a delay of 25–35 min (hereafter referred to as the Day of Conditioning). After a 72-hr recovery period, rats were again presented with the milk solution during extinction sessions. These reexposures to milk were single bottle tests presented under conditions in which rats had continual access to food and water (free extinction) or in which food and water intake had been restricted (forced extinction). When necessary, animals were quickly anesthetized with ether and blood samples (.8 ml) collected in heparinized tubes by cardiac puncture. Serum was centrifuged as 2,000 rpm for 15 min, and the plasma extracted and frozen until assay by a fluorometric micromethod to determine plasma levels of corticosterone.

FIGURE 2 shows the consumption of the test solution (milk) by rats before and after CTA using the procedure described above. Rats increased milk intake across the sessions preceding LiCl injection. This injection resulted in a CTA, as evidenced by the 75–80% suppression in drinking. When free extinction procedures are followed, drinking recovers to preconditioning levels within 10–12 days, given that extinction sessions occur daily.

P-A RESPONSE TO THE US

It has been well established that aversive unconditioned stimuli (US) activate the P-A system. Does the injection of LiCl act as an US in terms of the P-A system? Injection

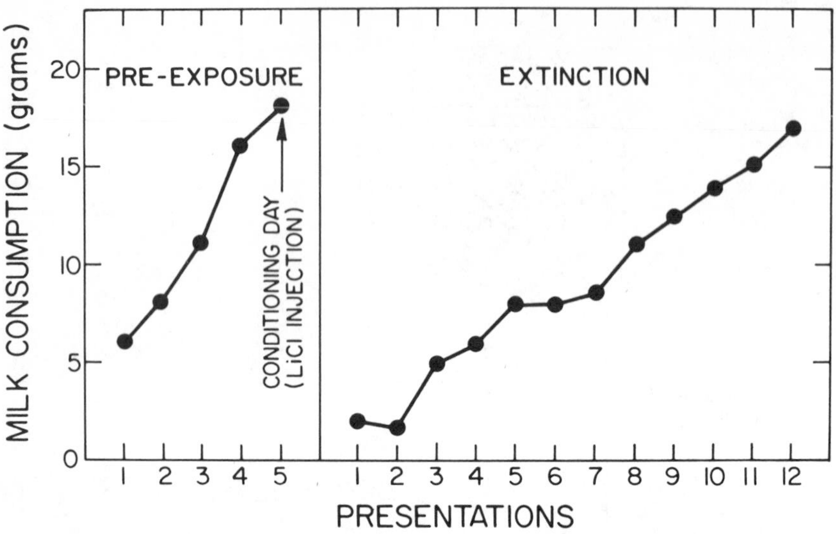

FIGURE 2. CTA acquisition and extinction in rats that received an i.p. injection of LiCl (0.40 M; 7.5 ml/kg) after intake of a sweetened milk solution on presession Day 5. After an initial suppression in intake of 90%, extinction (recovery) was complete within 12 days.

of LiCl in a dosage and concentration sufficient to produce CTA increases plasma levels of corticosterone.[3] While the magnitude of the pituitary-adrenal response is unaffected by LiCl concentration, the duration of the response is sustained longer with greater concentrations (FIGURE 3). There is no evidence that the response to LiCl attenuates as a function of prior US presentation. There is no evidence of novelty-induced activation of the P-A system when tastes are encountered for the first time. Preexposure to the CS has no effect on the pituitary-adrenal response to the US. These data show that ACTH and corticosterone are elevated at the time of CTA learning, and that preexposure to the US or CS does not affect the magnitude of the response to the US. Further, the data indicate that LiCl treatment activates the P-A system, elevating plasma ACTH and corticosterone.

P-A RESPONSE TO THE CS DURING FREE EXTINCTION

The observation that LiCl causes a sustained increase in plasma corticosterone suggests that corticosterone changes could be conditioned to stimuli that are initially paired with shock. Would such stimuli later be effective alone in eliciting a conditioned activation of the P-A system? In other words, might a similar early pairing with LiCl enable a CS to elicit elevations in corticosterone on the first day of extinction? To answer this question, individual groups of rats were conditioned to avoid a sweetened milk solution. Following the fifth milk (CS) presentation they were treated with LiCl (conditioned group) or an equal volume of isotonic saline (control group), which does not produce a taste aversion. Three days after these injections, during which food and water were continuously available (free extinction), the milk was again presented and the blood of rats in both groups was sampled 20 min after the end of the extinction session. Plasma from these samples was then assayed for determination of corticosterone levels (FIGURE 4). Clearly, the conditioned animals developed an aversion to the milk; they showed a 90% suppression in drinking. However, this CTA was not accompanied by an elevation in plasma levels of corticosterone. Under free extinction test conditions corticosterone levels remain low.

P-A RESPONSE TO THE CS DURING FORCED EXTINCTION

In the preceding experiment, the conditioned rats apparently sampled the milk after the formation of CTA, because milk drinking was not completely suppressed. Thus, the rats had re-exposed themselves to the CS. With knowledge of this information, another experiment was designed that was intended to increase consumption of the CS during extinction. Following a conditioning trial and a single free extinction session, rats were placed on food deprivation for three days. Water was withheld for the last two of these three days. This procedure was designed to force the rats to consume either a neutral substance, in this case tap water, or the aversive CS (milk). Blood was sampled after the forced extinction session and assayed to determine plasma levels of corticosterone. The forced extinction deprivation conditions reversed the aversion to some extent. Under these conditions, rats increased their intake of the CS and showed

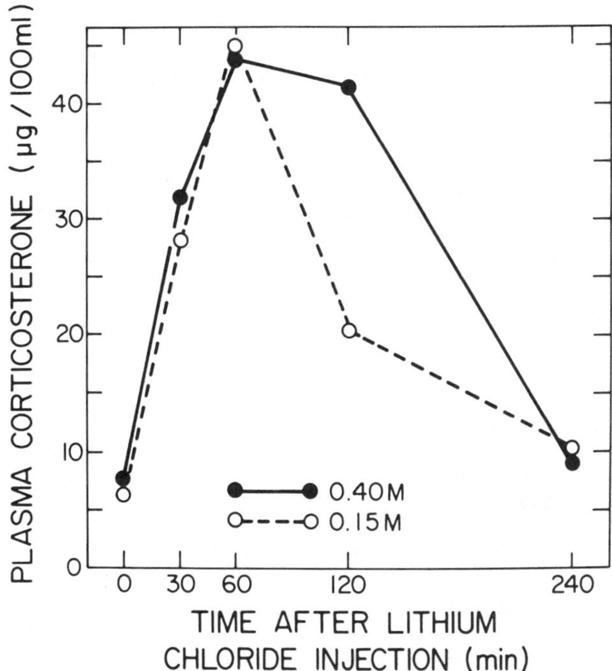

FIGURE 3. A time course of plasma corticosterone changes following injection of rats with 0.40 or 0.15 M lithium chloride (LiCl). Entries represent mean values (N = 6 rats at each time point for each concentration).

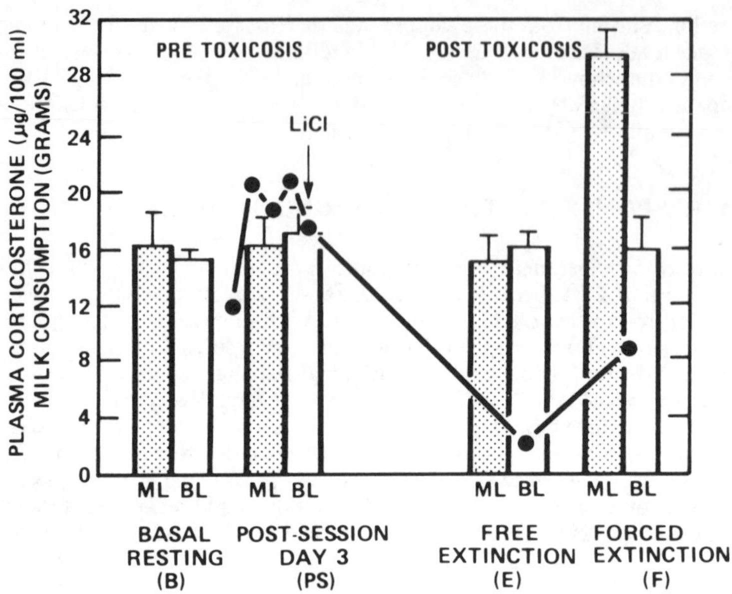

FIGURE 4. Solid line connects mean milk drinking for the five preconditioning days and the days of free and forced extinction (ML group). Vertical bars represent mean plasma levels of corticosterone (± S.E.M.). Rats in the ML group had milk paired with LiCl, while rats in the BL group had tap water paired with LiCl.

higher levels of corticosterone than animals experiencing the same deprivation regimen and drinking tap water. With this procedure, conditioned activation of the P-A system—elevation in plasma corticosterone—was demonstrated.

In both the free and forced extinction conditions, rats consumed a sweetened milk solution that had earlier been paired with LiCl. However, only under the conditions of forced extinction did a conditioned activation of the P-A system occur.[3,4] Ader[5] reported similar conditioned elevations in plasma corticosterone when rats consumed a saccharin solution that had been paired with either LiCl or cyclophosphamide.

The effectiveness of LiCl in establishing CTA changes strikingly as the number of CS preexposures increases. After two or five preexposures, LiCl injection is still effective in establishing an aversion, but after 10 preexposures LiCl is ineffective in conditioning an aversion (FIGURE 5).[6] To more systematically analyze this preexposure effect and to determine whether the preexposure manipulations would produce similar effects on the hormonal and behavioral indices of CTA, the number of milk preexposures was increased in a step-wise fashion from five to 10 before pairing with LiCl. Milk intake and corticosterone levels were measured after a forced extinction session (FIGURE 6). These data show that the nine- and 10-preexposure groups drank significantly more than groups preexposed five, six, seven, or eight times. The effect of preexposure on the behavioral index of CTA was evident when nine or 10 preexposures preceded LiCl injection, but the pattern of corticosterone elevation did not exactly coincide with the behavioral measure. Only the five- and six-preexposure groups showed elevated plasma corticosterone. Groups exposed seven, eight, nine, or 10 times did not show elevated corticosterone when reexposed after conditioning. While the suppression of drinking was accompanied by elevated plasma levels of corticosterone in groups preexposed five or six times, a similar suppression in the drinking of groups preexposed seven or eight times was not accompanied by elevated plasma levels of corticosterone. The nine- and 10-preexposure groups, which showed significantly less aversion, also failed to show elevated plasma levels of corticosterone.

Apparently, manipulation of preexposure alters the signal characteristics of the taste CS. One might speculate that the attention-eliciting capacity of the CS, as indexed by corticosterone change, is affected by fewer stimulus preexposures than is the behavioral response. This attention-eliciting function of the CS is diminished by several preexposures that have no effect on behavior. With more preexposures, the taste CS becomes safe or irrelevant as a signal associated with later illness (i.e., a poor predictor of illness) and the effect on behavior is seen.[6]

In summary, LiCl in a dosage and concentration effective in producing CTA activates the P-A system. When subjects have *ad libitum* access to food and water (free extinction) and control the intake of milk, endogenous ACTH/corticosterone levels do not elevate. However, promoting the animal to consume an aversive CS (forced extinction) results in conditioned elevations in ACTH/corticosterone. Preexposures to the CS before its pairing with LiCl affect both behavioral and endocrine response

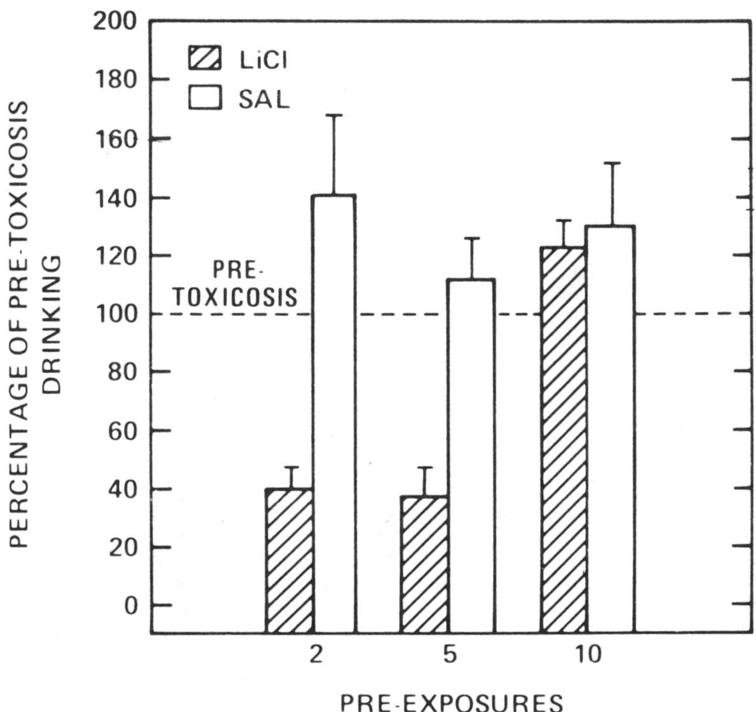

FIGURE 5. Milk drinking during forced extinction sessions for rats injected with LiCl or saline (SAL) after two, five, or 10 preexposures. Data are expressed as a percentage of the individual subject's drinking on the day of conditioning. Entries represent group means (± S.E.M.). (Copyright (1980) by the American Psychological Association. Adapted from Smotherman *et al.*[6] By permission of the publisher.)

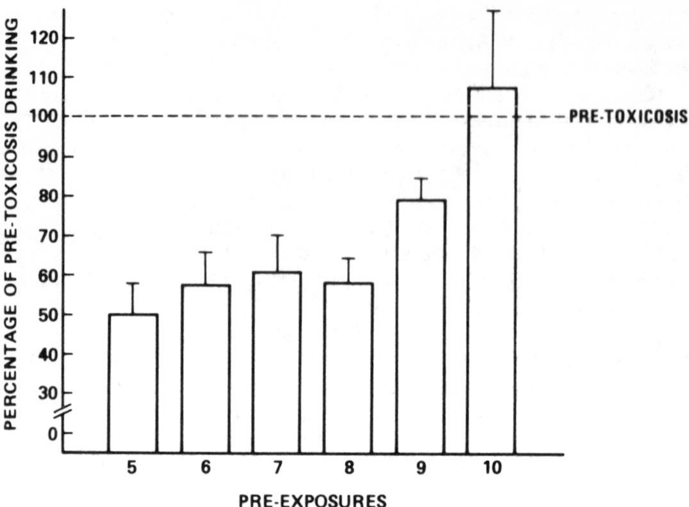

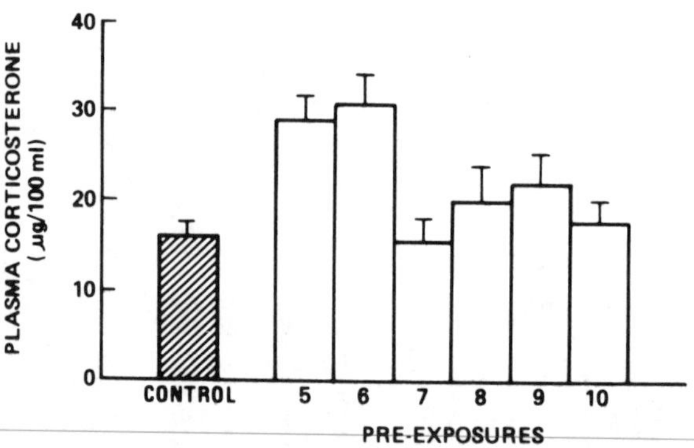

FIGURE 6. (Top) Milk drinking during the forced extinction session expressed as a percentage of the individual rat's drinking on the day of conditioning, and plotted separately for groups with five, six, seven, eight, nine, or 10 preexposures. Entries are means (± S.E.M.). (Bottom) Plasma levels of corticosterone on the day of forced extinction for the six preexposure groups and a control group that had eight preexposures to milk; the eighth preexposure was followed by LiCl. This group was sampled before reexposure on the day of forced extinction to provide a basal control group. (Copyright (1980) by the American Psychological Association. Adapted from Smotherman *et al.*[6] By permission of the publisher.)

systems upon reexposure to the aversive CS. Within a certain range of CS preexposures, there is a coupling of behavioral and adrenocortical responses where CTA is characterized by suppressed drinking and by elevated plasma levels of corticosterone. With further preexposures there is a dissociation of the two response systems. CTA is characterized by suppressed drinking, which is not accompanied by conditioned adrenocor-

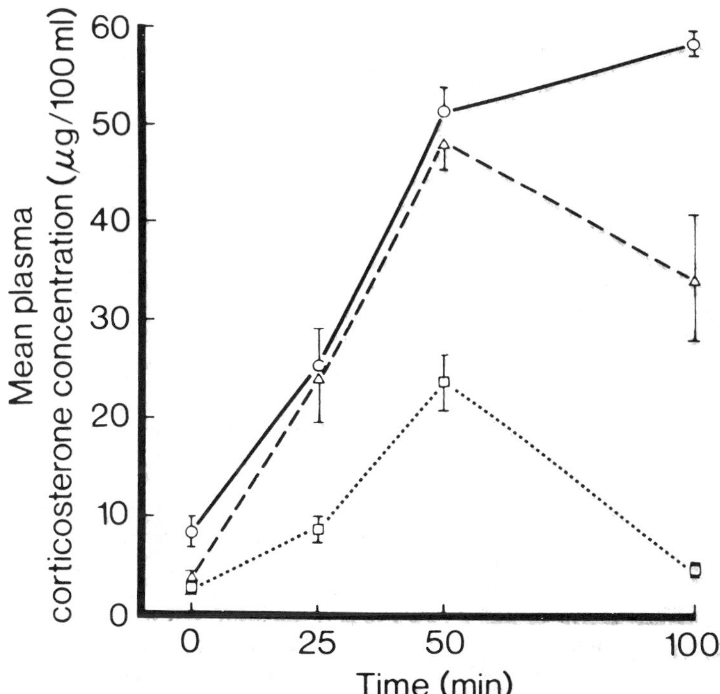

FIGURE 7. Postsession corticosterone concentrations for different session durations after different durations of prior water deprivation (N = 6 rats/time point). Entries represent means (± S.E.M.). (Copyright (1980) by the American Psychological Association. Adapted from Hart *et al.*[8] By permission of the publisher.)

tical activity. With yet further preexposures there is no evidence of CTA—no suppression in drinking and no elevation in plasma corticosterone.[6]

CONDITIONS NECESSARY/SUFFICIENT FOR CTA

Is activation of the P-A system a sufficient condition for the acquisition of a taste aversion?[7] Hart, Coover, Shnerson, and Smotherman[8,9] have shown that intake of a concentrated (23%) sucrose solution by water-deprived rats results in large and prolonged activations of the pituitary-adrenal system. The magnitude of the response is dependent upon the duration of deprivation (2, 24, or 48 hr) that precedes the drinking (FIGURE 7). To follow up on these findings, Smotherman (unpublished) exposed rats to 23% sucrose solution after 48 hr of deprivation. Exposures were repeated every third day for a 30-day period. TABLE 1 summarizes the sucrose intake and plasma levels of corticosterone, which were measured at the end of the first, fifth, and tenth 1-hr drinking sessions. Plasma corticosterone levels were markedly elevated at all three determinations. There was no evidence that pituitary-adrenal activation in response to the 48-hr deprivation and sucrose intake had changed over the course of presentations. Furthermore, there was no evidence that rats decreased their sucrose intake.

TABLE 1. Consumption of a 23% Sucrose Solution in 48-hr Water Deprived Rats across 10 Experimental Sessions

	Session Number		
	1	5	10
23% sucrose consumed (g)	15.2 ± 1.7	14.8 ± 2.2	16.2 ± 3.8
Plasma corticosterone at the end of the 1-hr session (μg/100 ml)	50.3 ± 3.7	48.5 ± 5.0	51.8 ± 3.3

N = 10 rats sampled after the first, fifth, and tenth exposure to the 23% sucrose solution. Entries represent mean values (± S.E.M.).

In other words, there was no indication of CTA formation. If large and prolonged (and repeated) activation of the P-A system was a sufficient condition to establish CTA, rats would have shown a decrease in sucrose intake. Such was not the case.

Clearly, activation of the P-A system is not a sufficient condition for CTA to occur. Furthermore, neither ACTH nor corticosterone, when injected after drinking, is highly effective as an aversive US to produce CTA.[10] ACTH can cause a slight suppression in intake but does so only after repeated taste/ACTH pairings and only in rats that have consumed small amounts of the CS before hormone injections begin.[10] In contrast to ACTH and corticosterone, the adrenal medullary hormone norepinephrine (NE) can function as a US to induce CTA. Aversions induced by NE are more easily conditioned to a highly preferred solution and depend upon the degree of discriminability between endogenous and exogenous epinephrine levels.[11]

Is activation of the P-A system necessary for the establishing of CTA? One way to answer this question is to prevent the elevation of ACTH and circulatory corticosteroids during formation of CTA. This can be accomplished by peripheral injection of the synthetic glucocorticoid dexamethasone phosphate (DEX).[4,12] While DEX treatment prior to the time of conditioning attenuates the CTA, it does not eliminate it. (These data are discussed in more detail below.) Therefore, even though the P-A system is activated at the time conditioning occurs and again (under certain conditions) when rats consume aversive tastes, pituitary-adrenal activation is neither sufficient nor necessary for the establishment of CTA.

ALTERATIONS IN ENDOGENOUS STEROID LEVELS

As outlined earlier, LiCl causes an activation of the P-A system that elevates plasma ACTH and corticosterone levels. Given that these hormones are elevated at the time conditioning occurs, a series of experiments was conducted to examine the effects of changes in pituitary-adrenal function on CTA acquisition and performance. Peripheral injection of DEX was again used in this series to block release of ACTH.

As a first step, the effects of DEX pretreatment and LiCl injections upon pituitary-adrenal activity were assessed. Pretreatment DEX injections were administered 2.5 hr prior to LiCl injection; one-half of the subjects received 400 μg of DEX while the other half received the volumetric equivalent of isotonic saline. Blood samples were taken from all subjects 1, 2, or 4 hr after LiCl injection, yielding six experimental groups: D-1, D-2, D-4, S-1, S-2, S-4. Plasma was separated from the serum and corticosterone levels determined. For the saline-pretreated groups, plasma corticosterone levels were elevated for 2 to 4 hr following LiCl administration. As was expected, DEX pretreatment uniformly suppressed these corticosterone elevations.

With the knowledge that DEX pretreatment blocks ACTH/corticosterone release in response to LiCl, we utilized a factorial design where four groups of rats received DEX or saline 2 hr prior to drinking on either the conditioning day, or throughout recovery, or both. Thus, four independent groups were employed: (1) those pretreated with DEX prior to both conditioning and during recovery (D-D); (2) those receiving DEX prior to conditioning and saline during recovery (D-S); (3) those receiving saline pretreatment before conditioning and DEX during recovery (S-D); and (4) those pretreated with saline throughout (S-S). The results (FIGURE 8) indicated that both groups pretreated with DEX on the conditioning day (D-D and D-S) showed an attenuated CTA relative to those treated with saline (S-D and S-S). The effect was present on the first day of testing and lasted throughout extinction. Thus, blockade of the P-A system at the time of conditioning appears to attenuate the aversion and facilitate recovery.[12]

Following a similar rationale, Cairnie and Leach[13] have reported that DEX also is a potent blocker of radiation-induced CTA in rats. However, they interpret their

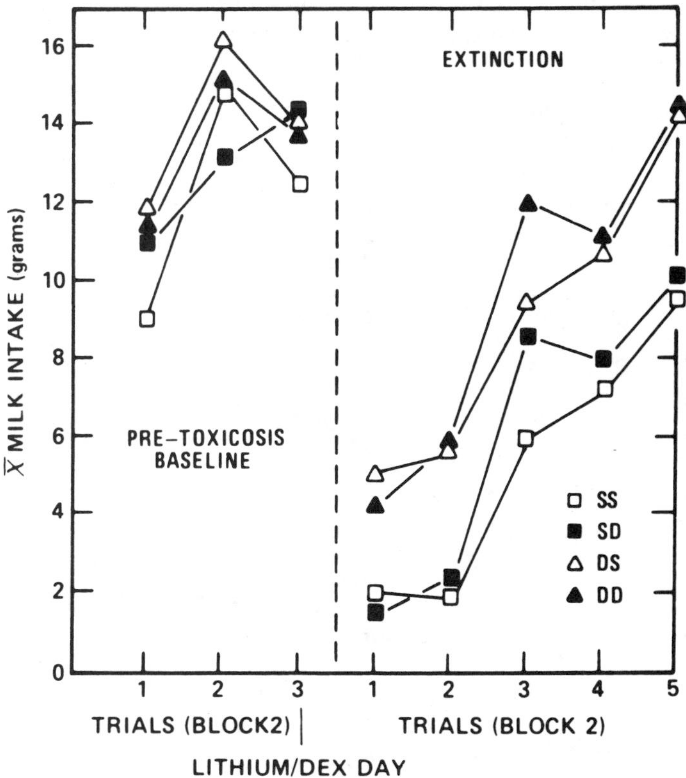

FIGURE 8. The effects of dexamethasone pretreatment during conditioning and/or extinction upon CTA to a sweetened milk solution.

TABLE 2. Response of Implanted Rats to Lithium Chloride Injection (corticosterone in μg/100 ml)

	Base (0) Time of Injection	+1 hr	+2 hr	+4 hr
Hydrocortisone implant	8.7	10.1	9.5	8.3
Cholesterol implant (control)	7.7	44.0	30.6	14.4

Drinking on Day 1 of Extinction in Implanted Rats (% of Test Day Consumption)

Cholesterol before conditioning	37.8
Cholesterol before extinction	40.0
Hydrocortisone before conditioning	63.4[a]
Hydrocortisone before extinction	42.1

[a]Significantly different from other means (Neuman Keuls test; $p < .01$)

results as suggesting that DEX functions as an antinauseant and antiemetic. In this way, rather than acting through the P-A system, DEX pretreatment could reduce the aversive properties of the LiCl and thereby attenuate CTA. But DEX pretreatment is not the only manipulation of the P-A system that blocks ACTH release at the time of conditioning and attenuates CTA acquisition. CNS implants of hydrocortisone in the median eminence also block the release of ACTH/corticosterone in response to

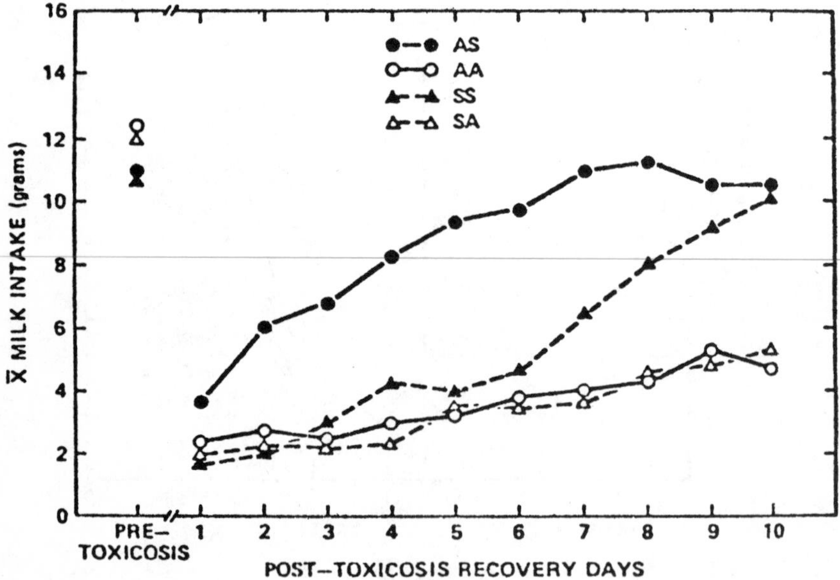

FIGURE 9. The effects of presession ACTH injections during conditioning and/or extinction upon CTA to a sweetened milk solution. (Adapted from Kendler *et al.*[14] By permission of the publisher.)

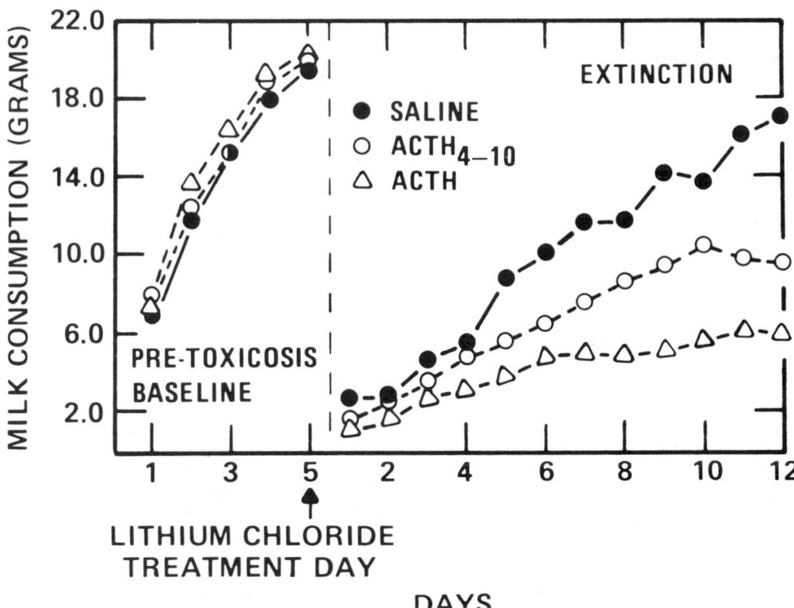

FIGURE 10. Milk consumption before conditioning and during extinction for groups of rats receiving ACTH, $ACTH_{4-10}$, or saline (N = 8 rats/group) 15 min before each extinction session. (Copyright (1978) by the American Psychological Association. Adapted from Smotherman & Levine.[10] By permission of the publisher.)

LiCl. When such implants are performed prior to acquisition, the resulting CTA is attenuated. Implants of this type are without effect when performed after acquisition but before extinction (TABLE 2). These data suggest that ACTH release and the elevation in plasma levels of corticosterone that follow are indeed important components of CTA. Manipulations that block the release of ACTH/corticosterone affect CTA acquisition. However, they do not eliminate the possibility that the CNS implants could also have had anti-emetic effects.

In another series of experiments, the possibility that manipulation of the ACTH-steroid levels, via exogenous administration, might also affect CTA learning and/or performance was investigated. Preliminary evidence had shown that ACTH injections (8 IU) administered prior to both conditioning and extinction sessions tended to prolong recovery, i.e., ACTH-injected rats drank less milk during extinction.[12] In a more detailed investigation of this finding, a factorial design was employed to measure the effects of presession ACTH injections during either conditioning or recovery.[14] Again, it was found that ACTH injections, when given prior to recovery sessions, affected performance and prolonged the extinction process (FIGURE 9). Since ACTH injections produce elevations in both ACTH and corticosterone levels, the possibility exists that ACTH injections may prolong extinction of CTA by elevating corticosterone levels. Rigter and Popping[15] reported that the peptide $ACTH_{4-10}$, which is devoid of corticotropic activity, also prolongs the recovery from CTA.

In an experiment that directly compared the peptide $ACTH_{4-10}$ with its parent molecule $ACTH_{1-39}$,[10,16] the $ACTH_{4-10}$ produced a recovery curve that was intermediate

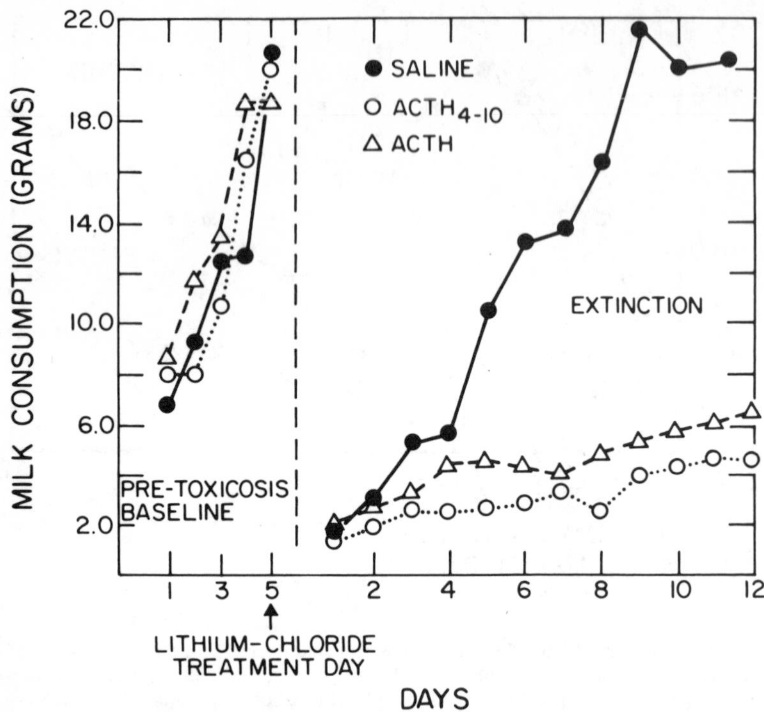

FIGURE 11. The effects of intracerebroventricular infusions of ACTH or $ACTH_{4-10}$ (N = 12 rats/group) 15 min prior to free extinction sessions on a CTA to a sweetened milk solution.

to that shown by ACTH and saline-treated rats (FIGURE 10). It is interesting to note that injecting rats before extinction sessions with the combination of $ACTH_{4-10}$ and corticosterone does not further prolong extinction compared with a group of rats receiving $ACTH_{4-10}$ alone.

Evidence collected recently in my laboratory suggests that ACTH is acting at sites in the central nervous system to affect CTA extinction and can do so independently of any action on the adrenal cortex. After rats had been conditioned to avoid a milk solution, they underwent a surgical procedure where a stainless steel guide cannula was implanted into the lateral ventricle. Polyethylene tubing was inserted through this cannula so that ACTH or $ACTH_{4-10}$ could be delivered directly into the brain. Experimental subjects received 15 μg of ACTH or $ACTH_{4-10}$ in 5 μl of buffered physiological saline 15 min prior to CTA extinction sessions; controls received just the 5 μl of saline. As shown in FIGURE 11, both ACTH and $ACTH_{4-10}$ infused into the CSF prolonged extinction. By the twelfth recovery session, rats in the ACTH and $ACTH_{4-10}$ groups were drinking only 20–30% as much as the saline-infused controls. In comparison with the data from peripheral ACTH administration (FIGURES 9 and 10), intracerebroventricular administration of ACTH and the peptide $ACTH_{4-10}$ produces more dramatic effects on the extinction of CTA.

It appears that ACTH/$ACTH_{4-10}$ are modulating, in some way, the brain circuitry that is reactivated when rats recall memories of the taste/LiCl association. Likely structures for this modulatory influence would include the limbic structures of hippocampus and amygdala. Hippocampal lesions can promote more rapid extinction from CTA[17] and eliminate the conditioned elevation in corticosterone triggered by the consumption of an aversive solution.[18] Amygdala lesions[19] eliminate the ACTH effect on extinction of CTA. ^{14}C-2-deoxyglucose metabolic neural mapping techniques are currently being adapted in my laboratory to characterize CNS structures and pathways involved in CTA acquisition and extinction.

The effectiveness of both DEX and ACTH injections is consistent with measures of pituitary-adrenal activity during the different phases of conditioning. DEX is effective at the time of conditioning, because endogenous pituitary-adrenal activity is high in untreated animals. Since the manipulation studies reported here used animals that had free access to food and water (free extinction), endogenous activity during recovery is low. ACTH injections are effective only when administered during recovery, presumably by elevating plasma levels of ACTH at that time.

The data from studies of pituitary-adrenal manipulation suggest that this system can affect both learning and performance in a CTA paradigm. Our initial interpretation of these data has focused on the importance of elevated levels of ACTH at the time of conditioning. Because a DEX block of ACTH release during illness can reduce the degree of aversion, we have concluded that ACTH participates, in some unspecified manner, in learning that ingestion of some substances may result in illness. This notion is certainly compatible with a reinforcement-memory function hypothesis. In a similar manner, the effects of ACTH injections can be related to the high levels of pituitary-adrenal activity at the time of conditioning. If high ACTH levels act as a salient component of the stimulus complex associated with illness, then treatment of the subjects with ACTH prior to recovery sessions may facilitate the retrieval of memories associated with the aversive event.

The interaction between the DEX and ACTH effects has also been investigated[20] to serve as a test of a "memory-retrieval" hypothesis. A factorial design was employed where four groups of rats received either DEX or ACTH during either conditioning or extinction. An additional group received saline injections throughout conditioning and recovery. The data from this experiment are presented in FIGURE 12. The DEX-DEX group showed an attenuated aversion and the most rapid extinction. The ACTH effect on extinction was shown by the ACTH-ACTH group; they showed prolonged extinction relative to the SAL-SAL controls. The data from DEX-DEX and ACTH-ACTH groups replicate the findings reported earlier in this review. The most interesting result of this experiment is the performance of the animals receiving DEX prior to conditioning and ACTH prior to extinction sessions. The behavior of this group closely paralleled that of the group receiving ACTH throughout and was significantly below that of the group receiving DEX prior to conditioning (DEX-DEX). Treatment with ACTH during extinction was sufficient to overcome the aversion-attenuating effect of the DEX given prior to conditioning.

The behavioral effects of the DEX-ACTH treatment provide one test of the memory-retrieval hypothesis as it relates to the ACTH effect. If ACTH promotes memory retrieval by reinstating some particularly significant stimulus attribute(s) associated with the illness, then animals that received a DEX blockade of ACTH release at the time of illness should not be particularly susceptible to the effects of ACTH injections during recovery. These animals did not experience an elevation of ACTH at the time of conditioning, so that the reinstatement properties of ACTH injections should not be effective and the DEX attenuation of the aversion should have been observed. However, the ACTH injections were effective in reversing the DEX effect upon extinction of the CTA, so that it is more likely that ACTH injections facilitate the retrieval process itself.[21]

The behavior of the DEX-ACTH group also speaks to questions concerning the

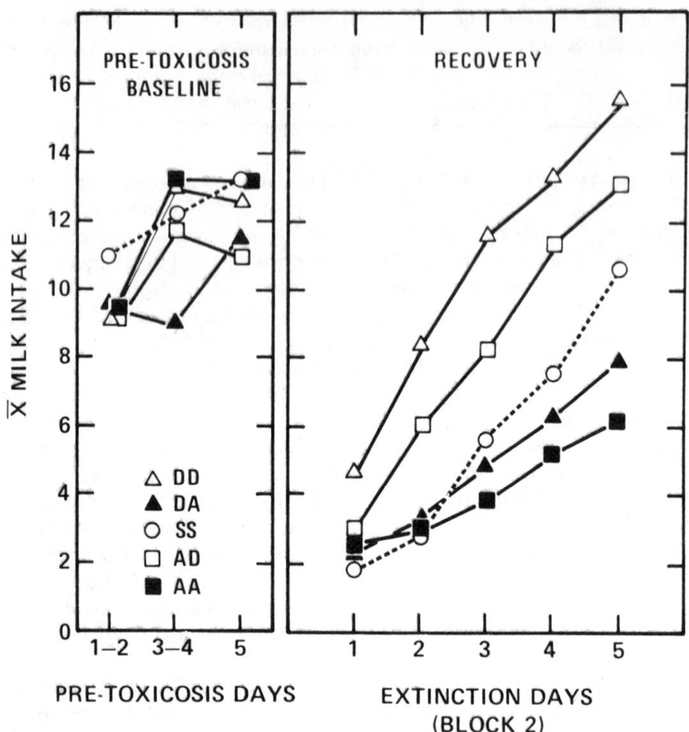

FIGURE 12. Taste aversion acquisition and extinction for groups of rats (N = 8 rats/group) receiving dexamethasone (D), ACTH (A), or saline (S) prior to conditioning and/or extinction trials. (Adapted from Hennessy *et al.*[12] By permission of the publisher.)

nature of the DEX effect upon the conditioning process. While it is quite reasonable to posit that hormonal consequences of conditioning events may serve a reinforcement-memory function, the nature of this process is often difficult to specify. It is possible that the pituitary-adrenal system is involved in the memory consolidation process. For example, Gold and van Buskirk[22] have shown that postsession ACTH injections can enhance or disrupt memory in a dose-dependent fashion. However, the term post-trial memory "consolidation" may refer to a number of events, including the storage of memory (consolidation) and some process that allows the retrieval of the stored memory (cataloging). It has been argued that many experimental manipulations, e.g., electroconvulsive shock, which were thought to affect the storage process may actually be affecting the ability of the animal to retrieve the information in subsequent test situations. The basic data supporting this statement are that a variety of reactivation treatments have been found effective in reversing amnestic effects. Since animals thought to be amnestic can, under some conditions, behave as though the memory had been stored, it is dubious to conclude that a particular treatment alters consolidation.

This logic can also be used when discussing the DEX-ACTH effect upon taste aversion recovery. Because the DEX-ACTH animals are quite capable of showing a normal, or possibly augmented, taste aversion, it is unlikely that DEX treatment disrupts consolidation or memory storage. Rather, it would seem that DEX produces a deficit in the ability to retrieve memories of the taste-illness association upon subsequent presentation of the milk. In this manner, one can relate both the DEX and ACTH effects to memory retrieval processes. This interpretation is also consistent with apparent state-dependent effects exhibited by the ACTH-DEX group in this experiment. The rats experience a shift, in terms of ACTH/corticosterone levels, between training and testing that could produce a decrement in learned performance, i.e., an attenuated aversion. As Spear[21] has pointed out, state-dependent effects of drug, and presumably hormone, administration can be viewed in terms of memory retrieval failure. It would not be surprising, then, to find a state-dependent phenomenon related to the injection of substances that may alter retrieval.

SUMMARY AND CONCLUSIONS

Results of research reported in this paper show that lithium chloride (LiCl) injection causes a marked and prolonged elevation of adrenocorticotropic hormone (ACTH) and corticosterone. Peak elevations occur within 30 min after injection and continue for 60 to 120 min depending upon the molarity of the LiCl solution. CS preexposures do not alter the pituitary-adrenal response to LiCl. Although this response occurs, evidence argues that pituitary-adrenal activity is neither a sufficient nor essential condition for CTA to occur. It is possible that this prolonged ACTH secretion, which would be essential to maintain corticosterone levels elevated for one to two hours, is acting as a component of the unconditioned response associated with LiCl injections.

Under certain types of extinction (forced extinction) the P-A system is activated. Thus, when an animal drinks an aversive solution following deprivation, intake of the solution causes a conditioned elevation of plasma corticosterone.

Two measures of CTA, behavioral and hormonal, do not always coincide with one another. Preexposure to the CS alters both behavioral and corticosterone indices of CTA. These two systems will show either a coupling (e.g., parallel change) or a dissociation depending on the number of preexposures prior to conditioning.

Manipulating the hormones associated with the pituitary-adrenal system also affects the acquisition of CTA and influences extinction. Thus, if one pretests with dexamethasone phosphate (DEX) prior to the administration of LiCl, CTA is attenuated. It would appear that ACTH is involved in the acquisition of CTA since a central block of ACTH also affects the magnitude of the aversion. If ACTH is injected during recovery, animals show a prolonged suppression of drinking. These data appear to be best explained using a memory-retrieval model.

The manipulation of hormones and their effects on CTA appear to follow the effects observed endogenously. Thus, ACTH administered to rats during the conditioning phase does not appear to have any effect upon the learning of the aversion. Since LiCl markedly elevates ACTH, as indicated by prolonged elevations of corticosterone, the additional ACTH given exogenously at the time of conditioning does not appear to add to the effects already attributable to endogenous ACTH. Conversely, DEX given during recovery appears to have no effect upon the recovery function. Because endogenous levels of ACTH are already low during the free extinction procedure, DEX treatment does not appear to further reduce ACTH and has no effect upon recovery.

The effects of ACTH appear to be due to the behaviorally active 4-10 sequence of amino acids of the parent molecule $ACTH_{1-39}$. It is hypothesized that ACTH is functioning in the CNS in a modulatory role to promote retrieval of memories for

TABLE 3. Hormone and Hormone-like Substances Investigated in Relation to Conditioned Taste Aversions and Neophobia

Hormone	Reference	Neophobia	Acquisition	Extinction	Unconditioned Stimulus
Thyrotropin-releasing-releasing hormone (TRH)	23				+
Testosterone	24		–	+	–
Estrogen	24			–	
Alpha-melanocyte stimulating hormone (alpha-MSH)	15, 25			+	–
MSH-release inhibiting hormone	15			–	
Arginine vasopressin (AVP)	26				+
Bombesin	27				–
Calcitonin	28				–
Cholecystokinin (CCK)	29				+
Histamine	30				+
Melatonin	31, 25	+			–
Norepinephrine (NE)	32, 11	+			+
ACTH	*	+	+	+	–
Corticosterone	*			–	–

+ = demonstrated effect, – = no effect, * = presented in the present article.

the taste-illness association. While peripherally administered ACTH has a greater effect than $ACTH_{4-10}$ on extinction, $ACTH_{4-10}$ and ACTH are equally effective in prolonging extinction when administered by intracerebroventricular infusion in microgram amounts.

TABLE 3 presents data on other hormone and hormone-like substances that influence neophobia, CTA acquisition, CTA extinction, or US function. It is evident that the table is incomplete, but the existing entries indicate that a number of the endocrine systems are involved in the establishment and expression of CTA. Clearly, further work is warranted to characterize the range of substances as well as their type(s) of influence.

Finally, it appears that CTA may be especially well suited for the study of pituitary-adrenal hormone influences on behavior. During the free extinction procedure, in which endogenous levels of ACTH and steroids are not elevated, hormone influence(s) upon the extinction of CTA can be studied without concern that endogenous hormone levels will interfere and override the effects of exogenously administered hormones.

REFERENCES

1. GARCIA, J., W. G. HANKINS & K. R. RUSINIAK. 1974. Behavioral regulation of the milieu interne in man and rat. Science **185**: 824–831.
2. LEVINE, S., W. P. SMOTHERMAN & J. W. HENNESSY. 1977. Pituitary-adrenal hormones and learned taste-aversion. *In* Neuropeptide Influences on the Brain and Behavior. L. Miller, C. A. Sandman & A. Kastin, Eds.: 163–177. Raven Press. New York.
3. SMOTHERMAN, W. P., J. W. HENNESSY & S. LEVINE. 1976. Plasma corticosterone levels during recovery from LiCl produced taste aversions. Behav. Biol. **16**: 401–412.
4. SMOTHERMAN, W. P., J. W. HENNESSY & S. LEVINE. 1976. Plasma corticosterone levels as an index of the strength of illness induced taste aversions. Physiol. Behav. **17**: 903–908.
5. ADER, R. 1976. Conditioned adrenocortical steroid elevations in the rat. J. Comp. Physiol. Psychol. **90**(12): 1156–1163.
6. SMOTHERMAN, W. P., A. MARGOLIS & S. LEVINE. 1980. Flavor preexposures in a conditioned taste aversion situation: A dissociation of behavioral and endocrine effects in rats. J. Comp. Physiol. Psychol. **94**: 25–35.
7. BRAVEMAN, N. S. 1977. What studies on preexposure to pharmacological agents tell us about the nature of the aversion-inducing agent. *In* Learning Mechanisms in Food Selection. L. M. Barkler, M. R. Best & M. Domjan, Eds.: 511–532. Baylor University Press. Waco, TX.
8. HART, R. P., G. D. COOVER, A. SHNERSON & W. P. SMOTHERMAN. 1980. Plasma corticosterone in rats in response to consumption of concentrated sugar solutions. J. Comp. Physiol. Psychol. **94**(2): 337–345.
9. COOVER, G. D., G. T. SATTERFIELD, W. P. SMOTHERMAN, D. STEINKE & D. M. DORSA. 1983. Endocrine activation, but not tail flick latency alteration, induced by consumption of concentrated sucrose solution. Soc. Neuro. Abstr. **9**: 1123.
10. SMOTHERMAN, W. P. & S. LEVINE. 1978. ACTH and $ACTH_{4-10}$ modification of neophobia and taste aversion responses in the rat. J. Comp. Physiol. Psychol. **92**(1): 22–33.
11. CAZA, P. A., L. BROWN & N. E. SPEAR. 1982. Epinephrine-induced conditioned taste aversion. Horm. Behav. **16**: 31–45.
12. HENNESSY, J. W., W. P. SMOTHERMAN & S. LEVINE. 1976. Conditioned taste aversion and the pituitary-adrenal system. Behav. Biol. **16**: 413–424.
13. CAIRNIE, A. B. & K. E. LEACH. 1982. Dexamethasone: A potent blocker for radiation-induced taste aversion in rats. Pharm. Biochem. Behav. **17**: 305–311.
14. KENDLER, K., J. W. HENNESSY, W. P. SMOTHERMAN & S. LEVINE. 1976. An ACTH effect on recovery from conditioned taste aversion. Behav. Biol. **17**: 225–229.
15. RIGTER, H. & A. POPPING. 1976. Hormonal influences on the extinction of conditioned taste aversion. Psychopharm. (Berl.) **46**: 255–261.

16. Smotherman, W. P. & S. Levine. 1980. $ACTH_{4-10}$ affects behavior but not plasma corticosterone levels in a conditioned taste aversion situation. Peptides **1**: 207–210.
17. Smotherman, W. P., G. Burt, D. P. Kimble, G. Stickrod, R. Bre Miller & S. Levine. 1981. Hippocampal lesions alter plasma corticosterone elevations and behavior during retention of a conditioned taste aversion. Physiol. Behav. **27**: 569–574.
18. Smotherman, W. P., L. A. Kolp, S. Coyle & S. Levine. 1981. Hippocampal lesion effects on conditioned taste aversion and pituitary-adrenal activity in rats. Behav. Brain Res. **2**: 33–48.
19. Burt, G. & W. P. Smotherman. 1980. Amygdalectomy induced deficits in conditioned taste aversion: Possible pituitary-adrenal involvement. Physiol. Behav. **24**: 651–655.
20. Hennessy, J. W., W. P. Smotherman & S. Levine. 1980. Investigations into the nature of the dexamethasone and ACTH effects upon learned taste aversion. Physiol. Behav. **24**: 645–649.
21. Spear, N. E. 1973. Retrieval of memory in animals. Psychol. Rev. **80**: 163–194.
22. Gold, P. E. & R. B. Van Buskirk. 1976. Enhancement and impairment of memory processes with posttrial injections of adrenocorticotropic hormone. Behav. Biol. **16**: 387–400.
23. Takulis, H. 1983. Thyrotropin-releasing hormone (TRH) potentiates pentobarbital-based flavor aversion learning. Behav. Neural Biol. **39**: 135–139.
24. Chambers, K. 1985. Sexual dimorphisms as an index of hormonal influences on conditioned food aversions. Ann. N.Y. Acad. Sci. (This volume.)
25. Golus, P., R. McGee & M. King. 1981. Melatonin and melanocyte-stimulating hormone (MSH) do not produce conditioned taste aversions. IRCS Med. Sci. **9**: 437.
26. Ettenberg, A., D. Van Der Kooy, M. Le Moal, G. F. Koob & F. E. Bloom. 1983. Can aversive properties of (peripherally-injected) vasopressin account for its putative role in memory? Behav. Brain Res. **7**: 331–350.
27. Deutsch, J. A. 1980. Bombesin: satiety or malaise? Nature **285**: 592.
28. Deutsch, J. A. 1981. Calcitonin: Aversive effects in rats? Science **211**: 733–734.
29. Deutsch, J. A. & W. T. Hardy. 1977. Cholecystokinin produces bait shyness in rats. Nature **266**: 196.
30. Sessions, G. R. 1975. Histamine and radiation-induced taste aversion conditioning. Science **190**: 402–403.
31. Golus, P., R. McGee & M. King. 1979. Attenuation of saccharin neophobia by melatonin. Pharm. Biochem. Behav. **10**: 367–369.
32. Mason, S. T., D. C. S. Roberts & H. C. Fibiger. 1978. Noradrenaline and neophobia. Physiol. Behav. **21**: 353–361.

Neurotransmitter Control of Carbohydrate Consumption

JUDITH J. WURTMAN

Department of Applied Biology
Massachusetts Institute of Technology
Cambridge, Massachusetts 02139

The ability of animals or humans to control their consumption of energy has been recognized for several decades.[1] Considerably less is known about how the intake of specific macronutrients such as protein and carbohydrate is regulated. Although Richter pointed out over 40 years ago that the selection of dietary constituents conducive to normal growth and reproduction was not receiving adequate research attention,[2] studies on feeding behavior still tend to focus largely on the animal's consumption of calories rather than of macronutrients. Food consumption is regarded as motivated solely by the individual's need for energy. Although the roles of protein, carbohydrate, and fat in the body have been described and the daily needs for these nutrients established, the ability of the animal to control its intake of these nutrients independent of its consumption of energy is usually not examined. This lack of attention to the regulation of macronutrient intake is due in part to the way that feeding experiments are designed. Traditionally, such experiments are carried out by manipulating the animal's hunger and measuring its consumption of a single test diet containing macronutrients in a fixed ratio (chow, for example). Although the animal's hunger for calories can be measured by this method, what cannot be measured is its hunger for specific macronutrients. The animal is unable to modify its intake of one macronutrient without also modifying proportionately its intake of the other two. Thus, if an experimental treatment has changed the animal's hunger for say, protein, there is no way that the animal can demonstrate this change.

A new paradigm that enables the investigator to distinguish between an animal's ingestion of a specific nutrient for its nutritive value or for its caloric value was developed recently by Musten *et al.*[3] Animals were allowed to choose their foods from a pair of diets whose calorie contents were identical but which contained different amounts of the macronutrient being examined. This type of feeding experiment has demonstrated separate regulations of protein[3] and carbohydrate[4,5] independent of calorie consumption.

Our interest in studying carbohydrate intake stemmed from earlier studies showing that the synthesis and release of brain serotonin are dependent on the relative proportions of carbohydrate and protein consumed in the previous meal.[6,7] When a carbohydrate-rich, protein-poor meal is consumed, major changes occur in the pattern of amino acids in the plasma. This is brought about by the action of insulin: the pancreatic hormone facilitates the uptake of most of the amino acids into tissues like skeletal muscle. The levels of plasma tryptophan, the amino acid precursor to serotonin, do not fall, and the ratio of plasma tryptophan to the plasma concentrations of the other large neutral amino acids (LNAA), leucine, isoleucine, valine, tyrosine, and phenylalanine, rises markedly. This ratio is critical in determining the concentration of tryptophan within the brain,[6,7] because all the LNAA are carried competitively by a single transport system into the brain. Thus this insulin-mediated fall in the other LNAA elevates brain tryptophan levels[6,7] and subsequently the synthesis and release of serotonin increase.

However, if the meal consumed is, instead, rich in protein, a similar increase in the ratio of plasma tryptophan to LNAA does not occur.[6,7] Although tryptophan levels rise, so do the levels of the other LNAA. Since the relative proportion of tryptophan to the other LNAA in protein is small (tryptophan constituting only about 1 to 1.5% of the amino acid content of protein) the actual plasma tryptophan/LNAA ratio falls in response to protein ingestion. Brain tryptophan and serotonin levels show a similar decline.

When animals are allowed to choose their daily food intake from two diets that differ in their content of carbohydrate but not calories or protein, they choose among the two food dishes so as to obtain a desired proportion of carbohydrate. This amount is independent of the sweetness of the carbohydrate being tested.[4,5] Serotonin-releasing neurons appear to be involved in regulating this food choice. When animals are treated with any of a large number of drugs that act at different loci to enhance serotonin-mediated neurotransmission, they specifically decrease their consumption of a diet high in carbohydrate but not of a diet considerably lower.[4,5,8] Moreover when rats are given a carbohydrate-rich pre-meal containing sufficient carbohydrate to elevate brain serotonin levels and increase its release, the animals respond by consuming a lower proportion of carbohydrate to protein in the subsequent meal. Their calorie intake, however, is the same as that of control rats given a pre-meal of the same caloric value that contains protein as well as carbohydrate.[9]

Conversely, dietary manipulations (like the chronic consumption of a carbohydrate-poor diet) that diminish the plasma tryptophan/LNAA ratio and thus reduce brain tryptophan and serotonin levels, sharply elevate the proportion of carbohydrate that the animal subsequently eats when it is given the opportunity to consume this nutrient.[9]

It seems likely that humans also regulate the proportion of protein to carbohydrate in their daily diet, especially since national nutrition surveys indicate relatively constant intakes of these nutrients.[10,11] We extended our studies on a specific appetite for carbohydrate to human subjects, especially those who described themselves as having a strong urge to snack on carbohydrate foods. A pilot study with subjects who were normal in weight was done first.[12] (In this and the subsequent human studies to be described, all volunteers signed consent forms that had been formally approved by the MIT Committee on Use of Humans as Experimental Subjects and by the Clinical Research Center Committee, which oversees studies on human volunteers.)

Eleven subjects participated in this first study as outpatients. They kept a record of their meal and snack food consumption for eight days. All of the subjects consumed 60% or more of their snacks as high-carbohydrate foods and they ate these snacks at very specific rather than random times of day or night.

Subsequently they were asked to restrict their carbohydrate snack intake to a prechosen high-carbohydrate food (such as crackers or candy) and to eat only this snack food during the four-hour period when their cravings tended to be most intense. They were with treated DL-fenfluramine (20 mg; a drug that releases serotonin into synapses), tryptophan (1 g; serotonin's precursor), and their placebo in a double-blind crossover schedule. Each treatment period lasted five days and was followed by a five-day washout period. The designated pills were taken one hour before the onset of the snack period, and the subjects recorded the number of snacks they ate. Fenfluramine reduced significantly the number of carbohydrate snacks consumed by the group as a whole; tryptophan lacked a significant group effect but did reduce snack intake in three of the subjects.

As this pilot study revealed that some individuals have a definite need to snack on high-carbohydrate foods and that this need seems to involve brain serotonin, it seemed possible that this need might be exaggerated in some obese people and might account for their excess calorie intake. This possibility seemed even more likely because of the abundance of anecdotal reports from obese subjects who claimed that their failure to lose weight or maintain weight loss was due to their inability to control their carbohydrate intake.

A second clinical study[13] was designed to see whether obese adults who consider themselves carbohydrate cravers would indeed snack preferentially on high-carbohydrate foods if allowed 24-hour access to an assortment of isocaloric carbohydrate-rich and protein-rich foods. We predicted that if these obese individuals suffered from a general inability to control their calorie intake, i.e., consumed too much food regardless of its nutrient content, then they would consume, indiscriminately, both the protein-rich and carbohydrate-rich snack foods. However, if their hunger for carbohydrates was specific, then they should snack primarily on the carbohydrate-rich foods and ignore the others. Finally, we allowed the subjects to choose from a variety of both sweet and non-sweet carbohydrate snacks to observe whether there was a particular preference for only sweet carbohydrates among the obese.

The study lasted four weeks and was conducted on an inpatient basis. A controlled but non-hospital like environment was created by using a floor of an unoccupied MIT dormitory during the summer. A variety of on-campus educational, crafts, athletic, and social activities were available to the subjects; however, they could not be away from the study facility for more than 90 minutes at a time.

Subjects were allowed no choice of foods at meals; the daily menu provided about 1000 calories and the required daily nutrients. Since this was below the usual calorie intake of the subjects, they were encouraged to snack freely from ten isocaloric protein-rich and carbohydrate-rich snack foods, i.e., potato chips, bagel and cream cheese, chocolate candies, a chocolate or cranberry muffin, ham and cheese, meatball, salami and cheese, barbecued pork chops, and miniature frankfurters. (The fat contents of the snacks were similar so that if the subjects had a preference for high-fat foods, no consistent pattern of snack choice would be seen.) Snacking was encouraged by insisting that the subjects maintain their weight and preventing them from dieting until the completion of the study. The snacks were dispensed in a refrigerated vending machine operated by a microcomputer. Subjects gained access to the snacks by typing a personal code that opened up all doors of the vending machine. Once a snack was removed, the computer recorded its calorie and protein or carbohydrate content, the name of the subject who took it, and the time of day.

Twenty-three subjects completed this study. The first two weeks were used to obtain baseline food intake information and the second, to test the effect of administration of DL-fenfluramine (15 or 20 mg/dose), L-tryptophan (800 mg/dose), or placebo, three times a day.

The group consumed significantly more carbohydrate than protein snacks per day (4.1 ± 0.4 vs. 0.8 ± 0.3). No consistent pattern in their choice of sweet or starchy snacks was observed; indeed the sweet chocolate cupcake initially provided was found to be too "sweet" and was replaced with the cranberry muffin. As with our normal weight subjects, these volunteers also consumed their snacks at very characteristic times of the day or evening and also tended to eat a relatively constant number of snacks a day.

Fenfluramine reduced their carbohydrate snack intake significantly while tryptophan decreased carbohydrate snack intake among three of the six subjects in its treatment group.

It was not possible to measure the voluntary choice of nutrients at meals among these carbohydrate cravers because meal choices were fixed in this study. Thus a third clinical study was carried out to determine whether obese carbohydrate snackers would choose a high proportion of carbohydrate to protein at meals as well as snacks. This inpatient study was shorter and conducted at the MIT Clinical Research Center. [14] Subjects spent two days a week for four consecutive weeks at the Center. They were admitted on the evening before the first baseline day of the study and food intake measurements were made over the subsequent 48 hours. D-Fenfluramine (15 mg at 7 a.m. and 4 p.m.) or its placebo was administered for eight days in a double-blind crossover schedule. Food intake was measured in the Clinical Research Center on days 1, 7, and 8 of each treatment period and subjects were allowed to live at home during days 2-6. To determine how much protein and carbohydrate the obese carbohydrate-craving subject would choose to eat from both meals and snacks, a variety of isocaloric high-carbohydrate and high-protein foods was offered at meals. As in the second study, five isocaloric protein and five isocaloric carbohydrate snacks were dispensed in a computer-driven vending machine. (Fat was added as an ingredient to make the foods isocaloric; there is no information as to whether or not appetite for fat is also regulated.) The choice of foods provided at each meal remained the same throughout the study to minimize the possible effects of novelty. The foods represented those commonly eaten in this geographical area. Three high-protein and three high-carbohydrate foods were offered at every meal. They were served in small preweighed containers and several of each item were available for each subject. Subjects took what they wanted to eat on their trays; when they left the dining room, the containers on their trays were weighed. (Dinner choices were for example: scalloped potatoes, Spanish rice, macaroni with garlic butter sauce, chicken a la king, beef Stroganoff, and baked haddock.)

The results of this study pointed out significant differences between the nutrient choices made at mealtimes and as snacks (TABLE 1).[14] The subjects, as in previous studies, ate only the carbohydrate-rich foods as snacks in the same proportions as found previously. However, their choices of meal foods were quite different. Contrary to our expectations, they ate similar amounts of protein and carbohydrate at meals. Their carbohydrate intake (about 120 g from meals) would be considered moderate by U.S. standards of food intake and their protein intake (about 104 g from meals) slightly high. Clearly, the overconsumption of carbohydrate claimed by our subjects was true only of their snack intake; their choice of nutrients at meals does not reflect any abnormality in the pattern of nutrient choice.

Although D-fenfluramine is known to have general anorectic effects, it did not depress appetite for meals and for snack foods to the same degree. D-Fenfluramine caused our subjects to decrease their intake at meals by 16% and their calories from snacks by 41%. This selective effect on food intake was also seen in the choice of nutrients; D-fenfluramine significantly reduced carbohydrate intake from meals but did not have a significant effect on decreasing mealtime protein intake. (Our subjects ate too few protein snacks to assess the effects of D-fenfluramine on protein intake from snack foods.) These results suggest that the need to snack on carbohydrate and the consumption of carbohydrate and protein at meals may be motivated by different regulatory mechanisms. Perhaps the desire to consume a certain proportion of carbohydrate to protein at meals involves a regulatory mechanism concerned with maintaining adequate nutrient intake, while the desire to consume carbohydrate snacks unaccompanied by any protein in the mid-afternoon or evening reflects the brain's "desire" for serotonin, unrelated to the body's nutritional needs. The release of serotonin is known to increase drowsiness, to facilitate the onset of sleep, and to diminish pain sensitivity.[15] Moreover, carbohydrate consumption in the afternoon as opposed

TABLE 1. Effect of D-Fenfluramine on Meal and Snack Consumption

	Meals			Snacks		
	Calories	Protein (g)	Carbohydrate (g)	Calories	Protein (number/day)	Carbohydrate
Placebo	1940	104	121	707	0.7	5.8
D-Fenfluramine	1630[a]	93	94[a]	414[a]	0.5	3.4[a]
% Reduction	16	10	23	41	28	41

Twenty obese carbohydrate-craving subjects received D-fenfluramine (15 mg/kg, twice daily) or a placebo for consecutive eight-day periods. Food choice was measured on days one, seven, and eight of each. Subjects chose from among six isocaloric foods at meals and from among ten foods for snacks; half of the foods available at any time were rich in protein and half were rich in carbohydrate.

[a] $p < 0.01$ differs from placebo group.

to the morning has been shown, recently, to increase feelings of calmness and relaxation and drowsiness among 184 normal men and women.[16] Protein consumption had no such effects. Thus it is possible that these changes in mood states reflect an increase in brain serotonin synthesis and release after carbohydrate consumption.

Most antidepressant drugs, moreover, share with dietary carbohydrates the propensity to enhance serotonin-mediated neurotransmission (either by blocking serotonin's intracellular metabolism by monoamine oxidase or by suppressing its reuptake into the presynaptic terminals that release it). The subgroup of obese people who claim to be carbohydrate cravers may, in reality, consume carbohydrate snacks for their psychopharmacologic effects.

If this proves to be so (studies to measure the effects of consuming a protein or carbohydrate meal on mood in this population are under way), then measures used to assist the obese carbohydrate craver to reduce should take into account this pharmacological-like need to consume carbohydrates. Reserving a specific number of carbohydrate calories to be consumed as a snack food at the appropriate time of day or evening may be the most effective therapy in producing weight loss in this population. It will also be of interest to see whether supplemental tryptophan can replace the need to snack on carbohydrate, especially since the tryptophan/LNAA plasma ratio tends to be abnormally low in obese people (possibly as a consequence of peripheral insulin resistance).[17] Certainly avoidance of carbohydrate-rich foods would be an inappropriate weight loss therapy for this group of carbohydrate cravers: recent evidence suggests that a protein-rich, carbohydrate-poor diet, with which many obese people are treated, further lowers the tryptophan/LNAA ratio.[17] Regardless of which type of treatment is used, the type of overeating that defines the obese individual must first be identified. No longer can it be assumed that obesity is caused by a simple indiscriminate overconsumption of calories, regardless of the food source. Hungers for specific nutrients do exist and so too, abnormalities in regulating their consumption.

REFERENCES

1. KISSILEFF, H. & T. VAN ITALLIE. 1982. Physiology of the control of food intake. Ann. Rev. Nutr. **2**: 371-418.
2. RICHTER, C., L. HOLT & B. BARELARE. 1938. Nutritional requirements for normal growth and reproduction in rats studied by the self-selection method. Am. J. Physiol. **122**: 734-744.
3. MUSTEN, B.,D. PEACE & G.H. ANDERSON.1974. Food intake regulation in the weanling rat: self selection of protein and energy. J. Nutr. **104**: 563-572.
4. WURTMAN, J.J. & R.J. WURTMAN. 1979. Fenfluramine and other serotoninergic drugs depress food intake and carbohydrate consumption while sparing protein consumption. Curr. Med. Res. Opin. **6**: 28-33.
5. WURTMAN, J.J. & R.J. WURTMAN. 1979. Drugs that enhance central serotoninergic transmission diminish elective carbohydrate consumption by rats. Life Sci. **24**: 895-904.
6. FERNSTROM, J.D. & R.J. WURTMAN. 1972. Brain serotonin content: Increase following ingestion of carbohydrate diet. Science **174**: 1023-1025.
7. FERNSTROM, J.D., R.J. WURTMAN, B. HAMMERSTROM-WIKLUND, W.M. RAND, H.N. MUNRO & C.S. DAVIDSON. 1979. Diurnal variations in plasma concentrations of tryptophan, tyrosine and other neutral amino acids: effect of dietary protein intake. Am. J. Clin. Nutr. **32**: 1912-1922.
8. MOSES, P. & R.J. WURTMAN. 1985. The ability of certain anorexic drugs to suppress food consumption depends on the nutrient composition of the test diet. Life Sci. (In press.)
9. WURTMAN, J.J., P. MOSES & R.J. WURTMAN. 1983. Prior carbohydrate consumption affects the amount of carbohydrate that rats choose to eat. J. Nutr. **113**: 70-78.
10. CENTER FOR DISEASE CONTROL. 1972. Ten-State Nutrition Survey 1968-1970. DHEW pub-

lication no. (HSM) 72-8132, 72-8133. Health Services and Mental Health Administration, Washington, D.C.

11. NATIONAL CENTER FOR HEALTH STATISTICS. 1975. Preliminary findings of the first health and nutrition examination survey. United States 1971-1972. DHEW publication no. (HRA) 76-1229-1. Health Resources Administration. Washington, D.C.
12. WURTMAN, J.J. & R.J. WURTMAN 1981. Suppression of carbohydrate consumption as snacks and at mealtime by dl-fenfluramine or tryptophan. *In* Anorectic Agents: Mechanisms of Actions and of Tolerance. S. Garattini, Ed.: 169-182. Raven Press. New York.
13. WURTMAN, J.J., R.J. WURTMAN, J. GROWDON, P. HENRY, A. LIPSCOMB & S. ZEISEL. 1981. Carbohydrate craving in obese people: suppression by treatments affecting serotoninergic transmission. Int. J. Eating Disorders **1**: 2-11.
14. WURTMAN, J.J., R.J. WURTMAN, S. MARK, R. TSAY, W. GILBERT & J. GROWDON.1985. D-fenfluramine selectively suppresses carbohydrate snacking among obese carbohydrate craving subjects. Intl. J. Eating Disorders. (In press.)
15. WURTMAN, R.J. & J.J. WURTMAN. 1984. Nutrients, neurotransmitter synthesis and the control of food intake. *In* Eating and Its Disorders. A. Stunkard & E. Stellar, Eds.: 77-86. Raven Press. New York.
16. SPRING, B.,O. MALLER, J.J. WURTMAN, L. DIGMAN & L. COZOLINO. 1983. Effects of protein and carbohydrate meals on mood and performance interactions with sex and age. J. Psychiatr. Res. **17**: 155-167.
17. HERAIEF, E.,P. BURCKHARDT, C. MAURON, J.J. WURTMAN & R.J. WURTMAN. 1983. The treatment of obesity by carbohydrate deprivation suppresses plasma tryptophan and its ratio to other large neutral amino acids. J. Neural Transm. **57**: 187-195.

PART III. COMPARATIVE APPROACHES TO LEARNING, FORAGING, AND TOXIPHOBIA

Introduction: Conditioned Taste Aversion – Function and Mechanism

GEORGE H. COLLIER

Psychology Department
Rutgers University
New Brunswick, New Jersey 08903

The two prototypic models of learning, originally developed by Pavlov and by Thorndike, have endured without substantial modification since they were first advanced. Each model was developed within the framework of a specific situation: the salivation of a hungry dog receiving food in the presence of a distinctive stimulus and the escape of a hungry cat from a puzzle box to feed. The original situations have been elaborated and diversified to account for the variety and complexity of the effects of experience on behavior, but the basic paradigms have remained unchanged. These models present a reductionistic view of acquired behavior; that is, both assume that all learned behavior can be accounted for in terms of response strengthening, shaping, and chaining. Further, they assume that responses, unconditioned stimuli, and reinforcers can be described in physical language[1] without recourse to psychological and biological meaning. These models are assumed to be universal, holding for all instances of learning. They leave little room for the interaction of phylogeny with experience. Added to these models was the philosophy of the refinement experiment,[2] which argues that simple laws are discovered by reducing to the minimum the number of response possibilities and environmental stimuli affecting the phenomenon under study. Thus, the situations in which classical and instrumental conditioning were investigated were highly simplified and very different from those in which an animal might find itself in its niche. As a result investigators seldom asked to what use the acquired skills might be put. The unquestioned assumption was that understanding behavior in simple situations would generalize to complex ones. Unfortunately, this has not proven to be the case.

One of the first of a number of threats to these assumptions was the discovery of conditioned taste aversions. Here, both the time parameters and the rules of association of classical conditioning were violated. However, the usefulness of such a skill in an animal's avoidance of potentially noxious or toxic substances led to its eventual acceptance, even though this kind of functional criterion had not previously been invoked in support of learning models. These findings led to the concept of biological constraints on learning.[3] An earlier threat to the classical models, for the most part unnoticed, resulted from the work of the Brelands.[4] They discovered that the conditionability of responses or response patterns was species- and situation-specific. The strain on the classical learning models was further increased by the discovery of autoshaping[5] and species-specific defense reactions.[6] A potentially much greater challenge for classical models of learning, however, looms on the horizon in the form of behavioral ecology. This emerging field, stimulated by the theory of evolution, asks questions about function rather than mechanism. Recent findings developed in this framework suggest that it may not be possible to encompass the variety of ways that animals benefit from experience within the classical learning models. Each of the papers discussed below takes, to a greater or lesser degree, this functional point of view.

Let us first consider Bronstein's analysis of the behavior of the Siamese fighting fish (*Betta splendens*), whose behavior has long been thought of as controlled by social reinforcement. Consider the male fish's problem: intra-specific competition for a scarce resource, gravid females. This competition is conventional[7] or surrogate rather than direct. The male fish establishes a territory, builds a nest, and patrols for intruders of either sex. This behavior bears an immediate cost and a potential reproductive benefit. Consider next the problem of a male intruder. Competing with the resident male for ownership of the territory may yield a benefit in the form of capturing the territory and the possibility of courting females, but it also incurs costs in terms of energy, time, and potential injury. According to Bronstein, the function of the display behavior and abortive combat is to provide estimates of the fighting potential for both combatants. The decision either to stay or cut and run is based on these estimates. Conventional combat makes the breeding benefit less expensive; that is, the animal can optimally allocate its time and effort and minimize risk of injury. Following Bronstein's argument, the interpretation of this assessment-behavior in terms of reinforcement of aggressive behavior is an artifact of the testing situation; display and fighting are elicited by the constrained proximity of the test situation that the fish cannot escape. If this analysis is correct, there is no reinforcement, but one can still ask about learning. That is, how should one regard the assessment of combat potential? That is, how do the fish learn the values of the important variables—size, vigor of display, ownership of a territory, etc.? Is this learning? If so, what kind of learning is it?

The second paper, by Brower and Fink, poses a different problem: the decision to eat or not to eat made by a foraging predator. Again the setting is the animal's niche. Here, the predator is faced with reluctant prey that have evolved many different defense strategies, one of which is becoming emetic by consuming certain plants. The predator must distinguish between a succulent and nauseating prey. Because the prey is an important resource and because the amount of emetic gained from the plants varies among prey strains, among anatomical loci within the prey, and across habitats, it is not cost/benefit-effective for the predator species to use a simple avoidance rule (e.g. don't eat monarch butterflies) stored in the nervous system. Rather, each individual must acquire information abut the specific prey type to be avoided. This type of information acquisition is different from that reported by Bronstein. It is direct (the animal experiences emesis) not conventional (not a surrogate of emesis); it is stable not transitory; and it involves complex discriminations between prey types and prey parts. However, information is necessary in both cases to exploit a resource. Brower and Fink propose that the prey choice problem they study is a member of the class of conditioned taste aversions. Is this membership veridical or only analogous? The predator is "programmed" to pursue and consume butterflies, and it is apparently programmed to use many methods of learning to avoid noxious prey, e.g. observational learning, social transmission of preferences, etc. The extent to which this type of learning is species-specific[8] or is a case of conditioned taste aversion sharing the same mechanism studied in rats is still an open question.

Our third author, Shettleworth, after briefly reviewing song learning in birds and spatial learning in rats, brings to our attention a different resource-exploitation problem requiring information acquisition and storage. Resource availability and abundance fluctuate, and animals have evolved a number of strategies to buffer these fluctuations. Storage is an obvious one. Many animals assemble hoards of food at their nest sites that provide both short- and long-term buffering of resource fluctuations. Birds use their crops to store food for their nocturnal fast or for longer periods of scarcity.[9-11] Other animals use mouth pouches, and many carnivores[12] and ruminants[13] can store large reserves in their stomachs. Finally animals can store energy in their adipose tissue,[14] protein in their muscles, and minerals in their bones.[15] Shettleworth reviews a somewhat different storage mechanism in which small passerine birds store food in their environment by caching. During times of abundant resources, these birds will cache food in a number of different locations to which they subsequently return. This behavior requires an astounding ability to discover and remember a large number of cache sites. For some of the birds studied this is a short-term (daily) process, and for others, a long-term (seasonal) process. Here we have, at least at first glance, a different type of learning and forgetting. Neither of the conventional models seems to encompass these processes. There is no obvious conventional reinforcer, no simple association between stimuli, and no extinction. Is it learning? If so what kind?

The fourth paper, by Galef, discusses the social transmission of information, defined as the process by which the experience of one animal influences the behavior of a second. The paradigm discussed in detail in this paper involves a "demonstrator" rat and an "observer" rat. The demonstrator is given experience with one of a set of foods differing in sensory quality. The observer rat is then exposed to the demonstrator and subsequently given a choice of the set of foods. The relative amounts eaten of the different foods is determined. The results show that the observer rat prefers the food eaten by the demonstrator. Galef and his co-workers have explored both the route by which information is transmitted and its content. It seems that, at least in the case of the rat, minimal information is actually transmitted. Neither the consequences of the food for the demonstrator, nutritious or toxic, nor any information the demonstrator has acquired about the food's location, availability, or abundance appears to be passed along. Furthermore, the demonstrator does not act as a herald; rather, he seems to be passive in his role as an informer. What the observer appears to acquire is merely a transitory fondness for the food just eaten by the demonstrator when offered a choice. Barnett[16] and later Calhoun[17] also noted the fondness of rats for eating socially. Thus, the rat's capacities for social transmission of information in this situation appear to be at the low end of the spectrum of possible information transmission. As Galef points out, some birds are capable of acquiring an aversion by observation of a conspecific made sick by consuming an adulterated food, and the capacity of the eusocial honey bee to transmit location, quality, and abundance of a food source to her fellow foragers by her highly choreographed dance is an example of an even more complex process in this same realm.

Once again one might ask about the function of this preference. In spite of the rat's long association with humans and its economic and public health importance, the investigation of function is hampered by a lack of a detailed natural history of the rat.[18,19] The Norway rat is a colonial species and a generalist omnivore whose tastes run to human food. According to Canby[20] they consume over 20% of all the food grown. Many animals forage in groups as a way of optimizing the discovery of food,[21] but rats appear to use a strategy similar to that of the honey bees (albeit without their elaborate social structure, division of labor, and the resulting efficiency), in which the information gained from a solo foraging bout about food availability is transmitted to colony members. These sketchy and possibly questionable facts provide a hint of the possible function of social information transfer. This phenomenon of social transmission of the availability of a food appears to be a "prewired" phylogenetic mechanism that (may) improves the foraging efficiency of a rat colony.

Let us return to the question of how this modification of preference by the experience of a conspecific fits into the classical learning models. It is clearly not instrumental since there is no differential consequence. It is also difficult to force this phenomenon into the classical conditioning mode. There is a superficial similarity in that some sensory aspect of the demonstrator rat (US?) resulting from the ingestion of a specific food elicits eating of that food (CR?) in the observer rat. Two aspects of this process differ from the more mechanical character of the typical classical conditioning paradigm. First, the eliciting stimuli, the sensory properties of the demonstrator, are dependent upon what the demonstrator has just eaten. Second, the food eaten, that is the choice of food, is dependent upon the eliciting stimulus. The CR in classical conditioning is usually an autonomic response; choice is not.

Our fifth and final paper by Rozin and Zellner poses the most intractable problem of all: What controls human food intake? Rozin and Zellner approach this problem not with a functional analysis but from the point of culture and classical conditioning. They distinguish between liking-disliking and preference. They ask how previously neutral stimuli (foods) acquire either tendency (liking or disliking) and answer the question in terms of classical conditioning. The US acquires its associative strength either through phylogeny (e.g., sweet tastes) or through culture. The latter is presumably a form of higher-order conditioning, which at best is a relatively weak process. This conjecture is a programmatic hypothesis. However, few data have been gathered either to support or contradict it.

Methodologically, feeding has been central to the study of learning within both the classical and the instrumental paradigms. How might we reconsider Rozin and Zellner's problem within the functional context used by the first four authors?

The basic problem for any animal is to acquire the appropriate number of calories, the right mix of macronutrients (protein, fat, and carbohydrate) within a specific feeding cycle (e.g., 24 hr) and, over a longer time span, the right mix of micronutrients. At a first approximation the requirements are the same for all animals; the originality has come in terms of how these requirements are met. Animals can be arranged along trophic levels, i.e., herbivores, omnivores, carnivores; along the specialist-generalist dimension, i.e. diet breadth; and along the dimension of digestive-selective strategies. Where do humans fit into this three-dimensional space? Apparently, the most recent, rapid evolution of hominoids occurred during the late Pleistocene age. They hunted big game, ate mostly meat, and fed opportunistically. Their variable frequency and size of meals was buffered by storage, both physiological storage (adipose tissue) and by cultural storage (caches and hoards).[18] These considerations suggest a carnivorous biology that requires little in the way of diet choice since meat is of high, constant caloric density and is a good quality protein. However, in the post-Pleistocene era, the human diet became more catholic and, following the invention of agriculture, broader still. On the specialist-generalist dimension, humans surely are the ultimate generalists. They seem to have occupied almost every habitat and to have used any biological substance as food.

With regard to the digestive-selective strategies, many animals (e.g., herbivores) eat poor foods, low in caloric density and containing imbalanced amino acid and mineral ratios. By post-ingestive fermentation and selective absorption these animals can improve their diet. These strategies involve a large digestive cost: They require both the ingestion of large amounts of food as well as an intensive digestive effort. Typically, such animals have complex and/or long GI tracts. An alternative is to be selective, picking and choosing among various food items in such a fashion as to compose a calorically adequate and balanced diet. Here the costs are in the search for and discovery of the various food items and in the choosing among the quantitatively and qualitatively different items. Digestive effort is relatively low as reflected in the short, simple GI tracts of such animals. These two strategies have been discussed for herbivorous primates in an excellent, recent book by Milton.[23]

If one can judge by gut length and complexity, humans are found at the selective end of this dimension. Thus for humans we have the picture of a selective generalist, ex-carnivore. To be a generalist who occupies a wide range of habitats and eats a wide range of foods differing in caloric density and quality requires a phylogenetically acquired library of dietary rules, a buffered but sensitive physiological feedback system that eventuates in an experientally acquired library of dietary rules, or a culturally acquired library of dietary rules. It should be noted that the feedback loop in the last system is very long. Humans probably employ a mix of the above strategies. It seems likely that their niche requires choices among a very wide variety of potential food items in such a fashion as to compose a calorically sufficient, balanced diet with little help from phylogeny. That is, humans must benefit from either individual and/or cultural experience.

Two questions arise. First, how stringent are human dietary requirements? Second, how successful are they in meeting these requirements? A satisfactory answer to these questions is not available. Some older studies suggest that humans are competent at selecting diets. On the other hand, if one believes the current concerns about diets, the answer to the second question would be "poorly." Yet with the exception of certain areas where resources are restricted in quantity and/or quality, most people and cultures appear to thrive. Somehow they are composing an adequate diet. How? This most interesting problem has received little attention. Rozin and Zellner suggest a mechanism by which cultural rules become likes and dislikes. This difficult task is assigned to higher-order classical conditioning. However the question of whether individual or cultural rules, in appropriate settings, result in a calorically sufficient, balanced diet, or whether there are other strategies by which a good diet is achieved is not asked. What is lacking are good field studies of the pattern of amounts and kinds of different nutrients humans consume and the extent to which a "good" diet is achieved. More is known about the unsuccessful, i.e., malnourished populations than the successful.

Finally, because the theme of this conference is conditioned taste aversions, let us see if we can place acquired ingestive behaviors mediated by taste, olfaction, and vision into the functional framework. Plants and animals have interacted over the millenia. Pollination and seed dispersal are two of their shared activities. Here the plant offers energy (carbohydrates or fat) or protein as an attractant and the animal provides pollination and/or seed dispersal in return. On the other hand, plants are the reluctant prey of herbivores. As a result they have evolved a plethora of defense mechanisms that include toxic or noxious secondary compounds produced by diversion and modification of some of their metabolic products. The specificity, complexity, and economics of these interactions form a subject matter in and of themselves.[24,25] The animal, in order to ameloriate, avoid, or exploit these plant-animal interactions, must be able to detect by one or another of its sensory systems both the consequences of consuming a plant and the source of the consequences. Some of these problems have been solved phylogenetically, but some must be solved ontogenetically. It is to this problem that animals devote a large part of their visual, gustatory, and olfactory activity and the central representations of these systems. The variety of these interactions and the kinds of information acquisition and, in some cases, forgetting, that they require suggest that the two, current, simple models of how animals benefit from experience are insufficient and inadequate. Both are based on highly simplified situations and pose problems to the animal that are selected by the experimenter rather than by Mother Nature. Selection pressure may dictate similar solutions to similar problems, but it does not necessarily require similar mechanisms for similar solutions.

Historically, psychologists and biologists have been preoccupied with mechanism in studies of how animals profit from experience. Only the future will tell whether this preoccupation has obscured our ultimate understanding of the problems that animals face as well as their solutions. Perhaps we should discover the problem before we propose the solution.

REFERENCES

1. Carnap, R. 1934. The Unity of Science. *In* Psyche Miniatures. London.
2. Collier, G. H. 1982. Determinants of choice. *In* The Nebraska Symposium on Motivation. D. J. Bernstein, Ed. University of Nebraska Press. Lincoln.
3. Hinde, R. A. & J. Stevenson-Hinde, Eds. 1973. Constraints on Learning. Academic Press. London.
4. Breland, K. & M. Breland, 1961. Animal Behavior. MacMillan. New York.
5. Brown, G. & H. M. Jenkins. 1968. Autoshaping of the pigeon's keypeck. J. Exp. Anal. Behav. **11**: 1–8.
6. Bolles, R. C. 1970. Species-specific defense reactions and avoidance learning. Psychol. Rev. **77**: 32–48.
7. Wynne-Edwards, V. C. 1962. Animal Dispersion in Relation to Social Behavior. Oliver Boyd. Edinburgh.
8. Zahorik, D. M. & K. A. Houpt. 1977. The concept of nutritional wisdom: Applicability of laboratory learning models to large herbivores. *In* Learning Mechanisms in Food Selection. L. M. Barker, M. R. Best & M. Domjan, Eds. 45–67. Baylor University Press. Waco, TX.
9. Griminger, P. W., V. Villamil & H. Fisher. 1969. The meal eating response of the chicken: Species differences and the role of partial starvation. J. Nutr. **99**: 368–374.
10. Richardson, A. J. 1970. The role of the crop in the feeding behavior of the domestic chicken. Anim. Behav. **18**: 633–639.
11. Ziseiler, V. S. & D. S. Farner. 1972. Digestion and the digestive system. *In* Avian Biology. D. S. Farner & J. R. King, Eds. **2**: 343–430. Academic Press. New York.
12. Schaller, G. B. 1972. The Serengeti Lion: A Study of Predator—Prey Relations. University of Chicago Press. Chicago.
13. Bell, R. H. V. 1971. A grazing system in the Serengeti. Sci. Am. **225**: 86–93.
14. Dawson, W., R. L. Marsh & M. Yacoe. 1983. Metabolic adjustments of small passerine birds for migration and cold. Am. J. Physiol. (Regulatory Integrative Comp. Physiol.) **245**: R755–R767.
15. Belovsky, G. E. 1978. Diet optimization in a generalist herbivore: The moose. Theor. Pop. Biol. **14**: 105–134.
16. Barnett, S. A. 1963. The Rat: A Study in Behavior. Aldine. Chicago.
17. Calhoun, J. B. 1963. The Ecology and Sociology of the Norway Rat. Public Health Service Publication 1008. U. S. Government Printing Office. Washington, D.C.
18. Richter, C. P. 1968. Experiences of a reluctant rat-catcher. The common Norway rat-friend or enemy? Proc. Phil. Soc. **112**: 403–415.
19. Richter, C. P. 1985. A hidden mysterious permanent release of behavior. *In* Perspectives in Behavior. R. A. Gandelman, Ed. Lawrence Erlbaum. Hillsdale, NJ.
20. Canby, T. Y. 1977. The rat: Lapdog of the devil. Nat. Geogr. **152**: 60–86.
21. Pulliam, R. & T. Caraco. 1984. Living in groups: Is there an optimal group size? *In* Behavioural Ecology. 2nd edit. J. R. Krebs & N. B. Davies, Eds. Sinauer Associates. Sunderland, MA.
22. Geist, V. 1978. Life Strategies, Human Evolution, Environmental Design. Springer-Verlag. New York.
23. Milton, K. 1980. The Foraging Strategy of Howler Monkeys. Columbia University Press. New York.
24. Futuyma, D. J. & M. Slatkin. 1983. Coevolution. Sinauer. Cambridge, MA.
25. Heinrich, B. 1979. Bumblebee Economics. Harvard University Press. Cambridge, MA.

Toxiphobia, "Social Reinforcement," Comparative Psychology, and Patrick J. Capretta[a]

PAUL M. BRONSTEIN
Department of Psychology
University of Michigan
Flint, Michigan 48502

This paper begins with reminiscences about my absent friend, one of my teachers, Pat Capretta, and concludes with a description of some recent studies of taste and odor aversion. Most of the intervening material concerns social motivation in animals and illustrates the potential power of food-aversion studies and the functionalist thinking with which this phenomenon has been associated, e.g., to stimulate inquiries into other domains.[1] The present review also supports a perceptual-motivational view of behavior modifications, as suggested by Bindra.[2,3]

I view animals as having evolved to be functionally embedded in *n*-dimensional ecosystems and social networks, and, therefore, am skeptical about the adequacy of univariate laboratory designs to uncover the great range of multivariate dialectical realities in nature. These views and their application to my research are due in no small part to my association with Pat Capretta. Capretta was trained in the Hull-Spence tradition, but by the mid-1960s was changing his orientation. Pat's early empirical work led him to suggest that the details of learning were situation specific years before any widespread appreciation of this idea.[4] In addition, he came to agree with ethologists that it was necessary to study behavior in an ecological context. The failure of much work on animal learning to actively consider these concepts led Pat to the private conclusion that traditional approaches to learning could easily result in an incomplete and flawed understanding of animals. Thus, after writing a book on the history of psychology,[5] Capretta began to study foraging from the perspective of a behavioral ecologist.[6] My current work reflects a full measure of Pat's skepticism about behaviorism as well as some sensitivity to ecological considerations.

OPERANT AND SEMINATURALISTIC APPROACHES TO *BETTA SPLENDENS*

Siamese fighting fish (*Betta splendens*) are Asian teleosts and the species of choice for operant psychologists in alleging the existence of a "social-reinforcement process." These fish have also been studied by ethologists concerned with social communication and have provided data leading to theoretical accounts of aggression.[7,8] The basic

[a] Supported by grants from the Faculty Development Committee of the University of Michigan-Flint, by a Rackham Grant from the University of Michigan-Ann Arbor, and by grants from the National Institute of Mental Health (grants MH 38792-01 and MH 33389-01).

form of all the operant studies has been to present the visual image of a conspecific for, say, 30 seconds to a male betta following some change in behavior. When a conspecific image is presented in a particular locale contingent upon some behavior, increases in swimming speed and in the rate of approach to the site of stimulation occur. Also, when placed in a T maze, bettas turn toward a conspecific at levels far exceeding chance. Operant analysts have assumed that these behaviors are technical indicators of high motivation for fighting, and that fish change the direction and speed of their swimming in order to earn exposure to conspecific visual stimulation—the "social reinforcement." (See Hogan and Roper[9] for a thorough review of this operant literature.)

My own idea about these data, in spite of 25 years of totally consistent findings, was to distrust the reinforcement position. First, fish had always been studied in tiny vessels and in isolation from many potentially relevant ecological and social factors. Second, vertebrate aggression in nature appears highly selective, and associated with acquiring some reproductive advantage.[10,11] The operant interpretation of agonistic behavior in bettas has been that males are generally aggressive, lacking any hint of spatial or temporal selectivity. I suspected, therefore, that operant techniques had not adequately described these animals.

Ethological studies had shown that semitropical temperatures have a permissive effect on bettas' social behavior and the conspecifics are releasers of agonistic display.[7,12,13] The operant work with male bettas demonstrated that increased swimming behavior and changes in the direction of that movement are supported by conspecific visual stimulation.[9] My experiments have extended the ethological approach to an analysis of social systems, while also replicating the operant studies. These efforts have supported my general skepticism concerning the potential pitfalls of laboratory-based behavioristic studies of learning.

Agonistic and Reproductive Sequences

When a male betta is confronted for several hours either by its own mirror image or by another male displaying in a stationary container, a three-part ethogram is revealed.[14–16] Fish initially approach the site of stimulation, issue gill-cover displays when they are within about two body lengths (8 cm) of the stimulus, and then flee. Escapes (during which males can swim more than a meter per second) and further approaches and displays often last 30 minutes. The second stage of social interaction, attack, occurs when escape movements cease and males remain continually within one to two body lengths of the stimulus, displaying and biting all the while. Finally, often after hours of combat, fish retreat from the stimulation area and fail to reinitiate display for some hours.

The transitions in agonistic behavior—from conflict, to attack, to retreat—are determined by the duration of visual stimulation, as well as by individual differences. Intermittent stimulation results in conflict behavior from virtually all males. However, as the image of a displaying male becomes more persistent, a bimodal sample is revealed. Some fish are stimulated to attack, retaliating in direct proportion to available stimulation; others persist in escaping.[15] Agonistic behavior noted early in an encounter is also a reliable predictor of subsequent aggression. Fish that attack soon after being stimulated are the most tenacious fighters.[14,16,17] Further, ten minutes of conspecific stimulation leads to a threefold increase in the amount of personal space a male will defend.[18] Finally, males cease fighting when visual contact between combatants is interrupted, even briefly.[14,15]

Minor variations in this three-part ethogram are noted when a free-swimming opponent, rather than a spatially restricted image, is employed as the social stimulus. First, mobile and live opponents are attacked more intensely than are images of males visible at one fixed locale.[14] Second, the agonistic repertoire interacts with nest-building activity.[14,19,20] When a resident male and live intruder first encounter each other, they approach, display, and escape. The resident departs to its nest at which time further nest building occurs. The intruder also flees but if the animals continue to have visual contact, attack and then retreat by one or both fish is observed; display and attack occur throughout the tank.

When pairs of males are studied for several consecutive days the following results emerge:[20] First, mutual attack typically is initiated within 30 minutes of an encounter and is terminated within 12 hours. Second, subordinate males consistently escape from and fail to display at dominant males within 24 hours of the first encounter. Third, residents can gain an agonistic advantage over intruders due to their familiarity with the visual/tactile and chemical aspects of their environment. This familiarity results in fish that exhibit unusually rapid and persistent attack. Fourth, large body size also confers an agonistic advantage upon a male. Fifth, dominant males show a greater tendency to control space, build nests, court females, and display at a mirror than do subordinates. In short, if fertile females are available, victory in a male-male encounter is associated with relatively great reproductive opportunities during a time span at least adequate for one reproductive cycle—from courtship through the hatching of eggs.

When a female is added to a male's tank, copulation is usually noted within 30 hours.[21] Males initially respond as they do to male intruders—approaching, displaying, and then quickly retreating to elaborate their nests. However, females react to males with behaviors that lower the probability of injurious attack. First, females develop dark vertical bars; these reduce males' biting.[22] Second, females escape into crevices or clumps of vegatation where the bars can act as disruptive coloration.[21] Females also remain relatively immobile unless closely pursued by a male, at which time they escape rapidly. For the first day of cohabitation, males alternate between nest building and directing approach-display-escape sequences at females. Females then follow males to their nests and copulations occur intermittently for several hours. Males next chase females from their nests, and continue nest-building behavior, which now includes the mouthing of eggs and fry. Offspring are protected by males' attacks that drive off adult conspecifics; furthermore, fungi lethal to the young are destroyed by some as yet unknown aspect(s) of the paternal behavior.[21]

Social Reinforcement Reconsidered

Relative to the pattern of social behaviors just described, it is clear that the behaviorist picture of bettas was framed narrowly. Moreover, every operant situation involves the release of conflict behavior typical of the onset of aggression; and this relatively fixed sequence has consistently been distorted so as to engineer superficial support for "social reinforcement theory." I contend that there is no unambiguous evidence favoring this "reinforcement" concept in bettas.

Alleyway studies do not discriminate between approaches toward and escapes from social stimulation; and increases in swimming speed associated with the presentation of conspecific images are identical to movements elicited in male-male combat.[23] A re-analysis of T-maze data also supports the view that fish at the choice points were exhibiting species-specific attacks provoked by visible, displaying conspecifics alleged to be the reinforcers.[23] First, the distance between the subjects and stimulus fish confined in a goal arm always has been about one body length; at this distance bettas lunge and display at conspecifics. Second, no gradual acquisition or learning function has ever been revealed; fish perform at asymptotic levels from their initial trials. Third, turns toward the conspecific fall dramatically when either the subject or the alleged social reinforcer fail to display[24] or when animals cannot see each other prior to subjects' turning into a maze arm.[25]

Similarly, consider free-operant procedures.[9,23] These studies involve males moving to a specific locale (usually, through a tunnel) followed by a burst of social stimulation (say, a 30-second mirror exposure). Within-subjects comparison to periods when the mirror is unavailable and between-subjects comparison to yoked controls show that movement-contingent stimulation is associated with relatively high rates of return to the preselected locale. However, in the light both of bettas' ethogram and recent replications, all of these findings appear to be the systematic release and constraint of conflict behavior. First, the use of direct observations along with operant methods show that those procedures do not discriminate between approaches and escapes and that the alleged reinforcer does not differentially select for any particular movement with which social stimulation might be associated.[15,23,24] Subjects swim rapidly throughout test environments when exposed either to free-operant procedures, or to brief encounters with conspecific images that are not contingent upon any specific, antecedent movement. Second, differences between "reinforced" subjects and yoked controls seem due to spatiotemporal differences between these conditions,[23] controls being further away from the site of social stimulation. Third, the rapid fall in rates of movement associated with the removal of the mirror, i.e., "extinction,"[9] is predicted exactly by recent findings. The intensity of attack is a direct function of the duration of proximate social stimulation and quickly deteriorates in the absence of conspecific visual cues.[14,15] Morever, operant procedures confound the duration of stimulation with its frequency,[26] and have so greatly distorted, ignored, and mismeasured bettas' social behavior as to produce the false conclusion that swimming movement is unaffected by the duration of stimulation.[27]

Finally, one recent experiment fails to demonstrate any significant correlation between success in actual combat and rate of performance on what traditionally has been labeled a free-operant task.[17] That is, fish defined as highly motivated for aggression because of their high rate of approach to a mirror-stimulation site are somewhat less likely to dominate an opponent than fish portrayed by operant methods as having little interest in fighting. Operant techniques, as just shown, have lacked discriminant validity in separating learning from performance and in differentiating between elicited and reinforced movement. I now suggest that operant methods as applied to bettas also lack predictive validity and have produced decades of devotion to behaviors that have, at best, an uncertain relationship to actual aggression.

In this Orwellian year, especially, this episode with "social reinforcement" suggests caution in becoming attached to any particular operational definition. Academic psychology has traditionally emphasized operationalism and reliability in defining "processes" and "mechanisms." Problems of verisimilitude have received inadequate attention. Moreover, an active interest in behavioral ecology implies a reconsideration of the traditional psychological lexicon.

ANALYSIS, SYNTHESIS, HINDSIGHT, AND PROJECTIONS

In addition to raising questions about specific data, my proposed revision of the literature on bettas continues a strategic debate over the seeming inappropriateness of behaviorist concepts. The current thesis is that some of the assumptions associated with the misunderstanding of bettas are endemic to behaviorist approaches in general, and that the critique of "social reinforcement" includes lessons useful in understanding other behaviors. The remainder of this paper concerns some of these problematic assumptions, how these ideas are predispositions to create ambiguities and paradoxes, how ethology, comparative psychology, and behavioral ecology represent an alternative and potentially successful warrant for understanding behavior, and, finally, how these styles of thinking impact on some research on feeding.

Of the two conceptual or paradigmatic breakthroughs in the life sciences—the mechanical ideas of Descartes and Harvey and Darwin's notion of evolution—the behaviorist program for the study of learning in animals has pledged strong allegiance to the former and paid little attention to some implications of the latter. This theoretical orientation has involved attempts to take phenomena to pieces and to then reassemble these components to retrieve and understand the whole. However, this approach has also provided a license for enclosing subjects in restrictive environments in attempts to study hypothetical internal mechanisms without an adequate appreciation of how the assumptions and techniques of analysis might distort conclusions.

The traditions of classical and, especially, operant conditioning in psychology represent a minimalist strategy for understanding animal movement, sharing numerous similarities with the artistic movement bearing the same label. First, although many variations on these themes exist, operant researchers, like minimalist artists, have agreed traditionally to limit both their procedures and their interpretive activities:[28-30] Small numbers of subjects, a limited range of testing devices, and analyses of univariate digital codes (i.e., a movement rates) have been preferred, whereas extensive observations of subjects have been considered of but limited utility. Second, in deliberately choosing characterless, all-purpose, and indivisible elements (i.e., stimuli and responses) as the basis of explanation, behaviorists have divided action into small, hypothetical units, that is, to create a necessarily ambiguous formal calculus of behavior.[30,31] In essence, the decision was made to opt for Cartesian reductionism and to define the small unit as the most preferred; this decision also can be considered an inappropriate use of Occam's Razor.[32-35] Third, subjects have been separated from their ecosystems in attempts to isolate these uncontaminated behavioral specimens from the environments where they might usually be encountered.

The reasons for the failure of behaviorist techniques to decipher bettas' social behavior reside in the inappropriateness of these antecedent assumptions, and, in general terms, these problems were anticipated previously. First, Meehl[36] noted that the definition of "reinforcement" depends fundamentally on the existence of responses as verifiable entities. In reconsidering the social behavior of bettas there appear to be no individual responses as presupposed by operant investigators. Rather, different ways of measuring and distorting one ethogram presented the illusion of several different responses being strengthened. Failures to observe the animals permitted this error to persist and caused the actual character of the animals to remain obscure.

Second, Bindra[2,3] recommended a four-dimensional, spatiotemporal analysis of behavior change, and Bateson[37] has argued that explanations in fewer than those four dimensions make paradoxes and flaws inevitable. If one accepts these ideas, one-dimensional concepts, such as "contiguity" (CS-US) and "reinforcement" (R-US), must represent incomplete and potentially ambiguous accounts of animal movement. Two-dimensional principles, such as "contingency" ($p(US|CS)$) and "information" ($p(R_2|R_1)$) can present similar limitations.[38,39] The analysis of sociality in bettas requires a multidimensional and spatiotemporal approach even if subjects are severely restricted in their movement.[18,21] The absence of this perspective, especially the failure to recognize the importance of subject-to-stimulus distance in determining behavior, was crucial in creating errors typical of operant studies. Moreover, similar errors have occurred previously. The misapplication of "social reinforcement" to people[40,41] and Zuckerman's misrepresentation of social behavior in nonhuman primates are but two examples.[42,43] Each situation involved methodological distortions coupled with inappropriate limitations on the variety of data collected. (See Barber[44] for a general commentary on such "investigator errors.")

An alternative strategy for analyzing behavior is found in ethology and comparative psychology, wherein explanations usually have a foundation in zoological description, are multivariate (based upon syntheses of genetic, physiological, experiential, ecological, and evolutionary influences), and, by definition, include the existence of phenomena emerging from these different levels of analysis. Further, the *a priori* unit of analysis in comparative psychology is the molar, observable, and functional act (e.g., maternal behavior) rather than any hypothetical, molecular unit; also, the eliciting functions of stimuli are emphasized. The comparative/zoological approach met with rapid success in understanding bettas precisely due to these orientations. By including simulations of several ecologically important variables, it was discovered that domesticated bettas show behavioral similarities to wild-living teleosts.[45–47] The behavior of male bettas also supports Hinde's suggestions about communication.[48] First, display in males occurs in situations of social uncertainty, with male and female intruders initially provoking the same reactions from resident males. Second, and consistent with games-theory approaches to communication, a male's potential for engaging in a long-duration fight with another male is revealed at the start of combat,[16,49] while the precise, moment-to-moment style of aggression depends upon how one individual reacts to the prior movements of another.[7,15] Thus, a male betta that greets unknown conspecifics with persistent attack will soon stimulate those fish to reliably reveal their social potentials prior to the appearance of injurious aggression and to do so in a manner that the male is readily able to assess. Receptive females and subordinate males change their coloration and behavior so as to reduce the intensity of attack and cede control of the contested area to the attacking male. Males that will eventually retaliate, escalating the conflict into an intense fight, also reveal themselves early in the contest.

The recent literature on animal motivation contains numerous instances similar to my work with bettas, wherein psychological analyses have been displaced by zoological and ecological concepts. Species-specific revisions of avoidance learning,[50] general activity,[51,52] and food-related appetitive behaviors[53,53] are examples. Common to each situation is a history of failures, first, to predict that testing situations can contain multiple and interactive eliciting stimuli and second, to actively conceptualize behavior as a configuration or strategy for adjustments to ecosystems. Third, there has been some lack of appreciation of subjects' perceptual world. These themes exemplify a recurring epistemological problem in the study of animals. Huxley, for instance, showed that resistance to ecological and evolutionary thought delayed the understanding of animal coloration until well into this century.[55] Moreover, recent studies of human reasoning suggest that these examples are particular instances of our own species-specific bias; given the relative absence of background or contextual cues (in this case, ecological information) the variety of hypothetical solutions for problems is reduced.[56] In short, the academic tradition of isolating animal learning from ecology is a cognitive bias for trying to solve behavior problems within relatively closed cognitive systems and for eliminating from consideration many potentially fruitful explanations. Independent variables have regularly been viewed as causes of acquired behavior and less frequently thought of as catalysts for integrating animals into ecosystems.

Unlike Kenneth Patchen, I am not asserting that, "Truth is always what they don't say."[57] However, useful information appears regularly to have been overlooked and denied in attempts to discover general "processes" and "mechanisms." The understanding of behavior almost certainly will be improved by other detailed analyses of animals' physical and perceptual worlds in relation to their potentials for movement.[58] I turn now to expansions of the current argument about "social reinforcement" to other data sets.

To begin, many studies alleging the control of bettas' behavior by appetitive,[9,59] aversive,[60–62] and physiological[63] factors are ambiguous. All operant, appetitive work of which I am aware can be interpreted as fish approaching the highest concentration of food-related chemical cues, being more sensitive to those positive incentives following food deprivation[59] and searching (swimming on a tortuous path) in the vicinity of the feeding site for some seconds and then departing after food becomes unavailable.[27] Similar behavioral tendencies are known in other teleosts.[64–65] Also, the addition of electric shocks or physiological disruption to "social-" or "food-reinforcement" designs that are by themselves ambiguous cannot but lead to even more uncertainty. Furthermore, most of the "punishment" results with bettas seem explainable as low intensities of shock eliciting rapid swimming, with higher levels of shock reducing swimming behavior. For example, the high rates of "reinforcement" correlated with low levels of shock might be understood totally as the shock producing rapid locomotion that is channeled by a confining apparatus so that the fish are forced to approach the mirror-stimulation area, where conspecific images further potentiate swimming.[60–62] Thus, a plausible explanation for "punishment" can be couched in terms of different releasers and species-specific acts that are elicited and interact both with each other and with the restrictions of the chamber in which the action occurs.

Consider now Murray's contention that male bettas subjected to automaintenance procedures are able to produce or withhold one part of their agonistic repertoire in order to earn the appearance of a conspecific image.[66] There are several procedural problems that call this claim into question in spite of her dissertation being notably cited.[67,68] Murray's data actually provide little evidence that fish can adjust any particular movement independent of the other components of their behavior. Attempts to change the frequency of one behavior were nearly always accompanied by simultaneous changes in the frequency of other movements. The only exception to this conclusion was the animals' apparent ability to change the direction of their locomotion in order to gain subsequent stimulation. However, even this finding appears uncertain since Murray employed yoked controls as a standard for comparisons. The use of this procedure with bettas involves documented ambiguities and erroneous conclusions.[23,69,70] Murray's findings might have emerged from the particular spatiotemporal pattern of eliciting stimuli presented to her different groups. Finally, Murray tested her fish in their home tanks where bubble nests probably existed. Nests interact with conspecific cues, and it is necessary to know the location of an animal's nest in order to interpret the meaning of its swimming.[14,20] Murray failed to report nest-site data, however, leading to yet further ambiguity.

My conclusion about bettas is that none of the operant studies can be interpreted unambiguously, and, related to this species' ethogram, only two papers offer promising preliminary data suggesting either response or place learning.[59,71] Cross-species generalizations from the "social-reinforcement" work on bettas also might be revised following some comparative re-examination.[72–74] Furthermore, only one of the attempts at using Pavlovian procedures can make any claim to have differentiated between general agonistic arousal and stimulus-specific conditioning.[75] However, by current standards, even that success requires further elucidation with additional controls and with reference to bettas' ethogram. It seems certain that at least some bettas will exhibit agonistic behaviors at or near a light after the visual cue has regularly been followed by a conspecific image. However, it is not possible to determine how a potent

CS functions in altering a male betta's behavior. A light, once paired with social cues, may elicit attack, display, escape, nest building, courtship, or some combination of these—all acts elicited by a conspecific image. Because students of learning have not generally sought to determine how experientially modified behavior is dynamically embedded in an animal's species-specific repertoire, the available studies are silent on these issues. The required data have not been collected.

Consider, finally, some unpublished data on food-aversion learning. Ken Rusiniak, my friend and neighbor, has been exploring the interactions of tastes and odors, frequently finding that gustatory cues potentiate aversions to olfactory stimuli.[76-81] Impressed by suggestions that animal behavior is highly sensitive to changes in the spatiotemporal distribution of cues,[2,3,18,23] Rusiniak[82] recently altered the location of olfactory stimuli during the acquisition of an aversion.

For acquisition, thirsty rats were placed in individual cages where they drank quinine. An odorant, almond extract, was simultaneously present; however, independent groups had the scent placed either immediately adjacent to the drinking tube, or under the cage, directly beneath and approximately 8 cm from the spout. Injections of lithium chloride were administered 30 min following drinking. Control rats were poisoned after consuming plain water in the presence of either source of the almond scent. On the first day following recovery (Day 1), all subjects were offered plain water in the same olfactory environment encountered during acquisition. A second day of testing involved shifts in the location of the almond extract accompanying the water.

As seen in the left panel of FIGURE 1, the quinine taste, if present before poisoning, greatly enhances the odor aversion; this result replicates prior findings, and this enhancement occurs at each odorant location. However, the potentiation of the aversion for the almond scent is far greater if, during acquisition, the odor had been next to the drinking tube.

Futhermore, the actual behaviors of the two taste-odor groups were vastly different. With the odorant presented adjacent to the spout, all rats backed away from the water bottle; drinking was virtually eliminated. On the other hand, with the almond scent slightly displaced from the spout, most rats drank some water and spent a great deal of time in seemingly exploratory sniffing. It appears that a slight spatial disparity between the two chemosensory gradients results in considerable inability of the animals to localize, and hence, avoid the liquid. This conclusion is further emphasized by subsequent tests. On Day 2, with a switch in the position of the almond extract, the rats that had thoroughly abstained from drinking now showed no aversion, but consumed the water and also exhibited an elevation in sniffing behavior (FIGURE 1). In addition, all Day 1 behaviors were re-established when, on subsequent tests, the odorants were returned to their original sites.

These results might be accounted for, in part, on the basis of differences in chemosensory gradients or intensities between groups. However, granted the plausibility of that explanation, Rusiniak's findings indicate how motivation or performance can be altered by even slightly modifying spatial relations among stimuli. As indicated by the reliable taste potentiation of odor aversion in both odor-position groups, there was no lack of olfactory information for the animals in a two-dimensional sense. Yet, these data also show that toxiphobia is not adequately understandable in terms of temporally organized one- or two-dimensional conceptions of stimuli and action. Garcia's film records of lithium-treated carnivores also suggest this orientation.[83] Wolves and coyotes, for instance, engage in many different activities while not eating baits that previously have been paired with a poison. They appear to undergo a global, systemic reinterpretation of their food-related environment, affecting many behaviors. They seem not to learn only which substances are to be avoided. These bait-shyness data, along with my findings using bettas, suggest the necessity of establishing mul-

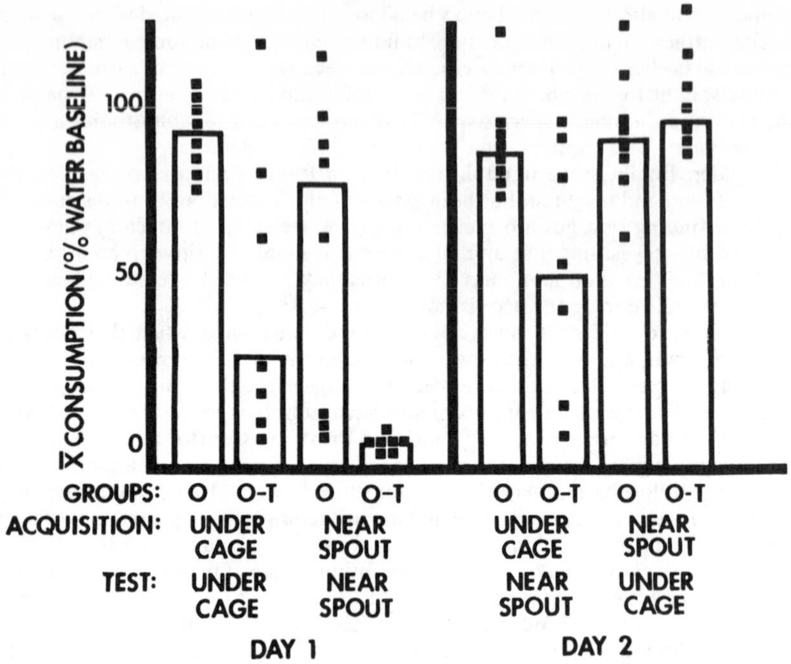

FIGURE 1. The mean consumption of water during two retention tests for rats poisoned either after drinking water in conjunction with almond odor (0 groups) or after consuming a quinine taste along with the almond odor (O-T groups). The position of the almond odor is given below the horizontal axis and the small squares represent the behavior of individual subjects.

tivariate spatiotemporal understandings of various motivational states, integrating several different behaviors in an ecological context. That is, the accurate study of motivation implies an adequate understanding of life histories.

CONCLUDING REMARKS

Beveridge[84,85] has shown that science regularly proceeds, not just by the gradual testing of hypotheses, but through the projection of highly personal analogies onto abstract areas of study. Gould,[86] Lehrman,[87] Skinner,[88] and Harlow[89] contribute many similar biographical anecdotes. There is no attempt here to dismiss any scientific arguments by labeling them "psychological." Rather, these observations represent personal explanations for Kuhn's descriptions of abrupt changes in scientific thought.[90] From this perspective, I conclude with some brief reminiscences.

My qualitatively ecological view of behavior takes as its metaphor childhood experiences watching animals on farms and observing people in their natural habitat, New York City. In such heterogeneous environments it seemed obvious that many behaviors change as subjects move between locales. Consequently, when first encountering the work of academic psychologists, I was impressed with the extent to which elaborate theoretical statements were based upon data collected in small and relatively homogeneous spaces. Omitted from these models were predictions about behavioral adjustments that might occur as animals shifted or were shifted among various habitats and life problems.

Pat Capretta and I shared some of the same skepticisms and Pat encouraged my interest in comparative psychology. He convinced me that if one couldn't quite buy the behaviorist program for studying animals, it was profitable, nonetheless, to rent temporarily with an option to renovate. Many of Pat's initiatives are extended in the papers of this volume; my own work certainly would have taken a different and less enriched path were it not for his insights and support.

ACKNOWLEDGMENTS

I am grateful to Larry Atherton, Jr. and William Mykolajenko for their excellent technical aid and to Colleen Pace for her secretarial assistance.

REFERENCES

1. Rozin, P. & J. W. Kalat. 1971. Specific hungers and poison avoidance as adaptive specializations of learning. Psychol. Rev. **78**: 459–486.
2. Bindra, D. 1974. A motivational view of learning, performance, and behavior modification. Psychol. Rev. **81**: 199–214.
3. Bindra, D. 1978. How adaptive behavior is produced: A perceptual-motivational alternative to response-reinforcement. Behav. Brain Sci. **1**: 41–91.
4. Capretta, P. J. 1961. An experimental modification of food preferences in chickens. J. Comp. Physiol. Psychol. **54**: 238–242.
5. Capretta, P. J. 1967. A History of Psychology in Outline. Delta. New York.
6. Farentinos, R.C., P. J. Capretta, R. E. Kepner & V. M. Littlefield. 1981. Selective herbivory in tassel-eared squirrels: Role of monoterpines in Ponderosa Pines chosen as feeding trees. Science **213**: 1273–1275.
7. Simpson, M. J. A. 1968. The display of Siamese fighting fish. Anim. Behav. Monogr. **1**: 1–73.
8. Caryl, P. G. 1981. Escalated fighting and the war of nerves: Games theory and animal combat. *In* Perspectives in Ethology. P. P. G. Bateson & P. H. Klopfer, Eds. **4**: 199–224. Plenum. New York.
9. Hogan, J. A. & T. J. Roper. 1978. A comparison of the properties of different reinforcers. *In* Advances in the Study of Behavior. J. S. Rosenblatt, R. A. Hinde, C. Beer & M.-C. Busnel, Eds. **8**: 155–255. Academic Press. New York.
10. Barrash, D. 1976. Sociobiology and Behavior. Elsevier. New York.
11. Dewsbury, D. A. 1982. Dominance rank, copulatory behavior, and differential reproduction. Q. Rev. Biol. **57**: 135–159.
12. Hess, E. H. 1952. Temperatures as a regulatory of the attack response in *Betta splendens*. Z. Tierpsychol. **9**: 379–382.
13. Goodrich, H. B. & H. C. Taylor. 1934. Breeding reactions in *Betta splendens*. Copeia. 165–166.
14. Bronstein, P. M. 1981. Commitments to aggression and nest sites in male *Betta splendens*. J. Comp. Physiol. Psychol. **95**: 436–449.
15. Bronstein, P. M. Agonistic sequences and the assessment of opponents in male *Betta splendens*. Am. J. Psychol. **96**: 163–177.
16. Bronstein, P. M. 1985. The prior-residency effect in *Betta splendens*. J. Comp. Psychol. **99**: 56–59.
17. Bronstein, P. M. 1985. Predictors of dominance in male *Betta splendens*. J. Comp. Psychol. **99**: 47–55.

18. Bronstein, P. M. 1983. Onset of combat in male *Betta splendens*. J. Comp. Psychol. **97**: 135–139.
19. Bronstein, P. M. 1980. *Betta splendens*: A territorial note. Bull. Psychon. Soc. **16**: 484–485.
20. Bronstein, P. M. 1984. Agonistic and reproductive interactions in *Betta splendens*. J. Comp. Psychol. **98**: 421–431.
21. Bronstein, P. M. 1982. Breeding, paternal behavior, and their interruption in *Betta splendens*. Anim. Learn. Behav. **10**: 145–151.
22. Robertson, C. M. & P. F. Sale. 1975. Sexual discrimination in the Siamese fighting fish (*Betta splendens* Regan). Behaviour **54**: 1–26.
23. Bronstein, P. M. 1981. Social reinforcement in *Betta splendens*: A reconsideration. J. Comp. Physiol. Psychol. **95**: 943–950.
24. Bols, R. J. 1977. Display reinforcement in the Siamese fighting fish, *Betta splendens*: Aggressive motivation or curiosity? J. Comp. Physiol. Psychol. **91**: 233–244.
25. Hogan, J. A. & R. J. Bols. 1980. Priming of aggressive motivation in *Betta splendens*. Anim. Behav. **28**: 135–142.
26. Bronstein, P. M. 1984. A confound in the application of fixed-ratio schedules to the social behavior of male Siamese fighting fish (*Betta splendens*). Bull. Psychon. Soc. **22**: 484–487.
27. Hogan, J. A., Kleist & C. S. L. Hutchings. 1970. Display and food as reinforcers in the Siamese fighting fish, *Betta splendens*. J. Comp. Physiol. Psychol. **70**: 351–357.
28. Sidman, M. 1960. Tactics of Scientific Research. Basic Books. New York.
29. Skinner, B. F. 1966. Operant behavior. *In* Operant Behavior: Areas of Research and Application. W. K. Honig, Ed. Appleton-Century-Crofts. New York.
30. Skinner, B. F. 1935. The generic nature of the concepts of stimulus and response. J. Gen. Psych. **12**: 40–65.
31. Nagel, E. & J. R. Newman. 1958. Godel's Proof. New York University Press. New York.
32. Bronowski, J. 1977. The logic of experiment. *In* A Sense of the Future. J. Bronowski, Ed.: 42–55. MIT Press. Cambridge, MA.
33. Dunbar, M. J. 1980. The blunting of Occam's Razor, or to hell with parsimony. Can. J. Zool. **58**: 123–128.
34. Holsinger, K. E. 1980. Comment: The blunting of Occam's razor, or to hell with parsimony. Can. J. Zool. **58**: 144–146.
35. Hutchinson, G. E. 1978. An Introduction to Population Ecology. pp. 2–4. Yale University Press. New Haven, CT.
36. Meehl, P. E. 1950. On the circularity of the law of effect. Psych. Bull. **47**: 52–75.
37. Bateson, G. 1979. Mind and Nature. E. P. Dutton. New York.
38. Rescorla, R. A. 1967. Pavlovian conditioning and its proper control procedures. Psychol. Rev. **74**: 71–80.
39. Shannon, C. E. & W. Weaver. 1949. The Mathematical Theory of Communication. University of Illinois Press. Urbana, IL.
40. Mahoney, M. 1974. Cognition and Behavior Modification. Ballinger. Cambridge.
41. Spielberger, C. D. & L. D. Denike., 1966. Descriptive behaviorism versus cognitive theory in verbal operant conditioning. Psychol. Rev. **73**: 306–326.
42. Zuckerman, S. 1932. The Social Life of Monkeys and Apes. Routeledge and Kagen Paul, Ltd. London.
43. Lancaster, J. B. & R. B. Lee. 1965. The annual reproductive cycle in monkeys and apes. *In* Primate Behavior. I. Devore, Ed.: 486–513. Holt, Rinehart & Winston. New York.
44. Barber, T. X. 1976. Pitfalls in Human Research. Pergamon Press. New York.
45. Chapman, D. W. 1966. Food and space as regulators of salmonid population in streams. Am. Nat. **100**: 345–357.
46. Myrberg, A. A. & R. E. Thresher. 1974. Interspecific aggression and its relevance to the concept of territoriality in reef fishes. Am. Zool. **14**: 81–96.
47. Thresher, R. E. 1978. Territoriality and aggression in the threespot damselfish (Pisces, *Pomacentridae*): An experimental study of causation. Z. Tierpsychol. **46**: 401–434.
48. Hinde, R. A. 1981. Animal signals: Ethological and games-theory approaches are not incompatible. Anim. Behav. **29**: 535–542.
49. Maynard-Smith, J. 1976. Evolution and the theory of games. Am. Sci. **64**: 41–45.

50. BOLLES, R. C. 1970. Species-specific defense reactions and avoidance learning. Psychol. Rev. **77**: 32–48.
51. SUAREZ, S. D. & G. G. GALLUP, JR. 1981. Predatory overtones of openfield testing in chickens. Anim. Learn. Behav. **9**: 153–163.
52. ROVEE-COLLIER, C., J. B. CAPATIDES, J. W. FAGEN & V. NEGRI. 1983. Selective habituation of defensive behavior: Evidence for predator-prey synchrony. Anim. Learn. Behav. **11**: 127–133.
53. COLLIER, G. H., E. HIRSCH & P. E. HAMLIN. 1972. The ecological determinants of reinforcement in the rat. Physiol. Behav. **9**: 705–716.
54. COLLIER, G. H. & C. K. ROVEE-COLLIER. 1981. A comparative analysis of optimal foraging behavior: Laboratory simulations. *In* Foraging Behavior: Ecological, Ethological, and Psychological Approaches. A. C. Kamil & T. Sargent, Eds.: 39–76. Garland STPM. New York.
55. HUXLEY, J. S. 1957. Introduction. *In* Adaptive Coloration in Animals. H. B. Cott, Ed. Methuen. London.
56. EINHORN, H. J. & R. M. HOGARTH. 1983. Diagnostic inference and causal judgment: A decision making framework. Center for Decision Research Memorandum. University of Chicago.
57. PATCHEN, K. 1968. 'Gentle and giving' and other sayings. *In* The Collected Poems of Kenneth Patchen. pp. 484–487. New Directions. New York.
58. VOGEL, S. 1981. Behavior and the physical world of an animal. *In* Perspectives in Ethology. P. P. G. Bateson & P. H. Klopfer, Eds. **4**: 179–198. Plenum. New York.
59. FANTINO, E., S. WEIGELE & D. LANCY. 1972. Aggressive display in the Siamese fighting fish (*Betta splendens*). Learn. Motiv. **3**: 457–468.
60. ADLER, N. T. & J. A. HOGAN. 1963. Classical conditioning and punishment of an instinctive response in *Betta splendens*. **11**: 351–354.
61. MELVIN, K. G. & J. E. ANSON. 1969. Facilitative effects of punishment on aggressive behavior in the Simense fighting fishing. Psychon. Sci. **4**: 89–90.
62. MELVIN, K. G. & D. H. ERVEY. 1973. Facilitative and suppressive effects of punishment on species-typical aggressive display in *Betta splendens*. J. Comp. Physiol. Psychol. **83**: 451–457.
63. HOLLIS, K. L. & J. B. OVERMIER. 1982. Effect of telencephalon ablation on the reinforcing and eliciting properties of species-specific events in *Betta splendens*. J. Comp. Physiol. Psychol. **96**: 574–590.
64. THOMAS, G. 1974. The influence of encountering a food object on the subsequent searching behaviour in *Gasterosteus aculeatus, L.* Anim. Behav. **22**: 941–952.
65. ZIPPEL, H. P., R. VOIGT & D. HAGER. 1980. Behavioural and electrophysiological effects of natural chemical stimuli in the goldfish (*Carassius auratus*). *In* Chemical Signals. D. Muller-Schwartze & R. M. Silverstein, Eds.: 409–410. Plenum. New York.
66. MURRY, K. A. S. 1973. Conditioning in *Betta splendens*. Ph.D. Disseration. University of Pennsylvania.
67. HOLLIS, K. L. 1982. Pavlovian conditioning of single-centered action patterns and autonomic behavior: A biological analysis of function. *In* Advances in the Study of Behavior. J. S. Rosenblatt, R. A. Hinde, C. Beer & M.-C. Busnel, Eds.: 1–64. Academic Press. New York.
68. WILLIAMS, D. A. 1981. Biconditional behavior. Conditioning without constraint. *In* Autoshaping and Conditioning Theory. C. M. Locurto, H. S. Terrace & J. Gibbon, Eds.: 55–59. Academic Press. New York.
69. GOLDSTEIN, S. R. 1967. Mirror images as a reinforcer in Siamese fighting fish: A replication with additional controls. Psychon. Sci. **7**: 331–332.
70. HOGAN, J. A. 1967. Fighting and reinforcement in the Siamese fighting fish (*Betta splendens*). J. Comp. Physiol. Psychol. **64**: 356–359.
71. ROITBLAT, H. L., W. THAM & L. GOLUB. 1982. Performance of *Betta splendens* in a radial arm maze. Anim. Learn. Behav. **10**: 108–114.
72. DAVIS, R. E., C. HARRIS & J. SHELBY. 1974. Sex differences in aggressivity and the effects of social isolation in the anabantoid fish, *Macropodus opercularis*. Behav. Biol. **11**: 497–509.

73. SEVENSTER, P. 1973. Incompatibility of response and reward. *In* Constraints on Learning. R. A. Hinde & J. Stevenson-Hinde, Eds.: 265–283. Academic Press. New York.
74. DELSAUT, M. & J. C. ROY. 1980. The effect of recorded contact calls on the reinforcing value of self-viewing among lovebirds. Behav. Neural Biol. **30**: 341–344.
75. THOMPSON, T. & T. STURM. 1965. Classical conditioning of aggressive display in Siamese fighting fish. J. Exp. Anal. Behav. **8**: 397–403.
76. RUSINIAK, K. W., W. G. HANKINS, J. GARCIA & L. P. BRETT. 1979. Flavor-illness aversions. Behav. Neural Biol. **25**: 1–17.
77. PALMERINO, C. C., K. W. RUSINIAK & J. GARCIA. 1980. Flavor-illness aversions: The peculiar roles of odor and taste in memory for poison. Science **208**: 753–755.
78. RUSINIAK, K. W., C. C. PALMERINO, A. G. RICE, D. L. FORTHMAN & J. GARCIA. 1982. Flavor-illness aversions: Potentiation of odor by taste with toxin but not shock in rats. J. Comp. Physiol. Psychol. **96**: 527–539.
79. RUSINIAK, K. W., C. C. PALMERINO & J. GARCIA. 1982. Potentiation of odor by taste in rats: Tests of some nonassociative factors. J. Comp. Physiol. Psychol. **96**: 775–780.
80. BERMUDEZ-RATTONI, F., K. W. RUSINIAK & J. GARCIA. 1983. Flavor-illness aversions: Potentiation of odor by taste is disrupted by application of novocain into amygdala. Behav. Neural Biol. **37**: 61–75.
81. GARCIA, J. & K. W. RUSINIAK. 1980. What the nose learns from the mouth. *In* Chemical Senses. Dr. Müller-Schwartze & R. M. Silverstein, Eds.: 141–156. Plenum. New York.
82. RUSINIAK, K. W. Taste-odor interactions in toxiphobia with rats. Unpublished data.
83. GUSTAVSON, C. R., D. J. KELLEY, M. SWEENEY & J. GARCIA. 1976. Prey-lithium aversions. I. Coyotes and wolves. Behav. Biol. **17**: 61–72.
84. BEVERIDGE, W. I. B. 1957. The Art of Scientific Investigation. Vintage. New York.
85. BEVERIDGE, W. I. B. 1980. Seeds of Discovery. W. W. Norton. New York.
86. GOULD, S. J. 1983. Hen's Teeth and Horse's Toes. W. W. Norton. New York.
87. LEHRMAN, D. S. 1971. Behavioral science, engineering, and poetry. *In* The Biopsychology of Development. E. Tobach, L. R. Aronson & E. Shaw, Eds.: 459–471. Academic Press. New York.
88. SKINNER, B. F. 1983. Origins of a behaviorist. Psychol. Today **17**: 22–33.
89. HARLOW, H. F. 1953. Mice, monkeys, men and motives. Psychol. Rev. **60**: 23–32.
90. KUHN, T. 1970. The Structure of Scientific Revolutions. University of Chicago Press. Chicago.

A Natural Toxic Defense System: Cardenolides in Butterflies versus Birds[a]

LINCOLN PIERSON BROWER AND LINDA SUSAN FINK

Department of Zoology
University of Florida
Gainesville, Florida 32611

INTRODUCTION

CFA in an Adaptive Context

The capacity to form a conditioned food aversion (CFA) under experimental conditions has been found in dozens of vertebrate species as phylogenetically and ecologically diverse as the garter snake, quail, and timber wolf,[1] suggesting that CFAs are extremely important in natural foraging encounters. From the earliest demonstration, CFAs have been attributed with the adaptive function of enabling individual animals to learn to avoid chemically noxious and/or physically harmful foods in their environments.[2-4] Conditioned food aversions are only one of several mechanisms shown to affect food acceptance and/or rejection by experimental subjects. Other associative and non-associative factors include observational learning,[5-9] social transmission of preferences,[10-12] neophobia,[13,14] and innate avoidance of bitter tastes.[16]

The presence of more than one mechanism does not diminish the potential value of conditioned aversions; an acceptable adaptive scenario can encompass the interplay of numerous food selection mechanisms. Most naturally occurring toxins are bitter in flavor,[16] and initial neophobia combined with an innate aversion to bitter often creates a wariness to any unknown food type. The predator may avoid the food or, if it does eat it, associate delayed effects, either negative or positive, with ingestion. An aversion may easily become conditioned after a single noxious experience, while after a single taste a palatable food will cease to stimulate a neophobic response, and may be incorporated into the diet. Familiar foods that an animal has learned are safe are less likely to become conditioned stimuli after an illness. Social foragers may learn which foods are safe to eat from parents, other conspecifics, or other species in mixed-species groups, and may learn aversions through watching another individual become sickened.

This scenario, while neatly packaging several food rejection mechanisms together in an intuitively satisfying manner, remains largely hypothetical and is overly simplistic. The majority of psychological CFA studies have used artificial foods, artificial conditioning agents, and/or artificial administration thereof,[1] since they were designed to explore the characteristics of the learning process itself rather than its

[a] Supported by National Science Foundation Grants to Amherst College and to the University of Florida with L. P. Brower as Principal Investigator.

ecological significance. Although we may have an accurate representation of the strategy used by the rat, upon which the majority of experiments have been conducted, the problems animals confront in nature vary widely and it is likely that different foraging challenges are solved with different combinations of these mechanisms. For example, Zahorik and Houpt[17,18] have pointed out that despite evidence that large mammalian herbivores can form CFAs under experimental conditions, the rat paradigm probably does not apply to this group due to their meal patterns and extended digestion. Indeed, the discrepancy between what a forager will do under experimental conditions and what it actually does when confronted with decisions in its natural environment may be considerable. Comparative ecological and phylogenetic exploration of the conditions under which these different mechanisms take precedence is needed and has yet to be done.[19] One distinct group in which comparative laboratory and field studies of food selection are both feasible and relevant is insect-eating birds.

Birds and Aposematic Insects

As a result of being food for many predators, insects have developed a diverse array of defenses.[20-22] Many rely on crypsis, retreats, or escape to avoid being observed or captured; once captured, however, they can be eaten without adverse effect on the predator. Other insects contain noxious compounds, such as cardiac glycosides, alkaloids, and histamines, that may be sequestered from plant foods or synthesized *de novo* and are capable of injuring or sickening predators.[23-25] The difference between palatable and unpalatable insects, however, is greater than just the physiological effect they have on an animal attacking or ingesting them. Those which are noxious usually advertise themselves by conspicuous appearance, sound, or odor prior to the first ingestive experience: they are aposematic. These aposematic cues act as a generalized warning during the very first encounter and also can promote rapid conditioning; they therefore benefit both predator and prey.

Although other arthropods (especially spiders and ants), lizards, and mammals eat many insects, historically most discussions of insect defense have focused upon birds as major predators. Birds are primarily visual rather than olfactory or auditory hunters, and are frequently cited as the most important selective force driving the evolution of cryptic and aposematic color patterns as well as visual mimicry. Since the probability of a bird encountering potentially noxious insect prey is considerable, this interaction offers a prime situation in which to understand the circumstances under which natural food items become conditioned stimuli of food aversions. Insectivorous birds feed on individually recognizable food items, take and digest discrete meals, and often feed in bouts of single food types. Unlike large herbivores therefore, they have meal patterns comparable to the rat, on which the original adaptationist scheme was based.

Despite the collective appellation, insectivorous birds are phylogenetically, morphologically, and physiologically diverse, with wide variation in such factors as prey capture and handling methods, social behavior, and preferred habitats. The group encompasses obligate insectivores, such as flycatchers, and others, such as icterids and corvids, which also eat substantial proportions of plant parts and non-arthropod animals.[26-28] This ecological diversity makes insectivorous birds ideal not only for studies of CFAs in natural interactions, but also for comparative investigations of their importance relative to other mechanisms of food selection.

The Blue Jay–Monarch Butterfly Laboratory Paradigm

Among insects, the most intensively studied in relation to its vertebrate predators has been the aposematic and chemically noxious monarch butterfly, *Danaus plexippus* L. Over the past 20 years the senior author's laboratory has been decoding the chemical signals used by monarchs to ward off potential avian predators and detailing how birds utilize this chemical information.

Using wild blue jays (*Cyanocitta cristata*) as predators, it was determined that monarchs are emetic, and it was also found that monarchs reared on one milkweed species caused all the birds to vomit, while monarchs reared on a different species were completely palatable.[29] By rearing monarchs on several species of milkweed and feeding them to jays, it was then found that the resultant butterflies ranged across a palatability spectrum from highly palatable to highly emetic.[30] As a result, palatability could be defined in terms of an emesis spectrum and quantitatively expressed as the number of blue jay emetic units per butterfly. Investigations of monarchs reared in their natural environments on two *Asclepias* species in California[31,32] determined a range of 0.28 to 26 emetic units per butterfly per 85 g jay. Other studies of monarchs collected in the wild from various migrating and overwintering populations indicated that the butterflies contained from 0 to more than 9 emetic units.[33,34]

Chemical and pharmacological analyses of the plants and butterflies have proven that emesis is caused by a class of natural toxic chemicals known as cardiac glycosides, or cardenolides.[31,35] Cardenolides also cause a general malaise syndrome, and most are extremely bitter at low concentrations.[25,36] While eating milkweed leaves, the monarch larvae digest and store the cardenolides and during metamorphosis the poisons become generally distributed throughout the tissues and organs of the adults, with highest concentrations occurring in the exoskeleton and wings.[25,36,37]

EXPERIMENTAL STUDIES

The cardenolide-based chemical defense of monarch butterflies offered an opportunity to explore several aspects of aversion behavior of blue jays from natural populations in controlled laboratory experiments. We housed wild-captured adult jays individually in cages provided with a rotating lazy susan feeder as described elsewhere[13] and shown in FIGURE 1. Each jay was presented with successive single insects, and its behavior observed from behind one-way glass. All insects were killed by freezing and thawed for presenting.

Experiment 1: Dosage-dependent Conditioned Visual Aversion

This experiment was designed to test the reactions of jays to monarchs that varied in their degree of emesis-based unpalatability.[38] These included completely palatable monarchs (reared on the cardenolide-free milkweed *Gonolobus rostratus*), highly emetic monarchs (reared on the cardenolide-rich *Asclepias curassavica*), and three categories of intermediate palatability obtained by feeding the monarchs for different proportions of time on these two plants (TABLE 1).

Sixty-three jays were trained to eat butterflies out of the lazy susan feeding cups

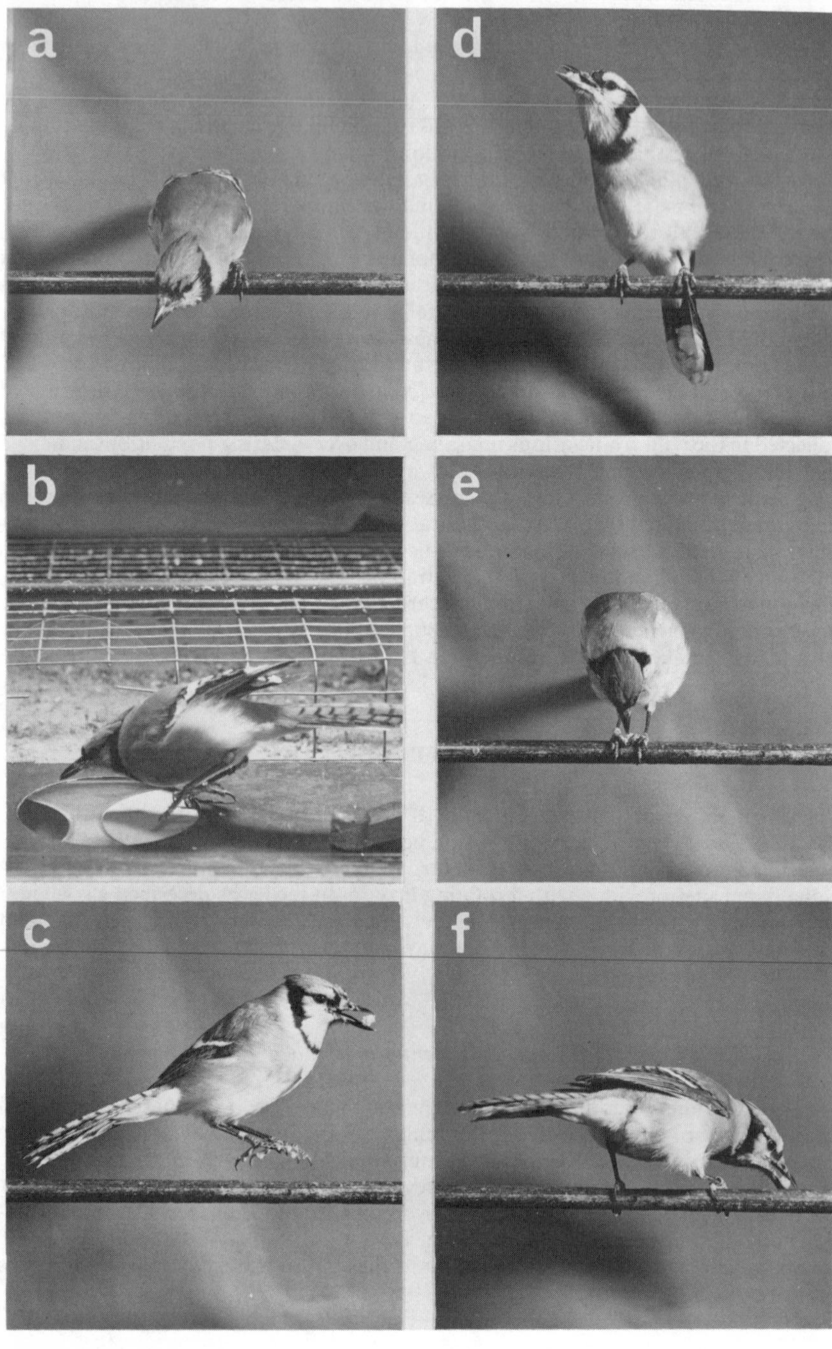
a
d
b
e
c
f

by first offering them palatable *Anartia jatrophae* butterflies until they accepted and ate them without hesitation. Then, after an overnight and morning food deprivation of 16 hours, each was offered its first monarch in a series of up to 10 passes of the lazy susan. If the bird did not attack and eat the monarch during one of these first 10 passes, it was eliminated from the experiment. If it did eat the monarch, its behavior (including vomiting) was recorded for the remainder of the hour and it was then fed laboratory chow for 30 minutes. Following food deprivation for 90 minutes, the same bird was presented with up to 10 passes of the second monarch (of the same palatability category as the first) over a one-hour period. If the bird refused to attack this second monarch, it was again fed lab chow for 30 minutes, deprived for 90 more minutes, and re-offered the second monarch for passes 11–20. If it again refused to attack, it was fed lab chow for the rest of the day, deprived overnight, and the regime continued on day 2 for blocks of ten passes from passes 21 to 50. This regimen was repeated for up to 30 passes per day on days 3, 10, 17, 34, and 41, for a maximum of 200 passes over the 41 days.

Experiment 1 established several points. (1) 35% of the jays refused to attack their first monarch on sight (TABLE 1). In a related experiment, eight of 40 jays similarly refused their initial monarch on sight (Brower and Glazier, unpublished data, Jan-Feb 1970).[39] Among the 65% that attacked, most did so on the first or second pass, their attack times ranged from 11–16 seconds, tasting times (mandibulating, pecking) ranged from 56–102 seconds, and their times to finish manipulating the butterflies ranged from 9.4 to 15.1 minutes. One-way ANOVA indicated no significant differences in any of these measures for the five cardenolide categories. Thus (2) the acceptor jays showed no initial taste discrimination among the butterflies of variable cardenolide content and emetic potencies. (3) No birds vomited after eating their monarch in the 0, 0.3, 0.4 emetic unit groups, 5 of 11 birds did in the 1.2 unit group (mean time to vomit = 16.6 minutes), and all 5 vomited in the 3.7 unit group (mean time = 9.0 minutes). The mean time to vomit in these two groups differed significantly (t = 3.03, d.f. = 8; $p < 0.02$). The data for the 1.2 emetic unit group suggested (4) that the recovery times from the cardenolide-induced malaise were greater for the birds that did not vomit than for those that did.

The birds' reaction to the second monarch (TABLE 1) showed (5) that the degree of visually conditioned aversive behavior was strongly dose-dependent upon the cardenolide content of the first monarch, with the most poisonous monarchs resulting in the birds' rejecting up to 200 passes over a total of 41 days. The vomiters in the highest dosage group showed greater conditioned visual aversion to their second monarch than did the non-vomiters in the 1.2 level group (the vomiters in the 1.2 group were not tested with a second monarch). This suggests (6) that vomiting *per se* may be a stronger unconditioned stimulus than drawn-out malaise.

Experiment 2: Conditioned Taste Discrimination

This experiment was carried out in February–March 1974 to investigate whether jays are capable of developing conditioned taste discrimination between cardenolide-

---

FIGURE 1. Representative behavioral sequence of a blue jay presented with a series of pieces of palatable and unpalatable (cardenolide-laden) dried bread. The piece that is about to appear was moderately unpalatable. The jay (A) anticipates the appearance of the bread, (B) jumps down to seize it out of the lazy susan cup, and (C) hops back to the perch. The jay (D) then tastes the bread, (E) pecks at it on the perch, and (F) places it on the perch, thereby rejecting it.

TABLE 1. Responses of Blue Jays to Initial Monarchs of Variable Emetic Potencies and Their Behavior to a Subsequent Monarch

Treatment of the First Monarch Butterfly by 63 Jays

Emetic units/butterfly	Number of Birds: Tested	Number of Birds: Eating	Minutes to Eat	Attack Latency[a]	Number of Birds Vomiting	Mean Minutes to Vomit[b]
0.0	17	10	12.9	1–4	0	–
0.3	13	10	10.0	1–3	0	–
0.4	7	5	15.1	1	0	–
1.2	17	11	11.4	1–2	5	16.6
3.7[c]	9	5	9.4	1	5	9.0

Treatment of Second Monarch Butterfly by 36 Jays[d] which Ate the First Monarch

	Number of Birds: Tested	Number of Birds: Attacking	Number of Birds: Eating	Minutes to Eat	Attack Latency
0.0	10	10	10	2.5	1–7
0.3	10	10	10	4.0	1–7
0.4	5	5	5	15.4	1–31
1.2	6[d]	5	1	16.0	2–>170
3.7	5	2	0	–	31–>200

Note: Variable emetic potencies are measured as number of emetic units per butterfly. Data are from Jaenike.[38]

[a] Number of times the lazy susan cup passed before the bird attacked the monarch.

[b] Minutes from when the butterfly was ingested.

[c] From Brower *et al.*[30]

[d] In the 1.2 emetic unit group, only the six birds that did not vomit in part A were tested in part B.

free monarchs (palatable) and cardenolide-laden monarchs (unpalatable) reared, respectively, on *G. rostratus* and *A. curassavica.* The butterflies were presented one at a time to the birds in the lazy susan cups for 30-second intervals. A bird could reject the monarch on sight; peck it in such a way that, had it been alive, it would have survived the attack; killed it, i.e. lethally pecked, dismembered and/or ate less than one fourth of the thorax or abdomen; or eaten it, i.e., ate more than one fourth of the abdomen or thorax.

All birds were deprived of food from 3:30PM of the previous day until approximately 8AM to assure a high level of hunger at the outset of each butterfly feeding sequence. During the screening period, each bird was presented with a sequence of palatable *Anartia amalthea* for as many passes as necessary until it consistently accepted and ate them without hesitation in a single pass of the lazy susan cup. Sixteen birds qualified for the experiment. Experimental day 1 was designed to induce the birds to eat palatable monarchs. Each bird was offered one *A. amalthea* butterfly until it ate it, followed by one palatable monarch butterfly, and then a second palatable monarch that they also had to attack and eat after one or more passes. Because the objective was to observe taste responses, birds that did not peck butterflies were reoffered for one or more passes with the result that only four butterflies were resolutely refused by two birds during two sequences in the entire experiment. Throughout the experiment, most birds pecked, killed, or ate each butterfly on its first pass.

Experimental day 2 continued familiarizing the birds with three palatable monarchs, and then duped them into eating one unpalatable monarch with consequent emesis. All 16 birds ate the unpalatable as well as the three palatable monarchs, 15 vomited at least once, and the sixteenth retched but did not vomit. Experimental days 3 through 5 included five feeding sessions that tested the birds' ability to taste-discriminate palatable from unpalatable butterflies. Each session lasted 30 minutes during which each bird was offered three palatable and one unpalatable butterflies in random order, for a total of 20 butterflies. Following a morning session, the birds were fed for 30 minutes, deprived for two hours and retested, fed and then deprived until the next morning's observation.

Prior to receiving the first emetic monarch, the birds' feeding behavior consisted of straightforward removal of the butterfly's wings with limited pecking of the body, followed by swallowing of the thorax and abdomen. After the emetic experience, most birds increased their attack latencies for all monarchs and also increased their times for dismembering, manipulating, and swallowing pieces or all of the thorax and/or abdomen. They also frequently regurgitated the body parts onto the perch before completely swallowing them and sometimes reinitiated the whole eating process of these regurgitated parts. At other times they flung the regurgitated pieces across the cage or attempted to store them. The individual behavior of nine birds indicated that they became consistent discriminators from the fourth to the eleventh monarch onward in the overall 20 butterfly test sequence (TABLE 2). (A discriminator was a bird that attacked and rejected all unpalatable monarchs and attacked and ate more than one-fourth of each palatable monarch.) Although the other seven birds did not develop consistent behavioral discriminations, they nevertheless also ate a higher percentage of the palatable butterflies. Overall, the birds ate 79% of the palatable butterflies and only 9% of the unpalatable butterflies (Sign test, in Siegel:[39] $N = 16, X = 0, p < 0.001$).

This experiment indicates that hungry wild-captured blue jays that have been trained to eat palatable monarchs will subsequently attack and ingest a sufficient amount of a toxic monarch to cause vomiting; that after one emetic bout, the jays can learn to distinguish between the two butterflies on the basis of taste; and, therefore that monarchs reared on the two foodplants have distinguishable gustatory properties, presumably as a result of the presence or absence of cardenolides.

TABLE 2. Taste Discrimination Based on Monarch Butterfly Palatability[a]

		Category and Treatments[b] of Butterflies					
		Palatable			Unpalatable		
Bird Number	Trial at which Discrimination = 100%[c]	Peck and Kill	Eat	% Eaten	Peck and Kill	Eat	% Eaten
50	–	10	5	33	5	0	0
57	–	7	8	53	5	0	0
84	15	6	9	60	5	0	0
66	–	5	10	67	4	1	20
52	–	4	11	73	5	0	0
91	–	4	11	73	4	1	20
83	8	3	12	80	5	0	0
38	–	3	12	80	3	2	40
73	4	2	13	87	5	0	0
43	–	1	10	91	3	2	40
75	12	1	14	93	5	0	0
60	4	1	14	93	5	0	0
4	2	1	14	93	5	0	0
36	5	1	14	93	4	1	20
18	1	0	15	100	5	0	0
20	5	0	14	100	5	0	0
Mean percent		23%		77%	89%		11%
Range in percent eaten:			33%–100%			0%–40%	

[a] Taste discrimination based on treatments of 15 palatable monarchs (reared on *Gonolobus rostratus*) and 5 unpalatable monarchs (reared on *Asclepias curassavica*) offered to each of 16 blue jays. The palatable monarchs lacked cardenolide, whereas the unpalatable ones contained more than three ED_{50} units of these bitter and emetic poisons.

[b] See text for detailed description.

[c] In the sequence of 20 tests, see text.

Experiment 3: Taste Rejection of Pure Cardenolides

The hypothesis that sequestered milkweed cardenolides are responsible for the emetic property of monarch butterflies was supported by dosage-response experiments[33] and later confirmed by force-feeding a purified milkweed cardenolide (labriformin) to jays.[31] This experiment[40] addressed three questions: (1) Do bitter cardenolides evoke taste rejection in the jays? (2) Can taste rejection protect a jay from ingesting an emetic dose of cardenolide? and (3) How are taste and emetic sensitivity related to cardenolide structure? Biochemical and pharmacological considerations predict that more polar cardenolides within any one group (such as the digitoxin series), because of their greater solubility in water, should be relatively more bitter than the less polar molecules. In contrast, the less polar cardenolides, which are more lipid soluble, should more easily cross cellular membranes and therefore be relatively more emetic.[41] These seemingly esoteric considerations are of potential ecological importance. When monarchs are reared on *A. curassavica*, there is a differential distribution of cardenolides in various body parts, with the more polar and therefore more easily tasted ones being relatively more concentrated in the wings (Plate 1A, Brower[25]).[32,42] Wild birds are known to capture and reject various species of aposematic butterflies in the field leaving them unharmed except for a tell-tale beakmark upon their wings.[25,36] The hypothesis is that natural selection has resulted in the most easily tasted cardenolides being stored in the wings, which the bird can sample and taste-reject without killing the butterfly.

In order to eliminate unknown chemical variability resulting from rearing butterflies on the different milkweeds, we trained the jays to feed upon a novel experimental food to which various concentrations of pure cardenolides were added. Pieces of dried whole wheat bread measuring about 9 × 6 × 5 mm were prepared such that 20 pieces weighed 1 g. Fifty μl of cardenolide solution were pipetted onto each bread piece, and control pieces were treated similarly with 95% ethanol. The highest concentration was based on that found in the wings of monarchs reared on *Asclepias curassavica* (equivalent to 5.29 mg of digitoxin per gram of wing, dry weight basis).[36,45] The cardenolide solutions were prepared with 95% ethanol and contained natural log increments in concentrations (in moles per liter) of three cardenolides in the digitoxin series. These were digoxin (mw = 781), digitoxin (mw = 765), and digitoxigenin (mw = 374). It was determined[43] through thin layer chromatography that the relative R_f values of these three compounds are similar in 14 separate solvent systems. The most polar is digoxin, digitoxin is intermediate, and digitoxigenin is least polar.

Individually caged wild captured blue jays were acclimated for three days in the lazy susan feeder cages, during which they were offered pigeon pellets in the rotating cups. Following food deprivation from 8:30PM until 11AM, they were repeatedly offered control bread pieces, which they learned to eat over two days. On days 6–7 each bird was offered a sequence of 10 control bread pieces, with each being available to the bird for up to 90 seconds. They were then deprived and observed for 30 minutes, and then fed pigeon pellets until 8:30PM. The cardenolide test feedings began on day 8 when each of four birds was offered a randomized sequence of 10 single pieces of bread, including five control and five minimal concentration pieces, over a period of one hour. Each subsequent day the concentration of cardenolide on the experimental bread was raised, and the procedure was repeated for up to seven days, i.e. up to seven concentration categories. Different sets of four birds were used for each of three cardenolides. Emetic-dose-fifty determinations of the pure cardenolides were made following the procedure in Brower *et al.*[31] for labriformin.

The tasting tests are summarized in TABLE 3. The digoxin birds appeared to taste this polar cardenolide at even the lowest concentrations, and showed a strong shift at the fourth level where the cardenolide bread eaten dropped from 80% to 37%. At level five the jays rejected all the cardenolide bread. The birds that were offered digitoxin bread did not appear to be deterred at levels one to three and ate all bread offered. However, as in the digoxin birds, their acceptance of the cardenolide bread dropped at level four to 53%, at level five to 19%, and at level six to 7%. The birds showed the least sensitivity to digitoxigenin, appeared to taste it at level five, became strongly deterred at level six where they accepted only 20% of the cardenolide bread, and at level seven accepted only 5% of the cardenolide bread.

The behavior of these birds was similar to other jays' reactions to cardenolide-laden monarchs. They exhibited extreme distaste, annoyance, and frustration when presented with the high (level six) digoxin and digitoxin bread.[42] They flew about the cages, often with the bread in their beaks, until they finally dropped or stored it on a perch for subsequent testing (FIGURE 1). Extensive bill wiping and water drinking were additional evidence of the aversive nature of the stimulus. Moreover, at concentrations above four for digoxin, above five for digitoxin, and above six for digitoxigenin, the jays began rejecting some of the control bread after taking it (TABLE 3). This is evidence of gustatory confusion at the higher concentration levels.

The emetic dose data are in TABLE 3. Digitoxin proved most emetic but did not differ significantly from digoxin, and digitoxigenin, contrary to prediction, was least

TABLE 3. Mean Reactions of 12 Birds (4 per Cardenolide) to Bread Treated with Successively Increasing Concentrations of Three Pure Cardenolides.

Numbers and Percent of Cardenolide-treated (E) and Control (C) Bread Pieces Eaten of those Pieces Taken by 4 Birds in <90 Seconds

Cardenolide Level[a] (10^{-9}moles)		Digoxin			Digitoxin			Digitoxigenin		
		µg[a]	%	N[b]	µg	%	N	µg	%	N
(1) 0.9	E	0.7	82	14/17	0.7	100	20/20	0.3	100	20/20
	C	0	100	18/18	0	100	20/20	0	100	20/20
(2) 2.3	E	1.9	88	14/16	1.8	100	20/20	0.9	100	20/20
	C	0	100	16/16	0	100	20/20	0	100	20/20
(3) 6.4	E	5	80	12/15	5	100	20/20	5	100	20/20
	C	0	100	15/15	0	100	18/18	0	100	20/20
(4) 17	E	14	37	7/19	13	53	10/19	7	100	20/20
	C	0	100	20/20	0	100	19/19	0	100	20/20
(5) 47	E	37	0	0/20	36	19	3/16	18	95	19/20
	C	0	94	16/17	0	100	15/15	0	100	20/20
(6) 130	E	99	0	0/17	98	7	1/15	48	20	4/20
	C	0	94	17/18	0	75	9/12	0	100	20/20
(7) 350	E	270	—	—	265	—	—	130	5	1/20
	C	0	—	—	0	—	—	0	90	18/20
ED_{50} Determinations										
ED_{50} [c] actual µg			133			118			380	
95% confidence limits			87 to 201			85 to 166			266 to 542	
ED_{50} digitoxin equiv.[d]			130			118			776	
95% confidence limits			85 to 197			85 to 166			543 to 1108	

[a] Quantity of cardenolide per 0.05 g piece of bread (successive levels are in natural log increments).

[b] For each test a total of 20 experimental and 20 control pieces of bread (5 experimental and 5 control pieces per bird × 4 birds) were offered; the fraction represents the number eaten of the number taken by the 4 birds. Fewer than 20 in the denominator indicates that the balance of bread pieces was rejected visually.

[c] µg of cardenolide per 85 g jay; the number of birds tested for digoxin = 11, digitoxin = 11, and digitoxigenin = 12.

[d] The µg values are adjusted by molecular weights to equivalent amounts of digitoxin (mw of digoxin = 781; mw of digitoxin = 765; mw of digitoxigenin = 375).

emetic. This is possibly because it is a genin rather than a cardiac glycoside. The relative thresholds for taste discrimination correspond to the polarities as predicted, with digoxin rejected at the lowest concentration and digitoxigenin at the highest. Taste thresholds in terms of μg of cardenolide per piece of bread were well below the emetic doses of each of the respective cardenolides. Thus the taste rejection threshold for cardenolides in the blue jays is sufficient to allow them to avoid ingesting an emetic dose without prior emetic conditioning.

Summary of the Three Laboratory Experiments

The first experiment established that food-deprived jays will attack variably emetic monarchs, show no difference in their treatment of them, and ingest a sufficient amount of a butterfly to vomit one or more times. As a result of eating the first butterfly, the jays develop a conditioned visual aversion of monarchs with the strength of the aversion proportional to the emetic potency of the monarchs. The second experiment extended the findings of the first by forcing previously conditioned jays to attack both palatable and emetic monarchs and demonstrating that the birds can in fact discriminate between them on the basis of taste alone. Experiment 3 confirmed the hypothesis that taste discrimination can be based on cardenolides *per se* and further demonstrated the birds are capable of taste rejection of cardenolide-tainted food at concentration levels substantially below that which would lead to emesis.

FIELD INVESTIGATIONS AND IMPLICATIONS

Together with previously published data,[21,25,32,44] the first experiment established that cardenolide-caused emesis can condition visual rejection of monarch butterflies by the blue jay. The prediction that monarch butterflies should be substantially protected from avian predators in their natural environments therefore seems eminently reasonable. However, the second experiment determined that jays are capable of taste-rejecting food that contains cardenolides and the third experiment established that they can do so at concentration levels sufficiently low to enable them to avoid becoming sickened. Given the fact that natural populations of monarchs vary in their cardenolide contents (FIGURE 2), taste discrimination provides a reasonable basis to explain how certain bird predators have succeeded in breaking through the cardenolide defense of the monarch in the large overwintering aggregations in Mexico.[34,45,46] Within these colonies, which form in the same general areas each year and are as large as five hectares in extent, many millions of butterflies aggregate for up to five months in dense clusters on the trees in a high altitude boreal fir forest.[47] Flocks of two species of birds, the blackheaded grosbeak (*Pheucticus melanocephalus*) and the blackheaded oriole (*Icterus galbula abeillei*) kill an average of 15,000 butterflies per day.[48] The grosbeak is able to feed upon the monarchs because it is insensitive to the emetic effects of cardenolides; the oriole, however, is sensitive.[34]

Orioles Foraging on Monarchs in Mexico

The birds feed upon the monarchs in large mixed- and single-species flocks and concentrate their predation in morning and late afternoon bouts. These coincide with the coolest times of day when the colony temperature is below the butterflies' minimum

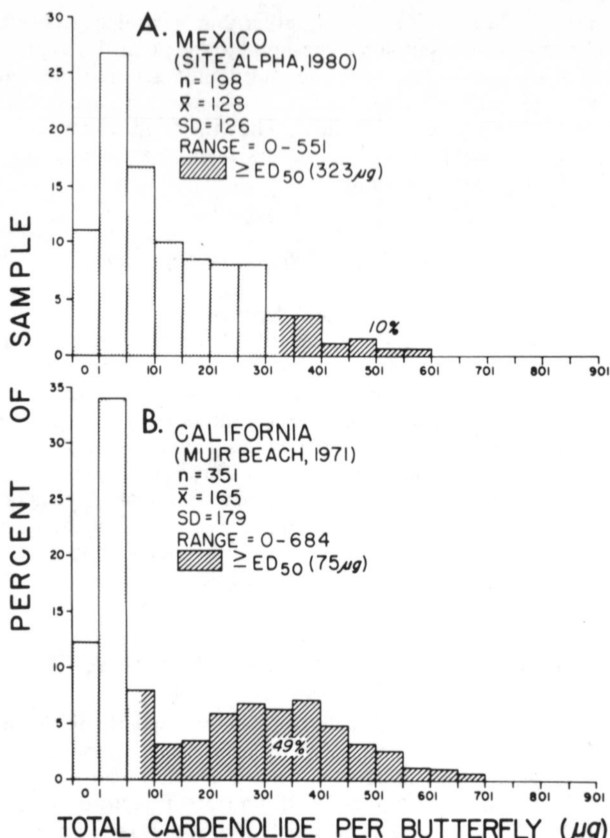

FIGURE 2. Comparison of the total amounts of cardenolides and the emetic potencies of monarch butterflies in overwintering populations (A) at Site Alpha, Michoacan, Mexico during 1980 and (B) at Muir Beach, California during 1971. The hatched area of each histogram represents that segment of the population of butterflies that contains enough cardenolide such that the ingestion of one butterfly would cause emesis in an 85 g blue jay. (Modified from Fink & Brower.[34])

flight temperatures so that the birds can forage upon effectively unlimited numbers of passive monarchs.

We have determined that the orioles kill monarchs in these Mexican overwintering colonies randomly with respect to cardenolide content but then proceed to eat them in ways that reduce the amount of cardenolide that is ingested.[34] Utilizing a modification of their normal fruit-eating behavior,[49,50] they insert their narrowly elongate bills into the abdomen and thorax, slit and pry them open, and pull out and eat only the internal tissues. Cardenolides are not uniformly concentrated throughout the monarch's body: the abdominal and thoracic contents comprise 59% of the dry weight of the butterfly (and an even higher percent of the wet weight) but contain only 21% of the total cardenolide.[37] By probing through the exoskeleton and eating only the soft parts, orioles are able to ingest substantially lower quantities of cardenolide per gram of food ingested than if they ate entire bodies.

Since the average cardenolide content of the Mexican monarchs was 128 μg (FIGURE 2A), non-discriminating orioles would on average ingest 27 μg (21% × 128 μg) per butterfly. Although we have shown that these orioles are sensitive to the emetic effects of monarchs,[34] we lack ED_{50} data for direct comparisons with the blue jays. On the assumption that orioles are equal in sensitivity to the jay, irrespective of the difference in the two species' body weights, they would, on average, have to eat the body contents of 12 monarchs to sicken (12 × 27 μg = 323 μg, the blue jay emetic dose). Adjusting for differences in their body weights, then an ingested dose of 133 μg of cardenolide from five monarchs should cause emesis (= 35 g oriole/85 g blue jay × 323 μg per emetic dose). If the monarchs produce physiological distress at subemetic doses as they do in the jay (experiment 1), then even fewer butterflies would need to be ingested to cause conditioned rejection.

The orioles' feeding strategy is even more refined: the amount of body contents consumed from each monarch is negatively correlated to cardenolide concentration so that a butterfly with a higher concentration has less of its contents eaten than one with a lower concentration of cardenolide. Thus by taste discrimination the orioles further reduce the quantity of cardenolides they ingest.[34] In fact, 35 Mexican oriole stomachs contained an average of only 7 μg of cardenolide and a range of 0 to 15 μg.[46]

These data raise the following question: Is the orioles' taste selectivity due wholly or in part to aversive conditioning based on one or more initial emetic experiences, or is it based on unlearned taste rejection of the bitter cardenolides in the butterflies? We will now explore these two alternatives.

The Conditioned Food Aversion Scenario

Let us assume that the butterflies have recently arrived at the same overwintering site as they do each November,[47] and further assume that the flocks of birds that will feed upon them contain older individuals experienced with the butterflies from having encountered them in previous years, as well as naive young birds. Although these naive individuals may initially be hesitant to attack and eat monarchs, social facilitation within the flock would probably rapidly induce them to attack the butterflies. If they initially ate the monarchs without regard to cardenolide contents (above experiments 1 and 2), then the young birds must eventually sicken. Such birds, if they foraged singly, might become visually conditioned against the monarchs for long periods of time (experiment 1). On the other hand, the presence of dozens of flockmates feeding on the monarchs would probably encourage their resumption of feeding and lead them to conditioned taste discrimination of palatable from unpalatable monarchs (experiment 2). In this way, the young birds could learn the margin of safety for individual butterflies through taste aversion and thereby exhibit the feeding patterns we have observed. The strength of conditioning would probably depend upon the severity and number of emetic experiences, as well as on the order with which the bird happened to encounter the variably poisonous monarchs.

The Non-conditioned Food Aversion Scenario

Within the monarch colony the orioles also take alternative food. Not only did we observe them gleaning among lichens on the butterfly roosting trees, but examination of the stomach contents of the 35 orioles collected in the area indicated that most birds had fed on representatives of two to four arthropod orders (unpublished data).[34] This availability of alternate food is evidence that the naive individuals need not be forced by hunger to attack and eat initial monarchs as the jays were in laboratory experiments 1 and 2, but can gradually attack them as their neophobic responses wane.

If the degree of the orioles' innate taste aversion to cardenolides is dose-dependent (as shown for jays in our experiment 3), this alone may suffice to regulate the quantity of monarch tissues consumed so that the birds need never ingest a sickening dose. The high emetic dose relative to the average cardenolide content of the Mexican butterflies means that there is little penalty for occasionally making a mistake in taste discrimination. The large proportion of low cardenolide butterflies assures that a bird has an abundance of palatable butterflies readily available, so that there is no incentive to eat more of the less palatable butterflies.

Conclusion from These Two Scenarios

Neither scenario contradicts any facts we now have concerning Mexican oriole behavior. Since similar selectivity can arise from more than one combination of mechanisms, need the ecologist be concerned with decision-making mechanisms (as distinct from decision outcomes) at all; is it ecologically important whether a bird rejects an aposematic insect because it has an unconditioned aversion or because it has been conditioned to do so? From both the oriole's and the monarch butterfly's point of view in Mexico, the answer initially appears to be no: each scenario suffices to protect the birds from poisoning, and each results in the death of monarchs since selectivity occurs only after their being killed.

The Situation in California Contrasted with Mexico

We are fortunate in being able to compare two natural populations of overwintering monarch butterflies that differ greatly in their cardenolide characteristics. In contrast to Mexico, California monarch overwintering sites appear to be relatively free from bird predation. Many hours of observations in several colonies indicated only occasional bird predation almost exclusively by chestnut-backed chickadees (*Parus rufescens*) feeding individually or in small flocks (Brower, personal observations).[51]

We hypothesize that the difference in predation intensity is largely based on two qualitative differences in the cardenolides in the butterflies from the two overwintering areas. Although the ranges in the amount of cardenolide in the butterflies from both areas are similar (FIGURE 2), the cardenolides in the California monarchs have on average 4.3 times the emetic potency (ED_{50} = 75 μg) of the cardenolides in the Mexican butterflies (ED_{50} = 323 μg). This results from the fact that the eastern population, which overwinters in Mexico, and western population of monarchs, which overwinters in California, feed on different species of milkweed plants that have very different arrays of cardenolides in them (Brower, Seiber, and Nelson, unpublished data).[32]

This difference in emetic strengths has three major populational consequences. First, if the California butterflies occurred in Mexico, an oriole that did not initially exhibit taste discrimination would have to eat only one or two monarchs to vomit compared to five or 12 Mexican butterflies. Secondly, whereas 90% of the Mexican population is subemetic to jays, only 51% is subemetic in the California population. As a result, the birds in Mexico[3] have the benefit of a broad range in cardenolide concentrations below the emetic dose, whereas in California this margin of safety is extremely narrow. Moreover, based on Rothkopf's data (experiment 3), a bird's ability to taste the cardenolides in the Mexican butterflies may be much greater because the overall polarities of the Mexican cardenolides are high compared to those in the California butterflies. Consequently, birds in California are confronted with a more difficult taste discrimination problem and if they fail, they face a substantially higher probability of emesis. Taken together, these populational and chemical data suggest that the cardenolides in the Californian monarchs, in contrast to those in the Mexican monarchs, are successful in preventing lethal attacks by birds upon the butterflies. It would be of great interest to observe the reactions of Mexican orioles to a California monarch population.

SUMMARY AND CONCLUSIONS

We have verified that wild birds can become conditioned to reject naturally toxic insects either visually (experiment 1) or by taste (experiment 2). We have also verified, however, that unconditioned taste rejection of noxious chemicals by wild birds also occurs (experiment 3). Such unconditioned responses to the aposematic visual and taste cues of many insects, in fact, often appear to be as important as, or more important than, conditioned responses. In a large number of laboratory feeding experiments with wild birds as predators of aposematic insects, initial and/or long-term rejection occurs without prior laboratory conditioning experience.[52–57] Although in some experiments the birds may have previously been exposed to (and therefore perhaps conditioned by) the aposematic prey in the wild, other experiments have used naive birds or insects whose ranges do not overlap those of the birds. Wiklund and Jarvi,[57] for example, tested the response of 47 naive hand-raised birds of four species to five aposematic insect species, and found that 69/136 (51%) insects were rejected visually without even tasting, while 63 were tasted and then rejected. Only four of the insects were actually ingested. Similarly, in Bowers' study[54] of the response of Massachusetts blue jays to aposematic western U.S. *Euphydryas* butterflies, several blue jays consistently rejected the butterflies visually or by taste without having eaten any. While these studies were not designed to separate neophobic effects from innate visual and/or taste aversions, they do differentiate between conditioned and unconditioned responses. Since both conditioned and unconditioned rejections can be demonstrated in the lab by insectivorous birds, and our available field evidence does not yet let us distinguish the mechanisms behind the observed patterns, our initial question, of the relative importance of conditioned versus unconditioned rejection mechanisms in different natural situations, is not yet answerable.

The most important requirement of a food-rejection strategy is that it prevents both poisoning and starvation. We have shown, however, that rejection of a noxious insect by a bird can take place at four distinct levels (visual, non-destructive taste sampling, destructive taste sampling, or post-ingestional physiological rejection), the first three of which may be either unconditioned or conditioned by a physiological reaction to ingestion. Rejection at each level has potential costs as a predator: visual rejectors can be fooled by a palatable mimic; taste rejectors must pursue and capture a number of inedible noxious insects in obtaining the edible; physiological rejection of toxic prey is clearly a useful ability if ingestion occurs, but it is safer and far more efficient to reject the prey before getting sick. For the noxious and/or mimetic insect, the level of rejection is of critical importance: the fact that Mexican orioles kill monarchs before taste-rejecting means that their discrimination does not provide any protection to high-cardenolide monarchs. We do not yet understand the factors that determine at which of the first three levels rejection will occur after conditioning, although clearly such factors as hunger level and proportion of toxic prey (California monarchs) are of major importance. The levels of rejection may be characteristic of different bird species, or of the same species faced with different types of noxious prey, or of the same individual at different stages in its life after different conditioning experiences.

ACKNOWLEDGMENTS

We are grateful to laboratory associate Susan Swartz for her many years of dedication to the monarch–blue jay research program while at Amherst College, and to former Amherst honors students John Jaenike and Douglas Rothkopf for their great efforts in carrying out the two learning studies reviewed in this paper. The original design of the Rothkopf experiment benefited greatly from advice from University of California colleagues Carolyn Nelson and James Seiber. We also thank Barbara Tiffany, the late George McIntrye, and Alan Krause for steadfast contributions to caring for the plants, butterflies, and birds, and helping in many other ways. We thank H. Jane Brockmann, C. Nelson, and J. Seiber for critical comments on the manuscript.

REFERENCES

1. Gustavson, C. R. 1977. Comparative and field aspects of learned food aversions. *In* Learning Mechanisms in Food Selection. L. M. Barker, M. R. Best & M. Domjan, Eds.: 23–43. Baylor University Press. Waco, TX.
2. Garcia, J. & R. A. Koelling. 1966. Relation of cue to consequence in avoidance learning. Psychonomic Sci. **4**: 123–124.
3. Garcia,J., F. R. Ervin & R. A. Koelling. 1966. Learning with prolonged delay of reinforcement. Psychonom. Sci. **5**: 121–122.
4. Rozin, P. 1976. The selection of food by rats, humans, and other animals, *In* Advances in the Study of Behavior. J. Rosenblatt, R. A. Hinde, C. Beer & E. Shaw, Eds. **6**: 21–76, Academic Press. New York.
5. Galef, B. G. 1976. Social transmission of acquired behavior: a discussion of tradition and social learning in vertebrates. *In* Advances in the Study of Behavior. J. Rosenblat, R. A. Hinde, C. Beer & E. Shaw, Eds. **6**: 77–110. Academic Press. New York.
6. Alcock, J. 1969. Observational learning by fork-tailed flycatchers (*Muscivora tyrannus*). Anim. Behav. **17**: 652–657.
7. Alcock, J. 1969. Observational learning in three species of birds. Ibis **111**: 308–321.
8. Klopfer, P. H. 1961. Observational learning in birds: the establishment of behavioral modes. Behaviour **17**: 71–80.
9. Mason J. R. & R. F. Reidinger. 1982. Observational learning of food aversions in red-winged blackbirds. Auk **99**: 548–554.
10. Galef, B. G. 1977. Mechanisms for the social transmission of acquired food preferences from adult to weanling rats. *In* Learning Mechanisms in Food Selection, L. M. Barker, M. R. Best & M. Domjan, Eds.: 123–148. Baylor University Press. Waco, TX.
11. Kawai, M. 1965. Newly acquired precultural behavior of the natural troop of Japanese monkeys on Koshima Islet. Primates **6**: 1–30.
12. Avery, M. L. 1983. Social transmission of an acquired dietary aversion among captive House Finches. 101st American Ornithological Union Meeting. New York. Poster session.
13. Coppinger, R. P. 1969. The effect of experience and novelty on avian feeding behavior with reference to the evolution of warning coloration in butterflies. Part I. Reactions of wild-caught adult blue jays to novel insects. Behaviour **35**: 4–60.
14. Coppinger, R. P. 1970. The effect of experience and novelty on avian feeding behavior

with reference to the evolution of warning coloration in butterflies. Part II. Reactions of naive birds to novel insects. Am. Nat. **104**: 323–335.
15. DOMJAN, M. 1977. Attenuation and enhancement of neophobia for edible substances. *In* Learning Mechanisms in Food Selection. L. M. Barker, M. R. Best & M. Domjan, Eds.: 151–179. Baylor University Press. Waco, TX.
16. GARCIA, J. & W. G. HANKINS. 1975. The evolution of bitter and the acquisition of toxiphobia. *In* Fifth International Symposium on Olfaction and Taste. D. A. Denton & J. P. Coghlan, Eds.: 39–45. Academic Press. New York.
17. ZAHORIK, D. M. & K. A. HOUPT. 1977. The concept of nutritional wisdom: applicability of laboratory learning models to large herbivores. *In* Learning Mechanisms in Food Selection. L. M. Barker, M. R. Best & M. Domjan, Eds.: 45–67. Baylor University Press. Waco, TX.
18. ZAHORIK, D. M. & K. A. HOUPT. 1981. Species differences in feeding strategies, food hazards, and the ability to learn food aversions. *In* Foraging Behavior. A. Kamil & T. Sargent, Eds.: 289–310. Garland Press. New York.
19. KAMIL, A. & S. YOERG. 1982. Learning and foraging behavior. *In* Perspectives in Ethology, (Ontogeny). P. P. G. Bateson & P. H. Klopfer, Eds. **5**: 325–364. Plenum Press. New York.
20. COTT, H. B. 1940. Adaptive Coloration in Animals. Methuen and Co. London.
21. BROWER, L. P. 1971. Prey coloration and predator behavior. *In* Topics in the Study of Life: The Bio Source Book, Section 6, Animal Behavior. pp. 360–370. Harper and Row. New York.
22. EDMUNDS, M. E. 1974. Defense in Animals. Longman Group, Ltd. Harlow, Essex.
23. EISNER, T. 1970. Chemical defense against predation in arthropods. *In* Chemical Ecology. E. Sondheimer & J. B. Simeone, Eds.: 157–217. Academic Press. New York.
24. BLUM, M. 1981. Chemical Defenses of Arthropods. Academic Press. New York.
25. BROWER, L. P. 1984. Chemical defence in butterflies. Symp. Royal Entomol. Society London **11**: 109–134.
26. BENT, A. C. 1942. Life histories of North American flycatchers, swallows, larks, and their allies. U.S. Nat. Mus. Bull. **179**. Washington, D.C.
27. BENT, A. C. 1946. Life histories of North American jays, crows, and titmice. U.S. National Museum Bull. **191**. Washington, D.C.
28. WELTY, J. C. 1982. The Life of Birds. 3rd edit. Saunders Publ. Co. Philadelphia.
29. BROWER, L. P., J. V. Z. BROWER & J. M. CORVINO. 1967. Plant poisons in a terrestrial food chain. Proc. Natl. Acad. Sci. USA **57**: 893–898.
30. BROWER, L. P., W. N. RYERSON, L. L. COPPINGER & S. C. GLAZIER. 1968. Ecological chemistry and the palatability spectrum. Science **161**: 1349–1351.
31. BROWER, L. P., J. N. SEIBER, C. J. NELSON, S. P. LYNCH & P. M. TUSKES. 1982. Plant-determined variation in the cardenolide content, thin-layer chromatography profiles, and emetic potency of monarch butterflies, *Danaus plexippus* reared on the milkweed, *Asclepias eriocarpa* in California. J. Chem. Ecol. **8**: 579–633.
32. BROWER, L. P., J. N. SEIBER, C. J. NELSON, S. P. LYNCH & M. M. HOLLAND. 1984. Plant-determined variation in the cardenolide content, thin-layer chromatography profiles, and emetic potency of monarch butterflies, *Danaus plexippus* L. reared on milkweed plants in California, 2: *Asclepias speciosa*. J. Chem. Ecol. **10**: 601–639.
33. BROWER, L. P. & C. M. MOFFITT. 1974. Palatability dynamics of cardenolides in the monarch butterfly. Nature **249**: 280–283.
34. FINK, L. S. & L. P. BROWER. 1981. Birds can overcome the cardenolide defence of the monarch butterflies in Mexico. Nature **291**: 67–70.
35. SEIBER, J. N., S. M. LEE & J. M. BENSON. 1984. Cardiac glycosides (cardenolides) in species of *Asclepias* (Asclepiadaceae). *In* Handbook of Natural Toxins Vol. I: Plant and Fungal Toxins. R. F. Keeler & A. T. Tu, Eds.: 43–83.
36. BROWER, L. P. & S. C. GLAZIER. 1975. Localization of heart poisons in the monarch butterfly. Science **188**: 19–25.
37. BROWER, L. P., C. J. NELSON & C. BOND. 1985. Distribution of cardenolides in the body and exoskeleton of adult monarch butterflies.
38. JAENIKE, J. R., JR. 1971. Parallels between the toxicity spectrum of monarch butterflies

and the behavior of their blue jay predators. Amherst College Senior Honors Thesis. Amherst, Massachusetts. pp. 1–75.
39. SIEGEL, S. 1956. Nonparametric Statistics for the Behavioral Sciences. McGraw Hill Book Co., New York.
40. ROTHKOPF, D. M. 1976. The taste rejection and emetic potency of several digitalis series cardenolides in the blue jay, *Cyanocitta cristata bromia* Oberholser. Amherst College Senior Honors Thesis. Amherst Massachusetts. pp. 1–95.
41. GOLDSTEIN, A., L. ARONOW & S. M. KALMAN. 1969. Principles of Drug Action. The Basis of Pharmacology. Harper and Row. New York.
42. ROESKE, C. N., J. N. SEIBER, L. P. BROWER & C. M. MOFFITT. 1976. Milkweed cardenolides and their comparative processing by monarch butterflies (*Danaus plexippus* L.). Rec. Adv. Phytochem. **10**: 93–167.
43. ZULLICH, G., W. BRAUN & B. P. LISBOA. 1975. Thin-layer chromatography for separation of digitoxin, digitoxigenin, and related compounds. J. Chromatog. **103**: 396–401.
44. BROWER, L. P. 1969. Ecological chemistry. Sci. Am. **220** (*2*): 22–29.
45. CALVERT, W. H., L. E. HEDRICK & L. P. BROWER. 1979. Mortality of the monarch butterfly (*Danaus plexippus* L.): avian predation at five overwintering sites in Mexico. Science **204**: 847–851.
46. FINK, L. S., L. P. BROWER, R. B. WAIDE & P. R. SPITZER. 1983. Overwintering monarch butterflies as food for insectivorous birds in Mexico. Biotropica **15**: 151–153.
47. BROWER, L. P. 1985. New perspectives on the migration biology of the monarch butterfly, *Danaus plexippus* L. *In* Migration, Mechanisms and Adaptive Significance. M. A. Rankin & H. F. Dingle, Eds. Suppl. to Vol. 27. (In press). University of Texas Contributions in Marine Science.
48. BROWER, L. P. & W. H. CALVERT. 1985. Foraging dynamics of bird predators on overwintering monarch butterflies in Mexico. Evolution **39**. (In press.)
49. BENT, A. C. 1958. Life histories of North American blackbirds, orioles, tanagers, and their allies. U.S. Museum Bull. **211**. Washington, D.C.
50. FORBUSH, E. H. 1929. Birds of Massachusetts and Other New England States. Norwood Press. Boston.
51. STECKER, R. E., H. T. HARVEY & J. DAYTON. 1981. Monarch butterfly monitoring study Natural Bridges and Moran Lake. Report to Harvey and Stanley Associates, Inc. Alviso, CA. pp. 1–42
52. BROWER, J. V. Z. 1958. Experimental studies of mimicry in some North American butterflies. I. The monarch *Danaus plexippus* and viceroy *Limenitis archippus*. Evolution **11**: 32–47.
53. BOWERS, M. D. 1980. Unpalatability as a defense strategy of *Euphydryas phaeton* (Lepidoptera: Nymphalidae). Evolution **34**: 586–600.
54. BOWERS, M. D. 1981. Unpalatability as a defense strategy of western checkerspot butterflies (*Euphydryas* Scudder, Nymphalidae). Evolution **35**: 367–375.
55. JARVI, T., B. SILLEN-TULLBERG & C. WIKLUND. 1981. The cost of being aposematic. An experimental study of predation on larvae of *Papilio machaon* by the Great Tit *Parus major.* Oikos **36**: 267–272.
56. SILLEN-TULLBERG, B., C. WIKLUND & T. JARVI. 1982. Aposematic coloration in adults and larvae of *Lygaeus equestris* and its bearing on mullerian mimicry: an experimental study on predation on living bugs by the great tit *Parus major.* Oikos **39**: 131–136.
57. WIKLUND, C. & T. JARVI. 1982. Survival of distasteful insects after being attacked by naive birds: a reappraisal of the theory of aposematic coloration evolving through individual selection. Evolution **36**: 998–1002.

The Role of Pavlovian Conditioning in the Acquisition of Food Likes and Dislikes[a]

PAUL ROZIN AND DEBRA ZELLNER

Department of Psychology
University of Pennsylvania
Philadelphia, Pennsylvania 19104

There are two things about human food preferences that dim the prospects for enlightenment from the perspective of animal food choice and animal conditioning. One is the fact that our relations to foods are dominated by affective responses; we like or dislike most of the foods we experience, and this hedonic response is a major determinant of our food choices. There is no reason to believe that animals don't share this hedonic response, but because we cannot use our language to communicate with them, it is very hard to get at. The second reason is the more daunting. Surely the primary determinant of human food preferences is culturally transmitted information or values. Although there is evidence of social transmission of information about foods in animals,[1] it is much more limited in complexity and extent than in humans. Furthermore, our world of food becomes an integral part of cultural institutions, and food comes to serve functions other than nutrition. It is a social vehicle, a way of stating one's closeness to or distance from another. And, through the development of cuisine, food has become part of an art form.

Nevertheless, we are animals and share the same pressing need for nutrients as chimpanzees, rats, and other homeotherms. As one among the many food generalists, we face the problem of identifying food sources, avoiding toxins, and eating a nutritionally balanced diet. Given the fundamental importance of nutrition, and in spite of the fact that it is a part of omnivore biology not to have a great many biological constraints on food choice, we expect that the human animal will show through the cultural overlay.

In this paper we explore one process common to humans and animals, Pavlovian conditioning, and see to what extent it can account for human food preferences and avoidances. We will define Pavlovian conditioning broadly, as changes in response or attitude to stimuli resulting from their contingent occurrence (temporally and/or spatially) with other, more potent stimuli. The potency of these other stimuli may be genetically programmed (the traditional US) or result from an acquisition process, as in higher order conditioning or sensory preconditioning. Many authors have thought of Pavlovian conditioning as particularly important in the acquisition of emotional responses by animals. Some have suggested that Pavlovian conditioning can account for evaluative responses by humans to objects or situations.[2–4] Since the problem of explaining human food preferences is in part the explanation of the acquisition of likes and dislikes for objects, we feel this enterprise has some hope.

[a] Some of the research described in this paper was supported by National Science Foundation Grant BNS76-80108 and National Institutes of Health Grant HD 12674. D.A.Z. was supported by a National Institute of Mental Health Training Grant 5-T32-MH150922. Preparation of this paper was supported by a MacArthur Foundation Grant.

We begin with a description of human motivations for food choice, and a food-oriented taxonomy of objects in the world. We then explicitly consider an issue central to animal-human comparisons: the distinction between preference and liking. Then, for the major part of this paper, we discuss categories of situations in which Pavlovian conditioning might lead to likes and dislikes.

THE END POINT—WHAT WE ARE TRYING TO EXPLAIN

Our aim is to account for the items that adults eat and those that they reject as food. We will limit ourselves to reactions to available foods. By doing so, we bypass two powerful determinants of actual food choice, literal availability and cost. Through questionnaires and interviews of American subjects, we[5-7] have identified three basic motivations for acceptance or rejection of foods. One is sensory-affective, basically liking or disliking the sensory properties (mostly naso-oral sensations). Items rejected primarily on these grounds are called distastes, those accepted primarily on these grounds are called good tastes. A second is anticipated consequences, that is, (instrumentally based) concern for the consequences (positive or negative) of ingestion. Items rejected primarily on these grounds are called dangerous, and those accepted, beneficial. A third motivation is uniquely human, and we call it ideational. It has to do with one's knowledge of the nature or origin of a potential food. It is, at least in part, culture mediated.

We discern two types of negative ideational rejections. One, inappropriate, encompasses items that are rejected as inedible, but do not have particularly negative affective properties as foods, such as certain leaves, sand, pencil erasers, etc. In fact, the majority of things in the world. A second, disgust, involves ideational rejections that are offensive and have negative sensory affective properties, such as feces, worms, and cockroaches.

Of course, many items fall between these categories, and so might be, for example, distasteful and dangerous. For example, most coffee drinkers accept it for multiple reasons, including good taste, a variety of positive physiological consequences (caffeine effects), and, for some, social ideational reasons (e.g. feeling grown up for an early teenager). Furthermore, our three current motivations may also be historical causes of one another, so that, for example, anticipated positive consequences may initially both support acceptance and be the cause of later acceptance based on sensory-affective grounds (liking for the taste).

PREFERENCE AND LIKING

In the contrasting pairings, distaste-danger, good taste-beneficial, and disgust-inappropriate, the first member of each pair has sensory affective (hedonic) value, while the second does not. While this distinction is easy to make with humans, it is hard to make with non-human animals. This forces us to examine a fundamental distinction that is often confounded in food selection research. It is the distinction between preference and liking.[8,9] Virtually all animal and much human choice data measure preference. Preference is a comparative term that simply indicates a greater intake of A than B in choice tests. Liking refers to an affective response to (the sensory properties of) a food. It can also be used as a comparative term, as when we say that A is liked better than B. Because (as indicated in the above taxonomy) liking is one, often predominant, determinant of preference, it is usually the case that the better liked choice is also preferred.

However, because there are other determinants of preference, preference and liking may be discrepant. For example, in humans, social context influences preferences. Sometimes, it is socially more appropriate to eat a less liked food, as when a person leaves a choice morsel for a friend or respected guest. Preferences also result from an instrumental relationship between some food and its effects, rather than liking for the food. For example, food A might be preferred over B even though B is liked more because the person is on a diet and A has fewer calories, or because the person suspects B of having some harmful effects (e.g. high in cholesterol). We also note that even if a food preference is based on liking, the preferred item is not necessarily liked. Instead, it could be that the preferred food is disliked less than the unpreferred one. Therefore, on two grounds, positive affect cannot be directly inferred from preference data.

When does a preference indicate liking? One can ask humans to make choices based on liking rather than other factors (e.g. with hedonic scales) or extract verbally expressed reasons for preference. But these techniques can't be used with animals. Yet, as P. T. Young[10] has forcefully argued, hedonic processes (manifested as palatability), are important aspects of the feeding behavior of animals. Fortunately, there are a few methods that can be used with both animals and humans, to at least support a weak inference of liking in animals.[8]

Appearance of Expressive Responses

Liking is suggested if ingestion of a food is accompanied by expressive behaviors that indicate positive and negative affect. There are well-documented pleasure (like) and disgust-distaste (dislike) facial expressions in humans,[11] including infants.[12] Grill and Norgren[13] have described what are probably corresponding negative facial and bodily gestures in rats consuming unpreferred substances, such as quinine. More recently, a pattern of "positive" expressions has been identified, elicited, for example, by sugar.[14] These rat facial expressions certainly suggest an affective response to the taste. We will elaborate on this later.

No Basis for Anticipated Consequences

Liking is suggested if, given the history of the subject, there is no reason to believe that consuming the preferred food has any instrumental value. (For example, ingestion of the food or flavor in question has not been followed by rapid satiation, illness, drug withdrawal, or recovery from vitamin deficiency). Alternatively, it may be possible to show that anticipated consequences that are in force are not necessary for the occurrence of a change in preference.

Stability across Different Physiological States or Environmental Contexts

A preference based primarily on liking may be more stable and longer lasting than a preference depending on consequences of ingestion. If an animal prefers A to B because A has previously been paired with greater satiation (or relief from drug withdrawal) and the animal seeks that state, then the preference should disappear in an energy-replete (or non-withdrawn) state. A similar logic has been applied to higher-order conditioning, in which the effect of devaluing the consequence (US) or extinguishing the linkage between a CS and its consequences has been explored.[15] Also, a change in social context (who is present, if it is a holiday) will certainly affect preferences based on social consequences in such contexts. In both social and physiological contexts, liking may or may not change; it is not necessarily related to these contexts. It does change with some shifts in physiological context, as in the alliesthesia phenomenon, where the hedonic properties of sweet tastes change in relation to state of energy deficit.[16] In a related formulation, Young[10] has emphasized the contrast between palatability and appetite, and argues that preferences manifested in brief exposures, with very small intakes, and in a need-free state are probably based on palatability.

Talking to Animals

It is conceivable that one might train an animal to make the distinction between liking of a flavor and ingestion based on consequences. Gleitman[17] has outlined experimental procedures that might accomplish this result. But, such studies have never actually been carried out.

Animal Situations that Parallel Human Hedonic Shifts

If conditions that produce hedonic shifts in humans induce preferences in animals, one may presume that a hedonic shift is produced in animals. Thus, graduated exposure to chili pepper in crackers, in a positive social context, leads to a preference for hot crackers in chimpanzees.[18] This exposure sequence mimics the sequence that gives rise to liking of chili pepper in humans. In the absence of any obvious anticipated consequence, it seems reasonable to presume an acquired liking in the chimpanzee.

Parallel with an Established Case of Hedonic Shift in Animals

If we establish, on some of the grounds indicated above, that a sensory-affective response is involved in an animal with respect to a particular object, then equivalent behavior toward other objects suggests a sensory-affective response as well. For example, an inference that thiamin-deficient diets come to taste bad in thiamin-deficient rats was supported by the observation that the rats' behavior to these diets was like their behavior to a known aversive substance, quinine.[19]

PAVLOVIAN CONDITIONING AND THE ACQUISITION OF GOOD TASTES AND DISTASTES

The animal data on food preferences rarely include measurements that allow us to distinguish preferences motivated by anticipated consequences (probably instrumentally based) from preferences motivated by liking. Since our major concern is with just this difference, we will sometimes be on shaky ground in establishing parallels between conditioning of hedonic changes in animals and humans. Furthermore, it is not always clear that the Pavlovian framework is the correct way to characterize an acquisition process; distinctions between Pavlovian conditioning and instrumental learning or association of "ideas" or non-associative processes are sometimes hard to make. We shall only consider cases in which we consider a Pavlovian construal reasonable and likely; we leave aside cases such as "mere exposure," where such a construal is possible but less likely.

We will consider in some detail two types of associations: flavor-postingestional consequence and flavor-flavor. We will then consider more briefly two other possible Pavlovian mechanisms, involving the role of social "USs" and conditioned compensatory (opponent) responses.

Flavor–Postingestional Consequence Relations

Preference changes resulting from pairing of a flavor with postingestional consequences can be framed as instrumental learning, in which case the preference is accounted for as a change in strength of a behavior (or, in our terms, motivation by anticipated consequences). A Pavlovian approach emphasizes a change in value of the stimulus itself. Both accounts might hold in any given case (i.e. cases of mixed sensory-affective and anticipated consequence motivation) and either can by itself account for some preferences.

Conditioned Taste Aversions

The paradigmatic and clearest example of hedonic change in the response to food is learned taste aversions. This phenomenon, in which rats rapidly come to avoid a flavor paired with "malaise," was first clearly described by Garcia and his colleagues.[20–22] The literature on this effect is now vast.[23] Although conditioned taste aversions show some special properties, in many respects they follow the general principles of Pavlovian conditioning.[24] A number of authors[17,22,25] suggested that this type of learning might involve a hedonic change. Following malaise, the animal may come to dislike the taste of the food, whereas following "exteroceptive" USs such as peripheral shock, one might see avoidance (based on anticipated consequences) as opposed to a hedonic change.

Following on the description of conditioned taste aversions in animals, parallel phenomena were reported in humans, based on results from questionnaires[26,27] and behavior therapy. Experimental evidence came from controlled studies in cancer patients receiving nausea-inducing chemotherapeutic drugs.[28,29] Pediatric and adult cancer patients reliably choose to eat a novel ice cream rather than the ice cream previously paired with illness, including nausea. Along with the animal studies, these studies focused attention on negative events in the upper gastrointestinal system as critical USs for the production of hedonic changes.

A special role for nausea was directly identified in a questionnaire study that collected hundreds of cases of ingestion of specific foods followed by any of a wide variety of negative events.[30] Hedonic changes (dislikes) were greatest, by far, when nausea or vomiting was a component of the negative events. Other negative postingestional events (e.g. lower gut cramps, fever, respiratory distress, skin rashes) often caused avoidance of foods, but usually did not lead to acquired dislikes. It was reported that people with food allergies that did not have a nausea component usually continued to like the allergy-inducing food, but, of course, avoided eating it.

This same distaste-danger distinction has now been demonstrated with rats, using expressive responses as the criterion for distaste. Grill[31] showed that following LiCl poisoning of sucrose solutions, a rat's normally positive facial response to sucrose solution was replaced by a set of facial gestures resembling those made to bitter quinine solutions. This finding suggested a hedonic change. But it remained to be shown that such a hedonic change was specific to nausea-inducing USs. This step was taken by establishing equal levels of avoidance of a sucrose solution in three groups of rats, by pairing drinking of the sucrose solution with either intragrastric LiCl (the standard US in conditioned taste aversions and presumed to produce nausea), intragastric lactose (producing lower gut bloating and, presumably, pain), or peripheral electric shock.[32] Hedonic change was assessed by examining changes in facial responses to sucrose solution (using the Grill and Norgren[13] procedure) before and after aversion training. The "quinine" facial pattern was observed reliably in the LiCl group and did not appear at all in the other two groups. Parker[33] demonstrated a similar distinction between lithium chloride and amphetamine-based avoidances in rats. Thus, the animal and human data point to a specific role for nausea in negative hedonic change.

The findings on conditioned taste aversions raise two interesting problems. One is, why should nausea, and no other postingestive event (under most circumstances) lead to a distaste? Lower gastrointestinal pain is as likely as nausea to result from something ingested. It is not because the delay of symptom onset is greater with lower gastrointestinal events or other types of negative events.[30] We don't have the answer to this. And we are puzzled as well by its adaptive significance. What is the functional reason for nausea producing different types of rejection than other negative events? A second problem has to do with the actual importance of conditioned taste aversions in the genesis of the many acquired food dislikes that most people have. Only about half of the people surveyed can remember one or more specific aversion (nausea) experiences. In order to account for most human distastes, we must either assume extensive forgetting or the occurrence of unnoticed effects of low levels of nausea. Or, it is possible that conditioned taste aversions are very well defined phenomena that account for only a small percentage of acquired distastes. In that case, we must look elsewhere for other mechanisms.

Acquired Likes

In animals, it has been much harder to establish acquired preferences than acquired aversions.[22,34] While a single trial with LiCl as the US reliably converts the innate sucrose preference into an aversion, it is almost impossible to convert a rat's aversion to bitter flavors or irritants into a preference with extended programs of exposure and reinforcement.[35] Animal studies are often confounded by two factors: the difficulty in measuring positive hedonic changes and the difficulty in distinguishing whether an enhanced preference for A with respect to B should be interpreted as an increased aversion to B or an enhanced preference for A.[19,34] Many studies that report enhanced preference associated with positive consequences can be interpreted as enhanced aversion of the alternative. Nonetheless, there are some studies[36] that demonstrated an enhanced positive preference. Interpreting the animal studies on preference liberally, a wide variety of USs or reinforcements, including termination of drug withdrawal,[37] brain stimulation, and recovery from vitamin deficiency have supported preference change. Even if these effects are smaller than the negative effects and require more trials, they do take place. There is no evidence that we are aware of for a specific potency for the reversal of nausea, the mirror image of the aversion effect. However, Booth and his colleagues[38,39] have shown substantial and rapid preference increases in rats using satiety as the reinforcement. This effect, which may (but need not) be expressed largely as an upper gastrointestinal phenomenon, may provide the parallel with conditioned taste aversions, but we believe it to be much less potent.

The question still remains whether these changes in preference are based on liking. There is one study that suggests a liking change for at least one preference acquired by rats.[40] Rats were raised from weaning on morphine as their only source of fluid. Morphine is bitter and is normally avoided by rats. Judged by their facial expressions, the morphine is disliked. After months of exposure to morphine, resulting in addiction, these rats showed a preference for the morphine solution over saccharin. This result, in itself, could be accounted for as instrumentally based, with relief of withdrawal and/or euphoria as the reinforcement. However, response of these rats to infusion of morphine into their oral cavity, measured in terms of the taste reactivity test,[13,14] showed ingestive responses to morphine, in contrast to the aversive responses in control animals. In this case, the evidence indicates that a positive hedonic change occurred as a result of pairing of the flavor of morphine with positive consequences. (The preference for morphine might be supported by an instrumental contingency, as well).

There are certainly ample opportunities for people to associate ingested items with positive aftereffects. While food can produce a wide spectrum of negative effects, the positive effect produced by most foods is satiation. Satiety is expressed in terms of both gastrointestinal and postabsorptive events. Ingested foods and medicines can also produce other effects, including relief of gastric pain, fever, vitamin deficiency symptoms, and drug withdrawal symptoms. But satiety is clearly the consequence of choice, based on both common sense and Booth's data on animals. Booth and his colleagues[39,41] have demonstrated clear enhancement in preference and liking for higher caloric density foods fed to hungry humans and evaluated when the subjects are hungry.

Is satiety specifically related to acquired liking, in the way that nausea relates to acquired dislike? The question has two components. First, is satiety a really potent force in acquired likings? Data from the animal literature are mixed, and data from humans are minimal but suggestive. Second, can similar effects be produced by other consequences? In one questionnaire study, humans rated their liking for medicines they had used that had distinctive tastes.[42] Analysis of these results reveals that no specific positive postingestional effects of medicines (relief of diarrhea, constipation, heartburn, fever, or pain) lead to substantial increases in liking. Since none of the medicines produced satiety, the fact that acquired likes for medicines was less common than for foods supports the idea of a special role for satiety. We[42] also tested directly for enhancement of liking for a flavor associated with recovery from drug withdrawal. Opiate addicts who had taken thousands of doses of (bitter) methadone in Tang® showed no enhancement in liking for either Tang,® or Tang® with bitter tastes simulating methadone. Furthermore, their rating for these substances was not higher than the rating of people not on a methadone program.

The opiate (and medicine survey) results suggest that humans tend not to get to like flavors paired with positive physiological effects other than satiety. This contrasts with the evidence for increased liking for the flavor of morphine by morphine-addicted rats.[40] However, there is a confounding in humans between context of ingestion (food or medicine) and type of postingestional effect (satiety or other). Both types of effect and context may contribute to the infrequent cases of acquired likes for medicine in humans. Note that although medicines such as antacids have positive, rapid and upper gastrointestinal effects, people rarely come to like their flavor. We suggested[42] that the medicinal context, that is, the explicit expectation of positive consequences may block hedonic changes in humans. This position has support both in general theory and in the food choice literature. Social psychologists[43] distinguish between intrinsic and extrinsic motivations. Intrinsic motivation refers to motivation deriving directly from interaction with an object (situation), while extrinsic motivation refers to motivation coming from anticipation of the consequences of interacting with the object. The parallel with our formulation of sensory-affective and anticipated consequence motivations is clear. Lepper[43] and others have shown that intrinsically valued objects or activities become less valued if extrinsic reward is introduced for engaging with these objects (activities). Thus, children's preference for an activity that they enjoy performing decreases if they are rewarded for performing this activity. Birch and her colleagues[44] have demonstrated this effect in the domain of food, using preschool children. When children are rewarded for consuming a food, the food (following termination of the reward phase of the study) drops in preference to a point lower than its initial preference. The explanation of this result, sometimes called the overjustification effect, is that reward from significant others for engaging with an object is a statement that these others do not value the object for its own sake. This perception devalues the object.

We[42] suggested an extension of this view that holds that the initial establishment of an intrinsically valuable object is interfered with if there are explicit rewards for engaging in the activity. Medicines may be viewed in this framework, because they are taken explicitly for their consequences. Hence, it is possible that social attributions block hedonic changes to the positive effects of non-foods.

Flavor-Flavor Associations

Association of a stimulus with another stimulus of either positive or negative hedonic value sometimes results in a change in the hedonic value of the first stimulus, in the direction of the value of the second stimuls. This has been called evaluative conditioning since what is conditioned is an affective response to the stimulus.[3] With flavors, the second (US) has generally been another flavor with strong hedonic properties. Animals and humans often consume, simultaneously or in sequence, a variety of separable food items that give rise to distinctive oro-naso-pharyngeal sensations. A single meal of mixed components allows many opportunities for flavor associations of the sort we are referring to. In addition, associations of neutral flavors would be very likely to occur in meals. These may also be involved in hedonic shifts, through prior or subsequent pairings of one of the flavors with hedonically potent USs by the processes of higher order conditioning or sensory pre-conditioning.[45,46] The two flavors in a flavor-flavor pairing are usually presented simultaneously (simultaneous conditioning[47]). There may be a role of special importance for simultaneous conditioning in hedonic change. This is especially appealing because preference changes resulting from simultaneous pairings cannot be explained in terms of anticipated consequences, since the CS does not "predict" the US.

Distastes Acquired by Flavor-Flavor Associations

Surprisingly, we know of no studies showing that flavor-flavor associations lead to acquired distastes in humans and are aware of only one relevant animal study. Although this rat study does not demonstrate a change in liking, it does show a clear negative change in preference for an initially preferred flavor following pairing of that flavor with quinine, an initially disliked flavor.[48] In the absence of an anticipated consequence, we suggest that this might be a hedonic change. A number of studies of sensory preconditioning demonstrate that associations between two originally neutral flavors can later result in preference (probably hedonic) change. When one of the flavors is paired with toxicosis, the other flavor becomes less preferred as well.[45,46] This result opens up the possibility of a wide range of acquired distastes.

Good Tastes Acquired by Flavor-Flavor Associations

In contrast to the situation with postingestional consequences, the data on flavor-flavor associations speak more clearly on the positive side. This is not because of the greater potency of positive flavor-flavor associations, but because there have been more attempts on this side of the problem. A few studies on rats report that neutral flavors simultaneously paired with sweet tastes (saccharin or sucrose) become more preferred.[48,49] Although from these data we cannot be sure that the increased preference results from an affective change, human data from our own laboratory suggest that flavor-flavor conditioning of this type does result in an affective change.

In our study,[50] subjects were exposed to two flavors, one flavor always in a 4% sucrose solution (simultaneous pairing) and a second presented an equal number of times in water without sucrose. Following pairing, the flavor previously paired with sugar increased in hedonic rating more than the flavor never paired with sugar. This effect appeared whether the two flavors were compared in a 4% sucrose base or in plain water. The effect was still present one week after conditioning.

Both the human and animal results seem very dependent on specific and subtle aspects of the training or testing situation, since there are difficulties in replicating the animal studies and in extending the human results to slightly changed situations. We do not know if this has to do with the general weakness or context sensitivity of positive conditioning, or a weakness or context sensitivity of flavor-flavor associations in general. There is not enough data on negative flavor-flavor associations to allow an evaluation of these alternatives.

We conclude that there is some evidence for flavor-flavor associations on both the positive and negative sides and that such associations could potentially explain a great many human likes and dislikes for foods and flavors.

Conditioned Opponent or Compensatory Responses

Preferences for innately negative substances are widespread among humans. These include bitter substances, such as coffee and tobacco, and irritant substances, such as chili pepper, horseradish or black pepper.[51] Such preferences are extremely rare in non-human omnivores.[18] The initial negativity of these items allows for the operation of preference mechanisms that generate positivity out of negativity. One example is Solomon's opponent process theory,[52] which, in the service of emotional homeostasis, postulates opponent responses on a non-associative basis. Siegel[53] and Schull[54] have hypothesized conditioned compensatory or opponent responses. These are Pavlovian conditioned responses that anticipate and oppose signalled events, in such a manner as to neutralize them. If one makes the additional assumption that with extended exposure, conditioned opponent responses can overshoot and hence reverse rather than neutralize the initial effect (US), one can account for acquired preferences for innately unpalatable substances. For example, in the case of chili pepper, cultural forces (in cultures that regularly consume this spice) maintain ingestion of the spice even though it produces oral pain.[51,55] Many experiences of piquant foods may allow conditioned opponent responses to the signalled arrival of oral pain to grow to the point where they generate a net pleasure.[55] This might be mediated by the conditioned secretion of endorphins in response to frequent ingestion of piquant foods, and an excess of endorphins might account for the chili eaters liking of the very same pain sensations that deter the uninitiated.[56]

Associations Between Foods and Social Stimuli

Social factors, such as the behavior of conspecific animals (age mates, parents) influence preferences for foods.[57] However, social effects are much more extensive in humans. Approval of elders or peers, or the perception that such people value a food, can enhance its preference.[58,59] Within the social domain, previous research addresses neither the preference-liking distinction nor the role of Pavlovian conditioning. However, it seems reasonable that positive facial expressions or other evaluative clues from others may function as unconditioned stimuli that lead to enhanced liking.

Tomkins[60] has suggested two possible pathways. A facial expression in another person may automatically cause a corresponding expression in the target person and hence (by Tomkins view) a corresponding reaction, which could condition a response to the object in question. An alternative involves voluntary modelling of the facial expression of the other. These ideas suggest that empathic responses may be involved, where the empathic response creates the US in the target person.

Disgust. Pairing of Food with Social Stimuli or with Ideas

Disgusting items are offensive because of their nature.[6,61,62] The sight, touch, odor, and taste are all undesirable, and they tend to induce nausea. Most critically, disgusting items are contaminants; when they come in contact with a good food (as when a fly falls in a glass of milk) they render it inedible or even offensive. Almost all disgusts are animals and animal products; feces is a universal disgust. The particular set of animals and animal products that are disgusting varies from culture to culture. Disgust represents a part of the acquisition of culture in which strong negative cultural values are "transferred" to youngsters. They represent a linkage between affect and cognitions (knowledge about the nature of objects).

We envision a role for Pavlovian processes at a number of points. We presume that feces is the primary disgust and that this disgust is created in the process of toilet training. Disgust for feces (and other items) could be produced with the intense disgust facial expression of others as the US (see discussion of Tomkins, above). Once disgusting items have been established for any individual, spatial co-occurrence (a condition of simultaneous associations) between neutral and disgust items may produce further disgusts. In surveys of negative or positive responses to objects or situations of any type caused by single, identifiable events, in about 400 students, we have come across eighteen cases that seem to involve disgust. These include experiences such as: rejection of M&Ms after hearing that the outside shell was made of fly droppings or rejection of spaghetti, after having a hand placed in what was described as a bowl of worms in a haunted house, and later discovering that it was spaghetti.[63]

The phenomenon of contamination may have a Pavlovian component. In one contamination situation, a disgust object (e.g. cockroach) is placed (falls into) a glass of juice. The juice is now rejected, even after the cockroach is removed.[64] This rejection could be motivated by cognitive factors; the realization that some trace of the disgust object might remain in the juice. But it could also result from an association between the juice and a disgusting object. There is evidence for the latter. For example, about half of the people we have interviewed say that would reject a glass of juice if it was stirred by a brand new fly swatter.[65] Now there is no possibility of a trace here. It is just the idea of the two together, and that falls well within an associational framework. The same explanation would hold for why the brand new fly swatter itself is disgusting.

Another paradigm that may illustrate this effect is as follows: a cockroach is dropped into a glass of apple juice. Now a second glass of apple juice is poured, into a clean cup. Rejection of this second glass (without any trace contamination), if it occurs, could be accounted for in Pavlovian terms.

Just as belongingness is a salient feature of affect related to food-illness associations, we can invoke it with disgust. The fact that almost all objects of disgust are animal in origin suggests that there is an associative predisposition to connect animals with disgust faces or with other disgust items.[62] There may well be a "preparedness" of disgust that parallels the preparedness of phobias[66] or the preparedness of food aversion learning.

Our claim at this time is simply that there is a possible place for conditioning in the acquisition of disgust, with facial or other expressions of others and already disgusting objects as the USs.

CONCLUSION

We believe that Pavlovian conditioning is alive and well, in the flavor-flavor associations of the billions of meals eaten each day, in the expressions of affect of billions of eaters as they eat away, each day, in the associations of foods and offensive objects, and in the associations of foods with some of their consequences. We see it as playing a special role in the hedonic realm, and being, perhaps, the major vehicle for producing hedonic shifts. But the evidence says only that such processes can occur. We don't know how often they do occur. We don't know why hedonic shifts, presumably of a Pavlovian nature, occur more rapidly and more powerfully in the negative direction. And we really don't know why there is liking and disliking at all. Why isn't anticipated consequences a sufficient basis for accepting or rejecting foods? We don't get a lot of explanatory power out of using likes and dislikes when we speak of animals. We can't avoid the terms when speaking about humans' relations to foods, but that doesn't mean we know why.

Why do humans, perhaps unique among food generalists, develop such strong likes for foods (and many other things, as well)? We have suggested[55] that this capacity of humans is an adaptation to culture. A particularly powerful form of enculturation is the internalization of the values of the culture; coming to like what the culture values and to dislike what it rejects. Such "intrinsic" values have one important advantage over extrinsic values. The motivation comes from within and does not depend on cultural sanction. When a child starts to eat chili pepper in Mexico, it may well do so to please others, look adult, and so on. But such extrinsic motivations are fallible; they don't operate when one is alone or when the payoff changes in the world. But the Mexican child comes, over months or years, to like the burn of chili pepper. It now likes it for its own sake, and does not need the external pressure of others.[51] The liking is in that sense more stable. If all this is true, it accounts for the great readiness of humans (in contrast to other animals) to come to like foods. And, ironically, it may harness one of the most simple and primitive of learning processes, Pavlovian conditioning, to the acquisition of cultural values, one of the highest accomplishments in the animal kingdom.

REFERENCES

1. GALEF, B. G. JR. 1977. Mechanisms for the social transmission of acquired food preferences from adult to weanling rats. *In* Learning Mechanisms in Food Selection. L. M. Barker, M. R. Best & M. Domjan, Eds.: 123–148. Baylor University Press. Waco, TX.
2. ARONFREED, J. A. 1968. Conduct and Conscience: The Socialization of Internalized Control Over Behavior. Academic Press. New York.
3. MARTIN, I. & A. B. LEVEY. 1978. Evaluative conditioning. Adv. Behav. Res. Therapy **1**: 57–102.
4. RAZRAN, G. 1954. The conditioned evocation of attitudes (cognitive conditioning?). J. Exp. Psychol. **48**: 278–282.
5. ROZIN, P. & A. E. FALLON. 1980. The psychological categorization of foods and non-foods: A preliminary taxonomy of food rejections. Appetite **1**: 193–201.
6. ROZIN, P. & A. E. FALLON. 1981. The acquisition of likes and dislikes for foods. *In* Criteria of Food Acceptance: How Man Chooses What He Eats. J. Solms & R. L. Hall, Eds.: 35–48. Forster. Zurich.
7. FALLON, A. E. & P. ROZIN. 1983. The psychological bases of food rejections by humans. Ecol. Food Nutr. **13**: 15–26.
8. ROZIN, P. 1981. Preference and affect in food selection. *In* Preference Behavior and Chemoreception. J. H. A. Kroeze, Ed.: 289–302. Information Retrieval. London.
9. AJZEN, I. & M. FISHBEIN. 1980. Understanding attitudes and predicting social behavior. Prentice-Hall. Englewood Cliffs, NJ.
10. YOUNG, P. T. 1948. Appetite, palatability and feeding habit: A critical review. Psychol. Bull. **45**: 289–320.
11. EKMAN, P. & W. V. FRIESEN. 1975. Unmasking the Face. Prentice Hall. Englewood Cliffs, NJ.
12. STEINER, J. E. 1977. Facial expressions of the neonate infant indicating the hedonics of food-related chemical stimuli. *In* Taste and Development: The Genesis of Sweet Preference. J. M. Weiffenbach, Ed.: 173–188. (DHEW Publication No. NIH 77-1068). U.S. Government Printing Office: Washington, D.C.
13. GRILL, H. J. & R. NORGREN. 1978. The taste-reactivity test. I. Mimetic responses to gustatory stimuli in neurologically normal rats. Brain Res. **143**: 263–269.
14. GRILL, H. J. & K. C. BERRIDGE. 1984. Taste reactivity as a measure of the neural control of palatability. *In* Progress in Physiological Psychology and Psychobiology. A. N. Epstein & J. M. Sprague, Eds. Academic Press. New York. (In press.)
15. RIZLEY, R. C. & R. A. RESCORLA. 1972. Associations in second-order conditioning and sensory preconditioning. J. Comp. Physiol. Psychol. **81**: 1–11.
16. CABANAC, M. 1971. Physiological role of pleasure. Science **173**: 1103–1107.
17. GLEITMAN, H. 1974. Getting animals to understand the experimenter's instructions. Animal Learning Behav. **2**: 1–5.
18. ROZIN, P. & K. KENNEL. 1983. Acquired preferences for piquant foods by chimpanzees. Appetite **4**: 69–77.
19. ROZIN, P. 1967. Specific aversions as a component of specific hungers. J. Comp. Physiol. Psychol. **64**: 237–242.
20. GARCIA, J., W. G. HANKINS & K. W. RUSINIAK. 1974. Behavioral regulation of the milieu interne in man and rat. Science **185**: 824–831.
21. DOMJAN, M. 1980. Ingestional aversion learning: Unique and general processes. *In* Advances in the Study of Behavior. J. Rosenblatt, R. A. Hinde, C. Beer, E. Shaw & M. C. Busnel, Eds. Vol. 7. Academic Press. New York.
22. ROZIN, P. & J. W. KALAT. 1971. Specific hungers and poison avoidance as adaptive specializations of learning. Psychol. Rev. **78**: 459–486.
23. RILEY, A. & C. CLARKE. 1977. Conditioned taste aversions: A bibliography. *In* Learning Mechanisms in Food Selection. J. Barker, M. Best & M. Domjan, Eds.: 593–616. Baylor University Press. Waco, TX.
24. LOGUE, A. W. 1979. Taste aversion and the generality of the laws of learning. Psychol. Bull. **86**: 276–296.
25. GARCIA, J., R. KOVNER & K. F. GREEN. 1970. Cue properties vs. palatability of flavors in avoidance learning. Psychonomic Sci. **20**: 313–314.
26. GARB, J. L. & A. STUNKARD. 1974. Taste aversions in man. Am. J. Psychiatry **131**: 1204–1207.

27. Logue, A. W., I. Ophir & K. E. Strauss. 1981. The acquisition of taste aversions in humans. Behavior Res. Therapy **19**: 319–333.
28. Bernstein, I. L. 1978. Learned taste aversions in children receiving chemotherapy. Science **200**: 1302–1303.
29. Bernstein, I. L. & M. M. Webster. 1980. Learned aversions in humans. Physiol. Behav. **25**: 363–366.
30. Pelchat, M. L. & P. Rozin. 1982. The special role of nausea in the acquisition of food dislikes by humans. Appetite **3**: 341–351.
31. Grill, H. J. 1975. Sucrose as an aversive stimulus Soc. Neurosci. Abstr. **1**: 525.
32. Pelchat, M. L., H. J. Grill, P. Rozin & J. Jacobs. 1983. Quality of acquired responses to tastes by *Rattus norvegicus* depends on type of associated discomfort. J. Comp. Psychol. **97**: 140–153.
33. Parker, L. A. 1982. Nonconsummatory and consummatory behavioral CRs elicited by lithium- and amphetamine-paired flavors. Learning Motiv. **13**: 281–303.
34. Zahorik, D. 1979. Learned changes in preferences for chemical stimuli: Asymmetrical effects of positive and negative consequences, and species differences in learning. *In* Preference Behaviour and Chemoreception. J. H. A. Kroeze, Ed.: 233–246. Information Retrieval. London.
35. Rozin, P., L. Gruss & G. Berk. 1979. The reversal of innate aversions: Attempts to induce a preference for chili pepper in rats. J Comp. Physiol. Psychol. **93**: 1001–1014.
36. Zahorik, D. M., S. F. Maier & R. W. Pies. 1974. Preferences for tastes paired with recovery from thiamine deficiency in rats: appetitive conditioning or learned safety. J. Comp. Physiol. Psychol. **87**: 1083–1091.
37. Parker, L., A. Failor & K. Weidman. 1973. Conditioned preferences in the rat with an unnatural need state: morphine withdrawal. J. Comp. Physiol. Psychol. **82**: 294–300.
38. Booth, D. A. 1972. Conditioned satiety in the rat. J. Comp. Physiol. Psychol. **81**: 457–471.
39. Booth, D. A. 1982. Normal control of omnivore intake by taste and smell. *In* The Determination of Behavior by Chemical Stimuli. ECRO Symposium. J. Steiner & J. Ganchrow, Eds.: 233–243. Information Retrieval. London.
40. Zellner D. A., K. C. Berridge, H. J. Grill & J. Ternes. 1985. Rats learn to like the taste of morphine. Behavioral Neuroscience. (In press.)
41. Booth, D. A., P. Mather & J. Fuller. 1982. Starch content of ordinary foods associatively conditions human appetite and satiation, indexed by intake and eating pleasantness of starch-paired flavors. Appetite **3**: 163–184.
42. Pliner, P., P. Rozin, M. Cooper & G. Woody. 1985. Role of medicinal context and specific postingestional effects in the acquisition of liking for tastes. (Manuscript).
43. Lepper, M. R. 1980. Intrinsic and extrinsic motivation in children: detrimental effects of superfluous social controls. *In* Minnesota Symposium on Child Psychology. W. A. Collins, Ed. **14**: 155–214. Lawrence Erlbaum. Hillsdale, NJ
44. Birch, L. L., D. Birch, D. W. Marlin & L. Kramer. 1982. Effects of instrumental consumption on children's food preference. Appetite **3**: 125–134.
45. Lavin, M. J. 1976. The establishment of flavor-flavor associations using a sensory preconditioning training procedure. Learning Motiv. **7**: 173–183.
46. Rescorla, R. A. & C. L. Cunningham. 1978. Within-compound flavor associations. J. Exp. Psychol. Animal Behav. Processes **4**: 267–275.
47. Rescorla, R. A. 1981. Simultaneous conditioning. *In* Advances in the Analysis of Behavior. P. Harzem & M. D. Zeiler, Eds. Vol. 2. Wiley. New York.
48. Fanselow, M. & J. Birk. 1982. Flavor-flavor associations induce hedonic shifts in taste preference. Animal Learning Behav. **10**: 223–228.
49. Holman, E. 1975. Immediate and delayed reinforcers for flavor preferences in rats. Learning Motiv. **6**: 91–100.
50. Zellner, D. A., P. Rozin, M. Aron & C. Kulish. 1983. Conditioned enhancement of human's liking for flavor by pairing with sweetness. Learning Motiv. **14**: 338–350.
51. Rozin, P. & D. Schiller. The nature and acquisition of a preference for chili pepper by humans. Motiv. Emotion **4**: 77–101.
52. Solomon, R. L. 1980. The opponent-process theory of acquired motivation. Am. Psychologist **35**: 691–712.

53. SIEGEL, S. 1977. Learning and psychopharmacology. *In* Psychopharmacology in the Practice of Medicine. M. E. Jarvik, Ed.: 61–72. Appleton-Century-Crofts. New York.
54. SCHULL, J. 1979. A conditioned opponent theory of Pavlovian conditioning and habituation. *In* The Psychology of Learning and Motivation. G. Bower, Ed. Vol. 13. Academic Press. New York.
55. ROZIN P. 1982. Human food selection: The interaction of biology, culture and individual experience. *In* Psychobiology of Human Food Selection. L. M. Barker, Ed.: 225–254. AVI. Westport, CT.
56. ROZIN, P., L. EBERT & J. SCHULL. 1982. Some like it hot: A temporal analysis of hedonic responses to chili pepper. Appetite **3**: 13–22.
57. GALEF, B. G. JR. 1976. Social transmission of acquired behavior: A discussion of tradition and social learning in vertebrates. *In* Advances in the Study of Behavior. J. S. Rosenblatt, R. A. Hinde, E. Shaw & C. Beer, Eds. **6**: 77–100. Academic Press. New York.
58. DUNCKER, K. 1938. Experimental modification of children's food preferences through social suggestion. J. Abn. Social Psychol. **33**: 489–507.
59. BIRCH, L. L. 1980. Effects of peer models' food choices and eating behaviors on preschooler's food preferences. Child Dev. **51**: 489–496.
60. TOMKINS, S. 1962. Affect, Imagery, Consciousness. Springer. New York.
61. ANGYAL, A. 1941. Disgust and related aversions. J. Abn. Social Psychol. **36**: 393–412
62. ROZIN, P. & A. E. FALLON. 1984. Disgust. (Manuscript).
63. ROZIN, P. 1984. Unpublished observations.
64. FALLON, A. E., P. ROZIN & P. PLINER. 1984. The child's conception of food. The development of food rejections, with special reference to disgust and contamination sensitivity. Child Dev. **55**: 566–575.
65. ROZIN, P., A. E. FALLON & R. MANDELL. 1984. Family resemblances in attitudes to foods. Dev. Psychol. **20**: 309–314.
66. SELIGMAN, M. E. P. 1971. Phobias and preparedness. Behav. Therapy **2**: 307–320.

Direct and Indirect Behavioral Pathways to the Social Transmission of Food Avoidance[a]

BENNETT G. GALEF, JR.

Department of Psychology
McMaster University
Hamilton, Ontario L8S 4K1
Canada

INTRODUCTION

During the past fifteen years my students and I have been examining the role of social factors in diet selection by wild and domesticated Norway rats. The results of our studies provide evidence of a number of discrete behavioral processes permitting a rat choosing between novel diets to make use of the learned feeding preferences of others of its social group. As a general rule, an individual rat tends to select for ingestion the same foods that others of its social group are eating.

In any two-choice situation there are, *a priori*, two motivational pathways that might lead an organism to ingest more of one diet than of another available to it. The subject might be directly motivated to ingest the selected food because of attraction to it or the animal might be indirectly motivated to ingest the selected diet because it is avoiding the available alternative.

Similarly, if an organism is observed to avoid ingestion of one of two accessible diets, such avoidance could be either directly or indirectly motivated: directly motivated in the sense that the animal avoids ingestion of the unselected food because of some aversion to it or indirectly motivated in the sense that the animal ingests little of one item in consequence of its greater liking for the other.

The somewhat surprising fact I will be focusing on below is that in 15 years of experimentation, while uncovering four independent socially mediated behavioral processes resulting in indirect avoidance of foods by rats, my co-workers and I have not been able to find any evidence of social influence acting directly to induce a food aversion. In each of our analyses of social transmission of diet selection, socially induced avoidance of one diet has been the indirect result of socially, directly induced preference for an available alternative.

Below, I first review data from my own laboratory that lead me to the conclusion that socially induced diet avoidance in rats tends to be indirect rather than direct. Second, I describe experiments by others indicating that direct social transmission of diet aversion occurs in at least one species, the red-wing blackbird. Last, I briefly discuss approaches to the question of why there might be interspecific differences in

[a] Preparation of this manuscript was greatly facilitated by funds provided by the Natural Sciences and Engineering Research Council of Canada (Grant A0307) and by the McMaster University Research Board.

the types of information socially transmitted about foods and implications of such interspecific differences for the study of social learning.

SOCIAL TRANSMISSION OF DIET PREFERENCE AT A DISTANCE FROM A FEEDING SITE

As a first illustration of the issue with which I'm concerned, I'll describe in some detail recent work in my laboratory on the use by rats of aggregation sites as "information centers"[1] at which members of a social group exchange information concerning foods they have ingested while on foraging expeditions away from the aggregation site itself. Our experimental procedures were designed to mimic a situation in which a foraging rat (a demonstrator) ingests a food at some distance from its burrow, returns to its burrow, and then interacts with a familiar burrow-mate (an observer). We were interested to know whether, as a result of such interaction, the observer could acquire information concerning the food the demonstrator had eaten and whether the observer would use this information when selecting a diet.[2]

Treatment of subjects during the experiment was as follows (FIGURE 1). (Step 1) Demonstrator and observer were first maintained together with *ad lib* access to Purina Laboratory Chow pellets for a two-day period of familiarization with both apparatus and pair-mate. (Step 2) The demonstrator was moved to the opposite side of a screen partition from the observer and food deprived for 24 hr to ensure that the demonstrator ate when given the opportunity to do so. (Step 3) Chow was then removed from the observer's side of the cage (in preparation for testing) and the demonstrator was moved to an enclosure in a separate room and allowed to feed for 30 min on either cocoa-flavored diet or cinnamon-flavored diet. (Step 4) The demonstrator was returned to the observer's cage and demonstrator and observer were allowed to interact for 15 min. (Step 5) The demonstrator was removed from the experiment and the observer was offered, for 60 hr, two weighed food-cups, one containing cinnamon-flavored diet and one containing cocoa-flavored diet.

The results of this experiment are presented in FIGURE 2, which shows the mean amount of cocoa-flavored diet (as a percentage of total amount eaten) ingested by observers whose demonstrators had eaten either cocoa-flavored or cinnamon-flavored diet during the 30 min they were removed to a separate room (Step 3 in FIGURE 1). As can be seen in FIGURE 2, those observers whose demonstrators ate cocoa-flavored diet ate a greater percentage of cocoa-flavored diet than did those observers whose

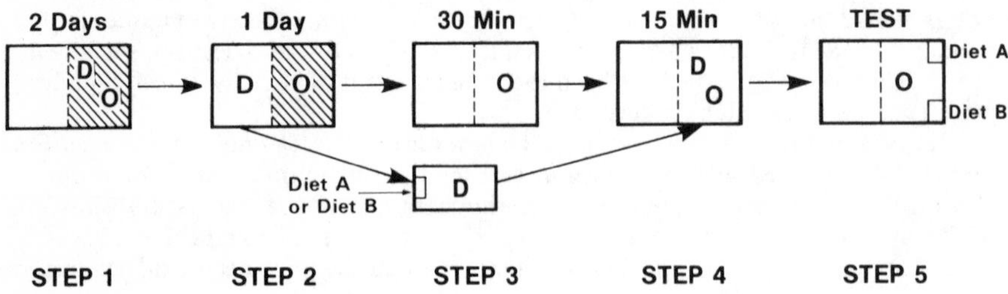

FIGURE 1. Schematic diagram of a procedure for investigating the ability of rats to communicate information concerning distant diets. D = demonstrator; O = observer; cross-hatching indicates Purina Laboratory Chow in cage. (From Galef and Wigmore.[2] Reproduced by permission of Baillière Tindall.)

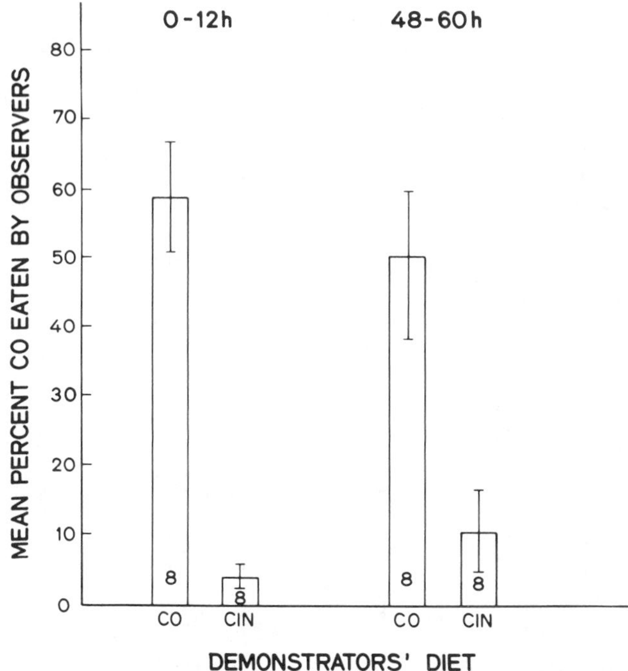

FIGURE 2. Mean amount of cocoa-flavored diet ingested, as a percentage of total amount eaten, by observers whose demonstrators had eaten either cocoa- or cinnamon-flavored diet. CO = cocoa-flavored diet; CIN = cinnamon-flavored diet. Bars indicate ± 1 S.E. Left-hand panel, 1st 12 hr intake; right-hand panel intake from the 48th-60th hr. (From Galef and Wigmore.[2] Reproduced by permission of Baillière Tindall.)

demonstrators ate cinnamon-flavored diet. Both the present data and similar findings by Strupp and Levitsky[3] and Posadas-Andrews and Roper,[4] clearly indicate that a demonstrator rat can influence conspecific observers to select the diet that the demonstrator ate at a distant time and place. Such preference for a demonstrator's diet may result in a reduced tendency to eat alternative diets, but as discussed above, this avoidance of alternative diets is only an indirect consequence of a socially induced preference for a demonstrator's diet.

What about food aversion? Can one rat communicate information about a distant diet to a naive conspecific that would cause that individual to directly develop an aversion to that diet. Suppose a rat leaves its burrow system, ingests some novel food that happens to be toxic, returns to its burrow, and while ill, interacts with a burrow mate. Will the burrow-mate of the sick individual subsequently avoid ingesting the food that made its companion ill?

There is some reason to believe that the naive individual might subsequently avoid ingesting the ill rat's diet. Coombes and Lavin[5] and their colleagues have reported data indicating that signals emitted by an ill rat can serve as unconditional stimuli in a taste aversion learning situation. If a naive rat ingests an unfamiliar diet and then interacts with a fellow who has been rendered ill by injection of a mildly toxic lithium chloride solution, the naive rat subsequently exhibits reluctance to ingest the novel diet it ate prior to interaction with the ill conspecific.

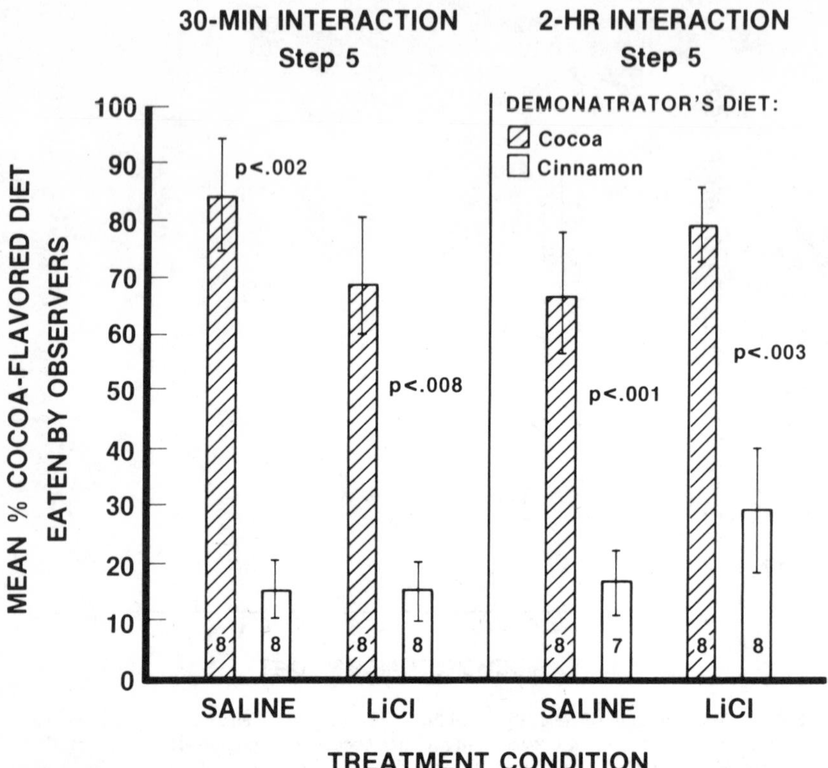

FIGURE 3. Mean amount of cocoa-flavored diet ingested by observers as a percentage of total amount eaten. Left-hand panel; observer and demonstrator interacted for 30 min; right-hand panel, observer and demonstrator interacted for 2 hr during Step 4 of FIGURE 1. (From Galef *et al.*[6] Reproduced by permission of the American Psychological Association.)

Our finding[2] that an observer can extract information from a demonstrator concerning the diet the demonstrator has recently eaten, taken together with Coombes *et al.*'s[5] observation that an ill rat can serve as an unconditional stimulus for taste-aversion learning, suggests that a rat made ill following ingestion of a novel food might provide two potentially useful signals to a conspecific: First, a signal containing information sufficient to permit identification of that food the signal-emitter has recently eaten, and second, a signal capable of inducing a learned aversion. Exposure to these two signals in temporal contiguity might produce in their recipient avoidance of the specific diet recently ingested by an ill conspecific.

We, therefore, repeated the experiment described in FIGURE 1, but with an important modification. Between the time the demonstrator was removed to a separate enclosure and fed either cinnamon- or cocoa-flavored diet (Step 3) and the time it was placed in its observer's cage (Step 4), it received an intraperitoneal injection. Demonstrators in experimental groups were injected with toxic LiCl solution, while demonstrators in control groups were injected with a benign saline solution.

The results of this attempt to demonstrate socially mediated direct taste-aversion learning are shown in FIGURE 3. Observers in all groups, regardless of whether they had interacted with poisoned or saline-injected demonstrators, exhibited a substantially enhanced preference for the diet their respective demonstrator had eaten. Poisoned demonstrators were as effective in promoting intake of the diet they had eaten (and which they would subsequently avoid) as were unpoisoned demonstrators.

Thus, results of recent work on social transmission of food preference in rats are consistent with the notion that direct social influence on preference is a more robust phenomenon than direct social influence on aversion.

SOCIAL TRANSMISSION OF DIET PREFERENCE AT A FEEDING SITE

The two studies discussed above are not the first of our experiments to reveal rats making use of information indicating that conspecifics are exploiting some food while, under similar circumstances, failing to make use of information that conspecifics have learned to avoid a diet.

In one of our earliest investigations of the role of social influence on diet selection, Mertice Clark and I[7] established colonies of adult wild rats in large enclosures and, by use of LiCl contamination, trained adults to eat only one of two simultaneously presented diets. We then looked at the food preferences of weanling young born to adults of our colonies. We found, as FIGURE 4 illustrates, that young rats ate the same food that the adults of their colony had been trained to eat. As can be seen in FIGURE 4, weanling wild rats born to a colony trained to avoid ingesting Diet A, ingested only Diet B and those born to a colony trained to avoid ingesting Diet B, ingested only Diet A.

As mentioned in the introduction, such a pattern of diet selection could be the result either of young learning to eat the food adults of their colony are eating or learning to avoid the food adults of their colony had learned to avoid. Clark and I[7] conducted a single experiment to determine which was the case. We established two different types of adult wild rat colonies. In the first type of colony, adults were again trained (by adulterating samples of Diet B offered to the colony with LiCl) to avoid ingesting the normally preferred Diet B and to eat Diet A. In the second, adults were forced to eat Diet A by making it the only food available. We waited till our adults had given birth to young and the young had grown to weaning and fed on solid food with the adults for ten days (those in the first type of colony eating no Diet B). We then removed the young to individual enclosures. In these individual enclosures each pup was allowed to choose between Diets A and B for nine days. As can be seen in FIGURE 5, there was no difference between pups from the two types of colony in rate of acceptance of Diet B. Pups from colonies of the first type (in which adults had learned to avoid ingesting Diet B) accepted Diet B as rapidly as those from colonies of the second type (in which pups had no information concerning Diet B). The fact that pups from colonies that had learned to avoid Diet B showed no greater reluctance to ingest Diet B than pups from colonies that had not learned an aversion to Diet B, suggests that pups from colonies of the first type learned nothing about avoiding Diet B as a result of social interaction.[7] Once again, through social interaction, rats are learning about what to eat, not about what to avoid.

It might well be argued that this single experiment is not sufficient to establish that pups in the first type of colony were learning nothing about the diet the adults of their colony were avoiding. In retrospect I would agree that we should have pursued the matter more diligently. However, the outcome of further analysis of factors

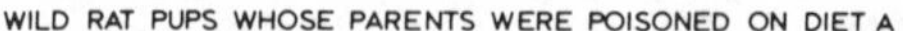

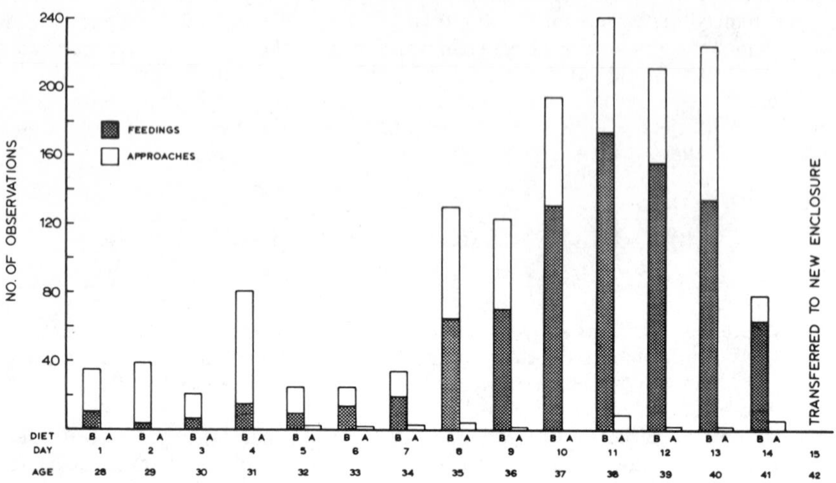

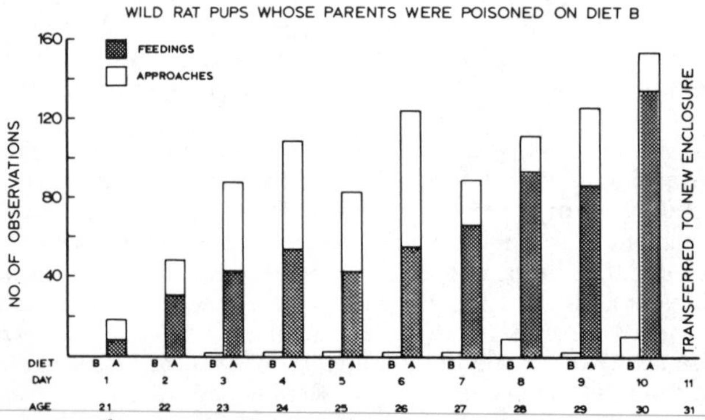

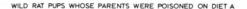

FIGURE 4. Number of observed approaches to and feedings on Diets A and B by wild rat pups the adults of whose colony had been poisoned when eating Diet A (upper panel) or Diet B (lower panel). (From Galef and Clark.[7] Reproduced by permission of the American Psychological Association.)

responsible for social transmission of acquired food preferences from adults to their young is entirely consistent with the view that it is only information about those foods that adults are eating that is transmitted to juveniles.

The primary behavioral process involved in the transmission of acquired adult food preferences to juveniles is a tendency of wild rat pups to approach adults, feed on the diet the adults are eating, become familiar with that diet, and subsequently exhibit a reluctance to ingest alternative foods. There is little place in such a scheme for the young to learn anything about foods that adults are not exploiting. In fact, during the time juvenile wild rats were with adults, they rarely approached adult-avoided foods and never tasted such foods (FIGURE 4). It is difficult to imagine how pups could acquire a socially induced aversion to adult-avoided foods to which they are never exposed.[8]

A further behavioral mechanism biasing rat pups to exploit foods that the adults of their social group are eating similarly offers little opportunity for the young to acquire knowledge of food that adults are avoiding. Linda Heiber and I[9] found that adult rats deposit residual olfactory cues in areas in which they feed. These olfactory markers are sufficient to bias pups to explore and eat in areas adults are utilizing for foraging. In this case, pup avoidance of adult-avoided feeding sites appears to be the result of the absence of conspecific olfactory signals in such areas. Once again the avoidance by pups of sites that adults are not utilizing seems to be indirect rather than direct.

ACTIVE DIRECT TRANSMISSION OF POISON AVOIDANCE: A FAILURE TO REPLICATE

In 1975 Danguir and Nicolaides[10] reported results of an experiment that suggested two rather surprising conclusions. First, that rats could directly transmit poison avoidance, and second, that the avoidance exhibited by naive individuals resulting from

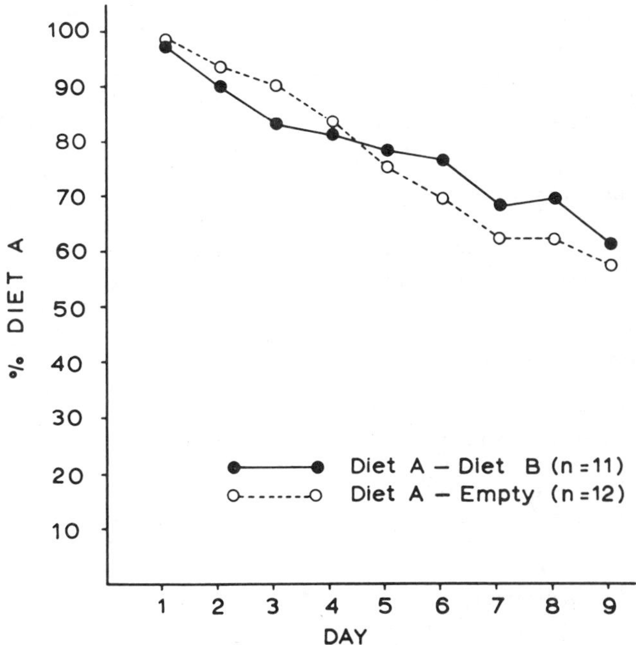

FIGURE 5. Amount of Diet A ingested, as a percentage of total intake, by pups in individual enclosures transferred from adult colonies eating only Diet A, either because it was the only diet available (Diet A- Empty Group) or because Diet B had been poisoned (Diet A-Diet B Group). (From Galef and Clark.[7] Reproduced by permission of the American Psychological Association.)

interaction with trained conspecifics was the result of active interference by knowledgeable animals in the ongoing behavior of their less knowledgeable fellows. The first conclusion was unexpected only in that it contradicted a generalization extrapolated from my own studies of social learning in rats and hence was more exciting than dismaying. The second implication of the Danguir and Nicolaides experiment, however, was contrary to generalizations based on fifty years of research on social learning processes in non-primate animals.

Reviews of the relevant literature[11,12] indicate that in a wide variety of social learning situations, the role of knowledgeable individuals in influencing the behavior of naive conspecifics is passive, not active. Rather than actively intervene in the behavior of naive individuals, knowledgeable conspecifics create, presumably unknowingly, a stimulus situation that causes naive individuals to match their behavior to that of the model. For example, an adult rat feeding at some location provides a stimulus complex that markedly biases orientation of the exploratory behavior of young conspecifics. It is the influence of such passively emitted stimuli that results in adult influence on diet preferences of their offspring. All examples of social learning in the literature, with the exception of two anecdotes,[12] can be understood in such terms. The finding that any nonprimate mammal would actively restrain a naive conspecific from approaching and ingesting a potential toxin suggested a previously unsuspected sophistication and complexity in the behavioral processes supporting animals social learning.

Danguir and Nicolaides[10] trained two members of trios of rats to avoid salt solutions by twice exposing them, when 24 hr water deprived, to a toxic 0.9 percent LiCl solution. To test for transfer of avoidance to naive trio members, trained pairs of subjects were reunited with their untrained trio mate, all were water deprived for 24 hr, and then allowed access as a group for 15 min to a single bottle containing NaCl solution. Trios in a control condition were treated identically to those in the experimental trios, treatment of which is described above, except that on the two training days trained subjects in control trios were exposed to a benign NaCl solution rather than toxic LiCl solution. The results of the experiment are presented in the left-hand panel of FIGURE 6. Naive subjects in experimental trios drank significantly less than naive subjects in control trios, indicating that the trained experimental pair had induced their naive trio-mate to avoid drinking the salt solution. This reduced intake of NaCl solution by naive members of experimental trios was attributed to overt behavior of trained individuals, which in seven of twelve cases were said both to hold down naive rats and to interpose themselves between naive rats and bottle spouts, blocking naive rats' access to NaCl solution.

There are two critical questions: first, whether naive subjects in experimental trios truly drank less NaCl solution during testing than did naive subjects in control trios. Second, if naive subjects in experimental trios did drink less than naive subjects in control trios, was this difference in intake the result of active intervention by trained members of experimental trios?

The answer to the first question was not as clear from Danguir and Nicolaides' data as one might hope. The problem arose in determining the amount of solution actually ingested by naive rats in control trios. During testing there were three animals potentially drinking from a single water bottle and it was only the intake of one of them, the naive animal, that was of interest. In the case of experimental trios, the problem was not particularly acute because trained members of such trios had learned to avoid salty solutions. Danguir and Nicolaides' observations revealed that trained members drank for only a few seconds and all intake could be safely attributed to the naive members of experimental trios. Control trios posed a greater problem. All members of each control trio were 24 hr water deprived at the time of testing. None

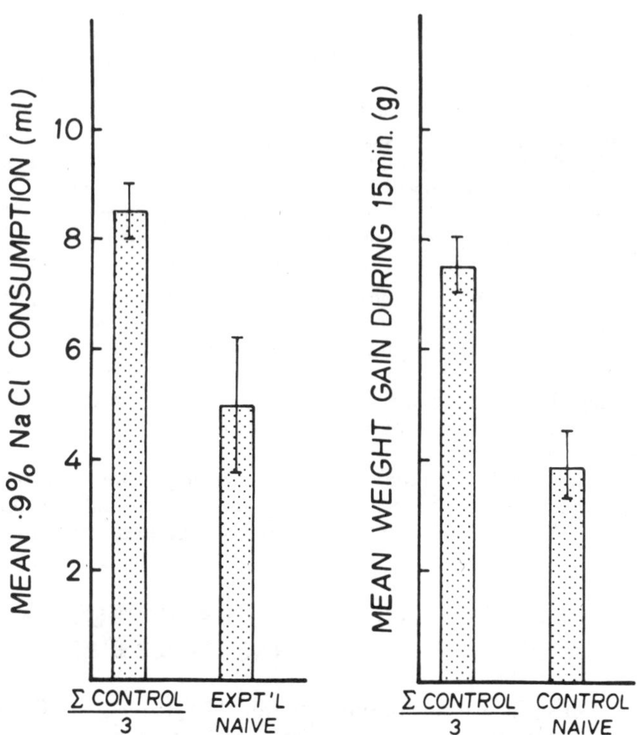

FIGURE 6. (Left) Prepared from data presented by Danguir and Nicolaidis.[10] Mean amount of .9% NaCl solution consumed by naive experimental subjects and naive control subjects. The latter amount was calculated by dividing the total amount consumed by control trios by 3. (Right) mean amount of .9% NaCl solution consumed by naive control subjects calculated by dividing the total weight gain of control trios by 3 and by directly measuring the weight gain of naive control subjects. (From Galef and Dalrymple.[13] Reproduced by permission of Academic Press.)

had learned to avoid ingesting salty solutions, and all drank avidly. How can one establish the proportion of the intake of a control trio attributable to its naive member? Danguir and Nicolaides determined the time each member of control trios spent in contact with the drinking spout. They found that trained and naive subjects drank an approximately equal length of time, and therefore, attributed one-third of the total intake of each control trio to its naive member. This is surely a reasonable procedure, but one open to some question.

There is reason to suspect that naive members of control trios, which had not previously experienced salt solutions, might be more hesitant to ingest such solutions than their trained fellows that had ingested NaCl solution on two previous occasions. If naive members of control trios were in fact more hesitant than their trained triomates to ingest NaCl solutions during testing, then the calculation of intake by naive control subjects employed by Danguir and Nicolaides (total amount drunk by control trios divided by 3) would have overestimated the intake of naive subjects in control trios. Apparent difference between the intakes of naive subjects in control and experimental groups could have been due to measurement artifact rather than differences in the behavior of naive subjects in control and experimental groups.

Andrew Dalrymple and I[13] attempted to replicate the Danguir and Nicolaides study as closely as possible while more directly measuring the intake of subjects in control trios. Rather than divide the intake of control trios by three to determine the intake of naive subjects in control trios, we weighed both trained and naive control subjects before and after the 15-min test session.

The right-hand panel of FIGURE 6 shows the intake of naive members of control trios calculated both by dividing the weight gain of all the members of control trios by 3 and by directly measuring individual weight gain. The two methods of calculating the intake of naive subjects in control trios produced the same difference in measured intake of naive subjects as Danguir and Nicolaides found between naive subjects in their control and experimental groups. Our data thus suggest that the apparent difference in intake of NaCl by naive subjects in control and experimental trios reported by Danguir and Nicolaidis was probably the result of measurement error in the determination of the amount ingested by naive subjects in control trios. Of course, in the absence of compelling evidence of social influence on avoidance in the situation under discussion, concern over the mechanisms by which such influence might proceed is unwarranted.

The conclusion I draw from the above is that the only instance of social learning of a direct avoidance by rats reported in the literature (and the only instance of active transmission of behavior) does not hold up under close examination.

SOCIAL TRANSMISSION OF FOOD PREFERENCES AND AVERSIONS BY RED-WING BLACKBIRDS

Understanding of social learning phenomena would be greatly simplified if information on social learning processes could be generalized across species with confidence. If, as the preceding sections suggest, I am correct in asserting that direct social transmission of taste aversions in rats is not an important factor in their diet selection, while direct transmission of diet preference is, one might hope to find similar patterns of the role of social interaction in diet selection in other species. Unfortunately this does not seem to be the case.

In a series of recent papers[14-16] Russell Mason and his co-workers have described the results of an integrated set of experiments on social learning of food preferences and aversions in red-wing blackbirds (*Agelaius phoeniceus*). Their data provide compelling evidence of direct transmission of both learned aversions and learned preferences in their avian subjects.

Demonstration of socially transmitted diet preference resulted from allowing five pairs of naive blackbirds to observe (for 1 hr/day on four consecutive days) pairs of demonstrators in an adjacent cage eat orange food and five additional pairs of naive blackbirds to observe demonstrators eat green food. Twenty-four hours following the last observation trial, all ten naive pairs were offered a choice between orange and green foods. It was found that each of the ten naive pairs of blackbirds exhibited a preference for that diet (orange or green) that it had observed a demonstrator-pair eat on the four preceding days.[14] Thus, red-wing blackbirds, like Norway rats, can directly influence the food preference of conspecifics.

Using similar procedures, Mason and Reidinger[15] have also been successful in demonstrating direct social transmission of a feeding-related avoidance. In this case, individually housed naive blackbirds watched a conspecific eat from a container marked with either a red or white rectangle. After each demonstrator had eaten for 1 hr, it was intubated with either toxic or control solution, and then returned to the feeding situation for a further hour. Naive birds were tested the following day, and for five days thereafter, with a simultaneous choice between two feeding containers, one labeled with a red and one with a white rectangle. Naive birds ate reliably less from the colored container from which their demonstrators had eaten if those demonstrators had been intubated with toxin, but not if they had been intubated with benign control solution. The naive observers clearly had learned to avoid a visual cue associated with the ingestive behavior of an ill conspecific.

Both of the above effects have been replicated and the aversion induced by watching a single trial in which a demonstrator becomes ill has been found more resistant to extinction than the preference induced by watching four trials in which a conspecific ate safely.[16] The evidence that red-wing blackbirds will directly learn aversions as the result of social interaction is compelling.

CONCLUSIONS

Data reviewed in preceding sections suggest the conclusion that there are qualitative differences in the role of social influence in diet selection by Norway rats and red-wing blackbirds. In blackbirds, direct transmission of diet aversion is at least as robust as transmission of diet preference. In rats, evidence of direct transmission of diet preference is easily found, while evidence of direct transmission of diet aversion has proven elusive. This contrast in the nature of the information communicated by members of different species concerning foods leads directly to the question of why such differences might exist. While I do not believe that the question can be answered from current knowledge, simply posing the question of why social learning should be employed in different species in different ways may prove a useful exercise.

Presumably, in those species and situations in which social transmission of information occurs, it increases the fitness of those individuals making use of the behavior of conspecifics in shaping their own behavior. One is thus led to ask in what situations the use of social learning by an individual might enhance fitness. There appear to be two sets of variables affecting the probability that social learning would be fitness enhancing in a population. The first has to do with the nature of the environment in which an organism lives and the second with the ability of the individual to cope with the demands of that environment in the absence of social learning.

In a provocative recent paper Boyd and Richerson[17] have examined the environmental conditions under which natural selection would favor social learning rather than "pure" individual acquisition of behavior. The results of Boyd and Richerson's modelling suggest that individual learning is favored in environments varying greatly over time, social transmission of behavior in moderately temporally variable environments, and genetic transmission in very stable environments. Social learning was also favored over individual learning in spatially varying environments, independent of the degree of environmental heterogeneity. Although the simplifying assumptions needed to render the problem tractable to mathematical analysis make it difficult to extrapolate with confidence Boyd and Richerson's conclusions to natural situations, their work suggests that the extent of trait-relevant environmental variability may prove to be an important determinant of the efficiency of social learning.

Similarly, Johnston and Turvey,[18] in their overview of adaptative behavior, have suggested that adaptation is achieved by behavioral mechanisms differing in the time scale over which they act. Johnston and Turvey propose that different rates of relevant environmental change require adaptive responses with different feedback characteristics (back-reference periods). Although Johnston and Turvey do not consider situations in which social learning might be an appropriate adaptive mode of response, Boyd and Richerson's analysis suggests that those environments varying spatially and those sufficiently autocorrelated to allow a back-reference period somewhat longer than that supporting individual learning might be particularly appropriate for social learning to occur.

Thus, one sort of answer to the question of why members of one species should socially transmit learned aversions and another should not, would lie in information about temporal and spatial variability in the distribution of toxins to which members of a species are exposed.

A second, and not totally unrelated, answer to the question of causes of differences in use of social learning as an adaptive response lies in consideration of alternative strategies available to an individual in coping with particular environmental challenges. The potential value to an individual of any behavioral tactic for coping with a challenge can only be evaluated in the context of alternative tactics available to that organism for dealing with that challenge. The psychological literature presents a picture of the individual wild rat as a highly specialized poison-avoider, possessing defenses in depth against the ingestion of lethal quantities of toxins: a very strong tendency to avoid ingesting novel foods, an inherent aversion to bitter foods, a tendency to sample novel foods suspiciously, and a capacity to learn toxicosis-induced taste-aversions in a single trial. Within such a behavioral complex, it is possible that social transmission of information concerning toxic foods would be of minimal benefit.

If the individual is capable of coping with the presence of toxins in its environment without the benefit of information acquired from conspecifics, there would be little selective pressure for the development of the capacity to exploit conspecifics as sources of information about potential toxins. As Lehrman[19] stated "Nature selects for outcomes not processes of development." If rats are adequately protected against ingesting deleterious substances by their individual behavioral repetoires, there would be little pressure to evolve social learning mechanisms to cope with the problem. Social learning may be more likely to evolve to fill a gap in an individual's capacity to cope with environmental challenges than as an addendum to a highly sophisticated system. If the above views of social learning is correct, one might well expect situational and species specificity of social learning to be the rule rather than the exception.

The study of individual learning has proceeded by analysis of phenomena conceptualized in abstract terms. Parallel attempts to formalize and reify social learning paradigms (e.g. observational learning, social facilitation, etc.) and to explore their properties at the level of abstraction that has characterized the study of operant and classical conditioning, have not proven particularly enlightening. The preceding discussion suggests that consideration of both ecological and organismic variables may be central to understanding of the distribution and use of social learning processes.

ACKNOWLEDGMENTS

I thank Deborah Kennett and Mertice Clark for their thoughtful comments on earlier drafts.

REFERENCES

1. WARD, P. & A. ZAHAVI. 1973. Ibis **115**: 517–534.
2. GALEF, B. G., JR. & S. W. WIGMORE. 1983. Anim. Behav. **31**: 748–758.

3. STRUPP, B. J. & D. A. LEVITSKY. 1984. J. Comp. Psychol. **98**: 257–266.
4. POSADAS-ANDREWS, A. & T. J. ROPER. 1983. Anim. Behav. **31**: 265–271.
5. COOMBES, S., S. REVUSKY & B. T. LETT. 1980. Learn. Motiv. **11**: 256–266.
6. GALEF, B. G., JR., S. W. WIGMORE & D. J. KENNETT. 1985. Anim. Learn. Behav. (In press.)
7. GALEF, B. G., JR. & M. M. CLARK. 1971. J. Comp. Physiol. Psychol. **34**: 341–357.
8. GALEF, B. G. JR. 1977. Mechanisms for the social transmission of food preferences from adult to weanling rats. *In* Learning Mechanisms in Food Selection. L. M. Barker, M. Best & M. Domjan, Eds.: 123–147. Baylor University Press. Waco, TX.
9. GALEF, B. G., JR. & L. HEIBER. 1976. J. Comp. Physiol. Psychol. **90**: 727–739.
10. DANGUIR, J. & S. NICOLAIDES. 1975. C. R. Acad. Sci. Paris (Ser. D.) **280**: 2595–2598.
11. EWER, R. F. 1969. Nature **222**: 698.
12. GALEF, B. G. JR. 1976. The social transmission of acquired behavior: A discussion of tradition and social learning in vertebrates. *In* Advances in the Study of Behavior. J. S. Rosenblatt, R. A. Hinde, E. Shaw & C. Beer, Eds. **6**: 77–99. Academic Press. New York.
13. GALEF, B. G. JR. & A. J. DALRYMPLE. 1978. Behav. Biol. **24**: 265–271.
14. MASON, J. R. & R. F. REIDINGER. 1981. Auk **98**: 778–784.
15. MASON, J. R. & R. F. REIDINGER. 1982. Auk **99**: 548–554.
16. MASON, J. R., A. H. ARZT & R. F. REIDINGER. Auk. (In press.)
17. BOYD, R. & P. J. RICHERSON. 1983. J. Theor. Biol. **100**: 567–596.
18. JOHNSTON, T. D. & M. T. TURVEY. 1980. A sketch of an ecological matatheory for theories of learning. *In* The Psychology of Learning and Motivation. G. H. Bower, Ed. **14**: 148–199. Academic Press. New York.
19. LEHRMAN, D. S. 1970. Semantic and conceptual issues in the nature-nurture problem. *In* Development and Evolution of Behavior. L. R. Aronson, E. Tobach & J. S. Rosenblatt, Eds.: 17–52. Freeman. San Francisco, CA.

Foraging, Memory, and Constraints on Learning

SARA J. SHETTLEWORTH

Department of Psychology
University of Toronto
Toronto, Ontario M5S 1A1 Canada

The discovery and analysis of food aversion learning was important to learning theory because the specificity of events that could be associated with illness and the long delays over which associations could be formed were unlike anything that had previously been studied. Moreover, the specificity and the long delays were just what would be expected of a system for associating the qualities of food with the consequences of ingesting it. Because food aversion learning was the first example of a learning paradigm with special properties matched to a special function studied intensively by psychologists, it raised general questions about the relationship between the study of animal learning and biological approaches to behavior. Although food aversion learning was studied mainly in the laboratory, the results led to suggestions that apparent anomalies in traditional paradigms can be understood in terms of possible natural functions of learning.[1] The study of food aversions thereby paved the way for the development of biologically oriented approaches to learning.[2-6] In this paper I discuss some approaches to learning that have been stimulated directly and indirectly by work on food aversion learning.

The most immediate implication of research on food aversion learning for the study of learning in general was that stimulus-stimulus (or response-reinforcer) "relevance" or "belongingness" might be characteristic of a wide range of associative learning situations. Investigations of this possibility have facilitated the incorporation of food aversion learning into mainstream conditioning work, since they establish that speed of learning in other preparations does indeed depend on the "belongingness" of the events to be associated. Domjan[7] has recently reviewed work along these lines from seven different kinds of learning situations. The issue of whether food aversion learning differs in any important way from other forms of associative learning seems closed. It does not so differ, although it is an especially vivid illustration of a general principle of causal relevance[8] or belongingness.

In this paper, two less direct general implications of conditioned food aversions for the study of learning in animals are illustrated. First, as an example of a form of learning with a clear function in the natural environment, food aversion learning challenged, and ultimately broadened and enriched, general conceptions of associative learning. Perhaps, then, we need to analyze other examples of naturally occurring learning and memory to determine whether they are amenable to analysis using principles known from the laboratory or whether, like food aversion learning, they demand a broadening of those principles. Second, the adaptiveness of the special properties of food aversion learning has been argued more or less post hoc. But if the ability to learn certain things in certain ways is an adaptation to the requirements of each species' niche, it should be possible to work backward from biological first principles to what the properties of learning and memory ought to be. Such an exercise may lead to greater understanding of phenomena that are already well studied. It can also lead to suggestions for investigations of new phenomena and a new sort of comparative approach to learning.

LEARNING IN THE WILD

Rozin and Kalat[1] suggested that analyzing examples of the learning animals do in the wild will reveal adaptive specializations of learning and memory. Analysis of such adaptive specializations, they suggested, involves not only a concern with learning processes but also an appreciation of the natural context in which they function. Although Rozin and Kalat did not offer a formal definition of adaptive specialization, it might be defined as learning that is specialized in differing quantitatively or qualitatively from learning in the same or a similar situation in a related species, or in a formally similar situation for that species. The differences between species in a single sort of situation or between situations within a species (i.e., the "specializations") would be adaptive if they match differences in ecological requirements.

The best examples of adaptive specializations come, not surprisingly, from the work of zoologists on song learning and imprinting in birds. Song learning is a particular good example because not only does it seem to involve a special kind of learning, but also the parametric features of that learning differ from one species to another in a way related to other aspects of life history.[9] For example, the sensitive period for song learning must occur during a time when the young bird will be exposed to the song of its species, and this time varies with the temporal organization of breeding and territorial behavior. Sensitive periods for song learning vary similarly. Sexual imprinting in precocial birds varies in a similar way and for similar reasons.[10]

Impressive though they may be, the examples of adaptive specializations from the ethological literature have had little impact on most psychologists' thinking about learning, probably because they do not readily fit into traditional paradigms. Food aversion learning began to be investigated when song learning and imprinting were already quite well studied. Its greater impact within psychology is probably due to the fact that it can easily be seen as an example of associative learning.

Work on rats' spatial memory is like work on conditioned food aversions in that laboratory studies are taken as a model of a natural situation where learning has an important function for the rat and the resulting data demonstrate a capacity well beyond what would be expected from data in formally similar situations. Olton and Samuelson's[11] now-classic paper on rats' behavior in radial mazes appeared when the surge of interest in food aversion learning and naturalistic learning more generally was already well developed. The rapid growth of research on spatial memory in old-fashioned mazes that it stimulated was undoubtedly facilitated by the zeitgeist created indirectly by research on food aversion learning.

In a radial maze task, a rat can get one piece of food in each arm of the maze. It has to remember which places it has already emptied of food in order to avoid fruitless revisits. Rats can remember places extremely well in this task, and just as with one-trial long-delay learning in conditioned food aversions, their good performance has been attributed to the resemblance of the task to a natural occurring foraging task.[11] Just as with conditioned food aversions, data on naturally occurring learning of this kind are quite limited. However, other species do appear to use spatial memory like the rat's while foraging in the wild. This has been demonstrated most spectacularly for food-storing birds, which are now being studied by several research groups.[12]

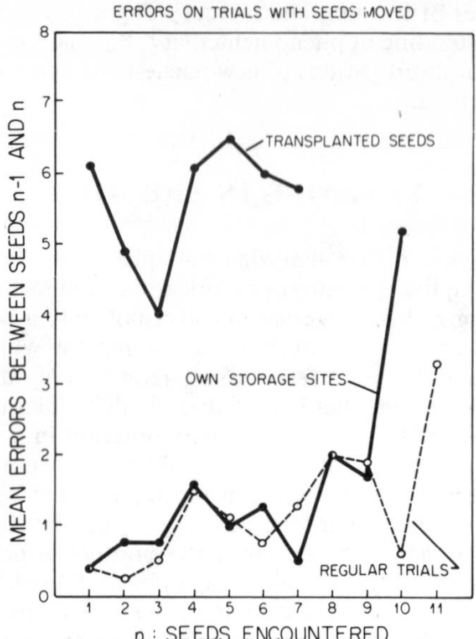

FIGURE 1. Mean errors for a group of four marsh tits recovering 12 stored seeds under two conditions: Regular trials in which seeds remained in the holes where the birds had stored them two hours earlier (dotted line); control trials, in which the seeds were moved by the experimenters before the birds were allowed to search for them (solid lines). The birds continued to visit the storage sites they had actually used ("own storage sites"), looking in many empty holes between visits to the transplanted seeds. Data from Shettleworth & Krebs.[14]

This research is a good example of a productive combination of laboratory and field work, interests in function, and interests in mechanisms of learning.

A number of species of birds, particularly parids (chickadees and titmice) and corvids (crows, jays, and nutcrackers), store food and recover it using memory. While some birds store up tremendous quantities of food for the winter, others use hoarding as a way to make the most of a temporary superabundance of food. For example, a marsh tit (*Parus palustris*) or black-capped chickadee (*Parus atricapillus*) will take many individual seeds from a bird feeder and store them, each one in a different place. The items are collected hours or days later. There is good evidence from the field that stored items are recovered by the bird that stored them using memory.[13]

Marsh tits and chickadees will also store food in the laboratory, so it is possible to study the properties of memory for storage sites in some detail. An experiment John Krebs and I did in Oxford with marsh tits[14] provides an example of what the memory is like. We allowed the birds to store hemp seeds in a 3×4 meter aviary that was furnished with sections of trees. The trees held a total of 100 storage sites (hemp seed-sized holes each concealed behind a flap of cloth that a bird had to lift when storing or recovering a seed). In each storage trial, a bird was allowed to store 12 seeds. Two hours later the hungry bird was allowed back into the aviary with no other food present but the stored seeds. Performance was scored as looks into holes where seeds were stored (recoveries) and looks into holes that had not been used for storage that day (errors). As can be seen from the group results in FIGURE 1, performance was far better than would be expected by chance, with less than one error per seed found over the first few recoveries. The birds were not detecting cues from the seeds themselves, since when we moved the seeds to new holes during the retention interval, the birds continued to go to the holes they had used for storage. They did not switch to the holes that actually contained seeds.

In our experimental situation, marsh tits tended to use some storage sites more than others. However, the probability of visiting given holes in recovery was always greater on days when those holes were used for storage than on days when they were not. Thus preference for going to certain storage sites plays a role in the low error rate, but memory is definitely involved too.

Marsh tits can use their memory of what sites contain seeds in a flexible, cognitive way. They are not, for example, just travelling a fixed route each time they enter the aviary on a given day. Instead of encouraging them to recover seeds two hours after storing them, we allowed them to store more seeds. We instructed them to do so simply by leaving the bowl of seeds in the room. Since each of the experimental storage sites was only big enough for one seed, if the marsh tits remembered where they had stored the first batch of seeds they should go to different sites when storing more seeds. This they did, although it was impossible to tell from the amount of data we were able to collect whether they were actually avoiding (i.e., going less often than would be expected by chance to) sites that already had seeds.

These experiments and others from further experiments by Krebs' group in Oxford and by David Sherry in Toronto (reviewed in Sherry[12]) show pretty clearly that marsh tits and chickadees can retain information about the location of many storage sites for periods of many hours and probably up to a week or more. Clark's nutcrackers, which store pine seeds in thousands of caches and recover them months later, also perform accurately in laboratory tests of memory.[15]

How does memory for stored food compare in capacity and persistence to other examples of animal memory that have been studied in the laboratory? Radial maze studies suggest that spatial memory is generally pretty good, at least when the animal visits the places to be remembered. But it is especially instructive to compare the results of food-storing experiments to the results from another paradigm used to study animal memory, the delayed matching to sample paradigm (or DMTS).

In DMTS tasks, the animal, often a pigeon, is given repeated trials a few seconds apart in which it is first shown a "sample," such as a particular key color, to be remembered. Then the sample is turned off and a few seconds later the subject is offered a choice between the sample and another stimulus, which may be the sample on other trials within the same series. The bird is rewarded for pecking the stimulus that matches the sample. For example, possible samples might be red or green key lights and the choice would always be between red and green. Thus the pigeon has to remember which color was the sample most recently. Performance in this kind of task varies with such things as the length of time the sample is present on each trial, but it typically falls to chance levels within 10–20 seconds. Wilkie and Summers[16] devised a spatial version of the matching task in which the possible samples were nine pecking keys differing only in location on the wall of the Skinner box. Here performance fell to chance after a retention interval of eight seconds.

It is tempting to see the comparison of delayed matching with food storing as suggesting that while some sort of memory-based performance can be squeezed out of animals in highly artificial situations, there must be something wrong with the DMTS situation, not with the pigeon's memory, to make memory appear so short-lived. However, there are some instructive points here regarding whether we want to say chickadee or marsh tit memory is adaptively specialized for a food storing way of life. There are many differences between food storage and DMTS, and most of them would be expected to make memory for stored food better than memory in the delayed matching paradigm. For example, unlike the unidimensional cues used in DMTS, storage sites are far apart (an average of seven meters in one study on marsh tits[13]) and differ in many physical characteristics. The food is in the site instead of being presented elsewhere after the site is found. And the subject visits the storage sites rather than being exposed to them in a passive way. These considerations seem to suggest that there may be nothing special about the memory of food-storing birds. Given that an animal stores food and chooses sites that differ somewhat from each other, memory for the storage sites is likely to be good.[12] That very large numbers of sites are apparently used (and presumably remembered) is also within the bounds of other examples of animal memory. According to Roberts,[17] radial maze data indicate that the number of places a rat can remember is limited only by the number of discriminable places it can be exposed to.

At the moment there is no evidence bearing on how spatial memory of any food-storing species compares in capacity and persistence to spatial memory of a close relative that does not store food. Both tits and corvids invite such comparisons because both groups include storers and non-storers. Corvids are likely to be especially instructive because there is so much inter-specific variation among them in morphological and behavioral specializations for a food-storing way of life.[18] It seems likely that this variation would be accompanied by variations in the ability to remember large numbers of storage sites for long periods of time.

Regardless of the eventual answer to the comparative question, what, if anything, can be learned about mechanisms of animal memory in general from studies on food-storing birds? The foregoing brief review might seem to suggest that the existing data do little more than document how a few unusual species, never before tested in psychologists' laboratories, use spatial memory to solve a real-life problem. There is nothing to suggest that memory for stored food is qualitatively different from a rat's memory for visited locations in a radial maze. With a few simple additions, the model developed by Dale and Staddon[6] for radial mazes and a variety of other memory tests can incorporate food-storing situations. However, these additions amount to a quantitative extension of the model. For example, Dale and Staddon suggest that a rat in a radial maze can be seen as temporarily tagging each visited arm and, in the usual radial maze task, avoiding revisits to arms emptied of food by choosing the arms with the least recent temporal tags. Marsh tits and chickadees recovering stored food in the laboratory also avoid going back to sites recently visited.[9,14] However, encompassing their behavior in the Dale and Staddon model requires that sites be tagged more than temporally. In the first place, a recently filled storage site must be identified in memory as such, to differentiate it from other places the bird visited while searching for a storage site. There is evidence that the particular type of contents of a given site is stored in memory and also that birds learn which types of sites are safe from predators and which unsafe.[12,19] Thus we might imagine that each storage site used is tagged with its contents and time of use; at the time of recovery or attempted recovery, the bird records a visit to that site and whether or not that visit was successful. Although this is not the place to develop the model further, this discussion does suggest that while perhaps not requiring a qualitatively different approach to spatial memory, studies of memory in food storing birds do force a quantitative extension of previous models in showing that the birds remember multiple attributes of the events involved in storing and recovering food. In this respect studies of food storing have a relationship to conventional laboratory studies of animal memory similar to the relationship of studies of conditioned food aversion to traditional associative learning experiments. In both cases a naturalistic example fitting a familiar paradigm has extended the boundaries of what was thought possible within that paradigm.

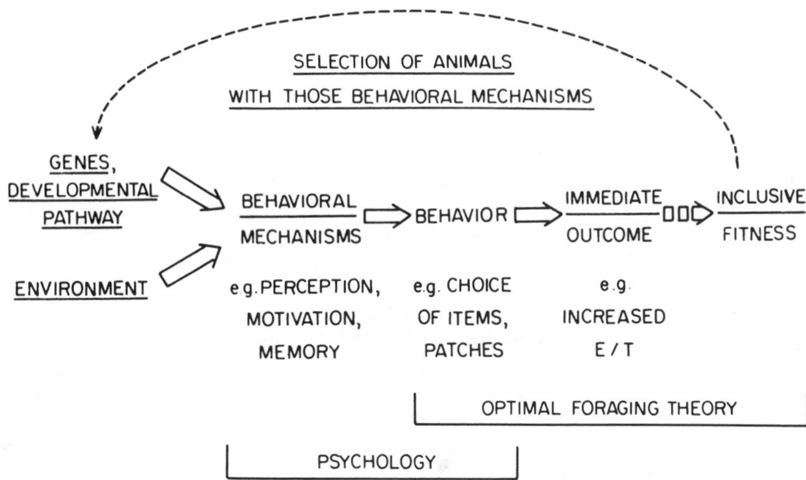

FIGURE 2. Schematic representation of the relationship between natural selection and behavioral mechanisms like learning and memory and of the relationship between the psychology of learning and optimal foraging theory.

LEARNING AND BIOLOGICAL FIRST PRINCIPLES

It is tempting to suggest that quantitative or qualitative variations in memory or learning are a product of natural selection, of increased fitness of individuals with certain behavioral or cognitive capacities. However, arguments from observations on behavior to the selective forces that produced it are necessarily somewhat loose and post hoc. One can never be sure whether a behavior with some definite present-day function is the product of selection pressures relevant to that or to another function. For example, it has sometimes been argued that food aversion learning is just the product of a general associative learning system applied to events that are especially associable because of their similarity to each other or because of the animal's prior history.[7] One implication of viewing learning as part of the animal's whole biology is that there is another and perhaps more satisfactory way of relating learning to selective pressures. We should be able to reason from theories about what promotes fitness to what the outcomes of behavior ought to be and then back one step more to what learning, perception, or motivation might be like (FIGURE 2).

In a general way, Andersson and Krebs[20] did just this for food storing. Most naturalists observing birds store food had found it incredible that such tiny creatures might remember hundreds or thousands of individual storage sites. Andersson and Krebs argued, however, that, in order for food storing to evolve, hoarders must be more likely to find stored items than non-hoarders. If this were not the case, "cheaters" that did not hoard would derive greater net benefit from the hoarders' efforts than would the hoarders themselves since they would collect stored food without incurring the costs of hoarding. Particularly in group-living species, greater probability of recovery by the hoarder is insured if the hoarder either remembers where it has hoarded or has idiosyncratic preferences for hoarding and foraging sites so that it is more likely than others in its area to revisit its storage sites. Thus, the existence of food storing implies the possibility of memory for storage sites. Interestingly, Krebs and I found that both memory and site preferences play a role in the recovery performance of marsh tits in the laboratory.[14]

This behavioral ecological approach to learning (discussed further in Shettleworth[21]) organizes learning phenomena according to the function they serve rather than the details of the mechanisms used. This can result in problem solutions that are not learned at all being lumped for comparative purposes with more cognitive solutions to the same sort of ecological problem. Again, a particularly straightforward example comes from food storing. One problem faced by a hoarder recovering its stores is how to avoid revisiting storage sites that it has already emptied or found to be pilfered. The problem is exactly the same as that faced by a rat in a radial maze with one item of food in each arm. Like rats, marsh tits[14] and chickadees[19] seem to solve the problem of avoiding revisits by remembering what sites they have already emptied or found to be empty. Clark's nutcrackers, however, may sometimes solve the same problem in a different way. These birds bury several pine seeds in each one of their caches. When they remove the seeds and eat them, they are likely to leave the shells lying near the hole where they have been buried. The empty shells and the empty hole therefore provide cues that a cache has been emptied. Memory would not normally be needed to avoid visiting such sites. In laboratory studies, nutcrackers do not avoid revisiting cache sites emptied in one bout of recovery when the experimenters smooth over the emptied holes between successive recovery tests.[15] However, there is some evidence that they may learn to use memory after repeated exposure to such a situation.[24]

LEARNING AND OPTIMAL FORAGING THEORY

Although it provides some illustrations of a behavioral ecological approach to learning, recovering stored food is not a problem that confronts more than a few species. Foraging behavior more generally, however, provides a particularly good area in which to explore the implications of working from biological first principles to properties of learning. This is because many aspects of foraging are encompassed by an explicit and fast-developing theory about what the outcomes of foraging ought to be, in the form of optimal foraging theory.[22]

Optimal foraging theory starts from the premise that animals have been selected to maximize a currency such as energy intake per unit time spent foraging. Such an immediate outcome of foraging is assumed to affect fitness. From such a premise the form of the optimal behavior for explicit foraging situations can be derived. Patch choice is a simple example of how these predictions overlap with psychologists' concerns. Animals feeding on prey that are distributed unevenly throughout the environment are assumed to be able to recognize "patches" where their prey occur. To forage optimally they must be able to choose the patches offering the greatest net energy intake per unit foraging time at a given moment. To do this the predator must "know" in some way such things as the energy offered by different food items, their abundance, and the travel time between patches. If patches deplete as the animal feeds, it must be able to track the current intake rate and compare it to a memory of the intake rate possible elsewhere in the habitat. Although foraging optimally depends on these sorts of information, the predator need not keep track of it cognitively. It need only be sensitive to some correlate of the variables that should influence rate of energy intake. For example, gut fullness may be used as a cue to current food abundance.[23] Size of food items may be used as a cue to energy value.[25] However, there is an obvious similarity between the patch selection problem and the problem faced by an animal working on a concurrent schedule. This similarity suggests that at least some species might select patches using the same mechanisms revealed by studies of behavior on such schedules.[6,25]

Thus, for patch choice the interaction between learning theory and foraging theory might amount to no more than learning theory supplying the (already understood) mechanisms by which animals solve a foraging problem. While this characterization is accurate to some extent, at the same time consideration of patch choice problems has inspired an interest in acquisition processes in choice situations that was not evident in the work on steady-state behavior that has dominated operant schedule research until recently.

The original optimal foraging models asked in effect what a forager ought to do if it had perfect information about all patches in its environment. Clearly, no animal can achieve this optimum unless the environment is completely stable. Foraging research therefore soon took up the problem of how animals might adjust to unknown or changing environments.[26] When the current state of the environment is unknown or changing rapidly, the forager must estimate availability in different patches on the basis of its past experience there and then act on the basis of some decision rule. If it is to be responsive to changing conditions, it should average over a sliding "memory window"[27] short enough to allow it to respond to change but long enough that it does not overreact to random fluctuations in the current average state. Ultimately, therefore, the memory window itself should be adjusted through evolution or through individual experience for degrees of fluctuation in the environment.

Such considerations, together with an interest in deriving schedule performance from more basic acquisition processes, has led to the development of a number of versions of a basic linear operator model for averaging reinforcement frequencies.[28-30] Nigel Lester[31] developed a particularly simple one that he applied to the problem of how a forager adjusts to two patches of unknown initial density that deplete as the predator feeds. While the averaging assumption is like that discussed by Killeen,[28] its particular application most closely resembles that developed by Harley.[30] In Lester's model, animals are assumed to form estimates of food availability (A_i) in given patches according to the following expression:

$$A_{i,n} = (1\text{-}b) \sum_{j=1}^{n} b^{n-1} R_{i,j} \qquad 0 < b < 1$$

$$\text{or } A_{i,n} = bA_{i,n-1} + (1\text{-}b)\, R_{i,n}.$$

The parameter b corresponds to the memory window. The R_i's are rewards. Note that although the first form implies that the animal stores all its past experience, the second equivalent form shows that present estimates depend only on the most recent past estimate and current experience. Estimates are assumed to be updated at regular intervals of time. The animal then allocates its time among patches by matching the proportion of time in a patch in a given time bin to the relative amount of food it estimated to be there at the end of the last time bin, as follows for two patches:

$$\frac{T_{1,n}}{T_{1,n} + T_{2,n}} = \frac{A_{1,n-1}}{A_{1,n-1} + A_{2,n-1}}.$$

Lester termed this decision rule dynamic matching. It predicts a gradual development of preference for the better of two new nondepleting patches. In the more interesting and realistic case where patches deplete as the animal feeds, it predicts that preference will first develop toward the initially better patch and will peak at the time when the initially better patch has been depleted to a level equal to that of the initially worse patch (FIGURE 3).

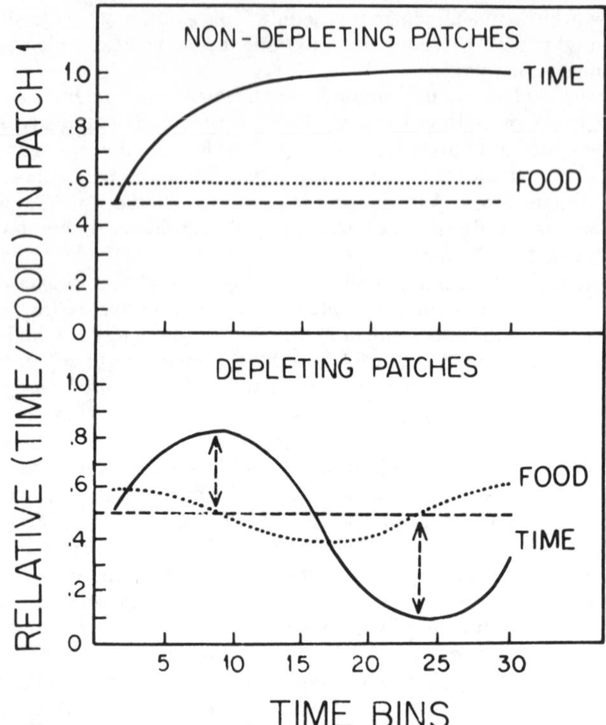

FIGURE 3. General form of the predictions of Lester's model for preference development when a forager confronts two patches and initially does not know which is better. Patch 1 is the patch with the initially greater density of food.

Lester and I, together with Mary-Ann Beeby, tested the model using pigeons feeding in two "patches" at opposite ends of a two-foot long shuttlebox.[32] The birds received single small food items on random ratio-like schedules as often as once every seven seconds. The initial densities were different at the beginning of every 30-minute session. Pigeons proved to be very good at detecting the better patch under these conditions, and when both patches depleted, their preferences cycled as predicted by Lester's model. In the majority of cases, however, peak preference for the initially better patch preceded the point at which relative food densities became equal. In the similar model developed by Harley[30] this can occur if an additive factor identified as "prior expectations" is relatively large. We are currently examining the effects upon adjustment to a standard pair of intermediate densities of the pigeons' previous experience of high versus low average densities.

In the preceding example of reasoning from first principles of behavioral ecology, foraging theory and observations of natural foraging behavior suggest a problem animals have to solve. The question for psychology is, "How do animals do it?" In this case the question has inspired a fresh look at some familiar problems, with an emphasis this time on acquisition processes rather than the steady state, but the more interesting kind of result of this kind of approach occurs when foraging theory predicts behavior that seems to fly in the face of known learning mechanisms. The data in this area are still quite limited, but a few examples are beginning to be studied. For instance, one pervasive idea in foraging theory is that animals should periodically sample the environment so that changes for the better in a currently rejected food item or patch will not go undetected. In effect, foragers should abandon a known best momentary alternative to gather information that may lead to greater intake in the long run.[22]

The best example of an experimental test of sampling involves selection among food items in the great tit (*Parus major*). In this case,[33] analysis of "errors"—deviations from the current optimum—showed that the birds were simply making mistakes in identifying the food items, not "deliberately" selecting suboptimal prey. Further investigations of the possibility that animals systematically sample in this and other situations remain to be done.

Another very cognitive notion from foraging theory is that animals should be sensitive to time horizon, the time available for foraging, since optimal choice sometimes depends on this variable. For instance, a small bird in winter has to have enough energy resources by the end of the day to survive the night. Near evening, if it has the choice between an option of constant value too small to make up its reserves and a variable option that has the same mean but that sometimes takes on a value high enough to keep it through the night, it should take the variable option. When time horizon is longer (say, in the morning) it should choose the other option. In terms of foraging theory, it should choose the risky option (be risk-prone) when time horizon is short and be risk-averse otherwise.[34] This kind of analysis throws new light on the problem of choice between fixed and variable schedules with the same mean. It also suggests that session length, rather than being a matter only of convenience, might sometimes influence the outcome of operant choice experiments.

CONCLUSIONS

Although food storing and patch choice are aspects of feeding along with food aversion learning the work I have been describing is pretty far afield from the theoretical analyses and practical applications of food aversion learning that are the material for most papers in this volume. However, theoretical and experimental research on foraging behavior partly owes its enthusiastic acceptance by learning psychologists to the way in which learning theory was shaken up by the discovery of food aversion learning in the mid-1960s. Food aversion learning has become an important tool for the analysis of associative learning. It has had broad practical applications. However, at least some of its long-term importance lies in its having been the first really powerful example of learning that cannot be completely understood outside its biological context.

REFERENCES

1. Rozin, P. & J. W. Kalat. 1971. Psych. Rev **78**: 459–486.
2. Domjan, M. & B. G. Galef. 1983. Anim. Learning Behav. **11**: 151–161.
3. Johnston, T. D. & M. T. Turvey. 1980. Psych. Learn. Motiv. **14**: 147–205.
4. Hollis, K. L. 1982. Adv. Study Behav. **12**: 1–64.
5. Timberlake, W. 1983. *In* Advances in Analysis of Behavior. M. D. Zeiler & P. Harzem, Eds. **3**: 177–222. Wiley. Chichester.
6. Staddon, J. E. R. 1983. Adaptive Behaviour and Learning. Cambridge University Press. Cambridge.

7. DOMJAN, M. 1983. Psych. Learn Motiv. **17**: 215–277.
8. DICKENSON, A. 1980. Contemporary Animal Learning Theory. Cambridge University Press. Cambridge.
9. KROODSMA, D. E. 1982. *In* Acoustic Communication in Birds. D. E. Kroodsma, E. H. Miller & H. Ouellet, Eds. **2**: 1–23. Academic Press. New York.
10. BATESON, P. P. G. 1979. Anim. Behav. **27**: 470–486.
11. OLTON, D. S. & R. J. SAMUELSON. 1976. J. Exp. Psychol.: Anim. Behav. Proc. **2**: 97–116.
12. SHERRY, D. F. 1984. Can. J. Psych. **38**: 304–321.
13. COWIE, R. J., J. R. KREBS & D. F. SHERRY. 1981. Anim. Behav. **29**: 1252–1259.
14. SHETTLEWORTH, S. J. & J. R. KREBS. 1982. J. Exp. Psychol.: Anim. Behav. Proc. **8**: 354–375.
15. KAMIL, A. C. & R. C. BALDA. 1985. J. Exp. Psychol.: Anim. Behav. Proc. **11**: 95–111.
16. WILKIE, D. H. & R. J. SUMMERS. 1982. J. Exp. Anal. Behav. **37**: 45–56.
17. ROBERTS, W. A. 1984. *In* Animal Cognition. H. L. Roitblat & H. S. Terrace, Eds.: 425–443. Erlbaum. Hillsdale, NJ.
18. VANDERWALL, S. B. & R. C. BALDA. 1981. Zeit. Tierpsychol. **56**: 217–242.
19. SHERRY, D. F. 1984. Anim. Behav. **32**: 451–464.
20. ANDERSSON, M. & J. R. KREBS. 1978. Anim. Behav. **26**: 707–711.
21. SHETTLEWORTH, S. J. 1984. *In* Behavioral Ecology. 2nd edit. J. R. Krebs & D. B. Davies, Eds.: 170–194. Blackwell. Oxford.
22. KREBS, J. R., D. W. STEPHENS & W. J. SUTHERLAND. 1983. *In* Perspectives in Ornithology. G. A. Clark & A. H. Brush Eds.: 165–216. Cambridge University Press. New York.
23. CHARNOV, E. L. 1976. Am Nat. **110**: 141–151.
24. TOMBACK, D. F., K. G. BUNCH & G. S. SULLIVAN. 1984. (Manuscript submitted.)
25. LEA, S. E. G. 1981. *In* Advances in the Analysis of Behavior. P. Harzem & M. D. Zeiler, Eds. **2**: 355–406.
26. KREBS, J. R., A. KACELNIK & P. TAYLOR. 1978. Nature **275**: 27–31.
27. COWIE, R. J. 1977. Nature **268**: 137–139.
28. KILLEEN, P. 1981. *In* Quantification of Steady-state Operant Behavior. C. M. Bradshaw, E. Szabadi & C. F. Lowe, Eds.: 21–34. Elsevier. New York.
29. DOW, S. & S. E. G. LEA. 1985. *In* Quantitative Analysis of Behavior. M. R. Commons, A. Kacelnik & S. J. Shettleworth, Eds. Vol. 6. Erlbaum. Hillsdale, NJ. (In press.)
30. HARLEY, C. B. 1981. J. Theoret. Biol. **89**: 611–633.
31. LESTER, N. P. 1985. Behaviour **89**: 175–199.
32. LESTER, N. P., M. A. BEEBY & S. J. SHETTLEWORTH. (In preparation.)
33. RECHTEN, C. M. AVERY & M. STEVENS. 1983. Anim. Behav. **31**: 576–584.
34. STEVENS, D. W. 1981. Anim. Behav. **26**: 628–629.

PART IV. PHARMACOLOGICAL AND TOXICOLOGICAL ASSESSMENTS USING CONDITIONED FOOD AVERSION METHODOLOGY

Introduction: Pharmacological and Toxicological Assessments Using Conditioned Food Aversion Methodology

SHEPARD SIEGEL

Department of Psychology
McMaster University
Hamilton, Ontario L8S 4K1

As indicated in these proceedings, the flavor-aversion preparation has had an enormous influence on theoretical interpretations of Pavlovian conditioning and has also been exploited for practical purposes, such as altering flavor preferences in animals (e.g., to control predation) and humans (e.g., as a therapy for alcoholism). In this section, we again see an interaction between learned flavor aversion theory and application.

An enduring enigma about flavor aversions concerns the wide variety of chemicals that can motivate such aversions. Indeed, as indicated in the contribution of Gamzu *et al.*, some drugs that are effective unconditional stimuli (UCSs) in the flavor-aversion situation appear not to be aversive in other situations—indeed, sometimes they seem to function as positive reinforcers. Because such an array of drugs, with such a large variety of effects, can be used to induce taste aversions, Gamzu *et al.* are pessimistic about the promise of any pharmacological insight into the mechanisms of flavor-aversion learning. Although there does appear to be a bewildering assortment of agents that are effective in altering flavor preference, it might be fruitful to examine in more detail the features of the aversions produced by the different substances. It is possible that there are qualitative differences in aversions motivated by drugs that do and do not cause upper gastrointestinal upset. For example, although the flavor aversions induced by both morphine and lithium are attenuated by preconditioning experience with these drugs, this drug preexposure effect is different with the two drugs; the deleterious effect of lithium preexposure on lithium-motivated taste aversions is pronounced only when preexposure and training occur in the same environment; in contrast, there is no such environmental specificity with respect to the UCS-preexposure effect in morphine-induced flavor aversion learning.[1-3] Such a functional difference raises the possibility of different mechanisms and suggests advantages to looking at aspects of flavor-aversion other than just the fact that alternative flavors are chosen in preference to the conditional stimulus (CS) flavor.

The advantages of going beyond mere intake measures are clearly documented in recent studies by Parker[4] and Pelchat *et al.*[5] Although rats may avoid flavors paired with a variety of agents, they nevertheless respond very differently to these flavors.

Following pairing of a normally preferred sweet solution with lithium chloride, rats not only avoid the sweet flavor, but respond to it with chin rubs[4] and orofacial responses[5] (gaping) similar to those seen in response to quinine, a manifestly unpalatable solution. Following pairing of a distinctive flavor with amphetamine,[4] or high concentrations of lactose,[5] the flavor is also avoided, but there is no display of chin rubbing or gaping. It would seem that the flavor aversions produced by different agents may be distinguished by behavioral measures other than mere ingestion—indeed, they may be mediated by different physiological pathways.[6,7] Such additional measures may well prove a valuable tool in the elucidation of the mechanisms of flavor aversions and the various types of associations that involve flavors as CSs.[8]

The fact that many agents can serve as effective UCSs has suggested to some investigators that the flavor-aversion procedure might be a useful assay of drug toxicity. The use of this preparation for toxicity is reviewed in the paper by Riley and Tuck. These investigators summarize the literature showing that many known toxins do serve as an effective UCS for flavor aversion learning, and many nontoxic agents do not readily serve as an effective UCS. However, as Riley and Tuck indicate, the use of the flavor-aversion situation as an assessment of toxicity is complicated by two categories of findings: some nontoxic agents are effective as UCSs (in the signal-detection terminology used by Riley and Tuck, these are "false alarms"), and some known toxic agents are ineffective as UCSs (these are "misses"). Riley and Tuck suggest that these apparent failures of the flavor-aversion assay to correctly identify drugs with respect to their toxicity may sometimes be understood as instances of the extreme sensitivity of the assay, or failures on the part of the experimenter to appropriately pair the flavor with the toxic effect of the chemical being assessed. Riley and Tuck further illustrate the utility of modified forms of the flavor-aversion technique in toxicity assessments. These investigators comprehensively and convincingly present the case for the role of flavor aversion methodology in screening potentially toxic substances. It is possible that additional evaluation of non-intake measures of the flavor-drug association, such as the evaluation of the previously mentioned orofacial responses, may further refine the technique. At present, a finding that a newly tested drug does or does not motivate a flavor aversion does not clearly address the issue of that drug's toxicity. Data indicating an aversion may be attributable either to the correct detection of the drug's toxicity or to a "false alarm." Similarly, data indicating no aversion may be attributable either to the drug's innocuousness or to a "miss." It would appear that we are just beginning to develop techniques that may potentially result in a simple and widely accepted evaluation of drug toxicity using the methodology of flavor aversion learning.

A further application of flavor-aversion methodology is indicated in Robert Ader's paper on "Conditioned Taste Aversions and Immunopharmacology." Ader's research also further demonstrates the importance of measures of the flavor-drug association other than mere intake of the flavored solution. Pairing saccharin with cyclophosphamide not only leads to an aversion of saccharin, but also to a saccharin-induced immunosuppressive response. Moreover, this saccharin-elicited conditional immunosuppressive response can be used to alter the course of immune disease, much as the unconditional immunosuppressive effect of cyclophosphamide. Thus, in certain regimens of drug administration, it may be feasible and therapeutically useful to occasionally administer drug-predictive cues, rather than the drug. The use of such a "partial reinforcement" schedule of drug administration (i.e., interspersing placebo administrations among drug administrations), which uses lower cumulative amounts of the drug than the usual "continuous reinforcement" schedule of drug administration, may well be a procedure for maximizing therapeutic efficacy while minimizing undesirable drug side effects. Although Ader presents a convincing case for the value of the partial reinforcement procedure in the case of cyclophosphamide administration, further research is needed to evaluate its value in the case of other, repeatedly presented drugs that affect CNS functioning (e.g., psychotropic drugs). In support of the generality of Ader's proposal, there is evidence that a deleterious effect of repeated opiate administrations (i.e., tolerance) can be minimized by a treatment regimen involving partial reinforcement procedures,[9–11] as well as other techniques derived from Pavlovian conditioning theory.[12]

A further important issue raised by Ader's research concerns the role of flavor as a cue for conditional immunosuppressive activity. Does flavor bear a special relationship to drugs affecting immunocompetence, as it apparently does to drugs with gastrointestinal effects? As Ader has indicated, there are many early studies concerning immunological conditioning that have used CSs other than flavors.[13] Although procedures used in many of these early studies raise methodological issues,[13] recent work concerning an immunological conditioning has demonstrated the effectiveness of a nongustatory CS (the environmental cues associated with a skin grafting procedure).[14]

Ader's psychoneuroimmunological insights resulted from an astute observation he made while engaged in flavor-aversion learning research for completely different reasons.[15] The value of such serendipity in flavor-aversion research is further illustrated by Revusky's research concerning drug-drug associations. In a series of experiments evaluating the associability of a drug-state with sickness (in an attempt to develop a more effective chemical aversion treatment of alcoholism), a two-phase, higher-order conditioning paradigm was used: (1) one drug (the CS drug) was paired with lithium (the UCS drug); (2) saccharin was then paired with the CS drug. The expected finding was that the initial drug-drug pairings would result in CS drug acquiring the aversive properties of the UCS drug, and thus the subjects would display a saccharin aversion as a result of pairing the saccharin with the CS drug. This did not occur; rather, the initial drug-drug pairings seem to decrease the ability of the CS drug to subsequently serve as a UCS for flavor-aversion learning. This failure of aversion learning (the "Avfail" phenomenon) stimulated additional research by Revusky and colleagues, who conclude that the relevant effect of the drug-drug associations is to train an "antisickness" response—the CS drug comes to elicit a conditional response that counteracts the lithium-induced distress. The evidence in support of the antisickness interpretation of the Avfail phenomenon is reviewed by Revusky, as are the practical implications of the procedure. If the Avfail technique could be exploited to minimize the distress caused by the therapeutically necessary administration of nausea-inducing drugs, it would be an important further demonstration of the practical utility of flavor-aversion methodology.

As Revusky indicates, the antisickness interpretation of the effects of drug-drug association are similar to compensatory CR interpretations of drug tolerance.[12] Further research on the Avfail effect may integrate this phenomenon with that of drug tolerance, and thus importantly contribute to knowledge in a number of areas.

A recent study by Greeley *et al.*[16] is relevant to the integration of antisickness and compensatory CRs. These investigators, like Revusky, studied drug-drug associations, but the same drug functioned as the CS and UCS—a small dose of ethanol (CS) signaled a large dose (UCS). Following such a schedule of drug administration, tolerance to the hypothermic effect of the large dose was seen only when it was preceded by the small dose. Furthermore, the small dose elicited an ethanol-compensatory CR of hypothermia. Thus, the drug-drug association formed by ethanol-ethanol pairings attenuated the effect of the UCS (i.e., the second, larger-dose of ethanol), a finding similar to Revusky's attenuation of the aversiveness of the lithium UCS by a pharmacological CS. Furthermore, in the Greeley *et al.* experiment, the CS (i.e., the first, smaller dose of ethanol) elicited a response opposite to the UCR, similar to Revusky's postulated antisickness function of the CS drug. Additional research will undoubtedly elucidate the relationship between Avfail and drug tolerance. Furthermore, as discussed by others, a gradual increase in the systemic concentration is an inevitable consequence of most drug administration procedures, thus drug-drug associations may play a heretofore unappreciated role in both flavor-aversion learning and drug tolerance.[17]

In summary, the papers in this section indicate the many uses of flavor-aversion methodology, not only in understanding fundamental issues in Pavlovian conditioning, but also in elucidating the relationships among learning, immunology, toxicology, and pharmacology.

REFERENCES

1. STEWART, J. & R. EIKELBOOM. 1978. Pre-exposure to morphine and the attenuation of conditioned taste aversion in rats. Pharmacol. Biochem. Behav. 639–645.
2. DECANAY, R. J. & A. L. RILEY. 1982. The UCS preexposure effect in food aversion learning: Tolerance and blocking are drug specific. Anim. Learn. Behav. **10**: 91–96.
3. DOMJAN, M. & S. SIEGEL. 1983. Attenuation of the aversive and analgesic effects of morphine by repeated administration: Different mechanisms. Physiol. Psychol. **11**: 155–158.
4. PARKER, L. A. 1982. Nonconsummatory and consummatory behavioral CRs elicited by lithium- and amphetamine-paired flavors. Learn. Motiv. **13**: 281–303.
5. PELCHAT, M. L., H. J. GRILL, P. ROZIN & J. JACOBS. 1983. Quality of acquired responses to tastes by *Rattus norvegicus* depends on type of associated discomfort. J. Comp. Physiol. Psychol. **97**: 140–153.
6. BERGER, B., C. WISE & L. STEIN. 1973. Area postrema damage and bait shyness. J. Comp. Physiol. Psychol. **83**: 475–479.
7. RITTER, S., J. J. MCGLONE & K. W. KELLY. 1980. Absence of lithium-induced taste aversion after area postrema lesion. Brain Res. **201**: 501–506.
8. PELCHAT, M. L. & P. ROZIN. 1982. The special role of nausea in the acquisition of food dislikes by humans. Appetite **3**: 341–351.
9. SIEGEL, S. 1977. Morphine tolerance acquisition as an associative process. J. Exp. Psychol.: Anim. Behav. Proc. **3**: 1–13.
10. SIEGEL, S. 1978. Tolerance to the hypothermic effect of morphine in the rat is a learned response. J. Comp. Physiol. Psychol. **92**: 1137–1149.
11. KRANK, M. D., R. E. HINSON & S. SIEGEL. 1984. The effect of partial reinforcement on tolerance to morphine-induced analgesia and weight loss in the rat. Behav. Neurosci. **98**: 79–95.
12. SIEGEL, S. 1983. Classical conditioning, drug tolerance, and drug dependence. *In* Research Advances in Alcohol and Drug Problems. Y. Israel, F. B. Glaser, H. Kalant, R. E. Popham, W. Schmidt & R. G. Smart, Eds. **7**: 207–246. Plenum. New York.
13. ADER, R. 1981. A historical account of conditioned immunobiologic responses. *In* Psychoneuroimmunology. R. Ader, Ed.: 321–352. Academic Press. New York.
14. GROCZYNSKI, R. M., S. MACRAE & M. KENNEDY. 1982. Conditioned immune response associated with allogenic skin grafts in mice. J. Immunol. **129**: 704–709.
15. ADER, R. 1974. Letter to the editor. Psychosom. Med. **36**: 183–184.
16. GREELEY, J., D. A. LE, C. X. POULOS & H. CAPPELL. 1985. Alcohol is an effective cue in the conditional control of tolerance to alcohol. Psychopharmacol. **83**: 159–162.
17. WALTER, T. A. & D. C. RICCIO. 1983. Overshadowing effects in the stimulus control of morphine analgesic tolerance. Behav. Neurosci. **97**: 658–662.

A Pharmacological Perspective of Drugs Used in Establishing Conditioned Food Aversions[a]

E. GAMZU, G. VINCENT, AND E. BOFF

Department of Pharmacology
Hoffmann-La Roche Inc.
Nutley, New Jersey 07110

INTRODUCTION

In a previous review of the then limited pharmacological studies of conditioned taste aversions (CTA), it was noted that modern psychology did not deal with the hedonic nature of reinforcers.[49] Rather the approach was, and continues to be, one of defining reinforcers operationally as those events that when appropriately paired with behavior have the ability to change the rate of occurrence of the behavior. Thus, positive reinforcers are events that an organism will seek out, try to maintain, and not avoid; negative reinforcers involve aversive stimuli that an organism will neither seek nor maintain, and will usually try to terminate. Although rigorous operational definitions can be given, the concept of a "reinforcer" carries with it a considerable amount of hedonic connotation.

To a large extent, pharmacological studies of CTAs, tacitly or otherwise, have addressed the issue of specifying the hedonic nature of the events that, when paired with a gustatory stimulus, produce a CTA.[5,19,49,55,56,117] There is general consensus among the numerous reviewers that the pharmacological literature does not give an answer to the specific nature of CTA producing events, but rather specifies limitations on previously postulated mechanisms. The conclusions are based on regarding CTA as a homogeneous process. Recent research has questioned this assumption by the introduction of measures other than consumption as indices of CTA[63,107] and this issue is addressed below. First, it is necessary to briefly review the history of explanations of CTA.

BRIEF HISTORY OF EXPLANATIONS OF CTA

Initial experiments on CTA paired a flavor with radiation, apomorphine,[52] or lithium chloride.[85] On subsequent exposure, compared to control treated animals, experimental rats showed either decreased consumption of the flavored solution or substantially

[a] In undertaking this review, we have selected among the very large number of studies using drugs to study CTA. A complete listing of these can be found in the bibliographic appendix of this volume.[101] Within the limitations of this chapter, it is impossible to do an exhaustive compilation and review of this material. Consequently, the specific papers cited were chosen to illustrate certain points and we ask for the understanding of those whose work is omitted.

lower preference for the flavor. These treatments produce severe gastrointestinal distress and emesis in man. This fact, coupled with the uniqueness of CTA with respect to its relative specificity for gustatory stimuli and its temporal robustness,[36] suggested a unique learning process by which an organism could rapidly learn to associate emesis, illness, or nausea with a prior taste in the mouth. The adaptive utility of such a mechanism for an omniverous organism is quite obvious. Consequently, it is easy to conceive of evolutionary pressures for such a specific learning process (see Garcia[50] for an eloquent elaboration of this proposal). In their classic paper, Garcia and Koelling[51] wrote about "agents which produce nausea and gastric upset." Indeed, the term conditioned taste aversion makes the plausible assumption that the agent used in the CTA produces an "aversive" event. When Nachman *et al.*[87] produced a CTA with ethanol and related compounds, they suggested that the CTA could be considered as a sensitive behavioral bioassay for toxic effects. Indeed, the term toxicosis to describe the agent producing a CTA is still widely used, as can be seen in a number of chapters in this volume. Cappell and LeBlanc[16] made similar assumptions when they proposed to study D-amphetamine and mescaline to observe the "aversive" properties of these drugs of abuse. However, Berger[5] showed that CTAs could be produced by relatively low doses of chlordiazepoxide, chlorpromazine, and lorazepam; such low doses that could not normally be considered to produce sickness. His conclusion that sickness was not a necessary feature of treatments that produce a CTA has been echoed by all reviewers of pharmacological perspectives of CTAs. Indeed, even the use of the word "aversion" in the nomenclature of CTA has been questioned.[116]

THE ROLE OF EMESIS IN CTA

Probably the most specific suggestion as to the mechanism of action is the postulated role of emesis as the major aspect of agents that produce a CTA. A series of experiments by Coil and co-workers first demonstrated that treatment with any of four chemically distinctive antiemetic agents (scopolamine, cyclizine, prochlorperazine, or trimethoxybenzamide) prior to testing animals that had already experienced a saccharin-LiCl pairing resulted in a significant attenuation of the CTA.[26] A second experiment[28] indicated that subdiaphragmatic vagotomy in rats disrupted the acquisition of a CTA to saccharin paired with either intraperitoneally or intragastrically administered copper sulfate ($CuSO_4$). When $CuSO_4$ was given intravenously, vagotomy was without effect, but lesions of the area postrema severely attenuated the ability of rats to acquire a CTA to saccharin paired with intravenous $CuSO_4$.[27] Since the area postrema had been identified by Borison and Wang[11] as a chemoreceptor site mediating emetic reflexes, it was suggested that two separate systems mediate CTA: a circulatory system acting through the area postrema and a vagal system responsive to peripheral stimulation. This argument is bolstered by the convergence in the nucleus solitarius of fibers subserving both gustatory afferents and the emetic pathway.[50] Furthermore, lesions of area postrema also abolish a CTA induced by LiCl (TABLE 1).

While the importance of emesis for establishing a CTA seems to have been established for $CuSO_4$, the utility of this particular mechanism as a global explanation for CTAs has to be questioned. A brief summary of research on this topic can be found in TABLE 1. Lesions of the area postrema, for example, can prevent a methylscopolamine-induced CTA, but do not effect a CTA based on amphetamine.[6,103,122] Moreover, area postrema lesions do not affect the ability of rats to acquire a CTA to saccharin paired with apomorphine,[122] a compound that is considered to be one of the most effective emetics in man. Furthermore, in an early study, Levy *et al.*[74]

TABLE 1. Effects[a] of "Anti-Emetic" Manipulations on CTAs Induced by Six Different Treatments[b]

Experimental Manipulation	CTA-inducing Treatment					
	Radiation	LiCl	$CuSo_4$	Apomorphine	Methyl Scopolamine	Amphetamine
Lesions of area postrema	↓:88	↓:82, 97 ↓:103	Ø:27 i.g. ↓:72 i.v.	Ø:122	↓:6, 103 122	Ø:6, 103
Anti-emetic drugs	Ø:15, 74 Ø:96	Ø:61, 96 ↓:26				Ø:17, 61
Vagotomy		Ø:80 i.p.	↓:28 i.p. ↓:28 i.g. ↓:28 i.v.			

[a] Ø = no effect, ↓ = attenuation or complete block.
[b] The numbers refer to the citation in the reference section.

demonstrated that pretreatment with the antiemetic drug trimethoxybenzamide had no effect on a CTA produced by radiation, but the CTA could be blocked with an antihistamine. While the latter effect is in some doubt, the failure of antiemetics to block radiation-induced CTAs has been replicated (TABLE 1), while the ability of antiemetics to affect a LiCl-induced CTA[61,96] or an amphetamine-induced CTA over a wide variety of conditions[61] has not.

There are other reasons for questioning the generality of an emetic response as the major event in CTAs. There is considerable agreement that amphetamine and nicotine CTAs are centrally rather than peripherally mediated (see the sections on catecholamines and cholinergics) while the area postrema is peripherally accessible. Even more challenging is the fact that CTAs can be obtained by application of compounds directly into some, but not other, brain loci. Thus, Δ^9-THC applied to dorsal hippocampus, but not caudate nucleus, can induce a CTA[1] and carbachol administered to the medial septum, but not to the ventral hippocampus, can produce a CTA.[84] These facts cannot easily be encompassed by a theoretical system that stresses the area postrema and the nucleus solitarius. Most damaging to the emesis interpretation is the fact that CTAs can be produced by agents that are quite clearly antiemetic in humans. This is true of cannabinoids,[31] chlorpromazine, and scopolamine.[5]

Recent evidence suggests that humans can avoid specific flavors for both hedonic and nonhedonic reasons.[94] In the former case, these seem to be associated with experiences of nausea, while in the latter case this is not so. Pelchat *et al.*[93] have shown that the orofacial response of rats, originally described by Grill and Norgren[64] as a method of classifying the rat's hedonic response to gustatory stimuli, can be used to distinguish between taste aversions based on upper GI distress (LiCl), presumed to be related to nausea and emesis, and aversions based on lower GI distress (lactose). In the former case the response to saccharin is transformed into the pattern normally seen in unconditioned rats when exposed to quinine. When the CTA is based on lactose there is no evidence of a change in the rat's response to the taste of saccharin. It has been postulated, and currently seems feasible, that only CTAs mediated through an emetic center will result in this "hedonic shift." However, an extremely broad range of compounds can be used to produce CTAs with the majority being devoid of emesis induction. Consequently, such compounds would not fit the "emetic-hedonic shift" category. Rather, Pelchat *et al.* suggested that the CTA in such cases would be based on a classification by the rat of "danger." Clearly, this initial classification of CTAs by an independent measure is an important advance, but explaining the residual class of CTAs as being based on "dangerous" events begs the question.

To summarize, the induction of emesis does not seem to be necessary to produce CTA, but it may well be sufficient.

ILLNESS, NAUSEA, OR TOXICOSIS AS THE BASIS FOR CTA

The same general arguments can be made to eliminate the possibility that a broader category of nausea, illness, or toxicosis may be the causal event in producing all CTAs. Symptoms of sickness need not occur while the animal is experiencing the event that produces a CTA.[86,112] More recently, Bernstein and Webster[7] reported that humans can develop a radiation-based CTA without reporting any symptoms of nausea.

A second consideration is that the doses that have been used to produce conditioned CTAs frequently are doses that are used standardly without side effects in various psychopharmacological tests[5] or are capable of enhancing behavior in non-CTA situations,[20] and can often be considered to be equivalent to the human therapeutic

TABLE 2. "Self-administered" Compounds that Produce a CTA[a]

Morphine (20)
Phencyclidine (42)
Cocaine (60)
Amphetamine (9)
Ethanol (20)
Nicotine (71)
Barbituarates (124)
Cannabinoids (31)
Nitrous oxide (59)
Benzodiazepines (49)
Caffeine (123)

[a] The numbers refer to the citation in the reference section

doses. Thus, for example, doses of benzodiazepines that have been used to produce CTAs[49] are equivalent to those doses which in rats and monkeys will release operant behavior that has been suppressed by electric shock.[108]

In addition, a number of agents which are clearly toxic do not produce CTAs when specifically paired with a flavored solution. A list of these compounds can be found in Riley's contribution in this volume. Based on these and other considerations, every reviewer of the CTA literature who has taken a pharmacological perspective has concluded that neither emesis, illness, nausea, sickness, nor toxicosis are necessary conditions to produce a CTA. Indeed, there has been some speculation as to whether or not the event has to be "aversive" at all.[49,56,117]

THE PARADOX OF SELF-ADMINISTERED DRUGS THAT PRODUCE CTA

An additional factor arguing against the interpretation that any CTA producing agent necessarily causes a hedonically aversive state is the fact that many compounds are capable of both producing a CTA and being self-administered by a variety of species. TABLE 2 lists some of these compounds and selected sources that demonstrate the CTA. In fact, the list is based primarily on compounds that most scientists would agree are self administered to a greater or less degree: ranging from the dangerous (morphine and phencyclidine) to the more innocuous (benzodiazepines and caffeine).

Operationally, the production of a CTA infers an aversive stimulus, while maintenance of self-administration infers a positive reinforcer. Although the early work on the two phenomena tended to use different routes of administration, this consideration is not crucial. Wise *et al.*[128] demonstrated that if saccharin were paired with apomorphine while the latter was being self-administered, the saccharin would subsequently be avoided. While there are some methodological problems with this particular study, a number of studies have demonstrated that rats injected with morphine in a specific location where they had drunk saccharin, would avoid the saccharin, but preferred the location (see Van der Kooy *et al.*[122] for a recent use of this procedure). Based on the multiple pharmacological actions of CTA inducing agents, it has been suggested that this paradox is more apparent than real.[19,49] Perhaps it is more accurate to state that this is a paradox for those psychological explanations that assume the hedonic baggage that is simply not stated in the operational definitions of reinforcers. Various attempts to solve this paradox have been relatively unsuccessful. An excellent review of the status of this issue can be found in Goudie.[56]

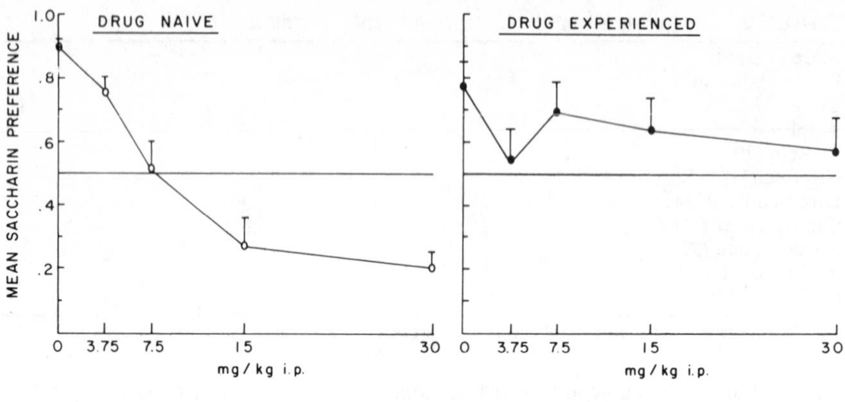

FIGURE 1. The effects of pre-exposure to chlordiazepoxide (CDAP) on saccharin preference after a single pairing of saccharin and various doses of CDAP. Saccharin preference (versus tap water) was measured in a two-bottle test 48 hours after the pairing. Drug naive rats (left panel) were given i.p. injections of isotonic saline on three consecutive days starting one week prior to the pairing of saccharin and CDAP. Drug experienced rats (right panel) were given i.p. injections of 15 mg/kg of CDAP on three consecutive days starting one week prior to the pairing of saccharin and CDAP.

LIMITATIONS ON INTERPRETING PHARMACOLOGICAL STUDIES OF CTA

Pharmacologists often employ drug interaction studies to elucidate the mechanism of action. For example, it is common to look at agonists, antagonists, and their interactions, or to use a precursor or transmitter-depleting agent in combination with a variety of compounds to ascertain which system is being activated. In the study of CTAs, the major complicating factor in using this type of analysis is the so-called UCS preexposure effect.

Prior exposure to a CTA-inducing agent can attenuate or eliminate the ability of that agent to produce a CTA when subsequently paired with a novel stimulus. Domjan and Best[37] identified two distinct preexposure effects: durable and proximal. The proximal preexposure effect occurs when a treatment closely precedes in time the pairing of a flavor with yet another treatment. Thus, a LiCl-saccharin pairing sufficient to produce a mild CTA (presumably through "backward conditioning"[4]) attenuated a saccharin-LiCl CTA in a LiCl-saccharin-LiCl paradigm. There clearly are a number of additional ways in which interpretation of drug pretreatment data is complicated, not the least of these is the fact that a wide variety of compounds, especially stimulants, have hypodypsic effects.[116] No less serious a problem is the fact that a wide variety of compounds, including benzodiazepines and barbiturates, can increase consumption directly.[29,30] Indeed, within limits, the amount of fluid consumption does affect the magnitude of a CTA.[14]

Probably a more difficult problem is the durable preexposure effect. An example of that is found in FIGURE 1.[49] On the left-hand side of the figure is shown the ability of different doses of chlordiazepoxide (CDAP) to produce a CTA in experimentally naive rats when paired with saccharin. On the right-hand side is the failure to produce a CTA in drug-experienced rats exposed to the identical paradigm. The only difference was that the drug-experienced rats had been exposed to three single injections of CDAP approximately one week prior to the pairing of saccharin and CDAP. This striking demonstration of the complete abolition of the agent's ability to produce a CTA is more extreme than the normal preexposure attenuation effect that has been demonstrated for amphetamine,[18] Δ^9-THC,[44] diazepam[49] ethanol,[38] LiCl,[12] meprobamate,[49] and morphine.[27,34,67] In addition, nonspecific effects have also been reported. For example, several studies have shown that preexposure to one type of compound has affected a CTA based on a pharmacologically unrelated agent[47,123] or on rotation.[12,13]

In reviewing compounds that have been used to produce a CTA, we have included agents that have been studied only at a single dose, because these studies are clearly important for this survey. Interpretation of such single-dose studies is subject to limitations, especially when the compound fails to produce a CTA. For this reason we would like to reiterate the importance of dose-response relationships in behavioral pharmacology, and the need to have equi-effective doses from other independent measures of drug effect when comparing compounds.[117]

CTA-PRODUCING COMPOUNDS BY THERAPEUTIC CLASS

With these warnings in mind, in TABLE 3 we have constructed a list of psychoactive components that produce CTAs by sorting them according to their therapeutic effect in man. It is obvious that a variety of stimulants, antidepressants, anxiolytic/hypnotics, and anesthetics are all capable of producing conditioned taste aversions. One can add to these categories antihistaminergics (e.g., chlorpromazine[5]), antibiotics,[10] antihypertensives (e.g. hydralazine[69]), and other therapeutic classes. Clearly the therapeutic effect of a particular agent in man is simply uncorrelated with its ability to produce a CTA in the rat.

CTA-PRODUCING COMPOUNDS BY TRANSMITTER CLASS

Another way of analyzing agents that produce a CTA from a pharmacological perspective is to examine their affects within and across different transmitter systems. Thus, for example, one can ask whether both agonists or antagonists are capable of producing CTAs or not. In doing so we will use a rather broad definition of agonists to include such things as precursors. Similarly, we will include depleting agents as well as antagonists. Where possible, we want to know whether or not the effect is stereospecific, since this is an important criterion of pharmacological specificity. Another question to be addressed is whether the CTA is centrally or peripherally mediated. Finally, we are interested in the degree of specificity to the particular transmitter system and its relationship to other phenomena mediated by the same transmitter.

Catecholamines and CTA

A partial list of compounds that affect catecholamine (CA) systems and have been used to produce CTAs is shown in TABLE 4. With respect to compounds that elevate CA function, it is quite obvious that a wide variety of such agents are capable of producing a CTA. This includes direct agonists such as apomorphine,[35] compounds

TABLE 3. Compounds that Produce a CTA by Psychoactive Class[a]

Stimulants	Anxiolytics/Hypnotics	Antidepressants	Anesthetics
Amphetamine and congeners (117)	Diazepam (49)	Amitriptyline (83)	Ketamine (42)
Cocaine (60)	Chlordiazepoxide (49)	Buproprion (83)	Nitrous Oxide (59)
Buproprion (83)	Flurazepam (124)	Desipramine (79)	
Methylphenidate (102)	Lorazepam (5)		
	Amobarbital (124)		
	Hexobarbital (124)		
	Pentobarbital (124)		
	Methaqualone (124)		
	Meprobamate (49)		

[a] The numbers refer to the citation in the reference section.

TABLE 4. Compounds Affecting Catecholaminergic Systems that Produce a CTA[a]

Agonists/Precursors	Antagonists/Depletors
D-Amphetamine (9)	Chlorpromazine (5)
L-Amphetamine (9)	AMPT (22)
Hydroxyamphetamine (9)	
Methamphetamine (9)	
p-Clormethamphetamine (9)	
Phenylpropanolamine (127)	
Cathinone (46)	
Cocaine (35)	
Methylphenidate (102)	
Amitriptyline (83)	
Apomorphine (35)	
Diisobutyrol-Apomorphine (35)	

[a] The numbers refer to the citation in the reference section.

that facilitate synaptic release such as amphetamine,[9] and compounds that inhibit reuptake of either dopamine (DA) or norepinephrine (NE), such as amitriptyline[83] or cocaine.[60] With the exception of cocaine, which will be discussed in a later section, all of these compounds have been shown to be capable of producing a CTA at doses that are clearly non-toxic.[100]

Of compounds that decrease CA function, only chlorpromazine, the dopamine antagonist, has been used to produce a CTA.[5] Given the importance of dopamine antagonism in the antiemetic effects of phenothiazine-related compounds,[53] the absence of research in this area is somewhat surprising. Indeed, a recently completed study[48] seems to indicate that a variety of dopamine antagonists, including haloperidol, chlorpromazine, and pimozide, do not function as CTA-inducing agents. Although the study did not employ dose-response evaluations of these agents, the single doses chosen (1, 20, and 1 mg/kg subcutaneous, respectively) were substantial. It is interesting, in this context, that it has been extremely difficult to use the DA-antagonist neuroleptic compounds to produce a discriminable drug stimulus state.[89] Clearly, this is one of the areas in which further CTA research with other types of agents might actually be helpful, rather than simply add to the mounting number of compounds that have been studied. Certainly, a comparison of such compounds with respect to their antiemetic and their CTA-inducing ability would be of some interest.

Alpha-methyl-para-tyrosine (AMPT) is a potent inhibitor of tyrosine hydroxylase and an effective depletor of brain catecholamines. For this reason it has been used rather extensively in the study of catecholaminergic specificity in CTA. However, the compound by itself is capable of producing a CTA.[22] To the best of our knowledge, no one has attempted to replicate this result. Since it is possible to selectively deplete either NE or DA by combining AMPT with other treatments, it is rather surprising that this particular finding has not been followed up, especially in light of the role of DA antagonism in controlling certain forms of emesis.

The issue of stereospecificity was first addressed by Carey and Goodall,[23] who demonstrated a fourfold difference between D- and L-amphetamine in their ability to produce a CTA. This corresponds with a similar potency ratio for these compounds in producing hypodypsia[23,115] and anorexia in rats.[2] However, this stereospecificity has been difficult to reproduce[9] despite attempts to magnify the effects by manipulating temporal parameters, and should be regarded as an unsettled issue.

The pharmacological specificity of CA systems in producing CTAs has been studied in at least three different ways. In the first, the compound 6-hydroxydopamine (6-

OHDA) has been used to selectively destroy CA-containing neurons. The second technique is the use of the CA depletor, AMPT, to likewise selectively decrease CA levels in the brain. A third technique has been to examine the effects of the dopamine receptor blocker, pimozide, on the acquisition of CTAs. Not surprisingly, there is considerable agreement that CA effects underlie the CTAs produced by amphetamine and related compounds, but not compounds whose pharmacological actions are mediated through non CA-systems.

In probably the first study of this type, Striker and Zigmond[119] showed that intraventricular injections of 6-OHDA had no effects on a CTA based on LiCl, although they did produce severe depletions of DA. This finding has been confirmed[81] and has also been shown following 6-OHDA lesions along the medial forebrain bundle.[111] In contrast, treatment with 6-OHDA severely attenuated a CTA based on amphetamine, but did not affect a CTA based on fenfluramine,[77] a compound whose activity is thought to be mediated more through serotonergic mechanisms. Since 6-OHDA lesions deplete both DA and NE, the question of specificity within the CA systems is important. Initially it was thought that amphetamine CTAs were mediated primarily through DA, since lesions that depleted NE while sparing DA[105] had no affect on either amphetamine or LiCl-induced aversions. However, the most recent work in this area questions the validity of this finding. Rats treated intraventricularly with 6-OHDA and desipramine (used to prevent the uptake of 6-OHDA into NE containing neurons) were able to learn a CTA based on amphetamine.[77] This study concluded that the effects of 6-OHDA lesions on amphetamine-induced CTA required a depletion of both DA and NE.

The data on the use of AMPT are consistent with those on 6-OHDA. Treatment with this agent decreases brain catecholamine levels and attenuates or blocks the CTA based on amphetamine or methamphetamine,[62,104,125] but has virtually no effect on LiCl-induced CTAs[104,110,125] or a Δ^9-THC–induced CTA.[110] It has also been reported that AMPT treatment attenuates CTAs based on morphine (but others have seen potentiation[32]) and ethanol,[110] although these compounds do not have direct effects on CA systems. Again, the issue of whether or not this effect is mediated through DA or NE has simply not been resolved.

Additional evidence for DA specificity was shown by Grupp[65] who was able to block the acquisition of an amphetamine-induced CTA with the DA blocker pimozide. In contrast, pimozide did not affect a CTA based on LiCl.[110]

These data, especially those from the 6-OHDA and AMPT studies, suggest that the amphetamine-induced CTA is a centrally mediated effect. Other evidence for this conclusion comes from the fact that para-hydroxyamphetamine (which penetrates the blood-brain barrier poorly) was much weaker than the parent compound in producing a CTA.[9] However, it should be noted that this "peripheral" agent was effective in producing a CTA.

As is obvious from this survey, most of the work showing CA specificity has focused on comparisons of CTAs based on amphetamine (and congeners) and lithium. A separate issue is how closely correlated is the CTA-inducing ability of CA compounds to their effects on other systems. This issue was first raised by Carey and Goodall[23] because of the anorectic and hypodipsic effect of compounds such as amphetamine. A series of elegant studies has been conducted by the Birmingham group and is summarized in the Stolerman and D'Mello review.[117] In general, there does not seem to be much correlation between the CTA effects of these compounds and their effects on hypodipsia, anorexia, or their ability to disrupt operant procedures. This finding has recently been confirmed by studies of the ability of the amphetamine analog DL-cathinone to produce a CTA.[45,57] While cathinone is as potent as amphetamine in many other behavioral measures, it is considerably less potent in its ability to pro-

TABLE 5. Compounds Affecting Various Transmitter Systems that Produce a CTA[a]

Agonist/Precursor	System	Antagonist/Depletors
5-HT (24) 5-HTP (131) Fenfluramine (10) Fluoxetine (79) MK212 (24) Quipazine (24)	Serotonergic	PCPA (87)
Carbachol (84) Nicotine (71) Physostigmine (92) Pyridostigmine (72)	Cholinergic	Scopolamine (5) Atropine (95) Methyl-Scopolamine (6) Methyl-Atropine (39) Mecamylamine (95)
Morphine (20) Methadone (25)	Opiate (mu)	Naloxone (118) Naltrexone (118) BC 2860 (118) Mr 1452 (118)

[a] The numbers refer to the citation in the reference section.

duce a CTA. Although there has been considerable progress in recent years in categorizing CA receptors into a variety of subclasses within both DA and NE domains,[114] little has been done within the area of CTA research to try to specify the causal events beyond a global invocation of CA. The one attempt to look at alpha and beta adrenergic effects[68] failed to show effects that were specific to CTA.

Effects on Serotonergic Systems and CTA

A list of agents that effect serotonergic transmission and have been used to produce a CTA is shown in TABLE 5. Serotonin (5-HT) itself can produce a CTA despite the fact that the compound does not cross the blood-brain barrier. The precursor, 5-hydroxy-tryptophan (5-HTP), does cross the blood-brain barrier and it too has been shown to produce a conditioned taste aversion.[24,131] Similarly, CTAs have been produced using 5-HT releasers such as fenfluramine[9] and specific 5-HT uptake inhibitors such as fluoxetine.[79] As was the case in the CA literature, there seems to have been little effort to attempt to use 5-HT antagonists to produce a CTA, but parachlorophenylalanine (PCPA), which depletes brain serotonin, is quite capable of producing a CTA.[87] Indeed, it seems quite reasonable that the effects of PCPA on alcohol consumption are mediated through a CTA.[126]

The issue of transmitter specificity to the 5-HT system of CTA-induced agents has been addressed in a series of experiments by Lorden and her colleagues. Electrolytic or chemically specific (by use of 5,7-dihydroxytryptamine) lesions of the dorsal and median raphe nuclei delayed extinction of a CTA based on LiCl[78] or fenfluramine.[76] Lesions of the raphe nuclei decrease telencephalic 5-HT; since CA lesions induced by 6-OHDA had no effect on a fenfluramine-based CTA, some degree of specificity is apparent. However, the fact that 5-HT depleting lesions have similar effects on both lithium- and fenfluramine-induced CTA suggests a more conservative approach to interpretation of these data. Moreover, the effects were obtained on the extinction rather than the acquisition of CTAs.

A variety of 5-HT agonists have recently been shown to be capable of producing a CTA.[24] Since these include serotonin itself, peripheral activation is sufficient to produce a CTA. The fact that CTAs based on 5-HT elevating compounds can be blocked by the peripheral serotonin antagonist, xylamidine tosylate, supports this position. Moreover, treatment with Ro 4-4602 (benserazide, an inhibitor of peripheral aromatic acid decarboxylase) blocked a 1-5HT—induced CTA, although this combined treatment prevented the elevation of 5-HT in the mesentery and elevated 5-HT in the brain.[40]

The work on the 5-HT system and CTA is relatively recent and might be fruitful in light of the suggestions by Wurtman[130] that "carbohydrate hungers" may be an important way that the body maintains homeostatic regulation of central levels of 5-HT. Since maintenance of the 5-HT system is so crucial to the organism's well-being, it could be interesting to study the 5-HT system and its relationship with CTA (presumably another mechanism for maintaining the well-being of the internal milieu).

Cholinergic Systems and CTA

The variety of cholinergic agonists and antagonists that have been effective in producing a CTA is also seen in TABLE 5. These include the muscarinic agonist, carbachol,[84] and the nicotinic agonist, nicotine.[71] Moreover, the cholinesterase inhibitors, physostigmine[92] and pyridostigmine,[72] are also quite capable of producing CTAs.[92] In the case of nicotine, 0.08 mg/kg subcutaneous was sufficient to produce a very robust CTA, putting nicotine among the most potent compounds to produce this effect.[71] Another intriguing factor is that the cholinergic antagonists (atropine and scopolamine), their tertiary analogs, and mecamylamine are no less effective than the agonists in producing a CTA.

In a series of elegant experiments, Kumar *et al.*[71] were able to demonstrate that the effect of nicotine on a CTA is stereospecific, with the (−)isomer being about 4.5 times more potent then the (+)isomer. Moreover, the nicotine-induced CTA was blocked by mecamylamine, a ganglionic blocker that penetrates the CNS, but not by hexamethonium, a ganglionic blocker that does not reach the CNS. This concurs with the earlier work of Myers and De Castro[84] showing that carbachol injected into some, but not other, brain areas was capable of producing a CTA. Nonetheless, it is also unequivocally the case that peripheral stimulation or antagonism of acetylcholine is also sufficient to produce a CTA. This can be seen from the fact that pyridostigmine (a cholinesterase inhibitor that penetrates the blood-brain barrier very poorly), and methylated scopolamine and atropine are capable of producing CTAs in relatively modest doses. Specificity to the cholinergic system has been demonstrated, since mecamylamine could block a nicotine-induced CTA but not an apomorphine-induced CTA.[71] An interesting study of inbred genetic strains of mice that differ in brain levels of various transmitters has shown an inverse relationship between endogenous cholinergic markers and the magnitude of an ethanol-induced CTA; there was no correlation between NE markers and CTA.[108]

The general finding that any perturbation in cholinergic transmission is capable of producing a CTA seems to argue against the use of this procedure for investigating the role of cholinergic activity in learning and memory and might explain some of the confusion in the literature.

Other Transmitter Systems

Other transmitter systems have not been studied as extensively as those cited above, but there is a reasonable amount of information with respect to the opiate mu receptor system (TABLE 5). Both morphine and methadone, mu agonists, can produce a CTA, but so can the mu antagonists, naloxone and naltrexone. In the latter case, this effect does seem to be stereospecific.[118] Blair and Amit[8] demonstrated that lesions in the periaqueductal gray could greatly attenuate a morphine CTA. Similarly, it has been shown that naloxone can attenuate a morphine[73,121] but not an amphetamine-based CTA.[58] While this would seem to indicate specificity, the very fact that the antagonists can induce CTAs seems to warrant some degree of reservation. It is also the case that pretreatment with either AMPT or pimozide has been shown to decrease the ability of morphine to produce a CTA.[110] Moreover, there is little correlation between opiate-mediated analgesia and opiate-induced CTA as shown by Bardo *et al.*,[3] who chronically treated rats with naloxone. This resulted in increased [^{3}H]naloxone binding in many brain regions and also potentiated morphine analgesia. However, there was no change in morphine-induced CTA.

Very little is known about CTAs and the histaminergic system. Histamine diphosphate itself can be used to produce a CTA.[74] We know of no studies of selective histamine antagonists as CTA-inducing agents, although it would be surprising if they were not active. Antihistamines have sometimes, but not always, been shown to block radiation-induced CTA, but do not alter the ability of LiCl to produce a CTA.[15,74]

Finally, there is some scattered information on the GABA-ergic system and CTAs. It has been known for many years that benzodiazepines and barbiturates are quite capable of producing CTAs at relatively low doses. There have been no attempts to investigate either stereospecificity or transmitter specificity with respect to these compounds. Pentylenetetrazole (PTZ, also known as metrazol) is a compound that has effects in the opposite direction from those of benzodiazepines[108] and interacts with the GABA-benzodiazepine receptor complex. It is, therefore, interesting that PTZ produces a CTA in rats.[54]

FAILURES TO PRODUCE A CTA

It is obvious from the above that most agents are quite capable of producing a CTA and, consequently, those few compounds that fail to do so turn out to be intriguing.[100] In a previous review[49] we identified cocaine and strychnine among those agents that failed to produce a CTA. There are now many demonstrations of cocaine's ability to produce a CTA,[46] but it should be emphasized that in all cases rather large doses are necessary to produce this effect. Strychnine also requires an extremely high dose to produce a CTA.

Of much higher visibility are the compounds that are clearly toxic and yet do not produce a CTA. Eleven of these compounds are listed in Riley's paper. Among the reasons offered for some of these failures is the possibility that the compound might interfere with an animal's ability to learn any new information. In this regard, we have recently discovered a possible addition to the list of compounds that failed to produce a CTA. However, in this case the compound, piracetam (2-pyrrolidinone acetamide), has demonstrable effects in protecting against disruption of memory.[33] We were interested in whether this class of nootropic drugs could be used to produce a discriminative stimulus. Although Overton had failed to do so with piracetam, we chose to use the CTA as a gross form of the animal's ability to indicate that it can discern a drug state. Rats were exposed to saccharin and then given 300, 600, or 1,000 mg/kg of piracetam (with a positive control group receiving 2 mg/kg of amphetamine) intraperitoneally. After a two-bottle choice test, and four days of water, the compounds

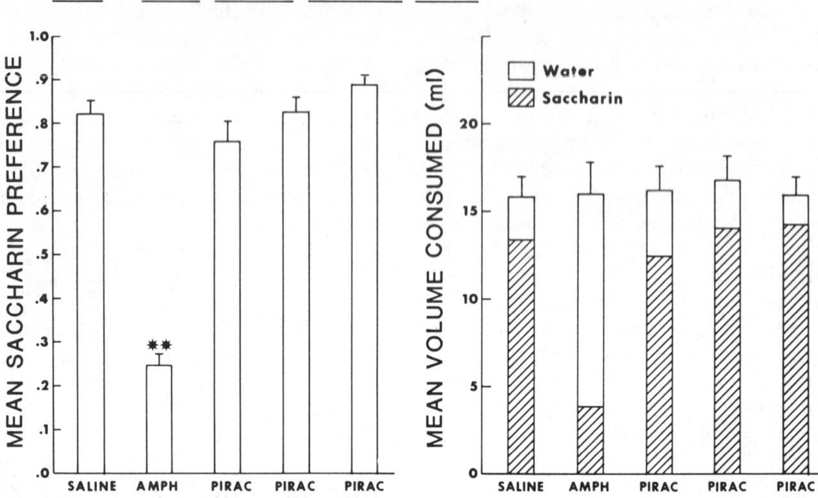

FIGURE 2. The effects of three pairings of saccharin with various i.p. treatments of piracetam and D-amphetamine on saccharin preference (versus tap water) in a two-bottle choice test. The numerical values in the abscissa indicate doses in mg/kg. See text for additional procedural details.

were again paired with saccharin on two consecutive days. The results of the two-bottle choice test two days later are shown in FIGURE 2. Despite the limitations of the procedure, the dose of amphetamine clearly produced a CTA, while none of the doses of piracetam did so. Since it is always difficult to prove the null hypothesis, these data require replication under more rigorous conditions. However, should this failure to produce a CTA be replicable, it probably is not attributable to an interference with learning and memory mechanisms (at least as measured in other paradigms). The failure of DA-blocking neuroleptics to produce a CTA also seems to be particularly interesting. However, these data also require replication under rigorous testing conditions.

INTERPRETATION OF THE FACT THAT A COMPOUND PRODUCES A CTA

While this review has shown that certain areas might warrant additional research, there is no common physiological substrate by which one can pharmacologically classify the ability of a compound to produce a CTA. CTA effects are often specific to the transmitter system through which compounds are known to exert their effects; anything else would be extremely surprising. However, within any given transmitter system the ability to produce a CTA is not clearly linked to the other known effects of these compounds.

It is our contention that the fact that a compound can be used to produce a CTA says very little about the nature of that compound, without a considerable amount of additional research. We would be loathe to conclude that the ability of a compound to produce a CTA at reasonable doses implies anything about the compound. Indeed, we feel that there are demonstrable over-interpretations of CTA results.

One example can be found in the literature on the so-called endogenous satiety peptides. These include such agents as cholecystokinin and bombesin. Both of these compounds have been used to produce CTAs, albeit in relatively high doses. This has been used by some authors to argue that their ability to decrease food intake is an artifact of sickness. This literature is reviewed by Kulkosky.[70] His work shows how careful dose response comparisons using equally effective doses and considerations of endogenous levels can render such an argument is invalid. Nonetheless, the ability of compounds to produce a CTA appears to have been given consideration in the development of therapeutic agents.[90,120,127] Clearly the ability of an anorectic or antiobesity agent to produce a CTA does not warrant the assumption that the compound's therapeutic effects are mediated through sickness. The fact that compounds that elevate food intake (e.g., benzodiazepines) are equally capable of producing CTAs raises serious questions about this conclusion.

A similar caveat seems to be warranted in the use of the CTA paradigm for studying the effects of endogenous peptides, hormones, or other substances on learning processes. Reviews of this part of the literature can be found in Rondeau *et al.*[106] and in Smotherman.[113] An interesting example seems to be the conclusion that the effects of vasopressin in a variety of learning paradigms are mediated through a peripheral stress response, because vasopressin can produce a CTA.[43] In the absence of a definitive interpretation of CTA experiments, this conclusion seems to be overstated, regardless of its veracity. A more promising approach to the use of the CTA paradigm to study learning processes might be to investigate the way in which treatments affect an animal's ability to learn CTAs over different delays between the pairing stimuli.[98] Manipulation of delays has proven useful in studying learning in aged rats in other behavioral paradigms.[75]

A third example of potential problem in interpretation is the use of a CTA baseline to study the anxiolytic-like effects of benzodiazepines and barbiturates.[106] Cappell and LeBlanc[17] demonstrated that pretreatment with CDAP would greatly attenuate an amphetamine-induced CTA. However, because the benzodiazepines increase fluid consumption, Riley and Lovely[99] were able to show, using a two-bottle testing procedure, that the phenomenon was probably a hyperdipsic artifact. The difference between the two experiments was the use of one-bottle versus two-bottle testing procedures. Recently, Ervin and Cooper[41] demonstrated that a variety of benzodiazepine and nonbenzodiazepine anxiolytic agents were able to reverse a CTA based on 5-HTP in a one-bottle test. Because the ED_{50}s in this particular test were highly correlated with the ED_{50}s based on other published conflict procedures, these results are particularly interesting. However, considerable care is required in the interpretation of one bottle tests.

CONCLUDING COMMENTS

The conclusion that behavioral pharmacology has been unsuccessful in unraveling the mysteries of the CTA paradigm seems warranted, but one might ask why. Progress in psychopharmacology over the last 10 years has been extensively reviewed by a number of different authors. Using behavioral pharmacological techniques, impressive advances have been achieved in demonstrating that the reinforcing properties of opiates are due to interactions at the mu, as opposed to the kappa or sigma, opiate receptors.[129]

Similarly, in the realm of drugs as discriminative stimuli, it has been shown that animals are quite capable of distinguishing between mu and kappa opiate receptor-mediated events.[66] Behavioral pharmacology has also had an important role in unraveling the role of the various components of the GABA-benzodiazepine ionic channel macromolecular receptor.[108] It seems to us, that the lack of success within the area of CTA evolves from the fact that the study of drug effects in CTA has been more directed to trying to understand the behavior than to understand the drug. Thus, for example, a wide variety of drugs can be used as discriminative stimuli. Most of the advances in psychopharmacology cited above focused on using behavior as a tool to understand the pharmacological mechanisms of drugs, rather than trying to use drugs to define the concept "stimulus." Where this approach has been taken within the CTA literature, remarkable successes have been achieved.[9,35,71] Thus, it is our contention that the study of drug effects in CTA has failed only to the extent that it was unable to clarify the hedonic connotations of reinforcement that are implied by psychological interpretations of the CTA paradigm. This is because the issue of hedonic interpretation of reinforcement is primarily a behavioral and not a pharmacological one. Until resolved within the discipline of psychology, it is unreasonable to expect that pharmacology will provide the answer. The recent work of a more purely psychological nature, defining the hedonistic responses of animals to various stimuli,[91,93] seems to be a far more promising avenue.

ACKNOWLEDGMENTS

We are particularly indebted to Anthony L. Riley for his help and comments, and to Domenica Iannicelli for typing and organizing the manuscript. We also thank Elias Schwam and Jerry Sepinwall for their editorial comments.

REFERENCES

1. AMIT, Z., D. LEVITAN, Z. BROWN & F. ROGAN. 1977. Neuropharmacology **16**: 121–124.
2. BAEZ, L. A. 1974. Psychopharmacologia **35**: 91–98.
3. BARDO, M. T., J. S. MILLER, D. F. MCCOY & M. E. RISNER. 1983. Soc. Neurosic. Abstr. **9**(2): 275.
4. BARKER, L., J. SMITH & E. SUAREZ. 1977. *In* Learning Mechanisms in Food Selection. L. Barker, M. Best & M. Domjan, Eds. Baylor University Press. Waco, TX.
5. BERGER, B. 1972. J. Comp. Physiol. Psychol. **81**: 21–26.
6. BERGER, B., C. WISE & L. STEIN. 1973. J. Comp. Physiol. Psychol. **82**: 475–479.
7. BERNSTEIN, I. & M. WEBSTER. 1980. Physiol. Behav. **25**: 363–366.
8. BLAIR, R. & Z. AMIT. 1981. Pharmacol. Biochem. Behav. **15**: 651–655.
9. BOOTH, D., G. D'MELLO, C. PILCHER & I. STOLERMAN. 1977. Br. J. Pharmacol. **61**: 669–677.
10. BOOTH, D. & P. SIMSON. 1973. J. Comp. Physiol. Psychol. **84**: 319–323.
11. BORISON, H. L. & S. C. WANG. 1953. Pharmacol. Rev. **5**: 193–230.
12. BRAVEMAN, N. 1975. Learning Motiv. **6**: 512–534.
13. BRAVEMAN, N. 1977. *In* Learning Mechanisms in Food Selection. L. Barker, M. Best & M. Domjan, Eds. Baylor University Press. Waco, TX.
14. BRAVEMAN, N. & J. CRANE. 1977. Behav. Biol. **21**: 470–477.
15. CAIRNIE, A. & K. LEACH. 1982. Pharmacol. Biochem. Behav. **17**: 305–312.
16. CAPPELL, H. & A. LEBLANC. 1971. Psychopharmacologia **22**: 352–356.
17. CAPPELL, H. & A. LEBLANC. 1973. J. Comp. Physiol. Psychol. **85**: 97–104.
18. CAPPELL, H. & A. LEBLANC. 1975. Psychopharmacologia **43**: 157–162.
19. CAPPELL, H. & A. LEBLANC. 1977. *In* Food Aversion Learning. N. Milgram, L. Krames, & T. Alloway, Eds. Plenum Press. New York.

20. Cappell, H., A. LeBlanc & L. Endrenyi. 1973. Psychopharmacologia **29**: 239–246.
21. Cappell, H., A. LeBlanc & S. Herling. 1975. J. Comp. Physiol. Psychol. **89**: 347–356.
22. Carey, R. & E. Goodall. 1974. Neuropharmacology **13**: 595–600.
23. Carey, R. & E. Goodall. 1974. Pharmacol. Biochem. Behav. **2**: 325–330.
24. Carter, R. & J. Leander. 1981. Fed. Proc. **40**: 172.
25. Chipkin, R. & J. Rosecrans. 1978. Psychopharmacology **57**: 303–310.
26. Coil, J., W. Hankins, D. Jenden & J. Garcia. 1978. Psychopharmacology **56**: 21–25.
27. Coil, J. & R. Norgren. 1982. Brain Res. **212**: 425–433.
28. Coil, J., R. Rogers, J. Garcia & D. Novin. 1978. Behav. Biol. **24**: 509–519.
29. Cooper, S., 1982. Neuropharmacology **21**: 483–486.
30. Cooper, S. 1982. Neuropharmacology **21**: 775–780.
31. Corcoran, M., I. Bolotow, Z. Amit & J. McCaughran. 1974. Pharmacol. Biochem. Behav. **2**: 725–728.
32. Coussens, W., W. Crowder & W. Davis, 1973. Psychopharmacologia **29**: 151–157.
33. Cumin, R., E. Bandle, E. Gamzu & W. Haefely. 1982. Psychopharmacology **78**: 104–111.
34. Dacanay, R. & A. Riley. 1982. Learning Behav. **10**: 91–96.
35. D'Mello, G., D. Goldberg, S. Goldberg & I. Stolerman. 1981. J. Pharmacol. Exp. Therapeutics **219**: 60–68.
36. Domjan, M. 1985. Ann. N.Y. Acad. Sci. (This volume.)
37. Domjan, M. & M. Best. 1977. J. Exp. Psychol. Anim. Behav. Proc. **3**: 310–321.
38. Eckardt, M. 1976. J. Studies Alcohol. **37**: 334–346.
39. Emmerick, J. & C. Snowden. 1976. J. Comp. Physiol. Psychol. **40**: 857–869.
40. Ervin, G., R. Carter, E. Webster, S. Moore & B. Cooper. 1984. Pharmacol. Biochem. Behav. **20**: 799–802.
41. Ervin, G. & B. Cooper. 1983. Soc. Neurosci. Abstr. **9**: 435.
42. Etscorn, F. & P. Parson. 1979. Bull. Psychonom. Soc. **14**: 19–21.
43. Ettenberg, A., D. Van der Kooy, M. LeMoal, G. F. Koob & F. E. Bloom. 1983. Behav. Brain Res. **7**: 331–350.
44. Fischer, G. & B. Vail. 1980. Behav. Neural Biol. **30**: 191–196.
45. Foltin, R. & C. Schuster. 1981. Pharmacol. Biochem. Behav. **14**: 907–909.
46. Foltin, R. & C. Schuster. 1982. Pharmacol. Biochem. Behav. **16**: 347–352.
47. Ford, K. & A. Riley. 1984. Pharmacol. Biochem. Behav. **20**: 643–645.
48. Gale, K. 1984. *In* Mechanisms of Tolerance and Dependence. C. Sharp, Ed. NIDA Monograph. Washington, DC. (In press.)
49. Gamzu, E. 1977. *In* Learning Mechanisms in Food Selection. L. Barker, M. Best & M. Domjan, Eds. Baylor University Press. Waco, TX.
50. Garcia, J. 1985. Ann. N.Y. Acad. Sci. (This volume.)
51. Garcia, J. & R. Koelling. 1966. Psychonom. Sci. **4**: 123–124.
52. Garcia, J. & R. Koelling. 1967. Radiation Res. Suppl. **7**: 439–450.
53. Goodman, L. & A. Gilman, Eds. 1980. The Pharmacological Basis of Therapeutics. Macmillan Publishing Co., Inc. New York.
54. Golus, P. & R. McGee. 1980. Psychopharmacology **68**: 257–259.
55. Goudie, A. 1979. Neuropharmacology **18**: 971–979.
56. Goudie, A. 1984. *In* Experimental Approach to Psychopharmacology. A. J. Greenshaw & C. T. Dourish, Eds. Humana Press. (In press.)
57. Goudie, A., J. Atkinson, T. Newton & C. Demellweek. 1984. Psychopharmacology. (In press.)
58. Goudie, A. & C. Demellweek. 1980. J. Pharmacy Pharmacol. **32**: 653–656.
59. Goudie, A. & D. Dickins. 1979. Pharmacol. Biochem. Behav. **9**: 587–592.
60. Goudie, A., D. Dickins & E. Thornton. 1978. Pharmacol. Biochem. Behav. **8**: 757–761.
61. Goudie, A., I. Stolerman, C. Demellweek & G. D'Mello. 1982. Psychopharmacology **78**: 277–281.
62. Goudie, A., M. Taylor & H. Atherton. 1975. Pharmacol. Biochem. Behav. **3**: 947–952.
63. Grill, H. 1985. Ann. N.Y. Acad. Sci. (This volume.)
64. Grill, H. & R. Norgren. 1978. Science **201**: 267–269.
65. Grupp, L. 1977. Psychopharmacologia **53**: 235–242.
66. Holtzman, S. G. 1984. *In* Behavioral Pharmacology: The Current Status. L. S. Seiden & R. S. Balster, Eds. Alan R. Liss. New York. (In press.)

67. JACOBS, W., D. ZELLNER, V. LOLORDO & A. RILEY. 1981. Pharmacol. Biochem. Behav. **14**: 779–785.
68. KRAL, P. & V. ST. OMER. 1972. Psychopharmacologia **26**: 79–83.
69. KRESEL, J. & I. BAROFSKY. 1979. Physiol. Behav. **23**: 733–736.
70. KULKOSKY, P. S. 1985. Ann. N.Y. Acad. Sci. (This volume.)
71. KUMAR, R., J. PRATT & I. STOLERMAN. 1983. Br. J. Pharmacol. **79**: 245–254.
72. LANDAUER, M. & J. ROMANO. 1984. Eastern Psychological Association Abstract.
73. LEBLANC A. & H. CAPPELL. 1975. Pharmacol. Biochem. Behav. **3**: 185–188.
74. LEVY, C., M. CARROLL, J. SMITH & K. HOFER. 1974. Science **186**: 1044–1046.
75. LIPPA, A., R. PELHAM, B. BEER, D. CRITCHETT, R. DEAN & R. BARTUS. 1980. Neurobiol. Aging **1**: 13–19.
76. LORDEN, J., M. CALLAHAN & R. DAWSON. 1979. J. Comp. Physiol. Psychol. **7**:97–101.
77. LORDEN, J., M. CALLAHAN & R. DAWSON. 1980. J. Comp. Physiol. Psychol. **94**: 99–114.
78. LORDEN, J. & D. MARGULES. 1977. Physiol. Psychol. **5**: 273–279.
79. LORDEN, J. & W. NUNN. 1982. Pharmacol. Biochem. Behav. **17**: 435–444.
80. MARTIN, J., F. CHENG & D. NOVIN. 1978. Physiol. Behav. **21**: 13–17.
81. MASON, S. & H. FIBIGER. 1979. Behav. Neural Biol. **25**: 206–216.
82. MCGLONE, J., S. RITTER & K. KELLEY. 1981. Pharmacol. Behav. **24**: 1095–1100.
83. MILLER, D. & L. MILLER. 1983. Pharmacol. Biochem. Behav. **18**: 737–740.
84. MYERS, R. H. & J. M. DECASTRO. 1977. Physiol. Behav. **19**: 467–472.
85. NACHMAN, M. 1970. Comp. Physiol. Psychol. **73**: 22–30.
86. NACHMAN, M. & J. ASHE. 1973. Physiol. Behav. **10**: 73–78.
87. NACHMAN, M., D. LESTER & J. LEMAGNEN. 1970. Science **168**: 1244–1246.
88. OSSENKOPP, K. 1983. Behav. Brain Res. **7**: 297–306.
89. OVERTON, D. 1982. Psychopharmacology **74**: 385–395.
90. PANKSEPP, J., A. POLLACK, R. MEEKER & A. SULLIVAN. 1977. Pharmacol. Biochem. Behav. **6**: 683–687.
91. PARKER, L. 1982. Learning & Motivation. **13**: 281–303.
92. PARKER, L., S. HUTCHISON & A. RILEY. 1982. Neurobehav. Toxicol. Teratol. **4**: 93–98.
93. PELCHAT, M., H. GRILL, P. ROZIN & J. JACOBS. 1983. J. Comp. Psychol. **97**: 140–153.
94. PELCHAT, M. & P. ROZIN. 1982. Appetite **3**: 341–352.
95. PRESTON, K. & C. SCHUSTER. 1981. Pharmacol. Biochem. Behav. **15**: 827–828.
96. RABIN, B. & W. HUNT. 1983. Pharmacol. Biochem. Behav. **18**: 629–636.
97. RABIN, B., W. HUNT & J. LEE. 1983. Radiation Res. **93**: 388–394.
98. RILEY, A., R. DACANY & J. MASTROPAOLO. 1984. Neurotoxicology (In press.)
99. RILEY, A. J. & R. LOVELY. 1978. Physiol. Psychol. **6**: 488–492.
100. RILEY, A. J. & D. L. TUCK. 1985. Ann. N.Y. Acad. Sci. (This volume.)
101. RILEY, A. J. & D. L. TUCK. 1985. Bibliography. Ann. N.Y. Acad. Sci. (This volume.)
102. RILEY, A. & D. ZELLNER. 1978. Physiol. Psychol. **6**: 354–358.
103. RITTER, S., J. MCGLONE & K. KELLY. 1980. Brain Res. **201**: 501–506.
104. ROBERTS, D. & H. FIBIGER. 1975. Neurosci. Lett. **1**: 343–347.
105. ROBERTS, D. & H. FIBIGER. 1977. Psychopharmacology **55**: 183–186.
106. RONDEAU, D., F. JOLICOEUR, A. MERKEL, & M. WAYNER. 1981. Neurosci. Biobehav. Rev. **5**: 279–294.
107. ROZIN, P. & D. ZELLNER. 1985. Ann. N.Y. Acad. Sci. (This volume.)
108. SEPINWALL, J. 1984. *In* Behavioral Pharmacology: The Current Status. L. S. Seiden & R. S. Balster, Eds. Alan R. Liss. New York. (In press.)
109. SHOEMAKER, H., V. J. NICKOLSON, S. KERBUSH & J. C. CRABBE. 1982. Brain Res. **235**: 253–264.
110. SKLAR, L. & Z. AMIT. 1977. Neuropharmacology **16**: 649–655.
111. SMITH, G. P., B. E. LEVIN & G. N. ERVIN. 1975. Brain Res. **88**: 483–498.
112. SMITH, J. 1971. *In* Progress in Physiological Psychology. E. Stellar & J. Sprague, Eds. Vol. 4. Academic Press. New York.
113. SMOTHERMAN, W. 1985. Ann. N.Y. Acad. Sci. (This volume.)
114. SNYDER, S. H. 1984. Science **224**: 22–31.
115. STOLERMAN, I. & G. D'MELLO. 1977. Pharmacol. Biochem. Behav. **8**: 107–111.

116. Stolerman, I. & G. D'Mello. 1978. Pharmacol. Biochem. Behav. **8**: 333–338.
117. Stolerman, I. & G. D'Mello. 1981. *In* Advances in Behavioral Pharmacology. T. Thompson & P. Dews, Eds. Vol. 3. Academic Press. New York.
118. Stolerman, I., C. Pilcher & G. D'Mello. 1978. Life Sci. **22**: 1755–1762.
119. Stricker, E. & M. Zigmond. 1974. J. Comp. Physiol. Psychol. **86**: 973–994.
120. Triscari, J. & A. Sullivan. 1981. Pharmacol. Biochem. Behav. **15**: 311-318.
121. Van der Kooy, D. & A. Phillips. 1977. Pharmacol. Biochem. Behav. **6**: 637–641.
122. Van der Kooy, D., N. Swerdlow & G. Koob. 1983. Brain Res. **32**: 2087–2094.
123. Vitiello, M. & S. Woods. 1977. Pharmacol. Biochem. Behav. **6**: 553–555.
124. Vogel, J. & B. Nathan. 1976. Psychopharmacology **49**: 167-172.
125. Wagner, G., R. Foltin, L. Seiden & C. Schuster. 1981. Pharmacol. Biochem. Behav. **14**: 85–88.
126. Walters, J. 1977. Pharmacol. Biochem. Behav. **6**: 377–383.
127. Wellman, P., P. McIntosh & E. Guidi. 1981. Physiol. Behav. **26**: 341–344.
128. Wise, R., R. Yokel & H. DeWitt. 1976. Science **191**: 1273–1275.
129. Woods, S. H. 1984. *In* Behavioral Pharmacology: The Current Status. L. S. Seiden & R. S. Balster, Eds. Alan R. Liss. New York. (In press.)
130. Wurtman, J. J. 1985. Ann. N.Y. Acad. Sci. (This volume.)
131. Zabik, J. & J. Roache. 1983. Pharmacol. Biochem. Behav. **18**: 785–790.

Drug Interactions Measured through Taste Aversion Procedures with an Emphasis on Medical Implications

SAM REVUSKY

Memorial University of Newfoundland
St. John's, Newfoundland A1C 5S7 Canada

We begin with the problem of what an animal learns when two internal states are each induced in sequence by means of drug injections. The first drug injected is called the CS and the second drug injected is called the US. The primary role of the CS drug is as a signal and it typically is administered at a low dose. The US drug has biological effects to which the animal ought to adjust and is injected after the CS drug is beginning to have an effect. Conditioning is demonstrated when the CS drug elicits a reaction that must be attributed to the prior occurrence of the CS→US pairings.

Pairing two drug states in this way probably mimics natural regularities in sequences of internal stimulation. If a later stimulus condition (US) elicits some sort of physiological adjustment, then a stimulus that precedes it (CS) might act as a cue to allow an anticipatory adjustment. As a heuristical example, suppose that blood pressure rises as a homeostatic response to the type of stimulation produced by the US drug. Pavlovian conditioning ought then to result in an anticipatory rise in blood pressure to a CS state that normally tends to precede this US. It is easy to imagine how such conditioning may participate in homeostatic regulation. It is a good general rule that conditioning occurs very readily if it is biologically useful,[1] the parade example being taste aversion learning.[2] Even under conditions that do not seem to me to be particularly biologically useful, drug states function as effective cues. I have in mind drug dissociated learning, the capacity of drug states to function as very effective discriminative stimuli for the direction in which to run to escape from shock.[3] This suggests that the far more natural drug-drug conditioning procedure ought to yield even more rapid conditioning.

Of course, the preceding analogical considerations are only suggestive, but they show that drug-drug conditioning is an interesting topic. If scientific progress always occurred in a rational orderly fashion, Pavlovians would have developed this area a half century ago as a byproduct of their interest in the role of conditioning in homeostatic regulation. The example of the conditioning of blood pressure in the preceding paragraph illustrates how neatly this method dovetails with traditional Pavlovian psychophysiology. But there was no organized use of the drug-drug paradigm by Pavlovians and I do not happen to know even of any particular studies. Instead, extensive drug-drug conditioning began as an offshoot of my taste-aversion conditioning work and similar independent work by Cunningham and Linakis.[4] The taste aversion approach to drug-drug conditioning is convoluted, but has led to the discovery of important phenomena that would not have been discovered as rapidly with the more straightforward approach of Pavlovian psychophysiology. Some work has been done recently in terms of the latter approach, but it is much less extensive than the taste aversion work and will not be reviewed here.[5,6]

THE AVFAIL EXPERIMENT

I began with ideas, based on truisms familiar to every student of conditioning, about how to improve the chemical aversion treatment (CAT) of alcoholism.[7,8] In CAT patients are made sick after the consumption of alcoholic beverages in order to induce a therapeutic dislike for the alcohol flavor. CAT is definitely useful,[9] but it has an important failing. It induces an aversion only to the flavor of alcohol, not to the state of being drunk. A determined drinker will drink in spite of the nausea resulting from the conditioned aversion and then the aversion may extinguish. Even without aversion treatment, many alcoholics have developed pronounced aversions to alcoholic beverages due to their hangovers and have learned to force booze down for the pleasure of intoxication. It seemed obvious to me that a true aversion to a drug state could easily be induced in rats by direct pairing of the drug state with lithium sickness. Not only did it seem that such methods might eventually improve CAT for alcoholics by creating an aversion to alcohol intoxication as well as the alcohol flavor, but they might also be useful for dealing with addictions to injected drugs. In these latter cases flavor aversion techniques are useless because the addict does not ingest the drug. Thus, for instance, first injecting a heroin addict with heroin and then sickening him with a high dose of lithium conceivably might attenuate the craving for heroin.

My first step was to try to make pentobarbital sedation aversive by pairing it with lithium sickness.[10] (I used pentobarbital instead of ethanol because pentobarbital is known to be an unusually effective discriminative stimulus.) The experimental procedure was to inject 5 mg of sodium pentobarbital into rats weighing 215–250 g followed, 30 min later, by injection of 50 mg of LiCl. The pentobarbital (Pent) dose was at a sedative level and the LiCl dose was very toxic, although not lethal. These drug-drug pairings were administered on five occasions spaced three days apart. I expected Pent→LiCl pairings to produce a Pent→LiCl association manifested in conditioned aversiveness to pentobarbital sedation. The test of this hypothesis involved allowing these experimental rats to drink saccharin solution prior to an injection of pentobarbital. If conditioned aversiveness to the pentobarbital were to develop, these pentobarbital injections ought to produce stronger saccharin aversions than they would in animals with a control history for the Pent→LiCl injections.

The theoretical basis of these ideas is summarized in TABLE 1. Its first column outlines Pavlovian higher-order conditioning and its second column shows how this is parallel to the drug-drug conditioning procedure. The pentobarbital is to function as CS1 and become associated with the LiCl US during Phase 1, the conditioning

TABLE 1. The Higher-Order Conditioning Paradigm Applied To Different Situations

		Experimental Situations		
	Paradigm	Drug-Drug	Tone→Light	Taste→Taste
Phase 1	CS_1→US	Pent→LiCl	light→shock	salt→LiCl
Phase 2	CS_2→CS_1	Sac→Pent	tone→light	Sac→salt
Phase 3	CR to CS_2	Unknown	fear of tone	Sac aversion

TABLE 2. Operational and Pavlovian Outlines of Procedures and Resulting Saccharin Preferences

	Groups				
	Pent→LiCl	Pent alone	LiCl alone	LiCl→Pent	Cont
Phase 1 five pairings	Pent→LiCl (CS_1→US)	Pent alone (CS_1 alone)	LiCl alone (US alone)	LiCl→Pent (US→CS_1)	does not matter
Phase 2 one pairing	Sac→Pent (CS_2→CS_1)	Sac→Pent (CS_2→CS_1)	Sac→Pent (CS_2→CS_1)	Sac→Pent (CS_2→CS_1)	Sac alone (CS_2 alone)
Sac Pref	0.36	0.28	0.27	0.26	0.38

phase. As a result of this Phase 1 conditioning, the pentobarbital CS1 is expected to function as a reinforcer in Phase 2 and induce an aversion to a previously consumed saccharin CS2 solution. The third and fourth columns show two paradigmatically similar situations in which higher-order conditioning has been demonstrated.[11-13] Column 3 shows the case in which audiovisual stimuli are the two CSs and shock is the US. Column 4 shows when two flavors are the CSs and sickness is the US.

TABLE 2 shows that the obtained results were opposite to those expected on the basis of the considerations outlined in TABLE 1. The test was 11 min of access to .75% saccharin solution some days after the Phase 1 pairing. (During conditioning, the drinking period had also been 11 min and the pentobarbital injection was administered 11 min after the saccharin bottle was removed.) Preferences (suppression ratios) were calculated as S/S+W, where S is the weight of saccharin solution consumed during the 11 min test and W is the weight of water consumed during a similar drinking session on the preceding day. Group Pent→LiCl received the experimental (putative higher-order conditioning) treatment illustrated in TABLE 1. The Pent-alone and LiCl-alone groups in TABLE 2 were subjected to Phase 1 procedures that traditionally ought not to produce conditioning; they got either the CS drug alone or the US drug alone. The LiCl→Pent group, subjected to another control procedure designed not to produce conditioning, was injected with LiCl 30 min before injection of the pentobarbital. Under some circumstances, backward pairings (such as LiCl→Pent) can produce inhibitory conditioning,[14,15] but we have not seen any in extensive experience with drug-drug conditioning. Even if it were to occur, it would not invalidate the use of that group as a control for the expected excitatory conditioning.

For the reasons outlined in TABLE 1, Group Pent→LiCl ought to have had the lowest saccharin preferences among the groups subjected to a Sac→Pent pairing in Phase 2. Instead exactly the opposite happened. The rightmost column of TABLE 2 shows the results for rats in Group Cont. These could not possibly have a learned aversion to saccharin because they were not drugged after drinking it. It is clear that the saccharin preferences for this group were not noticeably higher than those among the experimental rats (Group Pent→LiCl). Thus, the putative higher-order conditioning procedure had, in reality, virtually eliminated the capacity of pentobarbital to produce saccharin aversions.[a]

[a] Certain aspects of TABLE 2 may be confusing. I indicated that a preference ratio of 0.38 for Group Cont in TABLE 2 did not reflect a learned aversion to saccharin even though any ratio below 0.50 indicates less consumption of saccharin solution than of unflavored water on the preceding day. However, this low ratio is not due to a learned aversion but to intense neophobia produced by the use of a very strong solution of saccharin (0.75% w/vol). This concentration

The effect seemed paradoxical to me and I named it "Avfail," aversion failure, to reflect my befuddlement. The Pavlovian precedents for an intensified saccharin aversion as a result of Pent→LiCl pairings prior to conditioning had seemed so powerful that I could not conceive of a different result.

Pharmacological Generality

By the usual criterion of a difference in performance between an experimental group and appropriate control groups, the Avfail effect easily meets the definition of learning. However, the usual definitions fail to specify involvement of the types of biological mechanisms that are responsible for other types of learning and thus do not exclude the possibility that Avfail might be due to a specific pharmacological interaction between pentobarbital and LiCl. Such an interaction could not reasonably be considered an instance of learning because it is not produced by the same biological system(s) as traditionally studied types of learning.

However, Avfail does not seem to be due to a specific pharmacological interaction.[16] It is most pronounced under our original conditions, but it can be obtained when a wide variety of different drugs are substituted for pentobarbital as the CS drug. One of the CS drugs that produces Avfail is *d*-amphetamine, which is very different pharmacologically from pentobarbital. Chlordiazepoxide has produced an excellent effect also. Morphine and ethanol are CS drugs that yield a weakened Avfail effect. After being paired with lithium, they do not completely lose their capacity to produce a taste aversion, but the capacity is weakened. However, there are CS drugs that are not affected by the Avfail procedure or related procedures. These include atropine, chlorpromazine, and Δ^9-THC. In each of these cases, there have been a number of failures to obtain an Avfail effect. In contrast, I have used pentobarbital in six Avfail experiments under dose and delay conditions similar to those in TABLE 2[10,17-19] and in no case did the Pent→LiCl group exhibit significantly lower saccharin preferences than a group that drank saccharin solution without a later injection of pentobarbital. If pentobarbital is the CS and a very high dose of *d*-amphetamine is substituted for LiCl, Avfail is also obtained.[16] I do not know why the Avfail effect is not obtained under certain conditions, but it is produced by a wide enough variety of drug combinations to exclude a specific pharmacological interaction. Thus, by elimination, learning (or conditioning) seems responsible.

---

has the advantage of producing far more pronounced taste aversion learning than weaker concentrations. Since it turned out that our experimental effect was the failure of a weak saccharin aversion to occur, it was very important that taste aversions be obtained in control groups so that the negative experimental result could not be attributed to insensitivity. The weak taste aversions normally produced by pentobarbital were bound to be still further weakened by the drug habituation in Phase 1. So it was critical that all other parameters be set to maximize sensitivity. A related potentially bothersome question is why a barbiturate that might well be used recreationally by humans ought to produce any taste aversion whatsoever? However, as Gamzu's paper in this volume indicates, most drugs, even drugs that animals will administer to themselves by pressing a lever, are capable of producing flavor aversions if injected after consumption of a novel flavored solution.

The Conditioned Inhibition Theory

Harry Taukulis, who collaborated with me on the first Avfail experiments, suggested that we might have obtained conditioned inhibition instead of higher-order conditioning. Taukulis agreed with my supposition outlined in TABLE 1 that the rats tested under conditions outlined in column 2 formed associations between the pentobarbital and the lithium in Phase 1, but he thought they might have analyzed the Phase 2 situation more subtly than I originally considered possible. In Phase 2, they drank saccharin and then were sedated with pentobarbital and the lithium sickness that previously followed pentobarbital sedation failed to occur. According to Taukulis, the rats, as it were, concluded after these two phases that saccharin solution protected them from lithium sickness that would otherwise occur. In Pavlovian terms, the saccharin taste might have become a conditioned inhibitor (safety signal).

Higher order conditioning and conditioned inhibition are opposite effects that result from similar experimental procedures. However, conditioned inhibition is a more complex type of learning that is preceded by a higher order conditioning performance until the rat reinterprets the situation. I had carefully designed the original experiment to yield higher-order conditioning rather than conditioned inhibition. If I had desired inhibition I would have, following Pavlov,[14] modified the design in two important ways. First, instead of having a series of Pent→LiCl trials followed by a single Sac→Pent trial in Phase 2, I would have intermixed the two types of trials to make it easier for the rat to discern the difference between them. Second, I would not have waited until 11 min after removal of the saccharin bottle to inject pentobarbital. Instead, the pentobarbital sedation would have overlapped the saccharin taste since such an overlap strengthens conditioned inhibition at the expense of higher-order conditioning.

The difficulty of obtaining conditioning inhibition to saccharin by the method outlined in TABLE 1 is illustrated by an anthropomorphic description of how *rattus* would have to infer that saccharin is a safety signal. From a traditional vantage point, it should be easy for the rat to associate between pentobarbital sedation and lithium sickness in Phase 1. But in a single Sac→Pent trial in Phase 2 *rattus* must make some remarkable inferences. The initial pentobarbital sedation starts about 15 min after the saccharin solution has been removed and *rattus* begins to develop a slight aversion to the saccharin because the pentobarbital is secondarily aversive and it is expecting lithium sickness. (By Pavlovian rules, the pentobarbital would have to become secondarily aversive to support conditioned inhibition of the saccharin.) *Rattus* does not lose the expectation of lithium sickness for at least 30 min because that was the interval between the two injections in Phase 1. Finally *rattus* must realize that the expected lithium sickness is not occurring, change its mind about the saccharin solution, and credit it with the non-occurrence of lithium sickness. I would have been foolish to expect the slow conditioned inhibition process to yield the equivalent of such a complex chain of reasoning in one trial.

Despite its implausibility, we had no alternative to the Taukulis conditioned inhibition explanation. So we decided that the speed of Avfail conditioning was not a definitive argument against the involvement of conditioned inhibition since taste aversion learning is much faster than most other types of learning although it follows the basic principles.[20] We spent a year or so trying to find similarities between Avfail and conditioned inhibition in conventional Pavlovian experiments with no success.[19] It remained conceivable that Avfail had the same biological role as conditioned inhibition, but the mechanisms seemed different.

Another Anomaly

In the course of our efforts to detect conditioned inhibition, we devised a variant of the Avfail procedure.[19] The Phase 1 Pent→LiCl pairings were the same as in the Avfail procedure, but the Phase 2 procedure was changed to a Pent→Sac pairing in which the pentobarbital was injected 15 min prior to a 30 min saccharin drinking sessioin. The Phase 2 procedure among control rats was the same Pent→Sac pairings as for the experimental rats but Pent-alone or LiCl→Pent pairings in Phase 1. As previously indicated, the overlap between the CS drug effect and the taste CS produced by Pent→Sac pairings would be expected to strengthen the conditioning of inhibition to the saccharin at the expense of higher-order conditioning. Heuristically, association of the saccharin taste with the failure of lithium sickness to occur ought to be facilitated if the rat drinks saccharin solution at the time it wrongly expects lithium sickness to begin. In contrast, the Sac→Pent procedure of TABLE 1 requires the rat, at the time that lithium sickness fails to occur, to remember saccharin solution that it consumed an hour earlier. So I anticipated that after a number of Pent→Sac trials interspersed with Pent→LiCl trials, the saccharin would become such a powerful conditioned inhibitor that the rat would consume an unusually large amount of saccharin. Even after very prolonged training, nothing like that happened. However, on the very first Pent→Sac training trial in Phase 2, before the Phase 2 experience could have had any effect on saccharin preferences, the Pent→LiCl rats unexpectedly drank less

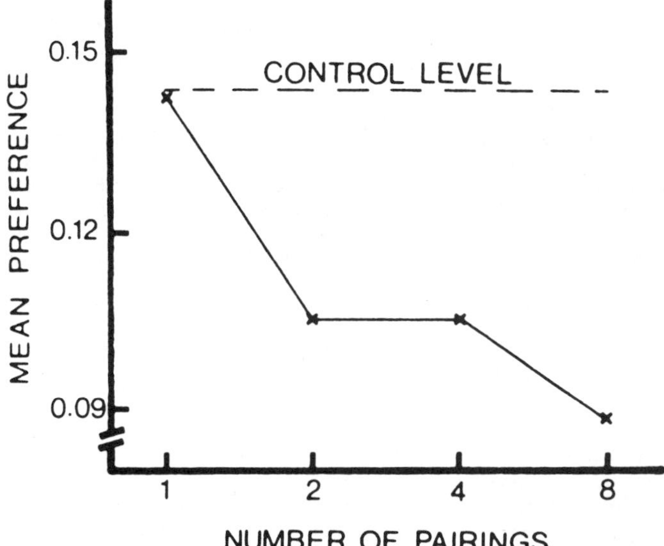

FIGURE 1. For the data indicated by crosses, the ordinate shows the number of pairings in which a sedative dose of pentobarbital was injected 30 min prior to a highly toxic dose of LiCl. The preference measure is a test of saccharin intake while under the influence of pentobarbital. The control level (dashed horizontal line) was obtained from rats subjected to reversed pairings (LiCl 30 min prior to pentobarbital). It is clear that after two or more forward pairings, the pentobarbital came to inhibit saccharin consumption.

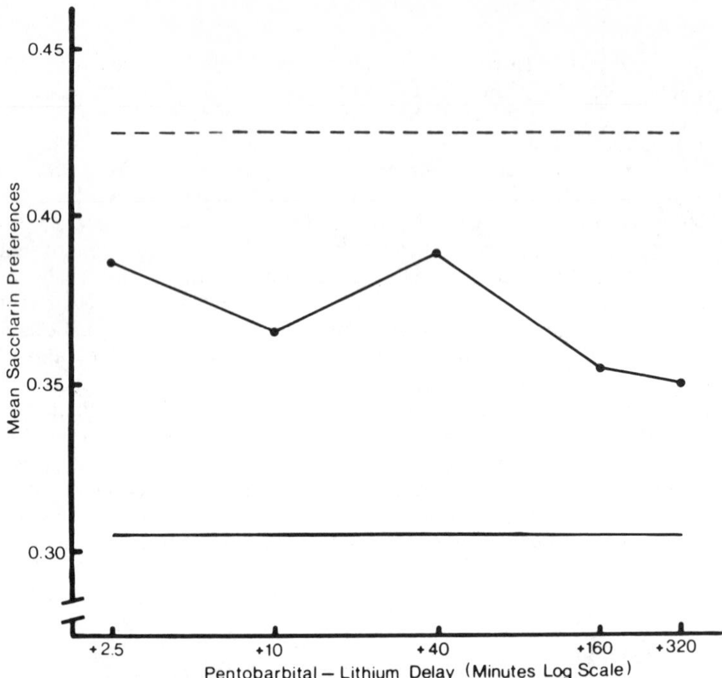

FIGURE 2. The middle curve shows saccharin preferences for experimental rats injected with a sedative dose of pentobarbital after they drank saccharin solution. These rats had been given five prior pentobarbital-lithium pairings in which the pentobarbital preceded the lithium by the indicated delay. The top dashed line shows preferences of rats that drank saccharin solution without any injection. The bottom solid line shows the lower preferences of rats that drank prior to injection with pentobarbital after backward pairings in which lithium was injected 40 min prior to pentobarbital. The backward pairings controlled for habituation to the pentobarbital.

saccharin than those in earlier control group. FIGURE 1 shows the results for experimental rats as a function of the number of Pent→LiCl pairings in Phase 1 as well as the result for pooled controls.

I reinterpreted the Pent→Sac procedure in light of FIGURE 1 and it looked like the first result to make sense in terms of well established conditioning procedures. A pentobarbital CS had preceded sickness in Phase 1 and inhibited consumption of saccharin solution by a thirsty rat in Phase 2. This is the same paradigm as that of conditioned suppression, in which presentation of an auditory or visual CS that has preceded shock in the past inhibits ongoing activity based on food or water reward.[21] This effect, called "conditioned sickness," looked like a way to detect drug-drug conditioning that would be congruent with the usual conditioning literature. Unfortunately, the conditioned sickness effect, readily obtained when pentobarbital was the CS, was not obtained when *d*-amphetamine, chlordiazepoxide, or ethanol were used instead. Such extreme pharmacological specificity made it seem implausible that conditioning was involved in this "conditioned sickness" effect, which remains unexplained.

Power and Importance of the Avfail Effect

Even though it made no sense to me, Avfail seemed important because it was learning produced by the occurrence of two internal states in sequence. Its robustness and reliability suggested that it reflected the operation of a biologically important process. An Avfail effect produced by pairings of pentobarbital and lithium is so pronounced that 13 successive pairings of saccharin consumption with pentobarbital sedation were not able to produce a saccharin aversion in rats subjected to four to eight prior Pent→LiCl pairings.[10] In TABLES 1 and 2, the delay between the pentobarbital and LiCl injections in Phase 1 was 30 min, but FIGURE 2 shows that Avfail effects can be obtained with delays of up to 320 min between these two injections.[17] (The pentobarbital dose was double that in earlier work.) This is almost as long as the delays over which learned taste aversions can be obtained. It indicates the strong involvement of selective association since the animal must have some criterion to associate between two specific events out of a large number of events that occur during a delay of several hours that easily includes thousands of events. However, it will be explained below how the selective association responsible for Avfail is very different from that responsible for long-delay taste aversion learning.

CONDITIONED ANTISICKNESS

Avfail made no sense to me because I had strong misconceptions that were to be corrected by Lett.[22] In explaining these, I will usually use the unqualified term "CS" to refer to the CS drug state and "saccharin" to refer to the taste CS. I had assumed throughout that the only relevant factor was learned associations between stimulus events: the CS and US drug states and the saccharin taste. I had completely failed to consider response factors. Lett did not fail to consider them. She postulated a homeostatic reaction to the sickness US that had the role of a Pavlovian unconditioned response (UR). She called it an antisickness response and assumed that it alleviates the sickness produced by the US injection (usually LiCl). CS→US drug pairings presumably resulted in elicitation by the CS of a conditioned response (CR) similar to the antisickness UR elicited by the US. This CR was called conditioned antisickness (CAS) and presumably alleviated sickness so effectively that it completely eliminated the slight capacity of the CS drug (usually pentobarbital) to produce a taste aversion. The original intellectual groundwork for these ideas was Siegel's[23,24] work on the role of conditioning in habitation to morphine, and, to a lesser extent, Solomon's[25] opponent process theory. At present, however, both Lett and I differ in many respects from these antecedents.

In Lett's[22] first experiment in support of her CAS theory, the CS drug was 20–25 mg/kg of sodium pentobarbital (a sedative dose) and the US drug was 200–250 mg/kg of lithium chloride (a very toxic but not a lethal dose). The experimental rats, called CAS, were given a history of five CS→US pairings identical to those administered to Group Pent→LiCl in Avfail experiments (TABLE 2) followed by what may be called a Sac→CS→US trial: Each rat drank 0.1% saccharin solution for 10–15 min, was injected with the CS drug immediately after the saccharin bottle was removed, and after 30 min was injected with the LiCl US at about 64 mg/kg (a dose about 30% of that used during the CS→US pairings). Lett expected the pentobarbital CS to elicit a CAS as a result of the CS→US pairings in Phase 1 and hence to attenuate the saccharin aversion produced by the lithium US.

TABLE 3. Saccharin Preferences after the CAS (Conditioned Antisickness) Procedure or Control Procedures

	Groups			
	CAS	Sac→US	US→CS	Cont
Phase 1 (five pairings)	Pent→LiCl	Pent→LiCl	LiCl→Pent	does not matter
Phase 2 (one pairing)	Sac→Pent→LiCl	Sac→30 min→LiCl	Sac→Pent→LiCl	Saccharin alone
Result	0.50	0.32	0.31	0.56

Comparison of the saccharin preferences of Lett's Group CAS with those of other groups in TABLE 3 confirms this. Group Sac→US (more exactly, a subgroup of concern to us here) had the same history of CS→US pairings as the Group CAS, but was not administered the CS drug during saccharin conditioning. Instead, the rats were subjected to a Sac→US trial in which the delay between removal of the saccharin solution and injection of the US drug was the same 30 min as in the Sac→CS→US trial administered to Group CAS. The Sac→US procedure produced stronger saccharin aversions than the CAS procedure; hence the presence of the CS drug during conditioning was required (presumably to elicit CAS) if Group CAS was to exhibit a weakened saccharin aversion. A second control group, Group US→CS, was subjected to US→CS pairings (the US injection 30 min prior to the CS) in Phase 1 so that (presumably) the CS would not become conditioned to elicit a CAS response. As Lett expected, Group US→CS did not exhibit the same weakened saccharin aversion as Group CAS. Note that if the antisicknesss effect in Group CAS had been due to unconditioned effects of pentobarbital, Group US→CS would also have exhibited an antisickness effect as compared to Group Sac→US. Group Cont was subjected to a procedure that could not produce a taste aversion and was statistically indistinguishable in its saccharin preferences from Group CAS, indicating how pronounced the CAS effect was. In passing, the preferences of Group Cont in TABLE 3 are higher than the corresponding preferences in TABLE 2 because a weaker concentration of saccharin was used for methodological reasons.

As far as is known, CAS is obtained with the same drug combinations that yield Avfail. The top data line of TABLE 4 contains Lett's data that were shown in TABLE 3 and the remaining lines show results when the CS drug is changed to morphine, ethanol, *d*-amphetamine, or chlordiazepoxide. It is clear that in every case, Group Cont exhibited the highest preferences and Group CAS was lower, but higher than Groups Sac→US and US→CS. There is no evidence in TABLE 4 for a significant difference among the latter two groups although I believe on the basis of extensive experience with other variants of the CAS procedure that the US→CS groups yield slightly lower

TABLE 4. CAS Effect for Different CS Drugs

	Procedures			
Drugs	CAS	Sac→US	US→CS	Cont
Pentobarbital	0.50	0.32	0.33	0.56
Morphine	0.43	0.27	0.27	0.55
Ethanol	0.47	0.27	0.20	0.59
d-Amphetamine	0.27	0.16	0.15	0.57
Chlordiazepoxide	0.36	0.30	0.18	0.61

preferences than the Sac→US groups because the mild aversion produced by the unconditioned CS drug summates with that produced by the US. As previously indicated, the CS drugs shown in TABLE 4 to produce CAS also produce Avfail. In unpublished work, I have found that chlorpromazine as well as Δ^9-THC CSs yield neither Avfail nor CAS. There is no known CS drug for which Avfail is obtained and CAS is not obtained or vice versa. This pattern makes it hard to doubt that Avfail and CAS each result from the same process.

Selective Association in CAS

When I started to work on drug-drug conditioning, my model had been taste-sickness conditioning in which the sickness US makes the taste CS aversive. By analogy, the sickness US in drug-drug conditioning capacity ought to produce something like an aversion to a drug CS (or other internal CS) that preceded it. Presumably, the drug CS would be able to control ingestion in much the same way as a taste. I had based a theory for the regulation of caloric intake upon these and related beliefs.[26] The Avfail effect contradicted these ideas since the drug CS did not seem to become aversive as a result of being paired with sickness. The following material is largely based on new ideas supplied by B. T. Lett in private conversations.

Two phenomena in addition to Avfail indicate that aversiveness does not transfer from a sickness US to a drug CS: (1) Internal states such as hunger, thirst, pentobarbital sedation, or amphetamine excitement[27,28] are poor cues for the regulation of the intake of different substances on the basis of a correlation of these internal states with whether lithium sickness would follow ingestion. There is some conditioning to these internal states, but it is negligible compared to conditioning to tastes. (2) Lithium chloride tastes so much like ordinary table salt that only an experienced rat can tell the difference between isomolar solutions of the two substances. The discrimination can be made still more difficult by means of masking substances. Thus, Rusiniak *et al.*[29] were able to devise a situation in which a rat could only discern that it was drinking the solution with lithium on the basis of the onset of lithium sickness. The rats drank so much lithium that they must have overshot considerably the onset of sickness, which was shown to be far inferior to a taste as a cue for cessation of drinking.

Thus internal stimuli do not seem to become unpleasant in the same way as tastes when they precede the same sickness. There are other instances in which the same US has different hedonic effects on different CSs. The same recreational drug that rewards motor behavior of rats also produces a taste aversion.[30-32] Also, since many alcoholics strongly dislike the taste of alcohol, the same alcohol state that so strongly motivates alcoholics can simultaneously produce an aversion to the alcohol flavor.

In light of such findings, two similar accounts of CAS (that probably overlap in practice) are tenable: (1) The drug CS does not primarily become associated with the sickness US. Instead it becomes associated with a homeostatic antisickness UR that is elicited by the US. (2) The drug CS becomes associated with the sickness US, but there is no transfer of affect from the US to the CS. With either interpretation, the drug CS comes to elicit CAS.

Hence CAS seems to be based on Pavlovian stimulus substitution, in which a CS comes to elicit a CR similar to the UR elicited by the US. Ten years ago, I and others believed that stimulus substitution was limited to special cases and emphasized more cognitive processes, like inhibition. But stimulus substitution now seems to be ubiquitous in phylogenetically older types of learning. There is a plausible theory that it is responsible for the conditioning of drug effects to environmental cues[33] and it also seems to be responsible for nearly all motor learning in nonmammalian vertebrates.[34,35]

In retrospect, it makes biological sense for CAS not to be aversive. Tastes must be selectively associated with the aversive aspects of sickness so that animals can avoid sickness by avoiding the tastes of substances that produce sickness. There is no adaptive reason for internal CSs to become aversive in the same way as tastes because the animal cannot directly avoid the contingent sickness by terminating the internal CS as it avoids sickness by terminating a taste. The proper role of the internal CS is to elicit anticipatory reactions to prepare for the sickness and thus Pavlovian antisickness responses readily become attached to it. Thus it is adaptive for tastes and drug CSs to have very different associative roles. It is even conceivable that CAS may be rewarding in much the same way in which conditioned antifear responses create a state of euphoria rewarding enough to motivate goofy behavior like sky-diving.[25]

Blocking Does Not Explain CAS

The paradigms in TABLE 3 superficially suggest a blocking explanation of CAS. Blocking occurs when one CS has preceded the US in the past. If the former CS and a novel CS are presented prior to the US, the former CS prevents the novel CS from becoming associated with the US. For instance, if vinegar solution is consumed prior to sickness in Phase 1 and both saccharin and vinegar are consumed prior to sickness in Phase 2, the subsequent saccharin aversion will be very weak because the vinegar-LiCl association will block the saccharin-LiCl association.[36] By analogy, a pentobarbital→LiCl association ought to have developed in Phase 1 of the CAS procedure outlined in TABLE 1 and interfered with association of the saccharin with the LiCl (and hence with the saccharin aversion). In mentalistic language, the rat ought to attribute the sickness in Phase 2 to the CS drug instead of to the saccharin because of its Phase 1 experience that the CS drug has been followed by sickness.

Critical to the blocking explanation is the assumption that there is strong concurrent interference between a taste CS and a drug CS when the US is sickness. Concurrent interference means that when two CSs precede the same US, the association of one CS with the US tends to prevent the other CS from becoming associated with the US.[36] Hence the blocking explanation presupposes a strong association between the CS drug state and the sickness US. As indicated in the preceding section on selective association in CAS, it is unlikely that the CS drug state becomes strongly associated with the sickness. Furthermore, even if there were a strong drug-sickness association, there probably would be little concurrent interference between the taste and drug CS. There seems to be almost no concurrent interference between two tastes presented prior to sickness if one taste is in solution and the second taste is in solid food.[37] By common sense extrapolation, there ought to be negligible concurrent interference between a drug state and a taste because their associations take different hedonic forms.

Transfer of CAS from One US to the Other

There is a parallel between the pairing of a CS drug with a sickness and the pairing of a conventional external CS with peripheral pain. The latter situation involves two types of conditioning: (1) Specific CRs made by the animal may reduce the particular injury produced by the specific pain US and hence alleviate the pain and (2) a general conditioned analgesia produced through the release of endogenous opiates that alleviate all types of pain, even types different from the US. The behavioral evidence for general analgesia is that a CS that alleviates pain in one situation is likely also to alleviate a different type of pain in a different situtation.[38] Analgesic alleviation of pain differs from the combined action of specific CRs that alleviate the condition that produces the pain.

Similarly, a drug US might conceivably produce a variety of CRs to counter the specific physiological effects of the US. One possibility was that Lett's CAS effect occurred because CRs in anticipation of these and other components of the lithium US countered specific elements of lithium sickness such as, for instance, hypothermia, bradycardia, and sodium depletion. But, it was also conceivable that, as is the case with peripheral pain, CAS might not depend on specific anticipatory CRs but on a general antisickness response similar to the general analgesia associated with fear of impending pain. If so, CAS based on one sickness US might alleviate an entirely different sickness.

I found that the CAS is a very general effect. My method was to change the US drug from Phase 1 (drug-drug pairings) to Phase 2 (saccharin aversion conditioning) of a CAS experiment. For instance, suppose a rat is trained by five pairings of 25 mg/kg of sodium pentobarbital with 250 mg/kg of LiCl. We know from previous work that the pentobarbital will produce an antisickness effect when LiCl is the US. But suppose that we use 20 mg/kg of *d*-amphetamine as the US during training so that the pentobarbital is conditioned to protect against amphetamine intoxication. Will the pentobarbital still protect against lithium sickness? Amphetamine intoxication is different enough from lithium sickness that it is implausible that specific CRs effective against one sickness (like blood pressure effects) alleviate the other. In fact, it is more plausible that specific CRs that alleviate lithium sickness exacebrate amphetamine intoxication. Furthermore, the two US drugs elicit different CRs[39] and area postrema ablations interfere with the capacity of lithium to produce taste aversion but have no such effect on amphetamine.[40] Nevertheless it will be shown below that the CAS is about as strong if the amphetamine or lithium US used in Phase 2 (Sac→CS→US) is different from the US used during the earlier CS→US pairings of Phase 1.

The design of the lithium-amphetamine transfer experiment was a horrendous 2 × 2 × 2 × 2 factorial within five male Sprague-Dawleys rats in each of 16 groups. The four factors were: (1) whether CS→US or US→CS pairings were administered during Phase 1; (2) whether the same US or different USs were used during Phase 1 and Phase 2; (3) whether Phase 2 consisted of Sac→CS→US trials (the CS drug administered 30 min after removal of the saccharin bottle and the US drug 60 min afterward) or Sac→US trials (only the US drug administered 60 min after drinking); and (4) whether *d*-amphetamine or LiCl was the US used during Phase 2. The saccharin solution was 0.3% weight/volume in tap water. The drug doses used during the five pairings of Phase 1 were 5 mg per rat of sodium pentobarbital diluted in saline to form 0.5 ml, 50.0 mg of LiCl in 2.5 ml of distilled water, or 4 mg of *d*-amphetamine sulfate in 0.5 ml of saline. All drugs were injected intraperitoneally. Note that drug doses are indicated per rat and not relative to body weight. The weight range of the rats on the day prior to drug-drug conditioning was narrow enough (215–229) to permit this and all groups were within 2 g of each other in mean weight. In Phase 2, the dose of pentobarbital was the same as in Phase 1 but the amphetamine and LiCl doses were lower and adjusted to body weight: 31.9 mg/kg of LiCl injected in a 0.674% solution and 4.0 mg/kg of *d*-amphetamine in 8 mg/ml of saline.

TABLE 5 shows the results. Each datum is the mean saccharin preference ratio during trials 2–5, where Trials 1 and 2 were acquisition trials and trials 3–5 were extinction trials. Each row of data refers to the indicated combination of Phase 1 and Phase 2 procedures. The two columns are differentiated by whether the US was the same or different in the two phases. For heuristical purposes, the results shown are pooled for the fourth factor of the 2 × 2 × 2 × 2 design, whether *d*-amphetamine or LiCl

TABLE 5. Amphetamine-Lithium US Crossover Experiment Saccharin Preferences: Means of Trials 2–5

Paradigm in Each Phase		US in Each Phase	
Phase 1	Phase 2	Same	Different
CS→US	Sac→CS→US	0.46	0.42
CS→US	Sac→US	0.36	0.34
US→CS	Sac→CS→US	0.16	0.14
US→CS	Sac→US	0.27	0.29

was the US used during Phase 2. An overall four-dimensional analysis of covariance (ANCOVA) with preference ratios from the first training trial as the covariate showed this factor exerted no effect relevant to the present interpretation of the results. Each mean in TABLE 5 is a mean of two groups and the comparison of any two means was made by performing *t*-tests based on the ANCOVA and combining them by the usual rules for combining normal deviates. The two-tail .05 significance level was used.

Whether the USs were the same or different in the two phases of the experiment did not affect the results shown in TABLE 5 since there was no significant difference between the two means in any row. Row 1 contains mean saccharin preferences produced by the CAS procedure and Rows 2 and 3 contain preferences produced by the Sac→US and US→CS control procedures shown in TABLE 3. In each column, the CAS mean was significantly higher than either control mean. Hence, CAS was demonstrated regardless of whether the US in Phase 2 was the same as or different from the US in Phase 1. The means in Row 4 in each column are significantly higher than the corresponding means in Row 3. This shows that after US→CS pairings, the Sac→CS→US procedure produced lower preferences than the Sac→US procedure and means that normally pentobarbital contributes to the saccharin aversion, exactly the opposite of the CAS effect. I have ignored the logical possibility that the pentobarbital contributed to the aversion in Row 3 due to the US→CS pairings in Phase 1 because it is known that such pairings actually reduce the capacity of pentobarbital to produce a taste aversion albeit to a less marked extent than CS→US pairings.[10]

Very recently completed work in my laboratory shows transfer of a CAS to cisplatin, dactinomycin, and mustargen when the CS drug is pentobarbital and the original US is LiCl. Preliminary work suggests a few cases in which such transfer is not obtained, but the possibility of an artifact due to a low Phase 2 US dose has not been excluded. In other work, I have found excellent transfer when the original CS is pentobarbital and the US is 15 mg/kg of atropine sulfate (a very high dose) to a CAS against both *d*-amphetamine and lithium sickness. Kent Harding (personal communication) has found that a CAS based on pairing pentobarbital either a lithium or an amphetamine US is effective against radiation sickness. Habituation to a sickness US diminishes its capacity to produce a taste aversion and, like CAS, this habituation effect transfers remarkably well from one US to the other.[11] These similarities suggest some commonality in underlying mechanisms although it is clear that Avfail is experimentally distinct from US habituation.[10]

The distress alleviated by the CAS is limited to the type of distress that produces taste aversions. Lett (personal communication) found that CAS could not mitigate the effects of peripheral pain. The CS was pentobarbital that had previously been paired with lithium sickness so as to yield a CAS. The test was how long it takes rats to remove themselves from a hot plate while affected by pentobarbital. There was no transfer of the CAS to the hot plate test although opiates are effective in such a test, as are fear stimuli that release endogenous opiates.[38] The specificity of antisickness

TABLE 6. Similarity of Imaginary Treatment for Alcoholism to Avfail

	Imaginary Treatment	Avfail Procedure
Phase 1	Alcohol state→Sickness	CS drug state→Sickness
Phase 2	Whisky→alcohol state	Sac→CS drug state
Result	No aversion to whisky (presumably)	No aversion to saccharin

to the distress produced by nausea is congruent with Garcia's [2,42] neuroanatomical model of taste aversion learning.[b]

Clinical and Theoretical Implications Related to the Addictions

Since Avfail is obtained if the CS drug is ethanol[10] or morphine,[16] the effect suggests that attempts to make such drugs of abuse aversive by pairing them with US drugs might actually be countertherapeutic. TABLE 6 outlines such a treatment for alcoholism so that its parallel with the Avfail procedure can be seen. If the alcohol state were to be paired with lithium sickness in Phase 1, the alcohol state would lose whatever capacity it might have to induce an aversion to the drinking of whisky in Phase 2.

It may be conjectured further that CAS is an etiological factor in the normal development of some types of alcoholism. Probably most people successfully regulate their alcohol intake partly because overindulgence causes sickness that leads to reduced intake as a result of conditioning. The Avfail and CAS effects imply that this regulatory system may have broken down for some alcoholics. Following the outline in TABLE 7, imagine a person who drinks too much sweet wine and, as a result, an alcohol state is followed by alcohol sickness. Presumably alcohol sickness is like a US in the Avfail paradigm while the earlier alcohol high is like the drug CS. Hence the pairing of the alcohol state with sickness in Phase 1 is parallel to Phase 1 of the Avfail procedure except that sweet wine is consumed prior to the pairing. It may be inferred from the work of Martin[43] that the addition of sweet wine will not prevent the Avfail effect from developing. The person then switches to whisky. If he does not

[b] One type of experiment did not confirm that the CAS effect indicates an alleviation of distress. I have already alluded to the fact that if lithium chloride solution is unfamiliar to a rat, the animal generalizes between it and ordinary saline solution and stops drinking the LiCl as a result of the onset of sickness rather than as a result of tasting the poison.[29] Lithium chloride was used as a salt substitute for humans until a number of patients died due to lithium intoxication. Lett suggested to me that CS→US pairings that produce the CAS effect might also cause greater intake of LiCl solution after injection of the CS drug than normally would be obtained. Presumably if the CS drug elicits a conditioned antisickness effect, it ought to delay perception of sickness by the rat and hence cause greater LiCl intake if injected before a LiCl drinking session. I could not use pentobarbital as the CS drug in any investigation of this possibility due to confounding by the so-called conditioned sickness effect shown in FIGURE 1. So I used chlordiazepoxide and *d*-amphetamine in different groups. The rats were given either five CS→US pairings with a LiCl US, five US→CS pairings, or five CS-alone administrations. Then they were habituated to drink 0.9% NaCl solution. Occasionally, a solution of 0.2% LiCl with 0.56% NaCl was substituted and the rats were injected either with the CS drug or with normal saline 15 minutes before being allowed to drink. Their consumption could be compared with their consumption of 0.9% saline after similar injections. I felt the experiment was sensitive enough to detect a reasonable effect and I could find no difference in the effect of the CS drug on drinking LiCl that could be attributed to prior CS→US pairings.

TABLE 7. How the Avfail Effect Might Make It Hard To Develop a Learned Aversion to Whisky

	Presumed Etiological Factor in Alcoholism	Avfail Procedure
Phase 1	Sweet wine→alcohol state→sickness	CS drug state→sickness
Phase 2	Whisky→alcohol state	Sac→CS drug state
Phase 3	No aversion to whisky (presumably)	No aversion to saccharin

drink very much because he has a generalized aversion to alcohol, he experiences the whisky flavor without getting sick. This parallels Phase 2 of the Avfail procedure; hence, the whisky becomes resistant to taste aversion learning because the initial stages of alcohol intoxication elicit CAS.

If so, CAS accounts for the inability of many heavy drinkers to develop aversions to the flavor of whisky. Furthermore, the distaste of many such drinkers for sweet wine may originate in something like the process outlined in Table 7. This cannot reasonably be considered a universal cause of alcoholism because, as mentioned earlier, many alcoholics have taste aversions to alcoholic beverages. But it may be an etiological factor for alcoholics without taste aversions.

Extension to Cancer Chemotherapy

The distress produced by drugs used in cancer treatment is often the dose-limiting factor. It also induces some cancer patients to forego treatment.[44] Most of the animal experimentation relevant to control of this distress has involved the study of vomiting and antiemetic drugs. However the taste aversion attenuation (TAA) method used by Lett[22] to validate her CAS effect is also useful. It was independently devised by Cairnie and Leach[45] to screen drugs for effectiveness against radiation sickness. By the TAA criterion, a drug is effective if the Sac→drug→US paradigm yields weaker saccharin aversions than the Sac→US paradigm, where "drug" is a putative antisickness drug and the US produces strong taste aversions.

Sickness distress is ambiguous even as a clinical entity and no single animal model of it will be entirely satisfactory. But TAA is certainly as useful as vomiting for this purpose. Like the taste aversions, vomiting is a biological adaptation to prevent sickness, but not an exact measurement of distress. The Romans were so undistressed by ordinary vomiting (not the pathological vomiting produced by cancer chemotherapy) that they induced it so they could feast more. McCarthy and Borison[46] reiterated the denial of Borison and Wang[47] that antiemetic effects demonstrated in animals imply relief from nausea and suggested that it might be possible to develop drugs that alleviate nausea without affecting vomiting.[46] In addition to the lack of any close correspondence between antiemesis and antisickness, there is substantial ambiguity about antiemetic drugs. Borison and McCarthy have gone so far as to claim that "it is usually impossible to determine" whether the clinical benefits of putative antimetics are due to antiemetic activity. They suggest that they are often side effects of sedation.[48] Thus, TAA defined through the Sac→drug→US paradigm is at least as good a measure of alleviation of distress as interference with vomiting.

The TAA method can be used to compare CAS with what may be called pharmacological antisickness (PAS), the capacity of a drug to attenuate a taste aversion without prior CS→US pairings. In fact, the usual controls for CAS include a test of PAS. That is, there is a Sac→drug→US group that had not had CAS pretraining (Group

US→CS) and a Sac→US group. If PAS were obtained, the former group would yield higher saccharin preferences than the latter. TABLE 5 not only shows no PAS for pentobarbital in the absence of prior CS→US pairings, but that it actually adds to the taste aversion. As already indicated, Lett's data (TABLE 4) show no PAS when *d*-amphetamine, chloridiazepoxide, ethanol, or morphine are the putative antisickness drugs. The failure of morphine to yield PAS is especially interesting since Borison and McCarthy[48] believe it is the most effective antiemetic, despite its use to elicit vomiting.

FIGURE 3 is of unpublished data that show that neither Δ⁹-THC nor chlorpromazine (CPZ) produces pharmacological antisickness by the TAA definition when 15.9 mg/kg of LiCl is the US. In fact, both these drugs have the opposite effect. The CPZ and Δ⁹-THC doses are expressed per 200–250 g rat rather than in terms of body weight. The left side shows that these drugs injected 60 min after a bottle of 0.4% saccharin solution is removed produce taste aversions by themselves as compared to Group NO-AV, a group that received no injections and thus is a baseline for the aversions produced by CPZ and Δ⁹-THC. The remainder of FIGURE 3 shows that the aversions produced by lower doses of CPZ and THC summate with the aversions produced by LiCl. (The CPZ or THC injections were administered 60 min after saccharin consumption, while the LiCl was administered 120 min later.) Thus both CPZ and THC intensify taste aversions even though they are used clinically to alleviate antisickness effects. Similarly, unpublished work in my laboratory shows that Δ⁹-THC, scopolamine, and haloperidol intensify taste aversions produced by 12 mg/kg of cyclophosphamide. It

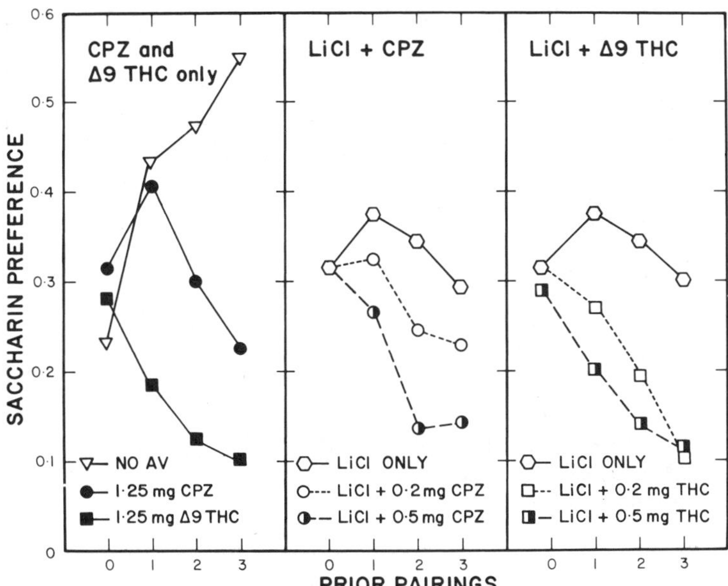

FIGURE 3. The left side shows that both chlorpromazine (CPZ) and Δ⁹-THC produce saccharin aversions if injected after saccharin consumption. Group NO-AV was not injected and served to supply a measure of saccharin preference in the absence of a learned aversion. The right side shows that aversions produced by these drugs summate with aversions produced by LiCl.

seems clear that most putative antisickness drugs actually strengthen taste aversions produced by the sicknesses they are supposed to alleviate. This effect is especially striking in FIGURE 3 because I deliberately spaced the antiemetics from the drinking so that the weak aversions they can produce would not easily become associated with the saccharin.

I grant that drugs that do not produce PAS may still be clinically useful since the TAA method does not measure everything that is important clinically. It is only particular types of distress produced by drugs that cause taste aversions to occur.[49] It may well be that the intensification of the saccharin aversion produced by putative antisickness drugs in the present PAS paradigm does not always reflect an increase in clinical distress. However, these limitations do not contradict the present hypothesis that attenuation of a taste aversions by a drug is very likely to indicate attenuation of distress. It is clear that such attenuation is not readily produced by common antiemetic drugs. The rarity of TAA resulting from the administration of such drugs makes the attenuation produced by CAS all the more interesting.

The rarity of TAA by drugs also makes it exciting that dexamethasone (DEX) yields TAA comparable to that obtained with CAS. An early report of the effectiveness of this drug by Hennessy *et al.*[50] had what I regarded as a procedural flaw. The procedure was DEX→milk→LiCl, with the DEX injected two hours before the milk was presented for drinking. This may introduce an artifact since the animal may perceive

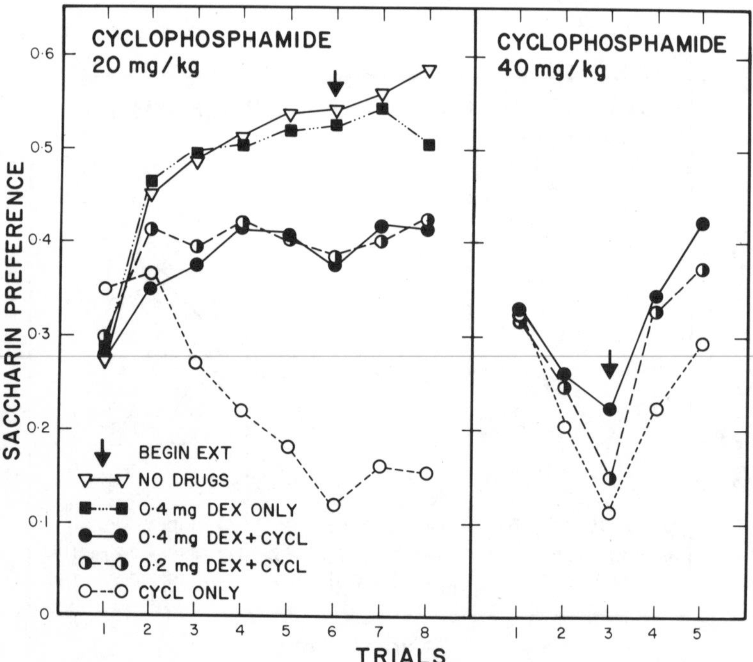

FIGURE 4. Dexamethasone attenuates the saccharin aversions produced by cyclophosphamide. The NO DRUGS group drank saccharin without contingent injections and it is clear that dexamethasone by itself does not produce a noticeable saccharin aversion. DEX doses shown per rat rather than in proportion to body weight.

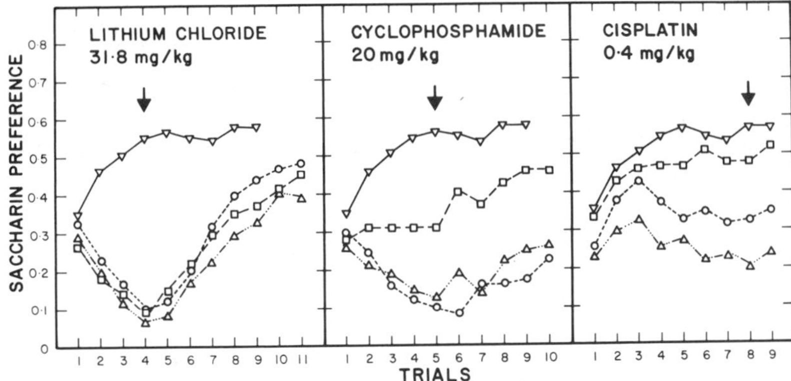

FIGURE 5. The top curves (inverted triangles) in each case show data for a group not injected with any drug after drinking saccharin solution. The circles refer to the case in which the indicated toxin was injected without being preceded by an antisickness injection. The squares refer to the rats injected with dexamethasone prior to injection with the indicated toxin. The upright triangles refer to the rats similarly injected with metoclopramide prior to toxin injection.

that his sickness began before the drinking. For instance, if a low dose of lithium is injected before drinking, a later dose will produce a weakened taste aversion because the animal believes its sickness began before drinking and hence is less likely to attribute it to what it consumed.[51] Such a weakened taste aversion is not evidence that lithium is an effective agent against lithium sickness. This analogy makes the drug →taste→US paradigm suspect as a measure of PAS. I also must say that I have not been able to replicate the Hennessy *et al.*[50] finding with a number of similar procedures and also failed with their original procedure and their high dose of LiCl. Nevertheless, the deficiency may be mine because we later found dexamethasone to be a potent antisickness drug by the TAA definition.

I became interested in DEX when Cairnie and Leach,[45] using the TAA method, found that DEX was effective in mitigating taste aversions induced by radiation. Insulin, domperidone, acetylsalicylic acid, naloxone, chlorpheniramine, and cimetidine were ineffective. Most of the latter drugs contributed to the saccharin aversion rather than attenuated it. Haloperidol yielded a statistically significant but very small TAA effect that Cairnie and Leach[45] did not seem to consider definitive probably due to the large number of antisickness drugs they tested and the resulting possibility of a Type-2 statistical error.

I found that DEX was an effective antisickness drug when cyclophosphamide was the US. The rats (12 per group) were maintained on 15 min per day of water that was flavored with 0.4% (w/vol) sodium saccharin every fourth day. The dose used of intramuscular DEX was either 0.2 mg or 0.4 mg per 200 g rat. The intraperitoneal cyclophosphamide dose was 20 mg/kg or 40 mg/kg. If used, the DEX was injected 30 min after the saccharin was removed. The cyclophosphamide was always injected one hour after the saccharin was removed. FIGURE 4 shows a potent antisickness effect resulting for dexamethasone when the US is 20 mg/kg of cyclophosphamide. This effect is less clear at 40 mg/kg of cyclophosphamide due to a floor effect.

Gerard Martin compared the PAS effects of DEX with those of metoclopramide, an antiemetic recommended for alleviation of distress due to cancer chemotherapy and considered particularly effective against cisplatin.[52] Each section of FIGURE 5 in-

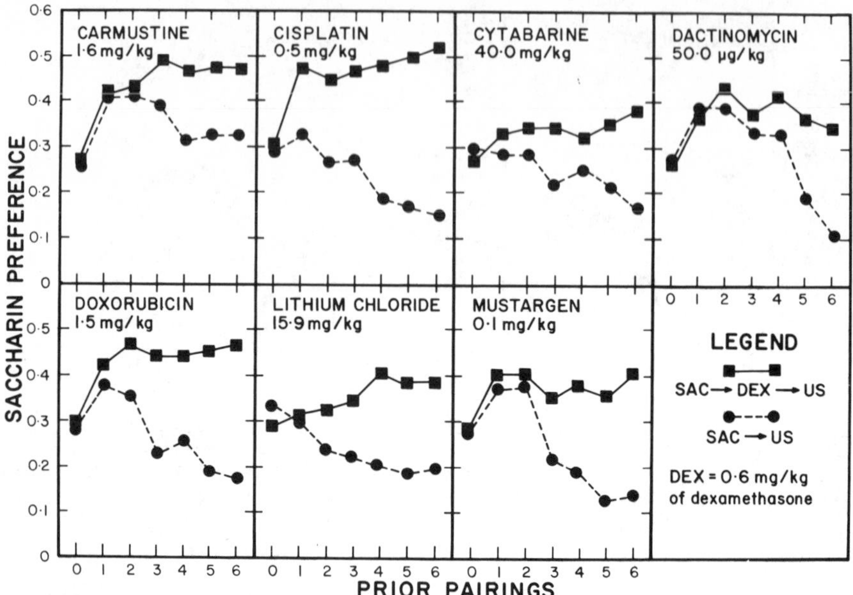

FIGURE 6. In each case injection of dexamethasone prior to the indicated toxin attenuated the resulting saccharin aversion.

volves use of a different drug (LiCl, cyclophosphamide, or cisplatin). In unspecified respects, the methods were like those for the experiment whose data are summarized in FIGURE 4. In no case did 1.0 mg/kg of metoclopramide attenuate the taste aversion. In fact, it seemed to make the aversion to cisplatin stronger, the effect being barely significant at the two-tail .05 level (ANCOVA) on the first extinction day. (The metoclopramide dose was selected on the basis of an insignificant trend in pilot data and is rather low.) In the case of LiCl, DEX was ineffective in agreement with my earlier work. However, DEX exhibited a strong TAA effect when used against either cyclophosphamide or cisplatin. In the case of cisplatin, the TAA effect of DEX was not statistically significant by the statistical criterion selected *a priori*, but ought to be considered a real effect nevertheless since it was confirmed in the experiment whose results are summarized in FIGURE 6. It is cautioned in passing that it would be wrong to conclude on the basis of a quick perusal of FIGURE 5 that cisplatin is more amenable to the PAS effect of DEX than cyclophosphamide because the cisplatin aversion was nearly eliminated by DEX. The cisplatin dose produced a weaker aversion than the cyclophosphamide dose and this flaws the comparison.

Both cyclophosphamide and cisplatin are alkylating agents used in cancer chemotherapy and related to nitrogen mustard, which may be radiomimetic.[53] To see if the effectiveness of dexamethasone was limited to alkylating agents, Martin and I tested it against the chemotherapies shown in FIGURE 6 as well as half the dose of LiCl shown in FIGURE 5. To our surprise, a PAS effect was obtained in every test. I believe, however, that DEX is more effective against cisplatin than against most of the other drugs shown in FIGURE 6 since that is the only case in which TAA was apparent after the first pairing.

I am able to conceive of only two potential alternatives to interpretation of TAA produced by dexamethasone as evidence for alleviation of sickness distress. One is the blocking possibility previously mentioned in discussion of the CAS. By this interpretation, the dexamethasone stimulus state becomes associated with sickness so that the rat effectively attributes its sickness to the dexamethasone state rather than the saccharin taste. This is even more unreasonable in the case of dexamethasone PAS than in the case of CAS since Gerard Martin has recently found (personal communication) that a series of dexamethasone injections (0.45 mg/kg every two days) that terminates a week before saccharin aversion training based on 12 mg/kg of cyclophosphamide substantially attenuates the resulting saccharin aversions. The other interpretation is that the dexamethasone somehow induces amnesia or memory blockade and that this has somehow not been noticed in the past even though dexamethasone is a widely used drug. If so, the rat does not remember the saccharin taste at the time it becomes sick. Given Martin's finding that dexamethasone injected a week prior to conditioning produces PAS, this explanation implies a one-week memory blockade. An additional point against the amnesia explanation is the orderly rise in saccharin preferences among the rats injected with dexamethasone alone after drinking saccharin as shown on the left side of FIGURE 6. This loss of neophobia is incompatible with the hypothesis that memory of the saccharin taste is disrupted.

TENTATIVE CONCLUSIONS

CAS seems to have more potent antisickness effects as measured by TAA than any drug used medically for that purpose except dexamethasone. This highlights the distinction between antiemesis and TAA as measures of antisickness since dexamethasone is not considered an antiemetic. I believe that CAS can produce more powerful antisickness than dexamethasone. For instance, FIGURE 4 shows dexamethasone is ineffective against the dose of LiCl routinely used in CAS experiments, including transfer experiments (TABLE 5). However, it remains to be seen whether CAS is effective against as wide a variety of toxins as DEX was shown to be in FIGURE 6. It would, of course, be nice to combine PAS and CAS by pairing dexamethasone with a high dose of LiCl. But when I tried this, I was not able to make dexamethasone effective against a 31.8 mg/kg dose of LiCl, the dose usually used in Phase 2 of CAS experiment. This suggests to me that dexamethasone and CAS produce different types of antisickness.

Medical treatment frequently involves the equivalent of pairing a CS drug with a sickness US and this carries the possibility that such elements of the treatment should be modified so as to condition a clinically useful CAS. But I am not sure this possibility is practical because, at least in the case of LiCl,[16] the US dose necessary to produce CAS as a result of CS→US pairings must be very high—well beyond a clinical range. But if, say, a neurochemical responsible for the CAS were to be isolated, it might be a potent antisickness drug.

REFERENCES

1. GANTT, W. H. 1973. Does teleology have a place in conditioning? *In* Contemporary Approaches to Conditioning and learning, F. J. McGuigan, Ed.: 111–126. John Wiley. New York.
2. GARCIA, J., W.C. HANKINS & K.W. RUSINIAK. 1974. Behavioral regulation of the milieu interior in man and rat. Science **185**: 823–831.
3. OVERTON, D.A. 1964. State-dependent or 'dissociated' learning produced with pentobarbital. J. Comp. Physiol. Psychol. **57**: 3–12.

4. CUNNINGHAM, C. L. & J. G. LINAKIS. 1980. Paradoxical aversive conditioning with ethanol. Pharm. Biochem. Behav. **12**: 337–341.
5. TAUKULIS, H. K. 1982. Attenuation of pentobarbital based hypothermia in rats with a history of pentobarbital-LiCl pairing. Pharm. Biochem. Behav. **19**: 695–697.
6. WILKIN, L. D. & C. L. CUNNINGHAM. 1982. Pavlovian conditioning with ethanol and lithium: Effects on heart rate and taste aversion in rats. J. Comp. Physiol. Psychol. **96**: 781–790.
7. REVUSKY, S. 1973. Some laboratory paradigms for the chemical aversion treatment of alcoholism. J. Behav. Ther. Exp. Psychiat. **4**: 15–17.
8. REVUSKY, S. & T. H. GORRY, 1973. Flavor aversions produced by contingent drug injections: Relative effectiveness of apomorphine, emetine, and lithium. Behav. Res. Ther. **11**: 403–409.
9. BOLAND, F. J., C. S. MELLOR & S. REVUSKY. 1978. Chemical aversion treatment of alcoholism: Lithium as the aversive agent. Behav. Res. Ther. **16**: 401–409.
10. REVUSKY, S., H. K. TAUKULIS, L. A. PARKER & S. COOMBES. 1979. Chemical aversion therapy: Rat data suggest it may be countertherapeutic to pair an addictive drug state with sickness. Behav. Res. Ther. **17**: 177–188.
11. BROGDEN, W. J. 1939. Sensory preconditioning. J. Exp. Psychol. **25**: 323–334.
12. BOND, N. W. & E. L. DIGIUSTO. 1976. One trial higher-order conditioning of a taste aversion. Aust. J. Psychol. **28**: 53–55.
13. BOND, N. W. & W. HARLAND. 1975. Higher order conditioning of a taste aversion. Anim. Learning Behav. **3**: 295–296.
14. PAVLOV, I.P. 1927. Conditioned Reflexes. G. V. Anrep, Trans. Oxford University Press. London.
15. SIEGEL, S. & M. DOMJAN. 1971. Backward conditioning as an inhibitory procedure. Learning Motiv. **2**: 1–11.
16. REVUSKY, S., S. COOMBES & R. W. POHL. 1982. Pharmacological generality of the Avfail Effect. Behav. Neur. Biol. **34**: 240–260.
17. REVUSKY, S. & S. COOMBES. 1982. Long delay drug-drug associations between drug states produced in rats by injecting two drugs in sequence. J. Comp. Physiol. Psychol. **96**: 549–556.
18. REVUSKY, S., H. K. TAUKULIS & S. COOMBES. 1979. Dependence of the Avfail effect on the sequence of training operations. Behav. Neur. Biol. **29**: 430–445.
19. REVUSKY, S., H. K. TAUKULIS & C. PEDDLE 1979. Learned associations between drug states: Attempted analysis in Pavlovian terms. Physiol. Psychol. **7**: 353–363.
20. REVUSKY, S. 1977. Learning as a general process with an emphasis on data from feeding experiments. *In* Food Aversion Learning. N. S. Milgram, L. Krames & T. M. Alloway, Eds.: 1–51. Plenum Press, New York.
21. ANNAU, Z. & L. J. KAMIN. 1961. The conditioned emotional response as a function in the intensity of the US. J. Comp. Physiol. Psychol. **54**: 428–432.
22. LETT, B. T. 1983. Pavlovian drug-sickness pairings result in the conditioning of an anti-sickness response. Behav. Neurosci. **97**: 779–784.
23. SIEGEL, S., R. E. HINSON & M. D. KRANK. 1978. The role of predrug signals in morphine analgesic tolerance: Support for a Pavlovian conditioning model of tolerance. J. Exp. Psychol.: Anim. Behav. Proc. **4**: 188–196.
24. SIEGEL, S. 1979. The role of conditioning in drug tolerance and addiction. *In* Psychopathology in Animals: Research and Clinical Implications. J. D. Keehn, Ed.: 143–163. Academic Press. New York.
25. SOLOMON, R. L. 1980. The opponent process theory of acquired motivation: The costs of pleasure and the benefit of pain. Am. Psychol. **35**: 691–712.
26. REVUSKY, S. & J. GARCIA. 1970. Learned associations over long delays. *In* The Psychology of Learning and Motivation: Advances in Theory and Research. G. H. Bower, Ed. **4**: 1–84. Academic Press. New York.
27. REVUSKY, S., R. W. POHL & S. COOMBES. 1980. Flavor aversions and deprivation state. Anim. Learn. Behav. **8**: 543–549.
28. REVUSKY, S., S. COOMBES & R. W. POHL. 1982. Drug states as discriminative stimuli in a flavor aversion learning experiment. J. Comp. Physiol. Psychol. **96**: 200–211.
29. RUSINIAK, K. W., J. GARCIA & W. G. HANKINS. 1976. Bait shyness: Avoidance of the taste without escape from the illness in rats. J. Comp. Physiol. Psychol. **90**: 460–467.

30. WISE, R. A., B. YOKEL & H. DEWITT. 1976. Both positive reinforcement and conditioned aversion from apomorphine in rats. Science **191**: 1273–1275.
31. REICHER, M. A. & E. W. HOLMAN. 1977. Location preference and flavor aversion produced by amphetamine in rats. Anim. Learn. Behav. **5**: 343–346.
32. WHITE, N., L. SKLAR & Z. AMIT. 1977. The reinforcing action of morphine and its paradoxical side effect. Psychopharmacology **52**: 63–66.
33. EIKELBOOM, R & J. STEWART. 1982. Conditioning of drug-induced physiological responses. Psychol. Rev. **89**: 507–528.
34. JENKINS, H. M. 1973. Effects of the stimulus-reinforcer relationship on selected and unselected responses. *In* Constraints on Learning. R.A. Hinde & J. Stevenson-Hinde, Eds.: 189–203. Academic. London.
35. MOORE, B. R. 1973. The role of directed Pavolvian reactions in simple instrumental learning in the pigeon. *In* Constraints on Learning. R.A. Hinde & J. Stevenson-Hinde, Eds.: 159–188. Academic. London.
36. REVUSKY, S. 1971. The role of interference in association over a delay. *In* Animal Memory. W. K. Honig & P. H. R. James, Eds.: 155–213. Academic. New York.
37. BERNSTEIN, I. L., M. V. VITIELLO & R. SIGMUNDI. 1980. Effects of interference stimuli on the acquisition of learned aversions to food in the rat. J. Comp. Physiol. Psychol. **94**: 921–931.
38. BOLLES, R. C. & A. FANSELOW. 1980. A perceptual-recuperative-defensive model of fear and pain. Behav. Brain Sci. **3**: 121–131.
39. PARKER, L. A. 1982. Nonconsummatory and consummatory behavioral CRs elicited by lithium and amphetamine-paired flavors. Learn. Motiv. **13**: 281–303.
40. BERGER, B., C. WISE & L. STEIN. 1973. Area postrema damage and bait shyness. J. Comp. Physiol. Psychol. **83**: 475–479.
41. BRAVEMAN, N. S. 1977. What studies on pre-exposure to pharmacological agents tell us about the nature of the aversion inducing treatment. *In* Learning Mechanisms in Food Selection. L. M. Barker, M. R. Best & M. Domjan, Eds..: 511–532. Baylor University Press. Waco, TX.
42. GARCIA, J. & F. R. ERVIN. 1968. A neuropsychological approach to the appropriateness of signals and specificity of reinforcers. Commun. Behav. Biol. Part A **1**: 389–415.
43. MARTIN, G. M. 1982. Examination of factors which might influence an association between pentobarbital and lithium chloride. Learn. Motiv. **13**: 185–199.
44. PENTA, J., D. POSTER & S. BRUNO. 1983. The pharmacological treatment of nausea and vomiting caused by cancer chemotherapy: A review. *In* Antiemetics and Cancer Chemotherapy. J. Lazslo, Ed.: 53–92. Williams and Wilkins. Baltimore.
45. CAIRNIE, A. B. & K. E. LEACH. 1982. Dexamethasone: A potent blocker of radiation induced taste aversions in rats. Pharm. Biochem. Behav. **17**: 305–312.
46. MCCARTHY, L. E. & H. L. BORISON. 1983. Animal models for predicting antiemetic drug activity. *In* Antiemetics and Cancer Chemotherapy. J. Lazslo, Ed.: 21–33. Williams and Wilkins. Baltimore.
47. BORISON, H. L. & S. C. WANG. 1953. Physiology and pharmacology of vomiting. Pharm. Rev. **5**: 193–230.
48. BORISON, H. L. & L. E. MCCARTHY. 1983. Neuropharmacologic mechanisms of vomiting. *In* Antiemetics and Cancer Chemotherapy. J. Lazslo, Ed.: 6–20. Williams and Wilkins. Baltimore.
49. LETT, B. T. 1985. The painlike effect of gallamine and naloxone differs from sickness induced by lithium. Behav. Neurosci. (In press.)
50. HENNESSY, J. W., W. P. SMOTHERMAN & S. LEVINE. 1976. Conditioned taste aversion and the adrenal pituitary system. Behav. Biol. **16**: 417–424.
51. DOMJAN, M. & M. R. BEST. 1977. Paradoxical effect of unconditioned stimulus preexposure: Interference with conditioning of a taste aversion. J. Exp. Psychol.: Anim. Behav. Proc. **3**: 310–321.
52. GRALLA, R. J. 1983. Antiemetic studies with metoclopramide in chemotherapy induced nausea and vomiting. *In* Antiemetics and Cancer Chemotherapy. J. Lazslo, Ed.: 129–141. Williams and Wilkins. Baltimore.

Conditioned Taste Aversions: A Behavioral Index of Toxicity

ANTHONY L. RILEY AND DIANE L. TUCK
Psychopharmacology Laboratory
Department of Psychology
The American University
Washington, D.C. 20016

Although over the past 25 years the major focus of research on conditioned taste aversions (CTAs) has been on its empirical assessment and theoretical implications,[1-4] only recently has the issue of the application of CTAs been addressed. For example, within the last ten years CTAs have been applied to the study of the dietary preferences of cancer patients,[5] the examination of the mechanisms underlying drug dependence and withdrawal,[6] the control of predation,[7] and the treatment of alcohol abuse.[8]

More recently, the conditioned taste aversion paradigm has been presented as one possible element in a battery of behavioral indices of drug toxicity.[9-11] As an index, it has been suggested that compounds that induce taste aversions are toxic. The basis for this consideration comes primarily from the fact that a wide range of known toxins (as indexed by other behavioral and pharmacological procedures) are effective in inducing taste aversions (TABLE 1). This consideration also comes from a more theoretical perspective. As noted by Garcia and Ervin,[1] conditioned taste aversions can be seen as an adaptive response in the normal feeding behavior of an animal.[4] An animal that can acquire information about the toxic potential of its food supply is likely to avoid subsequent toxicosis, an avoidance that could prevent the accumulation of a possibly debilitating or fatal dose of the toxin. From this perspective, the animal is its own biological toxin screen. The adaptive nature of this screen is further illustrated by the fact that animals learn this avoidance response primarily to foods (the likely source of toxins), with only a single pairing of the taste and toxicosis (a rapidity that limits the need for repeated samplings)—even when a long delay is imposed between consumption and the onset of toxicosis (a delay likely to occur as a result of the natural temporal characteristics of digestion). The use of the CTA design as an index of toxicity, therefore, appears to be a natural extension of its function in normal feeding.

The consideration of taste aversion as an index of toxicity, however, has not been without criticism.[12-15] These criticisms can best be discussed within a signal detection framework. As illustrated in FIGURE 1, if a compound is classified as a toxin by the CTA paradigm, i.e., it induces a taste aversion, but there is no corroborative evidence that it is a toxin, this would be termed a FALSE ALARM. On the other hand, if a compound is classified as a nontoxin by the CTA design, i.e., it does not induce a taste aversion, although there is substantial evidence from other designs that the compound is toxic, this would be termed a MISS. These two outcomes would represent failures of the CTA procedure to classify accurately the toxic status of a compound.

		CTA ASSESSMENT	
		TOXIN	NONTOXIN
COMPOUND	TOXIN	HIT	MISS
	NONTOXIN	FALSE ALARMS	CORRECT REJECTION

FIGURE 1. A signal detection analysis of the conditioned taste aversion procedure as an index of toxicity.

FALSE ALARMS

When an analysis is made of the various agents that condition taste aversions, it is clear that FALSE ALARMS and MISSES do occur. In relation to FALSE ALARMS, a number of agents (e.g., amobarbital, amphetamine, chlordiazepoxide, chlorpromazine, cyclophosphamide, ethanol, lorazepam, methaqualone, methylatropine, morphine, and scopolamine) induce taste aversions at doses that produce no observable signs of illness or distress.[12,15] Because of these apparent FALSE ALARMS, the usefulness of the CTA design has been questioned. This argument, however, rests upon the assumption that other behavioral measures are better indicators of a compound's toxicity than the conditioned taste aversion design. In other words, if the CTA procedure classifies a compound as a toxin when another measure does not, it has typically been concluded that the CTA procedure has erroneously classified the compound.[12] Another way of interpreting the same data, however, is to suggest that the taste aversion design is simply more sensitive than other procedures in detecting toxicity. This latter interpretation has received considerable support when known toxins have been examined for their efficacy in inducing aversions and in producing effects on more traditional measures of toxicity. As illustrated in TABLE 2, a number of compounds are effective in inducing taste aversions at doses that are a small fraction of the LD_{50} dose or of the dose that produces a measurable effect on food and water consumption and body weight. For example, Parker *et al.*[11] reported that the dose of the anticholinesterase agent physostigmine required to condition a taste aversion was .05 mg/kg, a dose 20% of that necessary to produce any change in general water consumption or rearing, i.e., .25 mg/kg (FIGURE 2). The sensitivity of the taste aversion design is also evident when taste aversions are compared with more complex indices of toxicity such as the radial arm maze and schedule-controlled behavior. For example, although taste aversions can be induced by the organotin compound trimethyltin chloride at doses as low as .75 mg/kg,[10] Mastropaolo *et al.*[16] have recently reported that performance under a differential-reinforcement-of-low-rate schedule of water reinforcement was unaffected until a dose of 7.0 mg/kg was given (FIGURE 3). These dose-response comparisons are important in that compounds that produce effects in more traditional toxicity designs (and as such are classified as toxic) generally do so at higher doses than are necessary to produce taste aversions. This greater sensitivity clearly offers an alternative interpretation of the issue of FALSE ALARMS.

TABLE 1. Toxins that Are Effective in Inducing Taste Aversions

Acetaldehyde (Brown *et al.*, 1978)
Acrylamide (Anderson *et al.*, 1982)
Aflatoxin B1 (Rappold *et al.*, 1984)
Alloxan monohydrate (Brookshire *et al.*, 1972)
Alpha naphthylthiourea (Rzoska, 1953)
Arsenic (Rzoska, 1953)
Bal (Peele, unpublished)
Barium carbonate (Rzoska, 1953)
Cadmium chloride (Wellman *et al.*, 1984)
Carbaryl (MacPhail, 1981)
Chloral hydrate (Kallman *et al.*, 1983)
Chlordimeform (MacPhail & Leander, 1980)
Cobalt chloride (Wellman *et al.*, 1984)
Cobra venom (Islam, 1978)
Copper sulfate (Nachman & Hartley, 1975)
Cycloheximide (Bolas *et al.*, 1979)
Cyclophosphamide (Ader *et al.*, 1978)
Deltamethrin (MacPhail *et al.*, 1981)
1,2-dichloroethane (Kallman *et al.*, 1983)
1,2-dichloroethylene (Kallman *et al.*, 1983)
Dichlorvos (Roney *et al.*, 1984)
Diethyldithiocarbamate (Peele & MacPhail, unpublished)
Diisopropylfluorophosphate (Roney *et al.*, 1984)
DMSA (Peele, unpublished)
Endosulfan (Peele & MacPhail, unpublished)
Lead acetate (Dantzer, 1980)
Lithium carbonate (McFarland *et al.*, 1978)
Lithium chloride (Archer *et al.*, 1979)
Mercuric chloride (Klein *et al.*, 1974)

MISSES

Although it is typically assumed that any drug can condition a taste aversion, a wide range of agents have been reported to be ineffective (TABLE 3). Of this list, several compounds are relevant to the issue of MISSES when the ability to produce conditioned taste aversions is presented within a signal detection framework (TABLE 4). As illustrated, a number of compounds with known toxicity are ineffective in conditioning taste aversions. Although such MISSES clearly present a problem for the use of the taste aversion paradigm as an index of toxicity, they may be more a problem of the specific taste aversion procedures used in assaying toxicity than of the general use of taste aversions as a behavioral index. Such variables within the taste aversion procedure as dose, number of conditioning trials, convulsant properties of a compound, duration of drug action, and delayed onset of drug action may affect the occurrence of MISSES.

Dose

An often-reported finding in taste aversion learning is that aversions are a direct function of the dose of the drug administered.[17,18] Such a relationship is illustrated in FIGURE 4, which depicts the amount of saccharin consumed as a function of the dose of LiCl administered during aversion conditioning.[17] As illustrated, aversions

(TABLE 1, *continued*)

Mesurol (Gustavson *et al.*, 1982)
Methyl bromide (Miyagawa, 1982)
Methylmercury (Braun & Snyder, 1973)
Metrazol (Golus & McGee, 1980)
Monosodium glutamate (Vogel & Nathan, 1975)
n-butyraldoxime (Nachman *et al.*, 1970)
Ozone (MacPhail & Hatch, unpublished)
Paraquat (Dey *et al.*, 1984)
Parathion (Roney *et al.*, 1984)
Physostigmine sulfate (Parker *et al.*, 1982)
Plant homogenates (Yokel & Ogzewalla, 1981)
Red squill (Nachman & Hartley, 1975)
Scorpion venom (Islam, 1980)
Sodium fluoride (Ionescu & Buresova, 1977)
Sodium fluoroacetate (Nachman & Hartley, 1975)
Sodium iodoacetate (Ionescu & Buresova, 1977)
Strychnine sulfate (Nachman & Hartley, 1975)
Thallium sulfate (Nachman & Hartley, 1975)
Thiabendazole (Gustavson *et al.*, 1983)
Toluene (MacPhail & Tomlinson, unpublished)
1,1,2-trichloroethane (Kallman *et al.*, 1983)
Trichloroethylene (Kallman *et al.*, 1983)
Trichloromethane (Kallman *et al.*, 1983)
2,4,5-trichlorophenoxyacetic acid (Sjoden *et al.*, 1979)
Triethyltin (MacPhail, 1982)
Trimethyltin (MacPhail, 1982)
Triphenyltin (MacPhail & Peele, unpublished)
Viper venom (Islam *et al.*, 1982)

Note: To be included in this table, a toxin had to have been reported by at least a single study to condition a taste aversion. For complete references see Riley & Tuck.[41]

were clearly a function of the dose of LiCl. It is important to note, however, that there was a threshold dose for LiCl (.60 mEq, .15 M) below which aversions were not conditioned. Similar findings of a threshold dose for inducing an aversion have also been reported for other compounds (e.g., lead, triethyltin, and trimethyltin) and hypnotics. That aversions are dose dependent is important in relation to interpreting the aforementioned failures of known toxins to induce taste aversions. For five of the eleven toxins noted as being ineffective in inducing taste aversions (gallamine triethiodide, pyrrolopyrimidine, sodium cyanide, sodium malonate, and warfarin; TABLE 4), only a single dose was examined.[13,14] Although it is difficult to determine where on the dose-response function the specific dose for any one of these compounds lies, it is certainly possible that had the dose of the compound been increased aversions may have been produced.

Number of Conditioning Trials

Although taste aversions are typically acquired following only a single conditioning trial,[19] there are cases in which aversions are weak or not evident after a single taste-drug pairing. Such an effect was illustrated in FIGURE 4 in which groups of rats were given a range of doses of LiCl following saccharin consumption. Although following a single conditioning trial low doses of LiCl did not induce an aversion, with repeated conditioning trials aversions were acquired (FIGURE 5).[20,21] These findings are impor-

TABLE 2. Assessment of the Relative Sensitivity of CTAs

Toxin	Procedure	Dose (%)	Reference
Alcohol	LD_{50}	15	Yokel & Ogzewalla, 1981
Amphetamine	LD_{50}	3	Yokel & Ogzewalla, 1981
Cadmium	FOOD	10	Wellman *et al.*, 1984
	WEIGHT	10	
Chloral hydrate	WATER	50	Kallman *et al.*, 1983
Chlordimeform	LD_{50}	16	Reiter, 1982
	FIG 8	100	
	RAM	100	
	SCHEDULE	> 100	
Chlordimeform	LD_{50}	5	MacPhail & Leander, 1980
	WATER	50	
Chlordimeform	LD_{50}	10	Landauer *et al.*, 1984
	AMB	33	
	REAR	33	
	SOCIAL	33	
Copper sulfate	LD_{50}	50	Nachman & Hartley, 1975
DCE-2	WATER	15	Kallman *et al.*, 1983
LiCl	LD_{50}	16	Nachman & Hartley, 1975
LiCl	LD_{50}	30	Yokel & Ogzewalla, 1981
Mercuric chloride	AA	50	Klein *et al.*, 1974
Methylbromide	WATER	50	Miyagawa, 1982
Physostigmine	REAR	20	Parker *et al.*, 1982
	WATER	20	
	OTHER	20	
Poinsettia	LD_{50}	40	Yokel & Ogzewalla, 1981
Red squill	LD_{50}	44	Nachman & Hartley, 1975
TCE-1,2	WATER	30	Kallman *et al.*, 1983
Trichloromethane	LD_{50}	5	Landauer *et al.*, 1982
	MOTOR	2	
	SCHEDULE	1	
Triethyltin	LD_{50}	13	MacPhail, 1982
	FIG 8	25	
Trimethyltin	LD_{50}	38	MacPhail, 1982
	RAM	42	
1080	LD_{50}	50	Nachman & Hartley, 1975

Toxin = The toxin being analyzed. Procedure = The procedure with which the taste aversion paradigm is being compared. Dose = The percentage of the dose used in the procedure listed in Procedure that is necessary to condition a significant taste aversion. (LD_{50} = Lethal dose 50, FOOD = Food consumption, WEIGHT = Body weight, WATER = Water consumption, FIG 8 = Figure 8 maze, RAM = Radial Arm Maze, SCHEDULE = Schedule controlled behavior, AMB = Ambulation, REAR = Rearing, SOCIAL = Social behavior, AA = Active avoidance, and MOTOR = Motor behavior.)

For complete references see Riley & Tuck.[41]

tant when considering the basis for the failure of known toxins to induce taste aversions. For five of the eleven toxins in TABLE 4 (gallamine triethiodide, pyrollopyrimidine, sodium cyanide, sodium malonate, and warfarin) only a single conditioning trial was administered. Had multiple conditioning trials been given, aversions may have been induced. It is interesting to note in this context that strychnine sulfate, a compound often reported to be ineffective in inducing taste aversions,[14,22] produces a substantial aversion with repeated conditioning trials.[14]

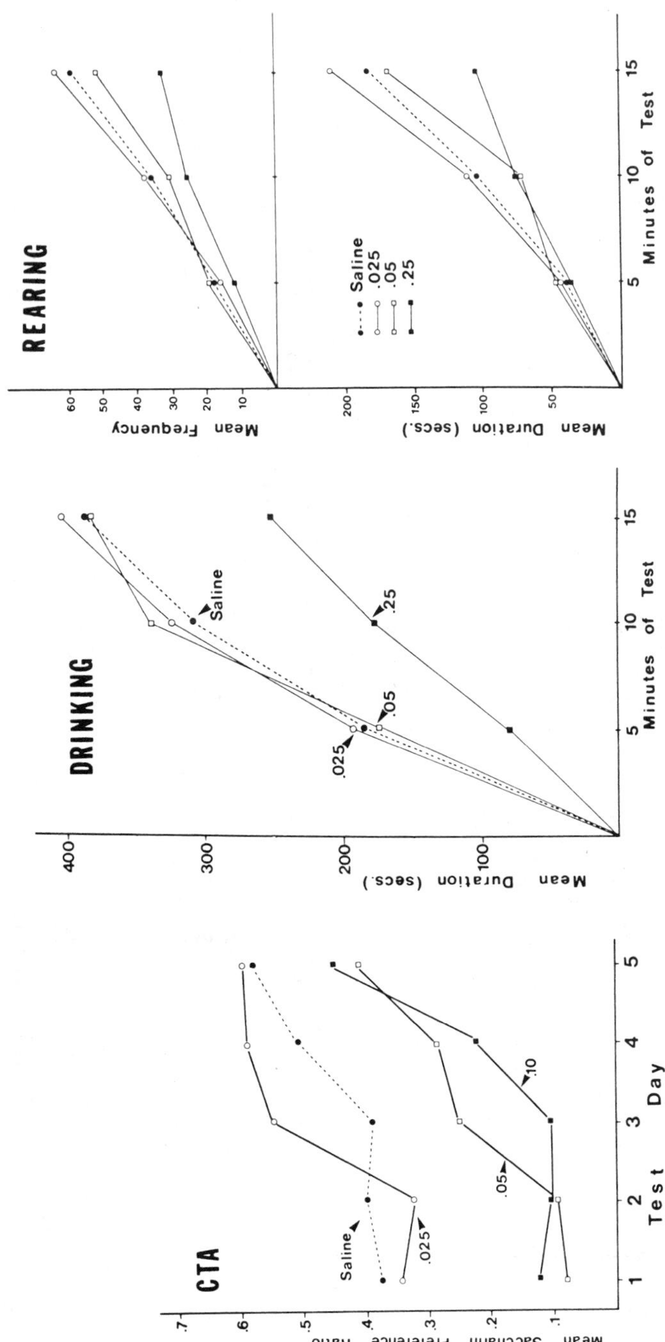

FIGURE 2. A comparison of the ability of physostigmine to produce taste aversions (left panel), suppress water consumption (center panel), and decrease rearing (right panel). (After Parker *et al.*[11])

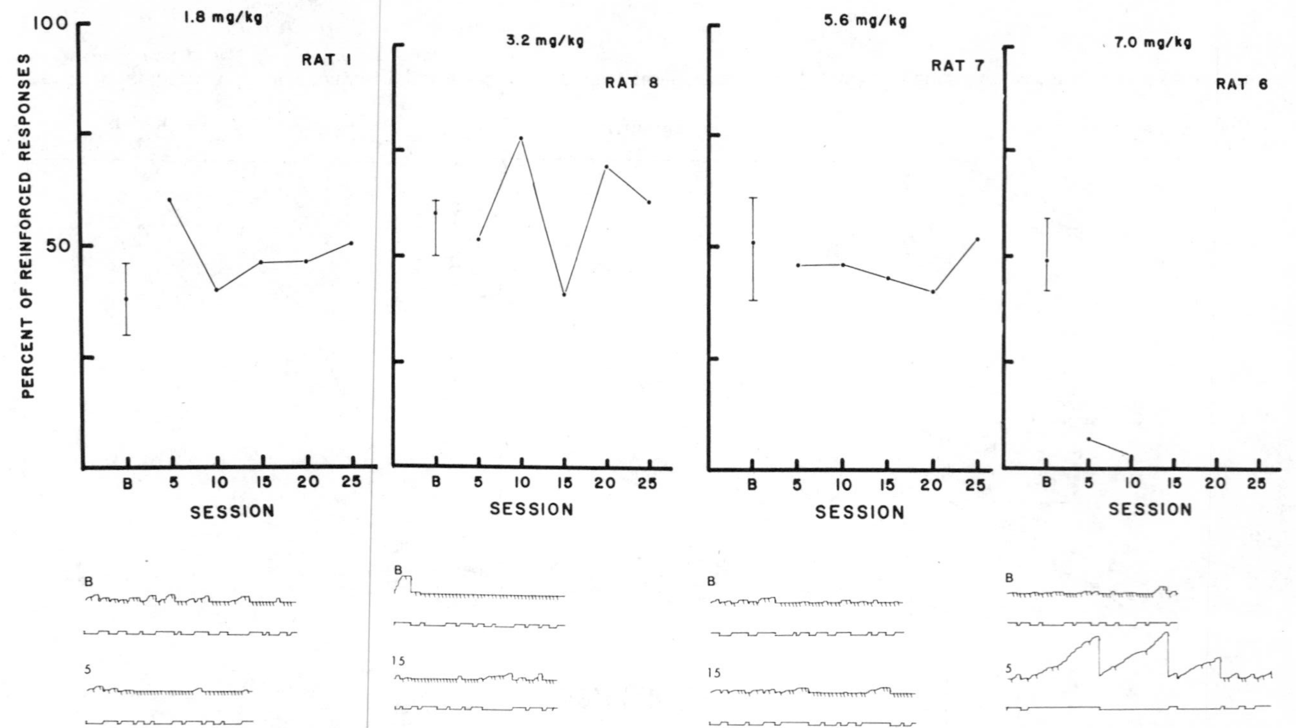

FIGURE 3. The effects of various dose of TMT on DRL performance. The top part of each panel illustrates the percent of reinforced responses at each dose. The lower panel illustrates cumulative records taken from sessions prior to (B) and following TMT exposure. (After Mastropaolo *et al.*[16])

TABLE 3. Agents that Are Ineffective in Taste Aversions

ACTH (Smotherman & Levine, 1978)
Ammonia (Gustavson & Gustavson, 1982)
Ammonium sulfate (Martin & Storlien, 1976)
Arabinoside (Bernstein *et al.*, 1980a)
Arginine HCl (Martin & Storlien, 1976)
Chloraphacinone (Marsh *et al.*, 1977)
Citric acid (Panksepp *et al.*, 1977)
Cytosine (Bernstein *et al.*, 1980)
Diphacinone (Marsh *et al.*, 1977)
Electroconvulsive shock (Berger, 1972)
Glucose (Martin & Storlien, 1976)
Haloperidol (Gale, 1984)
Heat (Green *et al.*, 1981)
Hot mustard (Gustavson & Gustavson, 1982)
Imipramine (Berger, 1972)
Melanocyte stimulating hormone (MSH) (Golus *et al.*, 1981)
Melatonin (Golus *et al.*, 1981)
Methaqualone (Jolicoeur *et al.*, 1977)
Methylprylon (Jolicoeur *et al.*, 1977)
Pimozide (Pfaus & Riley, unpublished)
Propranolol (Gale, 1984)
Quinine (Gustavson & Gustavson, 1982)
Saccharin (Kutscher *et al.*, 1979)
Sodium chloride (Kutscher *et al.*, 1977)
Sucrose-octa-acetate (Aravich & Sclafani, 1980)
Walker tumors (Bernstein & Fenner, 1983)
Vincristin (Bernstein *et al.*, 1980a)

Note: To be included in this table, the agent could not have been reported to condition a taste aversion. For complete references see Riley & Tuck.[41]

Convulsant Property of Drug

Although the basis for the failure of many of the MISSES to condition a taste aversion may be the dose examined or the number of conditioning trials administered, there are other possible explanations for some of the compounds, e.g., sodium cyanide.[13] Although cyanide has many effects, e.g., tissue asphyxiation, one well known characteristic is its convulsant property. It is quite possible that when a taste is paired

TABLE 4. Toxins that Are Ineffective in Inducing Taste Aversions

Aluminum chloride (Wellman *et al.*, 1984)
Baygon (Reiter, 1982)
Chloraphacinone (Marsh *et al.*, 1977)
Diphacinone (Marsh *et al.*, 1977)
Gallamine triethiodide (Ionescu & Buresova, 1977)
Methylchlorophenoxyacetic acid (MacPhail, unpublished)
Propoxur (MacPhail, 1980)
Pyrrolopyrimidine (Ionescu & Buresova, 1977)
Sodium cyanide (Nachman & Hartley, 1975)
Sodium malonate (Ionescu & Buresova, 1977)
Warfarin (Nachman & Hartley, 1975)

Note: To be included in this table, the toxin could not have been reported to condition a taste aversion. For complete references see Riley & Tuck.[41]

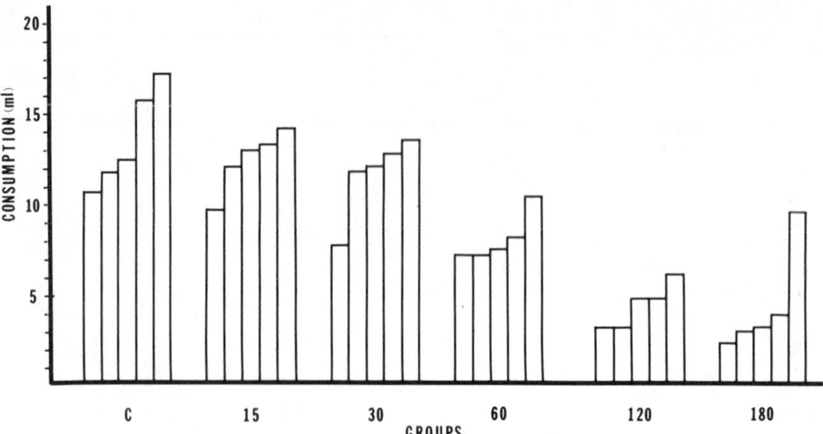

FIGURE 4. Consumption of saccharin for individual subjects previously injected with various doses (.15, .30, .60, 1.20, and 1.80 mEq) of 0.15 M LiCl following the consumption of saccharin. Subjects in Group C served as vehicle-injected controls. (After Dacanay *et al.*[17])

with cyanide, its convulsant property affects its association with the taste. In other words, the taste-cyanide association may be disrupted by the cyanide-induced convulsions (the weak aversions induced by strychnine could also be examined in this context). There have been several actual assessments of this possibility.[13,14] For example, following the demonstration that 4 mg/kg of cyanide did not condition a taste aversion, Ionescu and Buresova[13] gave this dose to rats receiving a pairing of a novel tasting saccharin solution and LiCl. Cyanide had no effect on the acquisition of the LiCl-induced taste aversion, suggesting that the convulsant property of cyanide was insufficient to affect conditioning with a second aversive agent (for a similar analysis with strychnine, see Nachman & Hartley[14]). Although the failure of cyanide to condition a taste aversion is unlikely to be a result of its convulsant property, it remains unclear if other MISSES are or could be a function of any associative disruption produced by the putative toxin. Given that a number of reports have demonstrated that associations between a taste and an established toxin can be disrupted by convulsant drugs, e.g., metrazol, or manipulations that affect cortical processing, e.g., electroconvulsive shock and cortical spreading depression,[23] this associative interference remains a possibility.

Duration of Drug Action

Another possible explanation for the weakness or failure of toxins such as strychnine and cyanide to condition aversions may be related to their duration of action. For each of these agents, the duration of their effects is very brief. Several reports have noted that drug duration may be an important variable in the conditioning of taste aversions.[24,25] Initial support for this hypothesis came from the finding that aversion-inducing drugs are typically more effective when administered intraperitoneally than intravenously, presumably because of the short duration of action associated with intravenous administration.[26] More recently, however, this hypothesis has been directly addressed. For example, Goudie and Dickens[25] demonstrated that although

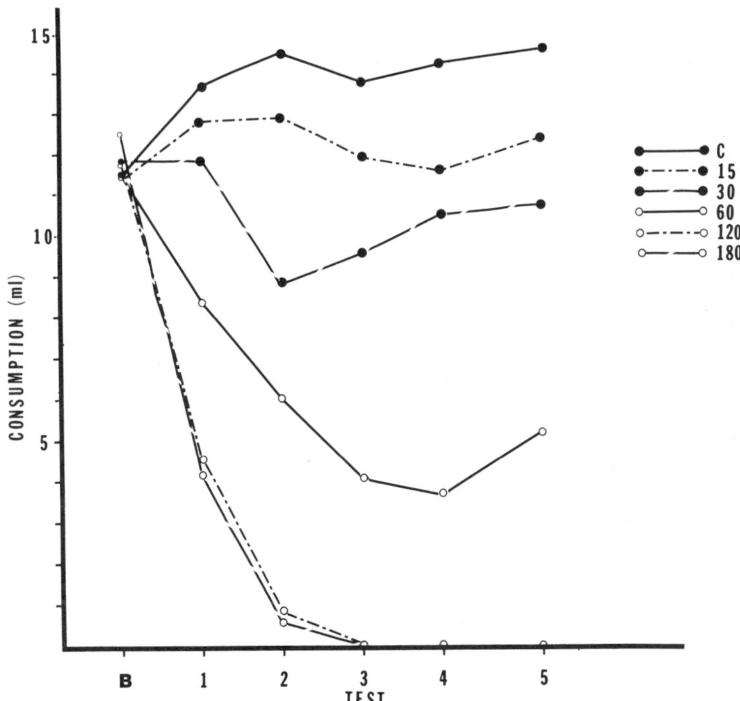

FIGURE 5. The effects of repeated conditioning trials on taste aversions induced by various doses of LiCl. (After Dacanay *et al.*[17])

a 30-min exposure to nitrous oxide induced only weak taste aversions, even when repeated conditioning trials were administered, nitrous oxide did induce taste aversions when the exposure was increased to one and four hours, a manipulation that increased the duration of the effects of nitrous oxide but not its overall dose. Similarly, the administration of the metabolic inhibitor, SKF 525A, to rats receiving a pairing of saccharin and *d*-amphetamine (a manipulation that slowed the action of amphetamine) potentiated aversions induced by amphetamine.[27]

Although this hypothesis has not been tested with any of the known toxin failures (see MISSES, TABLE 4), it has been examined with cocaine,[28] a compound that produces weak aversions, even when high doses are administered, repeated conditioning trials are given, or the more sensitive two-bottle aversion test is used. Instead of administering cocaine intraperitoneally following access to a novel taste solution, Gale[28] administered cocaine subcutaneously in a highly concentrated single bolus. Because of its concentration, cocaine induced vasoconstriction, an effect that substantially reduced the absorption of cocaine and consequently prolonged its duration of action. This procedure produced robust and clear dose-related taste aversions.

Delayed Onset of Drug Action

Although conditioned taste aversions have been reported to be acquired when there

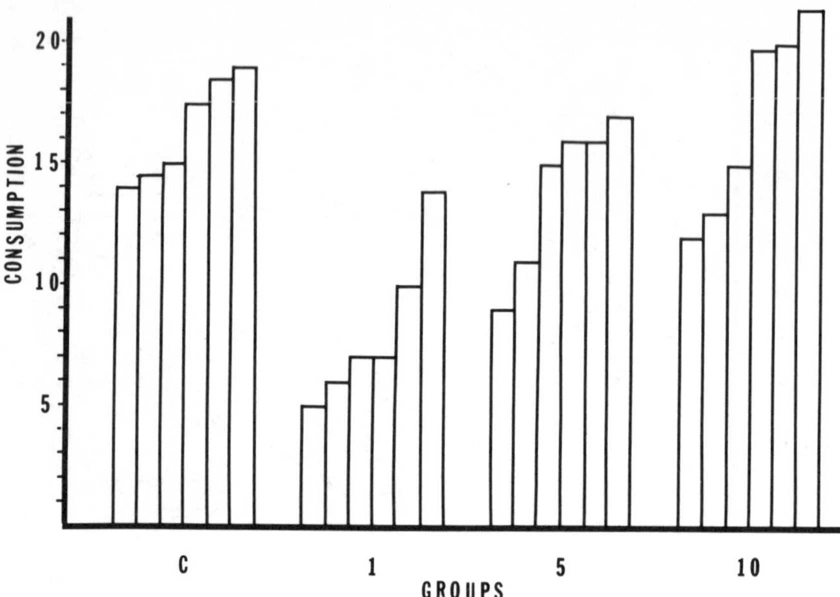

FIGURE 6. Consumption of saccharin for individual subjects previously given an injection of 1.8 mEq, 0.15 M LiCl 1, 5, or 10 hours following the consumption of saccharin. (After Riley *et al.*[31])

is a long delay between consumption of the taste solution and the onset of the drug's effects,[29] as illustrated in FIGURE 6 the longer the interval separating consumption and toxicosis, the weaker the aversion.[30,31] In fact, there is little evidence that any aversion is acquired with delays longer than 8–12 hours. This temporal constraint in associative learning with taste aversions may offer an explanation for the failure or weakness of several agents to condition aversions, e.g., warfarin and thallium sulfate.[13,14] For example, the effects of thallium sulfate are typically delayed between 30–36 hours post administration. Although on a typical taste aversion conditioning trial an animal may be given an injection of thallium sulfate immediately following consumption of a novel tasting saccharin solution, the effects of the toxin would be delayed beyond the point at which the animal could acquire an association, i.e., greater than 12 hours. Because of this delay, an aversion would not be acquired and the CTA paradigm would classify thallium as a nontoxin.[14]

Although a clear problem, Riley *et al.*[31] and Tuck *et al.*[32] have recently examined several modifications of the taste aversion design that may detect delayed-onset toxins. For example, instead of offering deprived animals limited access to a novel solution immediately before administering a toxin, Tuck *et al.*[32] examined the conditioning of taste aversions in nondeprived animals. In this procedure, different groups of nondeprived rats were given access to saccharin and injected with LiCl 12, 24, or 36 hours into the saccharin access period (the injection of LiCl was delayed as a simulation of a delayed-onset toxin that would have been given at the initiation of saccharin access but whose effects would be delayed 12, 24, and 36 hours). The logic underlying this modification was based on the fact that because nondeprived animals drink in multiple, discrete bouts throughout the day and night (FIGURE 7), they would likely be

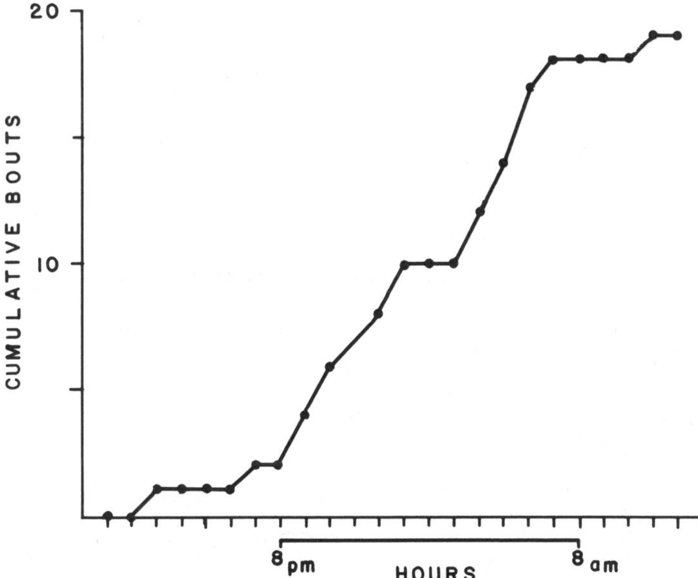

FIGURE 7. Cumulative number of drinking bouts over a 24-hour period for subjects given ad lib access to saccharin. (After Tuck *et al.*[32])

drinking or sampling the taste solution at the onset of the toxic effects of the compound, even though the effects of the toxin were delayed. This pattern of consumption would provide temporal contiguity between tasting the solution and toxicosis, a condition necessary for conditioning and under which aversions are maximally acquired.

As illustrated in FIGURE 8, nondeprived rats acquired robust aversions to saccharin (as compared to nonpoisoned controls) when the effects of the toxin were delayed 12 hours into the drinking period. Although weaker, aversions were also acquired when the effects of the toxin were delayed 24 and 36 hours (FIGURE 8). The weaker aversions at the longer delays presumably reflect the fact that these groups had 24 and 36 hours preexposure to the saccharin solution before the onset of the effects of the toxin (LiCl), a variable often reported to attenuate aversion learning.[21,33]

Although aversions can clearly be acquired when the effects of a toxin are delayed into the drinking period, it remains unclear if delayed-onset toxins such as warfarin and thallium sulfate will condition aversions in nondeprived animals. To date, the procedure has not been directly tested with such toxins. A design recently used by Bernstein and her colleagues, however, clearly suggests that this procedure could be effective. For example, Bernstein and Sigmundi[34] reported that rats implanted with pieces of PW-739 tumors and then given continuous access to a novel-tasting food for 10 consecutive days five to six weeks after tumor implantation subsequently avoided consumption of that food when given a choice between it and an alternative food that was not present during the growth of the tumor. In all cases, the rats avoided the food that had been present during the 10-day access period, i.e., the rats acquired a conditioned aversion to the tumor-associated food. Although there was no direct assessment of the onset of the toxic effects of the tumor, presumably the consumption of

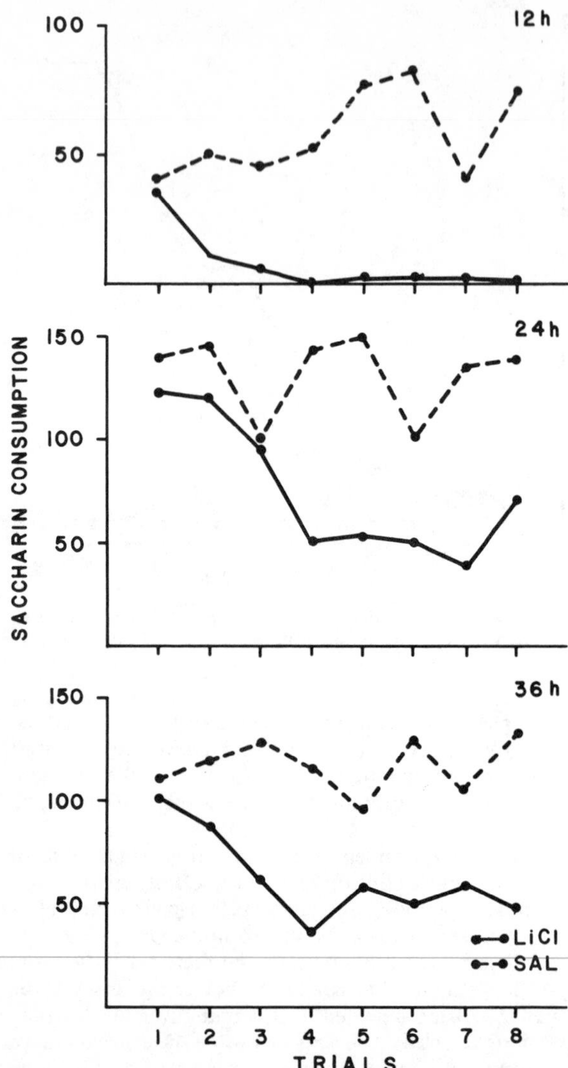

FIGURE 8. Consumption of saccharin over repeated conditioning trials by groups injected with LiCl 12, 24, and 36 hours into their saccharin access period. (After Tuck *et al.*[32])

the food was contiguous with the delayed effects. This assessment in animals subjected to the delayed toxicity of tumor growth does suggest that delayed-onset toxins could condition aversions under the nondeprived procedure.[4]

Although there clearly are examples of known toxins that do not induce taste aversions, the issue is how these apparent MISSES are interpreted. One interpretation is that the taste aversion paradigm is an inadequate index of toxicity. A second interpretation is that the taste aversion paradigm is in fact a sensitive index of toxicity and that

TABLE 5. Procedural Variations of the Taste Aversion Paradigm

Establish a dose-response function for the compound.
Give multiple conditioning trials with the compound.
Examine the compound for its effects on the conditioning of a taste aversion by a toxin that has been established to be effective as an aversion-inducing agent.
Examine the efficacy of the compound to induce taste aversions after its action has been slowed.
Examine the compound in nondeprived animals with continuous access to a taste solution.

the failure of compounds with known toxicity to induce taste aversions is a function of the specific paradigm in which the assessments are made. As described above, there were at least five variations of the typical taste aversion paradigm by which the failures could be examined for their efficacy in inducing taste aversions. According to this interpretation, when failures do occur the compound should be examined within these aforementioned procedural alternatives (TABLE 5).

It could be suggested that any model of toxicity can have some number of failures which is acceptable and that it is not necessary or possible to account for every instance in which the model fails. In addition, running the failures through the suggested "conditioned taste aversion battery" weakens the cost effectiveness of the taste aversion model. However, until it is clear that the CTA design does not account for the noted failures or that such procedural variations affect its cost effectiveness, these alternatives should be considered.

HITS AND CORRECT REJECTIONS

Thus far, the analysis of the utility of the taste aversion design as an index of toxicity has focused on the issues of MISSES and FALSE ALARMS. A reexamination of FIGURE 1, however, illustrates another concern. This involves the HITS and CORRECT REJECTIONS. A HIT occurs when a compound with known toxicity is classified as a toxin by the CTA design, i.e., it induces a taste aversion. Similarly, a CORRECT REJECTION occurs when a compound with no corroborative evidence of toxicity is classified as a nontoxin by the CTA design, i.e., it does not induce a taste aversion. The problem is not that taste aversions never produce HITS or CORRECT REJECTIONS, but how one interprets these findings. Although one might classify a compound as toxic if it induces a taste aversion, the taste aversion procedure does little in determining the effects of the toxin. The meaning of a HIT and a CORRECT REJECTION remains unclear. This failure to characterize the toxic effects of a compound is a severe limitation of the CTA paradigm, a limitation shared by many behavioral indices of drug toxicity. The question becomes, therefore, can the CTA design go beyond indexing a compound's toxicity to characterizing its effects.

One way to use the CTA design to characterize the toxic effects of a compound is by determining the mechanism underlying taste aversions. If this could be determined, it would be possible to speculate on some of the effects of the toxin. A brief examination of the myriad agents effective in inducing taste aversions (TABLE 6) suggests that although it is possible that there is some characteristic common to each of these compounds that underlies their ability to induce aversions, e.g., stress, disruption in homeostasis, or novelty, a more parsimonious conclusion is that each compound (or class of compounds) produces a specific effect, each of which is effective in inducing an aversion. What remains to be determined is what these effects are. If

TABLE 6. Agents that Are Effective in Inducing Taste Aversions

Acetaldehyde (Brown *et al.*, 1978)
Acrylamide (Anderson *et al.*, 1982)
Adriamycin (Bernstein *et al.*, 1980a)
Aflatoxin B1 (Rappold *et al.*, 1984)
Alloxan monohydrate (Brookshire *et al.*, 1972)
Allyl sulfate (Maruniak *et al.*, 1983)
Alpha-methyl-*p*-tyrosine (Carey & Goodall, 1974)
Alpha naphthylthiourea (Rzoska, 1953)
Amobarbital (Vogel & Nathan, 1975)
Apomorphine (Braun *et al.*, 1981)
Arsenic (Rzoska, 1953)
Bal (Peele, unpublished)
Barium carbonate (Rzoska, 1953)
Bombesin (Deutsch, 1980)
CI-628 (King & Cox, 1976)
Cadmium chloride (Wellman *et al.*, 1984)
Cannabichrome (Corcoran *et al.*, 1974)
Cannabigerol (Corcoran *et al.*, 1974)
Carbaryl (MacPhail, 1981)
Chloral hydrate (Kallman *et al.*, 1983)
Chlordiazepoxide (Cappell *et al.*, 1973)
Chlordiazepoxide + cocaine (Goudie, 1981)
Chlordimeform (MacPhail & Leander, 1980)
Chlorphentermine (Booth *et al.*, 1977)
Chlorpromazine (Berger, 1972)
Cholecystokinin (Deutsch & Hardy, 1977)
Cobalt chloride (Wellman *et al.*, 1984)
Cobra venom (Islam, 1978)
Cocaine (D'Mello *et al.*, 1979)
Copper sulfate (Nachman & Hartley, 1975)
Compound 48/80 (Persinger, 1978)
Cortical spreading depression (Freedman & Ward, 1976)
Cycloheximide (Bolas *et al.*, 1979)
Cyclophosphamide (Ader *et al.*, 1978)
d-amphetamine (Cappell & LeBlanc, 1971)
d-amphetamine + chlorpromazine (Cappell & LeBlanc, 1971)
Deltamethrin (MacPhail & Gordon, 1981)
1,2-dichloroethane (Kallman *et al.*, 1983)
1,2-dichloroethylene (Kallman *et al.*, 1983)
2-deoxy-*d*-glucose (Thompson & Zagon, 1981)
Delta-8-THC (Corcoran *et al.*, 1974)
Delta-9-THC (Amit *et al.*, 1977)
Desipramine (Lorden & Nunn, 1982)
Diazepam (Gamzu, 1977)
Dichlorvos (Roney *et al.*, 1984)
Diethyldithiocarbamate (Peele & MacPhail, unpublished)
Diisobutyrlapomorphine (D'Mello *et al.*, 1981)
Diisoprophylfluorophosphate (Roney *et al.*, 1984)
d-isoproxerenol HCl (Margules, 1970)
d,l-cathinone (Foltin & Schuster, 1981)
DMSA (Peele, unpublished)
Emetine (Revusky & Gorry, 1973)
Endosulfan (Peele & MacPhail, unpublished)
Epinephrine (Caza *et al.*, 1982)
Ergocornine hydrogen maleate (King *et al.*, 1979)

Ergocornine methane sulfonate (King & Cox, 1976)
Ethanol (Cannon *et al.*, 1977)
Ether (Vogel & Nathan, 1975)
Ethylenedine citrate (Panksepp *et al.*, 1977)
Ethylenediamine dihydrochloride (Panksepp *et al.*, 1977)
Fenfluramine (Booth *et al.*, 1977)
5-fluoroucil (Bernstein & Webster, 1980)
Fluoroacetate (Howard *et al.*, 1977)
Fluoxetine (Lorden & Nunn, 1982)
Formaline (Woods *et al.*, 1971)
Hashish (Corcoran, 1973)
Histamine diphosphate (Levy *et al.*, 1974)
Histidine-free amino acid load (Booth & Simpson, 1974)
(−)-hydroxycitrate ethylenedime (Panksepp *et al.*, 1977)
(−)-hydroxycitric acid (Panksepp *et al.*, 1977)
Hypertonic procaine (Mineka *et al.*, 1972)
Insulin (Domjan & Levy, 1977)
Ipecac (Baker & Cannon, 1979)
Irradiation (Garcia & Koelling, 1967)
Isotonic procaine (Mineka *et al.*, 1972)
Ketamine (Etscorn & Parson, 1979)
Lead acetate (Dantzer, 1980)
l-amphetamine (Carey & Goodall, 1974)
Leydig tumors (Bernstein & Fenner, 1983)
Lithium carbonate (McFarland *et al.*, 1978)
Lithium chloride (Archer *et al.*, 1979)
Lorazepam (Berger, 1972)
Mercuric chloride (Klein *et al.*, 1974)
Mescaline (Cappel & LeBlanc, 1971)
Mestranol (Howard & Marsh, 1969)
Mesurol (Gustavson *et al.*, 1982)
Methamphetamine (Booth *et al.*, 1977)
Methiocarb (Mason & Reidinger, 1983)
Methotrexate (Ader, 1977)
Methyl atropine nitrate (Emmerick & Snowdon, 1976)
Methyl bromide (Miyagawa, 1982)
Methylmercury (Braun & Snyder, 1973)
Methylnitrate (Clody & Vogel, 1973)
Methylscopolamine (Braveman, 1975)
Metrazol (Golus & McGee, 1980)
Monosodium glutamate (Vogel & Nathan, 1975)
Morphine (Cappell *et al.*, 1973)
Naloxone (Frenk & Rogers, 1979)
n-butyraldoxime (Nachman *et al.*, 1970)
Neutron exposure (Garcia & Kimeldorf, 1960)
Nicotine (Etscorn, 1980)
Nitrogen mustard (Bernstein & Webster, 1980)
Nitrous oxide (Goudie & Dickins, 1978)
Oxythiamine (Seward & Greathouse, 1973)
Ozone (MacPhail & Hatch, unpublished)
Paraquat (Dey *et al.*, 1984)
Parathion (Roney *et al.*, 1984)
p-chloramphetamine (Goudie *et al.*, 1976)
p-chloromethamphetamine (Booth *et al.*, 1977)
p-chlorophenylaline (Nachman *et al.*, 1970)
Phencyclidine (Etscorn & Parson, 1979)
Phenobarbital (Vogel & Nathan, 1975)

Phenylpropanolamine (Wellman *et al.*, 1981)
p-hydroxyamphetamine (Booth *et al.*, 1977)
Physostigmine sulfate (Parker *et al.*, 1982)
Pilocarbamide (Gay *et al.*, 1975)
Plant homogenates (Yokel & Ogzewalla, 1981)
Proferrin (Feinberg, 1973)
Pseudo-coriolis effect (Lamon *et al.*, 1977)
Red squill (Nachman & Hartley, 1975)
Rotation (Braun & McIntosh, 1973)
Scopolamine (Berger, 1972)
Scopolamine methyl nitrate (Berger, 1972)
Scorpion venom (Islam, 1980)
Serum from irradiated donors (Garcia *et al.*, 1967b)
Sesame oil (Deutsch *et al.*, 1976)
Shock (Krane & Wagner, 1975)
Skin secretions (Mason *et al.*, 1982)
Smoke (Etscorn, 1980)
Sodium chloride + polyethylene glycol (Kutscher *et al.*, 1977)
Sodium fluoride (Ionescu & Buresova, 1977)
Sodium fluoroacetate (Nachman & Hartley, 1975)
Sodium iodoacetate (Ionescu & Buresova, 1977)
Strychnine sulfate (Howard *et al.*, 1968)
1,2-trichloroethane (Kallman *et al.*, 1983)
2,4,5-trichlorophenoxyacetic acid (Sjoden *et al.*, 1979)
Thallium sulfate (Nachman & Hartley, 1975)
Thiabendazole (Gustavson *et al.*, 1983)
Thiamine deficiency (Maier *et al.*, 1971)
Toluene (MacPhail & Tomlinson, unpublished)
Trichloroethylene (Kallman *et al.*, 1983)
Trichloromethane (Landauer *et al.*, 1982)
Triethyltin (MacPhail, 1982)
Trimethyltin (MacPhail, 1982)
Triphenyltin (MacPhail & Peele, unpublished)
Tryptophan-deficient diet (Treneer & Bernstein, 1981)
Vagotomy (Bernstein & Goehler, 1983b)
Vasopressin (Ettenberg *et al.*, 1983)
Viper venom (Islam *et al.*, 1982)
Win 35.428 (D'Mello *et al.*, 1979)

Note: To be included in this table, an agent had to have been reported to condition a taste aversion by at least a single study. For complete references see Riley & Tuck.[41]

they can be determined, it would be possible to characterize the specific toxicity of the aversion-inducing agents.

One note of caution is necessary before attempting to determine the specific mechanisms underlying taste aversions. It may be inappropriate simply to determine the toxic effects of a compound in any one behavioral test and assume that this is the characteristic of the compound that induces aversions. For example, trimethyltin, a compound very effective in inducing taste aversions,[10] is a known neurotoxicant that does specific damage to the limbic system, primarily to the subfields CA1 and CA3 of the hippocampus. This hippocampal damage is corroborated behaviorally in that a single administration of trimethyltin disrupts performance in a number of behavioral designs thought to be mediated in part by the hippocampus, e.g., radial-arm maze, Hebb-Williams maze, and DRL. The difficulty with assuming that this damage to the hippocampus is responsible for trimethyltin-induced aversions is the fact that the

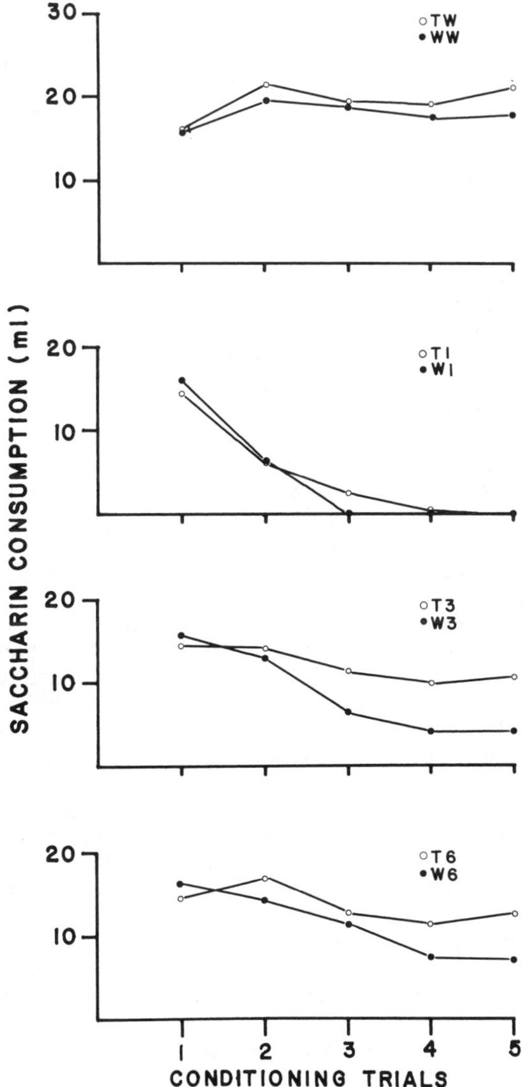

FIGURE 9. Consumption of saccharin by groups previously injected with 1.8 mEq, 0.15 M LiCl immediately, 3 or 6 hours following the consumption of saccharin. The groups labeled (T), e.g., Groups TW, TI, T3, and T6, were pretreated 21 days earlier with trimethyltin. The groups labeled (W), e.g., Groups WW, WI, W3, and W6, were pretreated with distilled water. (From Riley *et al.*[30] With permission from *Neurotoxicology*.)

dose producing the behavioral and anatomical effects is 500% greater than that needed to condition taste aversions.[10,30] However, even if the dose of trimethyltin that produces hippocampal damage was determined to be the same as that which induces taste aversions, it would still be unclear if the hippocampal damage was underlying the aversion.

This caution, however, does not mean that it is impossible to determine the mechanism underlying taste aversion learning with specific compounds. In fact, over the past 10 years considerable attention has been devoted to this question.[23,35–38] For example, to determine where a compound acts to induce an aversion, the aversion-inducing agent can be given centrally or peripherally or in various forms that differentially penetrate the blood-brain barrier. If it is determined that the compound works centrally, it can be infused into different brain areas to determine its specific site of action. Finally, various isomers of the same compound can be given to determine if its effects are mediated by a drug/receptor complex. Chemical interventions and electrolytic lesions can also be helpful in determining the neurophysiological mediation of taste aversions. For example, in relation to chemical infusions, the noradrenergic neurotoxicant DSP4 has been reported to have no effect on LiCl-induced aversions, suggesting that the noradrenergic system is not involved in aversions produced by LiCl.[39] Similarly, in relation to electrolytic lesions, destruction of the periaqueductal gray region of the midbrain attenuates aversions induced by morphine sulfate but has no effect on LiCl-induced aversions.[46]

Although none of these manipulations delineate the specific mechanism responsible for a specific agent to induce taste aversions, each of them restricts the range of systems involved and directs research towards elucidating the underlying system. The research does suggest that considerable attempts have been and are being made to determine the mechanism necessary for the formation of taste aversions induced by specific compounds. As such systems are defined, some specificity as to the toxic effects of the compound can also be determined.

Determining the mechanisms underlying taste aversions involves a physiological approach to assaying the effects of a toxin. Recently, another approach has been introduced that can be used to characterize the behavioral mechanisms underlying the toxicity of a compound. In this approach, the taste aversion design is used as a baseline on which a drug's effect can be examined.[13,14,30] For example, Riley *et al.*[30] gave water-deprived rats a single gavage of either physiological saline or the neurotoxin trimethyltin chloride. Twenty-one days later, these animals were given 20-min access to a novel saccharin solution and were injected with LiCl either immediately, three hours or six hours following the saccharin exposure. As illustrated in FIGURE 9, animals pretreated with trimethyltin did display taste aversions when the interval between saccharin consumption and the injection of LiCl was delayed by one hour but did not display aversions when the delay was three or six hours. These results suggest a memory deficit caused by the physiological effects of this toxin in the trimethyltin-pretreated animals. The long-delay taste aversion paradigm, therefore, was effective in characterizing (and corroborating) the memorial deficits that result from exposure to trimethyltin.

Research characterizing the toxicity of a compound is new. As illustrated, however, by attempting to determine the mechanism underlying taste aversions and by using the taste aversion paradigm as a tool, considerable information can be obtained regarding the physiological and behavioral effects of a toxin. The taste aversion procedure, then, becomes substantially more than a simple screen or index. The effects of the toxin may also be characterized by the taste aversion design.

CONCLUSION

This review has attempted to provide an overview of the issues surrounding the use of the conditioned taste aversion procedure in indexing drug toxicity. The major basis for considering the taste aversion design as an index is the fact that most known toxins do reliably condition taste aversions. As described, however, there are a number of criticisms with the use of this procedure, i.e., the occurrence of FALSE ALARMS and MISSES and the interpretation of HITS and CORRECT REJECTIONS. The present review has attempted to address each of these criticisms to illustrate that either the data on which the criticisms are based are subject to alternative interpretation (FALSE ALARMS), are a product of the specific designs used in the toxin assay (MISSES), or are just beginning to be analyzed (HITS and CORRECT REJECTIONS). Whether the responses to the criticisms will effectively substantiate its use as an index remains to be seen. Until then, however, the fact that taste aversions generally corroborate known toxicity and are relatively sensitive and very cost effective argues for its continued inclusion as one element in a broad battery of behavioral screens.

ACKNOWLEDGMENTS

The authors would like to thank R. J. Dacanay, J. P. Mastropaolo, and C. L. Wetherington for helpful comments on an earlier draft of this manuscript.

REFERENCES

1. GARCIA, J. & F. ERVIN. 1968. Commun. Behav. Biol. **1:** 389–415.
2. REVUSKY, S. & J. GARCIA. 1970. *In* Psychology of Learning and Motivation: Advances in Research and Theory. G. Bower & J. Spence, Eds. Vol. 4. Academic Press. New York.
3. RILEY, A. & C. CLARKE. 1977. *In* Learning Mechanisms in Food Selection. L. Barker, M. Best & M. Domjan, Eds. Baylor University Press. Waco, TX.
4. ROZIN, P. & J. KALAT. 1971. Psychol. Rev. **78**: 459–486.
5. BERNSTEIN, I. 1978. Science **200**: 1302–1303.
6. ZELLNER, D., R. DACANAY & A. RILEY. 1984. Pharmac. Biochem. Behav. **20:** 175–180.
7. GUSTAVSON, C. 1977. *In* Learning Mechanisms and Food Selection. L. Barker, M. Best & M. Domjan, Eds. Baylor University Press. Waco, TX.
8. ELKINS, R. 1975. Int. J. Addict. **10**: 157–209.
9. LANDAUER, M., M. LYNCH, R. BALSTER & M. KALLMAN. 1982. Neurobehav. Toxicol. Teratol. **4**: 305–309.
10. MACPHAIL, R. 1982. Neurobehav. Toxicol. Teratol. **4**: 225–230.
11. PARKER, L., S. HUTCHISON & A. RILEY. 1982. Neurobehav. Toxicol. Teratol. **4**: 93–98.
12. GOUDIE, A. 1979. Neuropharmacology **18**: 971–979.
13. IONESCU, E. & O. BURESOVA. 1977. Pharmac. Biochem. Behav. **6**: 368–371.
14. NACHMAN, M. & P. HARTLEY. 1975. J. Comp. Physiol. Psychol. **89**: 1010–1018.
15. RONDEAU, D., F. JOLICOEUR, A. MERKEL & M. WAYNER. 1981. Neurosci. Biobehav. Rev. **5**: 279–294.
16. MASTROPAOLO, J., R. DACANAY, B. LUNA, D. TUCK & A. RILEY. 1984. Neurobehav. Toxicol. Teratol. **6**: 193–199.
17. DACANAY, R., J. MASTROPAOLO, D. OLIN & A. RILEY. 1984. Neurobev. Toxicol. Teratol. **6**: 9–11.
18. NACHMAN, M. & J. ASHE. 1973. Physiol. Behav. **10**: 73–78.
19. GARCIA, J. & D. KIMELDORF. 1957. J. Comp. Physiol. Psychol. **50**: 180–183.
20. RILEY, A., W. JACOBS & V. LOLORDO. 1976. J. Comp. Physiol. Psychol. **6**: 96–100.
21. RILEY, A., W. JACOBS & J. MASTROPAOLO. 1983. Bull. Psychon. Soc. **21**: 221–224.
22. BERGER, B. 1972. J. Comp. Physiol. Psychol. **81**: 475–479.
23. BURES, J. & O. BURESOVA. 1977. *In* Food Aversion Learning. N. Miligram, L. Krames & T. Alloway, Eds. Plenum Press. New York.
24. CAPPELL, H. & A. LEBLANC. 1977. *In* Food Aversion Learning. N. Milgram, L. Krames & T. Alloway, Eds. Plenum Press. New York.

25. GOUDIE, A. & D. DICKINS. 1978. Pharmac. Biochem. Behav. **9**: 587–592.
26. COUSSENS, W. 1973. *In* Drug Addiction: Neurobiology and Influences on Behavior. J. Singh & H. Lal, Eds. Vol. 3. Symposium Specialists. Miami.
27. GOUDIE, A. & E. THORNTON. 1977. IRCS Med. Sci. **5**: 93.
28. GALE, K. 1984. *In* Mechanisms of tolerance and dependence. C. Sharp, Ed. U.S. Government Printing Office. Washington, D.C.
29. GARCIA, J., F. ERVIN & R. KOELLING. 1966. Psychon. Sci. **5**: 121–122.
30. RILEY, A., R. DACANAY & J. MASTROPAOLO. 1984. Neurotoxicology **5**: 291–296.
31. RILEY, A., J. MASTROPAOLO & J. PFAUS. 1982. Soc. Neurosci. **8**: 357.
32. TUCK, D., G. SHOENING, J. MASTROPAOLO & A. RILEY. 1984. Southern Society of Philosophy and Psychology. Columbia, South Carolina.
33. ELKINS, R. 1973. Behav. Biol. **9**: 221–226.
34. BERNSTEIN, I. & R. SIGMUNDI. 1980. Science **209**: 416–418.
35. ASHE, J. & M. NACHMAN. 1980. *In* Progress in Psychobiology and Physiological Psychology. J. Sprague & A. Epstein, Eds. Academic Press. New York.
36. GARCIA, J., K. RUSINIAK, S. KIEFER & F. BERMUDEZ-RATTONI. 1982. *In* Conditioning. C. Woody, Ed. Plenum Press. New York.
37. GASTON, K. 1978. Physiol. Psychol. **6**: 340–353.
38. KOLB, B., A. NONNEMAN & P. ABPLANALPH. 1977. Bull. Psychon. Soc. **10**: 389–392.
39. ARCHER T. 1982. Scan. J. Psych. **1**: 61–71.
40. BLAIR, R. & Z. AMIT. 1981. Pharmac. Biochem. Behav. **15**: 651–655.
41. RILEY, A. & D. TUCK. 1985. Ann. N. Y. Acad. Sci. (This volume.)

Conditioned Taste Aversions and Immunopharmacology[a]

ROBERT ADER

Division of Behavioral and Psychosocial Medicine
Department of Psychiatry
University of Rochester School of Medicine and Dentistry
Rochester, New York 14642

The present paper does not deal with the phenomenon of taste aversion learning, per se, but with an application of the taste aversion conditioning paradigm to the modification of immune responses. Considering what is known about the conditioning of pharmacologic effects,[1] conditioned immunopharmacologic effects might not be unexpected. However, the immune system is generally thought to be an autonomous agency of defense—a largely self-regulated network of cellular interactions functioning to discriminate between what is a part of itself and what is "non-self" and, in the latter instance, to defend the organism against foreign material. Thus far, relatively little attention has been directed to the role of the central nervous system in the modulation of immunity. Within the past few years, converging data from different disciplines have provided compelling evidence that the immune system is integrated with other physiological processes and subject to the influence of central nervous system function. Observations of conditioned alterations in immunologic reactivity are a part of this evidence.

The residual effects of some immunopharmacologic agents can be long-lasting. Similarly, the response to antigens are long-lasting. Moreover, the initial response to antigenic stimulation can not necessarily be precisely reproduced by subsequent stimulation with that same antigen. For these reasons, one-trial taste aversion conditioning has been an effective paradigm for studying the effects of behavior on immune responses. In the present paper, then, I propose to describe some of the data on the acquisition and extinction of humoral and cell-mediated immune responses, describe the application of this conditioning paradigm in modifying the development of autoimmune disease in New Zealand mice, and discuss the heuristic value of viewing some pharmacotherapeutic regimens as conditioning protocols.

CONDITIONED ALTERATIONS IN HUMORAL AND CELL-MEDIATED IMMUNITY

The hypothesis that conditioning could be applied to the modulation of immunity was derived from the serendipitous observation of mortality among animals being

[a] Preparation of this chapter and the author's research were supported by a Research Scientist Award (MHO6318) from the National Institute of Mental Health and by research grants from the National Institute of Neurological and Communicative Disorders and Stroke (NS 15071) and the Kroc Foundation.

tested in a taste aversion learning situation in which cyclophosphamide, a potent immunosuppressive drug, was used as the unconditioned stimulus.[2] In this study, different volumes of a saccharin drinking solution, the conditioned stimulus (CS), were paired with a constant dose of cyclophosphamide, the unconditioned stimulus (UCS). As expected, this single CS-UCS pairing resulted in an aversion of the saccharin-flavored solution when it was subsequently presented, and the strength of the aversion and its resistance to extinction were directly related to the volume of saccharin consumed on the single conditioning trial. Unexpectedly, several rats died during the course of extinction trials. Furthermore, mortality rate tended to vary directly with the amount of saccharin consumed on the single conditioning trial. In order to account for these observations, it was hypothesized that pairing a neutral stimulus with an immunosuppressive drug could result in the conditioning of an immunosuppressive response. If an immunosuppressive response was elicited when conditioned rats were repeatedly reexposed to such a CS, these animals might have become susceptible to any latent pathogen that existed in the laboratory environment. Based on these speculations, a study was designed to examine conditioned immunosuppression.[3]

Individually caged rats were adapted to drinking their daily allotment of fluid during a single 15-minute period at the same time each day. On the training day, conditioned rats received a sodium saccharin solution instead of plain water and drinking was followed by an intraperitoneal (i.p.) injection of 50 mg/kg cyclophosphamide (CY). Nonconditioned rats were given plain water as usual but were similarly injected with CY. (In subsequent studies, nonconditioned animals were exposed to saccharin as well as CY, but in a noncontingent manner.) A placebo group drank plain water and was injected with an equal volume of vehicle.

Three days after conditioning, animals were randomly assigned to subgroups. Thirty minutes after immunization with sheep red blood cells (SRBC), one subgroup of conditioned animals (Group CS) was given a single drinking bottle containing saccharin-flavored water and was then injected i.p. with saline. A second subgroup of conditioned animals (Group CSo) received plain water and was injected with saline. Group CSo was included to control for the effects of conditioning, per se. To define the unconditioned immunosuppressive effects of CY, a third conditioned subgroup (Group US) was given plain water and an injection of CY. Following immunization nonconditioned animals (Group NC) were provided with saccharin-flavored water and injected with saline while the placebo group (Group P) received plain water and remained unmanipulated. Independent subgroups of conditioned animals were reexposed to saccharin on the day they were immunized (Day 0), three days after the injection of SRBC, or on Days 0 and 3. Subgroups of nonconditioned animals were exposed to saccharin on a corresponding schedule. Blood samples were obtained six days after immunization for the assay of hemagglutinating antibody titer.

The effects of conditioning on antibody responses to SRBC are shown in FIGURE 1. Conditioned rats reexposed to saccharin on Day 0 or 3 did not differ and were combined into a single group characterized as having had a single reexposure to the CS. Nonconditioned subgroups also did not differ and were similarly combined. The relationship among the several groups were exactly as predicted. Placebo-treated animals had the highest antibody titers, and CY treatment at the time of immunization suppressed the immune response. Conditioned animals that were reexposed to saccharin at the time of immunization and/or three days later had lower hemagglutinating antibody titers than conditioned animals that were not reexposed to saccharin (group CSo), nonconditioned animals provided with saccharin, and the placebo-treated group. These original findings, then, supported the hypothesis that pairing saccharin consumption,

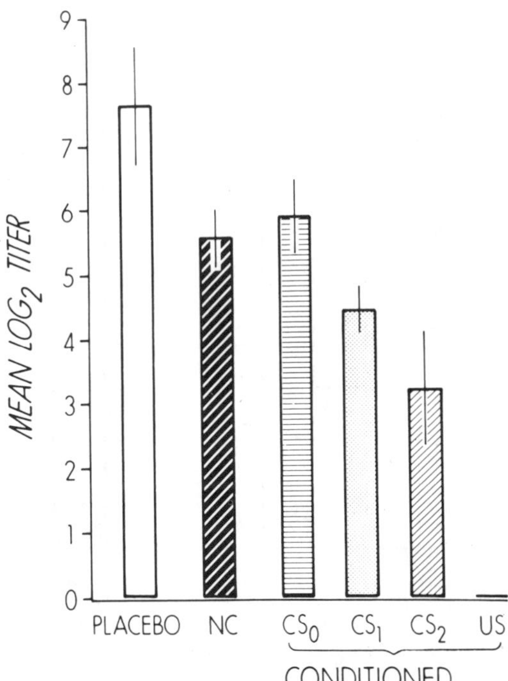

FIGURE 1. Hemagglutinating antibody titers (mean ± SE) measured six days after immunization with SRBC. NC = nonconditioned rats; CSo = conditioned animals that were not reexposed to the CS after SRBC; CS_1 = conditioned animals reexposed to the CS on one occasion; CS_2 = conditioned animals reexposed to the CS on two occasions; US = conditoned rats treated with CY at the time of antigen administration; P = placebo-treated animals. (From Ader and Cohen.[3] Reprinted by permission of Elsevier North-Holland, Inc.)

an immunologically neutral stimulus, with an immunosuppressive drug would enable saccharin to elicit a conditioned immunosuppressive response.

Although the magnitude of conditioning effects has not been large, the effects are quite consistent and independently reproducible under a variety of experimental conditions. We have, for example, increased the interval between conditioning and immunization in consideration of the residual effects of CY,[4] used sucrose instead of saccharin as the CS and methotrexate instead of CY as the UCS,[5] varied the dose of CY,[5] and varied the nature of the antigen using mice instead of rats.[6] A conditioned suppression of humoral immunity was observed in all these studies. Also, others[7,8] have independently verified our initial observations.

In order to control for the difference in fluid intake between experimental and control groups, reexposure to the CS has been accomplished using a preference testing procedure in which animals could choose between drinking plain or saccharin-flavored water. Under these conditions, the total fluid consumption of experimental and control groups does not differ, but conditioned animals still show an aversion to saccharin (FIGURE 2) and a conditioned immunosuppressive response (FIGURE 3).[9] The rats in this experiment were conditioned with 75 mg/kg CY and reexposed to the CS at different times before being injected with SRBC. These results indicate that an antigen-driven activation of the immune system is not a necessary condition for observing the effects of conditioning on the antibody response.

We had hypothesized[3] that the attenuated antibody response observed in conditioned animals was the result of a conditioned elevation in corticosterone level, which

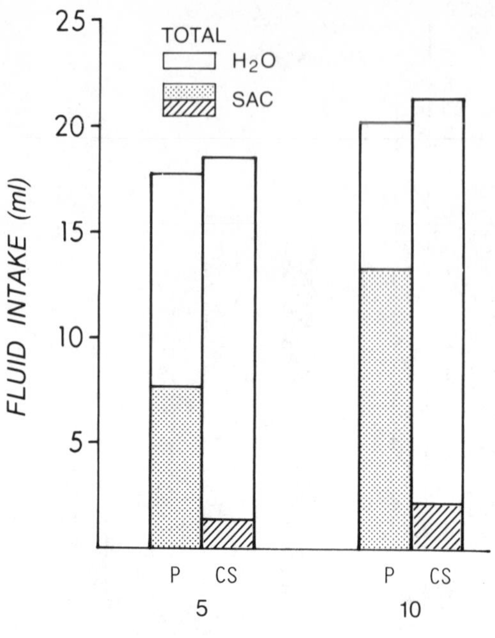

FIGURE 2. Mean consumption of a saccharin-flavored drinking solution and plain water under a two-bottle preference testing procedure in conditioned (CS) and nonconditioned, placebo-treated (P) rats. (From Ader *et al.*[9] Reprinted by permission of the American Psychological Association.)

can have immunosuppressive effects. Studies designed to evaluate this possibility failed to support the hypothesis.[3,4] Lithium chloride (LiCl), like CY, is an effective UCS for taste aversion learning and, like CY, elicits an elevation in adrenocortical steroids. However, LiCl does not suppress antibody titer in this paradigm, and rats conditioned with LiCl instead of CY do not show an attenuated antibody response to SRBC (FIGURE 4).[3] Additional experiments, designed to determine if an elevation in glucocorticoids superimposed upon the residual immunosuppressive effects of CY could account for the conditioned suppression of humoral immunity, also failed to support the hypothesis that the conditioned suppression of antibody response is mediated by experimentally induced elevations of corticosterone level.[4]

The generality of the phenomenon of conditioned immunosuppression is documented by observations of conditioned suppression of cell-mediated immune responses.[10–15] In our experiment,[10] Lewis × Brown Norway female rats were conditioned by pairing saccharin consumption with an injection of 50 mg/kg CY 48 days before immunogenic stimulation. Nonconditioned animals also received saccharin and CY, but these stimuli were not paired. A graft-versus-host (GvH) response was induced by injecting a suspension of splenic leukocytes obtained from female Lewis donors into a hind footpad of the hybrid recipients. That same day (Day 0), conditioned recipients were reexposed to saccharin and injected with saline. On the following day, they were again reexposed to the CS and injected with 10 mg/kg CY, and on the next day they were reexposed to the CS alone, for the third time. As can be seen in FIGURE 5, three low-dose injections of CY markedly reduced the weight of popliteal lymph nodes harvested five days after injecting antigen. A single, low dose of CY, however, yielded only a modest attenuation of the GvH response in nonconditioned animals (exposed to saccharin on Days 0, 1, and 2) and in conditioned animals

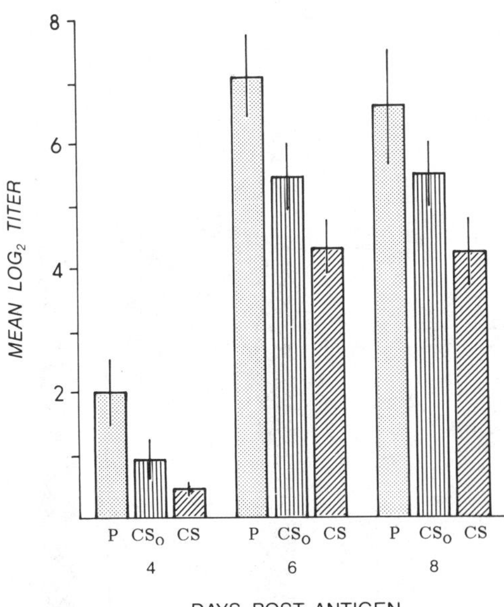

FIGURE 3. Hemagglutinating antibody titers (mean ± SE) measured 4, 6, or 8 days after immunization with SRBC in independent groups of nonconditioned (placebo-treated) rats (P), and in conditioned animals that were not reexposed to the CS (Group CSo) and those that were reexposed to the CS (Group CS) during the interval between conditioning and immunization. (From Ader *et al.*[9] Reprinted by permission of the American Psychological Association.)

that were not reexposed to the CS. In contrast, conditioned rats that received a single low-dose injection of CY and reexposure to the CS showed a significant suppression of the GvH response relative to the control groups and did not differ from rats that were given three injections of the immunosuppressive drug.

The conditioned suppression of a GvH response is also subject to experimental extinction.[11] Using the same experimental protocol, conditioned animals were divided into subgroups that received 0, 4, 9, or 18 unreinforced CS presentations between the time they were conditioned and the time they were exposed to antigen. Behaviorally, 4, 9, and 18 unreinforced CS presentations attenuated the conditioned aversion to saccharin measured seven weeks after conditioning, but there were no differences among these three groups. In terms of the GvH response (FIGURE 6), four extinction trials were not sufficient to attenuate the conditioned suppression of immunologic reactivity, but animals that received 9 or 18 extinction trials did not differ from controls and displayed a higher GvH response than animals that received either 0 or 4 extinction trials. The apparent dissociation between the behavioral and immunologic effects of extinction trials is a particularly interesting feature of these results. It is reminiscent of the dissociation between conditioned motor responses and physiological responses (schizokinesis) described by Gantt.[16]

These data are also the consistent with the results of a study of the acquisition and extinction of a conditioned enhancement of immune function in which antigen, itself, served as the UCS.[12] Mice were repeatedly grafted with allogeneic skin tissue at 40-day intervals. Subsequently, experimental mice responded to the stimuli associated with the immunogenic stimulation in the absence of the cellular graft. It was also noted that the conditioned response could be detected in only half of the mice tested in each of several replications of the experiment. "Responders" were divided into one group that experienced additional conditioning trials and a second group that was repeatedly reexposed to the CS plus sham grafts. When subsequently tested, all of the animals that experienced additional conditioning trials showed a conditioned en-

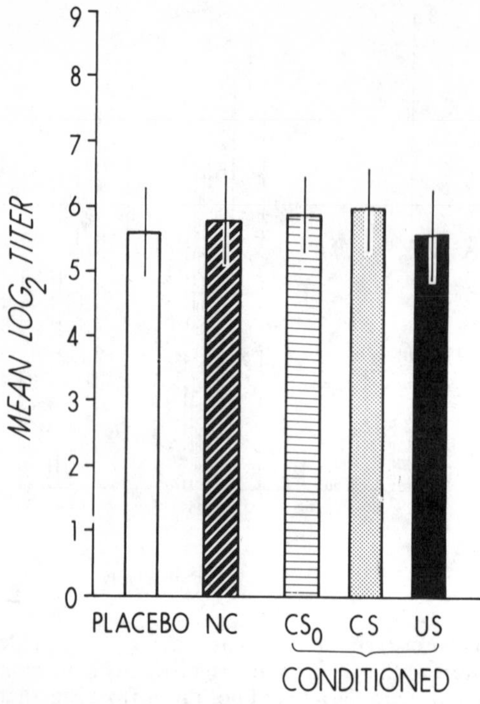

FIGURE 4. Hemagglutinating antibody titers (mean ± SE) measured 6 days after immunization with SRBC in animals conditioned with LiCl as the UCS. Group designations are as given in FIGURE 1. (From Ader & Cohen.[3] Reprinted by permission of Elsevier North-Holland, Inc.)

hancement of immunologic reactivity, whereas none of the mice that received extinction trials showed an increase in the immune response. These studies on different cell-mediated immune responses document the acquisition and extinction of a conditioned enhancement as well as a conditioned suppression of immunologic reactivity and sup-

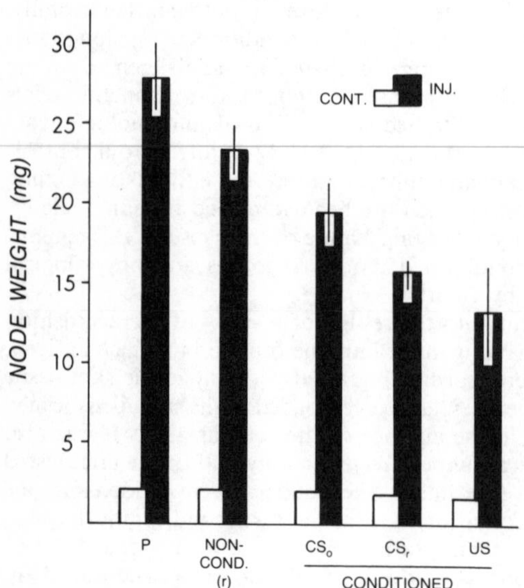

FIGURE 5. Popliteal lymph node weights in Lewis × Brown Norway female rats measured 5 days after inoculation with splenic leukocytes from female Lewis donors. Values for injected and contralateral footpads are shown for placebo-treated animals, for nonconditioned (NCr) animals given a single low-dose injection of CY, and for conditioned animals given a single low-dose injection of CY and provided with plain water (CSo), conditioned animals given a single low-dose injection of CY and reexposed to the CS (CSr), and conditioned animals given three low-dose injections of CY and provided with plain water (US). (From Ader & Cohen.[5] Reprinted by permission of Academic Press.)

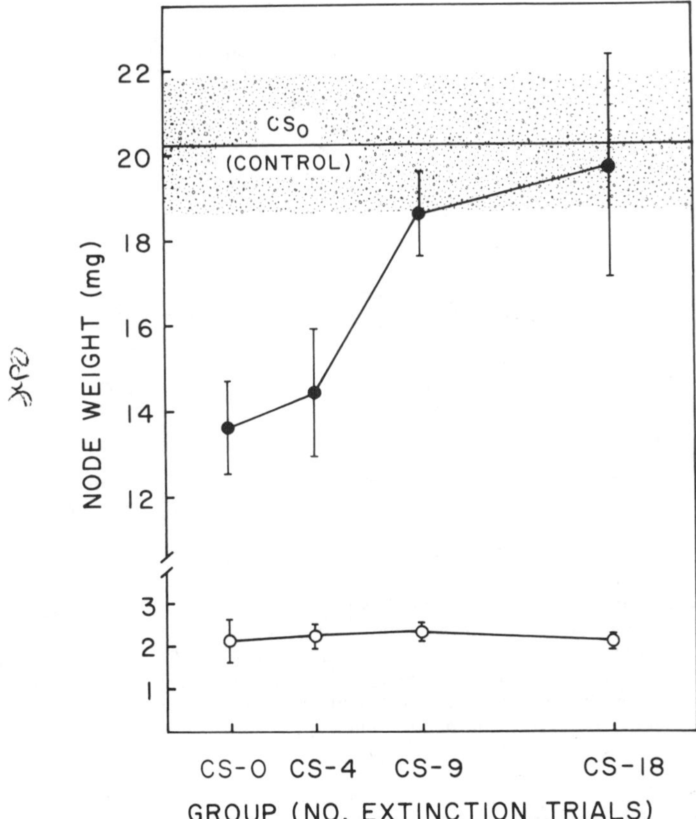

FIGURE 6. Effects of extinction trials on conditioned suppression of a graft-vs-host response. Results represent mean (+ SE) weights of draining (filled circles) and unstimulated (open circles) popliteal lymph nodes. (From Bovbjerg *et al.*[11] Reprinted by permission of the *Journal of Immunology.*)

port the proposition that associative processes are involved in the behavioral modulation of immunity.

CONDITIONED IMMUNOSUPPRESSION AND THE DEVELOPMENT OF AUTOIMMUNE DISEASE

In order to evaluate the biologic impact of conditioned alterations in immunologic reactivity, we chose an experimental model in which a suppression of immune function would be in the survival interests of the organism. New Zealand (NZB × NZW)F_1 mice develop a lethal glomerulonephritis at approximately 8 to 14 months of age and have become a standard model for the study of systemic lupus erythematosus (SLE).[17-19] Development of this autoimmune disease, however, can be delayed by treatment with cyclophosphamide.[20-23] Since immune responses can be suppressed by conditioning, we hypothesized that conditioned mice reexposed to neutral stimuli associated with

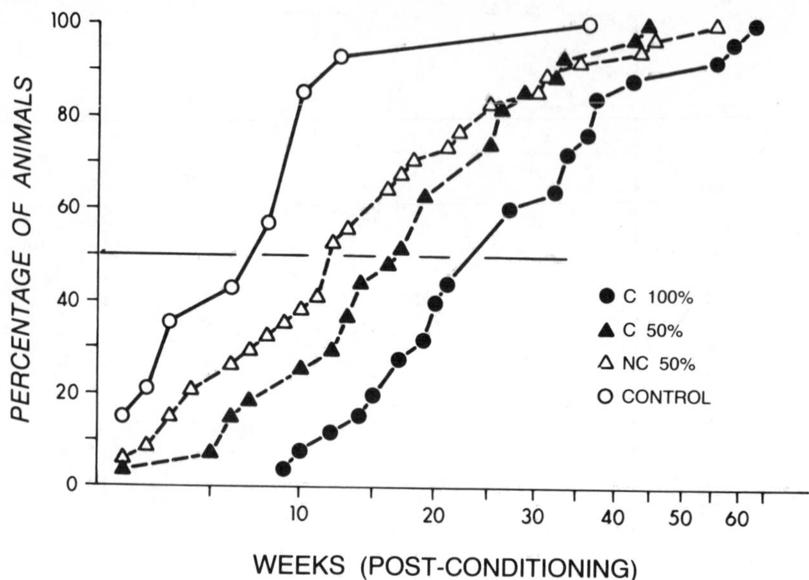

FIGURE 7. Rate of development of an unremitting proteinuria in (NZB × NZW)F_1 female mice under different chemotherapeutic regimens. Group C100% received saccharin followed by CY weekly; Group 50% received weekly saccharin presentations that were followed by CY on two of every four weeks; Group N50% received weekly saccharin presentations and unpaired injections of CY on two of every four weeks; Control animals received saccharin weekly but were not treated with CY. (From Ader & Cohen.[24] Reprinted by permission of the American Association for the Advancement of Science.)

immunosuppressive medication, CY, would show a suppression of immunologic reactivity that would delay the development of autoimmune disease. That is, it was hypothesized that exposure to a CS could be substituted for active drug in the course of a pharmacotherapeutic regimen and that such animals would be more resistant to the development of SLE than nonconditioned animals treated with the same amount of drug.[24]

An eight-week regimen of chemotherapy was begun when New Zealand hybrid mice were four months old. On the same day of each week, all mice were given the taste of a .15% solution of sodium saccharin by pipette (up to a maximum of 1.0 ml). Cyclophosphamide was injected immediately thereafter according to the following schedule:

Group C100% received an i.p. injection of 30 mg/kg CY after each exposure to saccharin. The CS-UCS pairing occurred at the same time of day and on the same day of each week. This sequence of events is, in effect, the standard pharmacotherapeutic protocol. The dose and duration of treatment proved to be effective in prolonging survival, but were not sufficient to prevent the ultimate development of disease.

Group C50%, another conditioned group, also received saccharin weekly, but injection of CY (30 mg/kg) followed saccharin on only two of each four weeks (in a random sequence). On the remaining half of the trials, mice in Group C50% received an injection of saline.

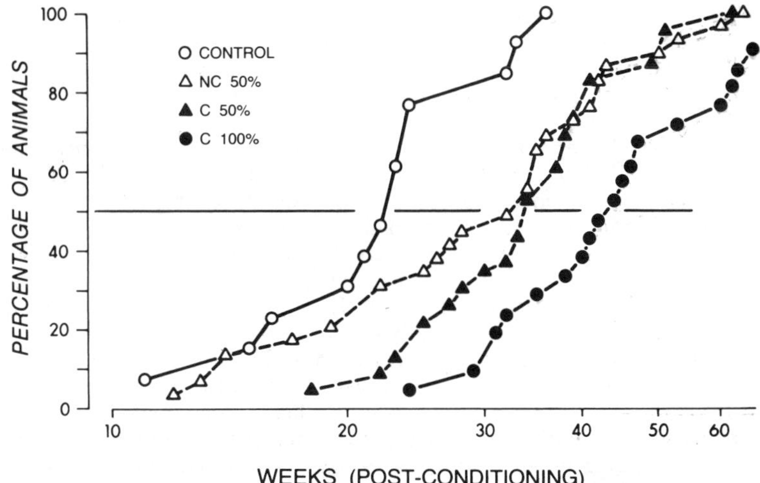

FIGURE 8. Cumulative mortality rate in New Zealand female mice following different chemotherapeutic regimens. Groups C100%, C50%, NC50%, and Control are defined as in FIGURE 6. (From Ader & Cohen.[24] Reprinted by permission of the American Association for the Advancement of Science.)

A nonconditioned group (NC50%) was also exposed to saccharin weekly and i.p. injections of CY or saline on two of each four weeks, but neither CY nor saline injections were paired with saccharin; they were administered on different days of the same week.

Control mice received weekly exposure to saccharin and injections of saline on a noncontigent basis, but they received no immunosuppressive therapy.

Pharmacologically, there was no difference between Groups C50% and NC50%; both groups received the same amount of and number of exposures to saccharin and CY. Since Group NC50% received only half the amount of drug administered to Group C100%, it was expected that these mice would show symptoms of SLE (proteinuria) and die sooner than animals in Group C100%. Group C50% also received only half the amount of drug administered to Group C100%. However, to the extent that reexposure to the CS paired with CY is capable of eliciting a conditioned immunosuppressive response, it was predicted that conditioned mice would show a greater resistance to the development of autoimmune disease than mice in Group NC50%, even though both groups were treated with the same amount of drug.

As expected, weekly treatment with CY delayed the onset of proteinuria and prolonged survival of these lupus-prone mice. The effects of the different treatment regimens on the development of proteinuria and mortality are shown in FIGURES 7 and 8. There were statistically significant differences among the groups, but inclusion of the total population of each group may underestimate the impact of conditioning since virtually all of these hybrid mice could be expected to develop SLE and die. Therefore, the longer one monitors the progression of disease, the more difficult it is to discern treatment effects.

Statistically significant differences were also obtained using as a reference point the rate of development of proteinuria in the initial 50% of the animals that developed SLE or the rate at which a 50% mortality was reached. Mice treated weekly with CY developed an unremitting proteinuria more slowly than animals in any of the other groups. Nonconditioned animals treated with half the amount of CY administered under the standard pharmacotherapeutic regimen did not differ from untreated controls. However, conditioned animals treated with the same cumulative amount of drug developed proteinuria more slowly than nonconditioned mice.

Mortality yielded essentially the same pattern of differences. Nonconditioned animals did not differ from animals that received no immunosuppressive therapy. In contrast, conditioned animals survived significantly longer than untreated controls and did not differ from animals in Group C100% (that received twice as much drug). Again, the critical comparison is between conditioned and nonconditioned mice that received the same amount of drug and, like the difference in the rate of development of proteinuria, Group C50% survived significantly longer than Group NC50%.

The differences observed in this study were consistent with the therapeutic effects of CY in murine SLE. Although this experiment did not provide direct evidence of altered immune function, per se, the results were also consistent with previous studies of conditioned immunosuppression and with predictions that might be derived from the application of conditioning principles to an analysis of a pharmacotherapeutic protocol. If a pharmacotherapeutic regimen can be structured as a conditioning paradigm, the conditioned pharmacotherapeutic response should be subject to experimental extinction, and resistance extinction should be a function of the schedule of reinforcement.[25] Preliminary data relevant to extinction were obtained in a second experiment.

During an initial period of drug treatment, the procedures were the same as those in the study described above, except that the critical experimental group (Group C33%) was injected with CY following saccharin on only one third of the weekly trials on which saccharin was provided. Nonconditioned animals (Group NC33%) received the same exposures to saccharin and injections of CY, but in an unpaired manner. At the end of the treatment period, Groups C100%, C33%, and NC33% were divided into three subgroups. One third of each group continued to receive saccharin and injections of saline (CS) or CY (UCS) on the same schedule that existed during the period of chemotherapy; one third continued to receive saccharin and injections of saline (CS), but CY treatment was discontinued; and one third received neither saccharin nor CY. Based on the conditioning effected by the pairing of saccharin and CY, it was predicted that unreinforced CS presentations would influence the development of autoimmune disease in conditioned animals but not in nonconditioned mice.

Although the number of animals per subgroup was relatively small, the results conformed to these predictions. Mortality was delayed in mice that continued to receive the immunosuppressive drug relative to mice that were taken off CY. Conditioned mice that continued to receive CS presentations (saccharin and injections of saline) after the termination of CY treatment, however, died more slowly than animals deprived of all "medication" (FIGURE 9). In fact, the mortality rate of animals that continued to receive the CS in the absence of the UCS did not differ from that in animals that continued to receive saccharin and CY.

As in our initial study, the critical comparison is between the effects observed in conditioned and nonconditioned animals that received the same amount of drug. These data are shown in FIGURE 10. For Groups C33% and NC33%, animals deprived of both saccharin and CY died relatively rapidly compared to mice that continued to receive drug therapy. Conditioned mice that were taken off CY but continued to receive weekly exposures to saccharin died more slowly than mice deprived of both saccharin and CY and, for the initial 50% of these populations, at least, the mortality rate among conditioned animals that were reexposed to the CS did not differ from

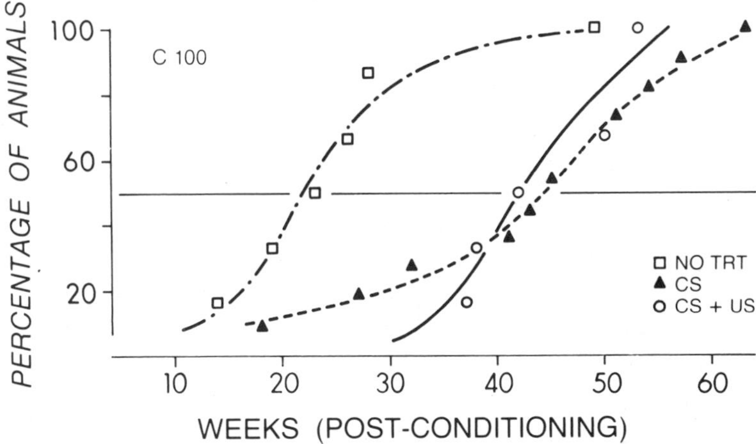

FIGURE 9. Mortality rate in New Zealand female mice treated with saccharin and CY weekly and then continued on a regimen of saccharin and CY (Group CS + US), continued on saccharin, alone (Group CS), or deprived of both saccharin and CY (No treatment). (From Ader.[26] Reprinted by permission of Guilford Press.)

mice that continued to receive CY treatment. In contrast, continued exposure to saccharin in nonconditioned animals originally treated with the same amount of immunosuppressive drug had no effect on survival. The mortality rate in these mice did not differ from that in animals that received neither saccharin nor CY.

As noted above, neither of these studies provide direct evidence of conditioned immunosuppression since we did not directly measure immune function. The findings are, nevertheless, consistent with the several experiments described above indicating that the pairing of saccharin and cyclophosphamide enables saccharin, the CS, to suppress humoral and cell-mediated immunity. Our results also support the hypothesis that the conditioning of immunosuppression could delay the development of autoimmune disease under a pharmacotherapeutic protocol that was not, in itself, sufficient to alter the course of disease in nonconditioned animals.

PHARMACOTHERAPEUTIC REGIMENS AS CONDITIONING PROTOCOLS

The data described above document the influence of behavioral factors in altering immune responses and suggest a role for the central nervous system in immunoregulation. Other neuroanatomical, neurochemical, neuroendocrine, and neuropharmacological data provide grounds for expecting such a relationship between behavior and immune function.[27] These data can also be viewed as an extension of the conditioning of drug-induced physiological responses.[1] As such, the data derived from our experimental paradigms have implications for the conduct of placebo research.[26]

Several writers have described the effects of placebo administration in terms of conditioning phenomena or alluded to the role of learning processes in attempting to account for the effects of placebo medication.[28–42] It has been proposed that the entire ritual that accompanies drug administration takes on the properties of a CS

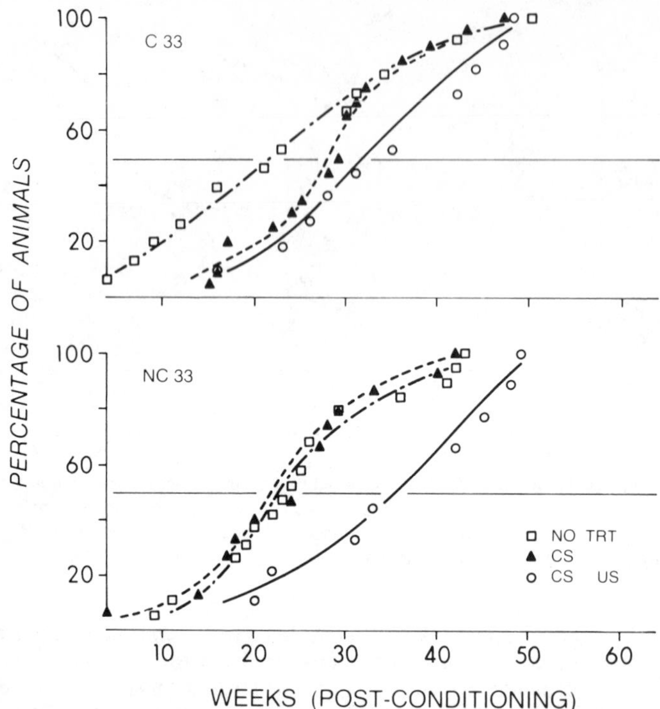

FIGURE 10. Mortality rate in conditioned (C33) and nonconditioned (NC33) female New Zealand mice that continued to receive saccharin and CY (Group CS + US), continued to receive only saccharin (Group CS), or received neither saccharin no CY (No treatment). (From Ader.[26] Reprinted by permission of Guilford Press.)

by virtue of the repeated association of such neutral events with the unconditioned effects of drug administration.[43] More recent analyses of placebo phenomena are provided in a forthcoming volume.[44] To argue that a placebo response is, in effect, a conditioned response, then, is not new. Despite the available literature dealing with the conditioning of pharmacologic and physiologic responses,[1,45–49] I am aware of no studies that have adopted a conditioning model for manipulating, controlling, or predicting placebo effects in pharmacotherapeutic situations.

The experimental evaluation of drug effects usually is based upon the comparison between an experimental group that is treated with active drug and a control group that is not treated with active drug but receives, instead, an inert or chemically irrelevant substance (placebo). In all other respects, the experimental and control groups are not supposed to differ. In conditioning terms, regimens of pharmacotherapy involve continuous reinforcement. The experimental group receives medication that is invariably followed (reinforced) by the unconditioned psychophysiologic and therapeutic effects of the drug. In the placebo group, administration of an inert substance is never pharmacotherapeutically reinforced. The experimental group, then, is treated under a 100% reinforcement regimen while the control group experiences a 0% reinforcement schedule.

Based on the pharmacotherapy of autoimmune disease in New Zealand mice described above, there is an alternative to the administration of either drug or placebo; namely, the administration of drug and placebo. By interspersing drug and placebo trials, it would be possible to manipulate the stimuli associated with the administration of drugs and evaluate the effects of partial schedules of pharmacologic reinforcement, i.e., reinforcement schedules in which the receipt of "medication" and the attendant environmental stimuli are pharmacologically reinforced on some occasions but not on others. Variation of reinforcement schedule (the active drug: placebo ratio) represents an alternative means of manipulating drug dose. In patients being treated with long-term pharmacotherapy, for example, the cumulative drug dose might be lowered by changing reinforcement schedule rather than the amount of drug that is received on each of the drug "trials."

In the studies described above, we found that the immunosuppressive effects of cyclophosphamide could be conditioned. In subsequent studies, we substituted CSs for immunosuppression for some proportion of the active drug administered in a pharmacotherapeutic regimen designed to protect animals against the development of autoimmune disease, and we found that we could delay the onset of lupus in conditioned animals using an amount of drug that was not, by itself, sufficient to alter the development of disease. The partial schedule of reinforcement was not as effective as continuous reinforcement, but the selection of a 50% reinforcement schedule was essentially arbitrary and the animals treated on the usual (continuous reinforcement) schedule received twice as much active drug. Based on studies indicating that behavioral responses conditioned under partial reinforcement are more resistant to extinction than responses acquired under continuous reinforcement,[25] it might also be hypothesized that the same would hold for conditioned pharmacologic responses. That is, pharmacologically unreinforced CS presentations might extend the pharmacotherapeutic effects of a partial schedule of pharmacologic reinforcement to a greater extent than a continuous reinforcement schedule. Again, this prediction needs to be examined among subjects treated with the same amount of drug.[50] Our preliminary examination of extinction does not satisfy this criterion and does not, therefore, adequately address the hypothesis. Animals treated under the continuous reinforcement schedule received three times as much drug as animals treated under the partial schedule of reinforcement. Comparing conditioned and nonconditioned animals that received the same cumulative amount of drug, we did observe different therapeutic outcomes. Substituting CSs for active drug yielded an effect that was "as if" the conditioned animals had received a greater amount of drug than was actually administered. Moreover, our preliminary data on extinction support the view that associative processes are involved in the (conditioned) immunopharmacologic effects that influence the development of autoimmune disease in New Zealand mice.

Capitalizing on conditioned pharmacologic effects could have important clinical implications for pharmacotherapies. It is conceivable that, by titrating reinforcement schedule (along with other parameters of a pharmacotherapeutic protocol), one could approximate the therapeutic effects of a continuous schedule of pharmacologic reinforcement using a lower cumulative amount of drug. If resistance to extinction is greater under partial schedules of reinforcement than under a continuous reinforcement schedule, it is also possible that pharmacotherapeutic effects could be extended or the gradual withdrawal of drugs facilitated by treating patients with a partial as compared to traditional, continuous regimen of pharmacotherapy. Of course, the conditioning of "side" effects must also be considered. These effects are discussed elsewhere[26] and, it is argued, do not necessarily constitute a deterrent to adoption of the research strategy proposed.

In addition to dose, route, frequency, and duration of medication, an active drug:

placebo ratio appears to be a relevant dimension of pharmacotherapeutic regimens and provides an alternative means for adjusting dose of drug. Based on a conditioning model, it is an alternative that leads to testable hypotheses regarding the acquisition and/or extinction of the response to placebo medication, and, as such, should suggest innovative strategies for psychopharmacotherapeutic interventions.

REFERENCES

1. EIKELBOOM, R. & J. STEWART. 1982. Conditioning of drug-induced physiological responses. Psychol. Rev. **89**: 507–528.
2. ADER, R. 1974. Letter to the editor. Psychosom. Med. **36**: 283–184.
3. ADER, R. & N. COHEN. 1975. Behaviorally conditioned immunosuppression. Psychosom. Med. **37**: 333–340.
4. ADER, R.,N. COHEN & L. J. GROTA. 1979. Adrenal involvement in conditioned immunosuppression. Int. J. Immunopharmac. **1**: 141–145.
5. ADER, R. & N. COHEN. 1981. Conditioned immunopharmacologic effects. *In* Psychoneuroimmunology. R. Ader, Ed. Academic Press. New York.
6. COHEN, N., R. ADER, N. GREEN & D. BOVBJERG. 1979. Conditioned suppression of a thymus independent antibody response. Psychosom. Med. **41**: 487–491.
7. ROGERS, M. P., P. REICH, T. B. STROM & C. B. CARPENTER. 1976. Behaviorally conditioned immunosuppression: Replication of a recent study. Psychosom. Med. **38**: 447–452.
8. WAYNER E. A., G. R. FLANNERY & G. SINGER. 1978. The effects of taste aversion conditioning on the primary antibody response to sheep red blood cells and *Brucella abortus* in the albino rat. Physiol. Behav. **21**: 995–1000.
9. ADER, R., N. COHEN & D. BOVBJERG. 1982. Conditioned suppression of humoral immunity in the rat. J. Comp. Physiol. Psychol. **96**: 517–521.
10. BOVBJERG, D., R. ADER & N. COHEN. 1982. Behaviorally conditioned suppression of a graft-vs-host response. Proc. Natl. Acad. Sci. USA **79**: 583–585.
11. BOVBJERG, D., R. ADER & N. COHEN. 1984. Acquisition and extinction of conditioned suppression of a graft-vs-host response. J. Immunol. **132**: 111–113.
12. GORCZYNSKI, R. M., S. MACRAE & M. KENNEDY. 1982. Conditioned immune response associated with allogeneic skin grafts in mice. J. Immunol. **129**: 704–709.
13. BOVBJERG, D. 1983. Classically conditioned alterations in two cell-mediated immune responses. Ph.D. Dissertation, University of Rochester. Rochester, NY.
14. KLOSTERHALFEN, W. & S. KLOSTERHALFEN. 1983. Pavlovian conditioning of immunosuppression modifies adjuvant arthritis in rats. Behav. Neurosci. **97**: 663–666.
15. KUSNECOV, A. W., M. SIVYER, M. G. KING, A. J. HUSBAND, A. W. CRIPPS & R. L. CLANCY. 1983. Behaviorally conditioned suppression of the immune response by antilymphocyte serum. J. Immunol. **130**: 2117–2120.
16. GANTT, W. H. 1953. Principles of nervous breakdown in schizokinesis and autokinesis. Ann. N.Y. Acad. Sci. **56**: 143–163.
17. STEINBERG, A. D., D. P. HUSTON, J. D. TAUROG, J. S. COWDERY & E. S. RAVECHE. 1981. The cellular and genetic basis of murine lupus. Immunol. Rev. **55**: 121–154.
18. TALAL, N. 1976. Disordered immunologic regulation and autoimmunity. Trans. Rev. **31**: 240–263.
19. THEOFILOPOULOS, A. N. & F. J. DIXON. 1981. Etiopathogenesis of murine SLE. Immunol. Rev. **55**: 179–216.
20. HAHN, B. H., L. KNOTTS, M. NG & T. R. HAMILTON. 1975. Influence of cyclophosphamide and other immunosuppressive drugs on immune disorders and neoplasia in NZB/NZW mice. Arth. Rheum. **18**: 145–152.
21. LEHMAN, D. H., C. B. WILSON & F. J. DIXON. 1976. Increased survival times of New Zealand hybrid mice immunosuppressed by graft-vs-host reactions. Clin. Exp. Immunol. **25**: 297–302.
22. RUSSEL, P. J., & J. D. HICKS. 1968. Cyclophosphamide treatment of renal disease in $(NZB \times NZW)F_1$ hybrid mice. Lancet **i**: 440–446.

23. Steinberg, A. D., M. C. Gelfand, J. A. Hardin & D. T. Lowenthal. 1975. Therapeutic studies in NZB/W mice: III. Relationship between renal status and efficacy of immunosuppressive drug therapy. Arth. Rheum. **18**: 9–14.
24. Ader, R. & N. Cohen. 1982. Behaviorally conditioned immunosuppression and murine systemic lupus erythematosus. Science **215**: 1534–1536.
25. Kimble, G. A. 1961. Hilgard and Marquis' conditioning and learning. Appleton-Century-Crofts. New York.
26. Ader, R. 1985. Conditioned immunopharmacologic effects in animals: Implications for a conditioning model of pharmacotherapy. *In* Placebo: Clinical Phenomena and New Insights. L. White, B. Tursky & G. E. Schwartz, Eds. Guilford Press. New York.
27. Ader, R., Ed. 1981. Psychoneuroimmunology. Academic Press. New York.
28. Beecher, H. K. 1959. Measure of Subjective Responses: Quantitative Effects of Drugs. Oxford Press. New York.
29. Evans, F. J. 1974. The placebo response in pain reduction. Adv. Neurol **4**: 289–296.
30. Gadow, K. D., L. White & D. G. Ferguson. 1984. Palcebo controls and double-blind conditions. *In* Applied Psychopharmacology: Methods for Assessing Medication Effects. S. E. Bruening, A. D. Pling, & J. L. Matson, Eds. Grune & Stratton. New York.
31. Gleidman, L. H. W. H. Gantt & H. A. Teitelbaum. 1957. Some implications of conditional reflex studies for placebo research. Am J. Psychiat. **113**: 1103–1107.
32. Herrnstein, R. J. 1962. Placebo effect in the rat. Science **138**: 677–678.
33. Knowles, J. B. 1962. Conditioning and the placebo effect. Science **138**: 677–678.
34. Kurland, A. A. 1957. The drug placebo: Its psychodynamic and conditioned reflex action. Behav. Sci. **2**: 101–110.
35. Lasagna, L., F. Mosteller, J. M. von Pelsinger & H. K. Beecher. 1954. A study of the placebo response. Am. J. Med. **16**: 770–779.
36. Petrie, A. 1960. Some psychological aspects of pain and the relief of suffering. Ann. N.Y. Acad. Sci. **86**: 13–27.
37. Pihl, R. O. & J. Altman. 1971. An experimental analysis of the placebo effect. J. Clin. Pharm. **11**: 91–95.
38. Ross, S. & S. B. Schnitzer. 1963. Further support for the placebo effect in the rat. Psychol. Rep. **13**: 461–462.
39. Skinner, B. F. 1953. Science and Human Behavior. MacMillan. London.
40. Stanley, W. C. & H. Schlosberg. 1953. The psychophysiological effects of tea. J. Psychol. **36**: 435–448.
41. Wikler, A. 1973. Dynamics of drug dependence: implications of a conditioning theory for research and treatment. Arch. Gen. Psychiat. **28**: 611–616.
42. Wolf, S. 1950. Effects of suggestion and conditioning on the action of chemical agents in human subjects—the pharmacology of placebos. J. Clin. Invest. **29**: 100.
43. Wickramasekera, I. 1980. A conditioned response model of the placebo effect: Predictions from the model. Biofeed. Self Regul. **5**: 5–18.
44. White, L., B. Tursky & G. E. Schwartz, Eds. 1985. Placebo: Clinical Phenomena and New Insights. Guilford Press. New York.
45. Harris, A. H. & J. V. Brady. 1974. Animal learning—Visceral and autonomic conditioning. Ann. Rev. Psych. **25**: 107–133.
46. Krank, M. D., R. E. Hinson & S. Siegal. 1984. The effect of partial reinforcement on tolerance to morphine-induced analgesia and weight loss in the rat. Behav. Neurosci. **98**: 79–95.
47. Lynch, J. J., A. P. Fertiziger, H. A. Teitelbaum, J. W. Cullen & W. H. Gantt. 1973. Pavlovian conditioning of drug reactions: Some implications for problems of drug addiction. Cond. Reflex **8**: 221–223.
48. Miller, N. E. 1969. Learning of visceral and glandular responses. Science **163**: 434–445.
49. Siegel, S. 1983. Classical conditioning, drug tolerance, and drug dependence. *In* Research Advances in Alcohol and Drug Problems. Y. Israel, S. B. Glaser, H. Kalant, R. A. Popham, W. Schmidt & R. G. Smart Eds. Vol. 7. Plenum Press. New York.
50. Humphreys, L. G. 1943. The strength of a Thorndikian response as a function of the number of practice trials. J. Comp. Psychol. **35**: 101–110.

PART V. APPLICATIONS OF CONDITIONED FOOD AVERSION METHODOLOGY

Introduction: Application of Conditioned Food Aversion Methodology

JAMES C. SMITH

Department of Psychology
The Florida State University
Tallahassee, Florida 32306

With the use of animal models and with data from human subjects, the contributors to this session discuss how learned taste aversions occur naturally in association with malaise that results from both short- and long-term diseases. Dr. Logue describes in detail the naturally occurring food aversions that can be observed in normal humans. She reports that the conditioning of food aversions in humans is quite similar to that described in the literature on conditioning of taste aversions in animals.[3] Two examples of this similarity would be that it is easier to condition an aversion to a novel taste and that aversions can be formed even if there is a considerable time delay between the taste and the aversive experience. Dr. Bernstein discusses the potential development of taste aversions in cancer patients. She points out that the taste experienced by the patient may not only be associated with the aversive aspect of the drug or radiation treatments but that symptoms of the disease itself may be potent unconditioned stimuli.

In addition, considerable attention is given in this session to the intentional conditioning of animals and humans in an effort to create aversions to specific taste targets. Dr. Gustavson reviews the literature on conditioned taste aversions for controlling predators that damage livestock and crops. These learned aversions are reported in a wide range of species that experience an extremely diverse diet. Dr. Nathan reports the use of chemical-aversion treatment of alcoholic patients. He discusses many of the problems in separating the role of the drug-induced aversion from the extra-therapeutic variables that may play a significant role in the outcome of this overall treatment.

A different kind of problem is presented by Dr. Kulkosky, i.e., differentiation between satiety and conditioned food aversions when an animal shows a diminished intake of certain tastants. He proposes a variety of tests to show that certain neuropeptides, such as cholecystokinin or bombesin, function as satiety signals and not as the aversive unconditioned stimuli in learned taste aversions. Dr. Bernstein encounters a similar problem in her work with animal models of cancer patients. Does the systemic effect of the disease itself totally result in the loss of appetite in the tumor-bearing animal, or can these symptoms of the disease serve as aversive unconditioned stimuli for the formation of learned taste aversions? Dr. Bernstein presents several well controlled experiments to support her argument that in this case learned food aversions are a most probable explanation for the reduction in eating and the subsequent loss of weight.

One additional idea is prevalent in this session, i.e., that in spite of the many similar-

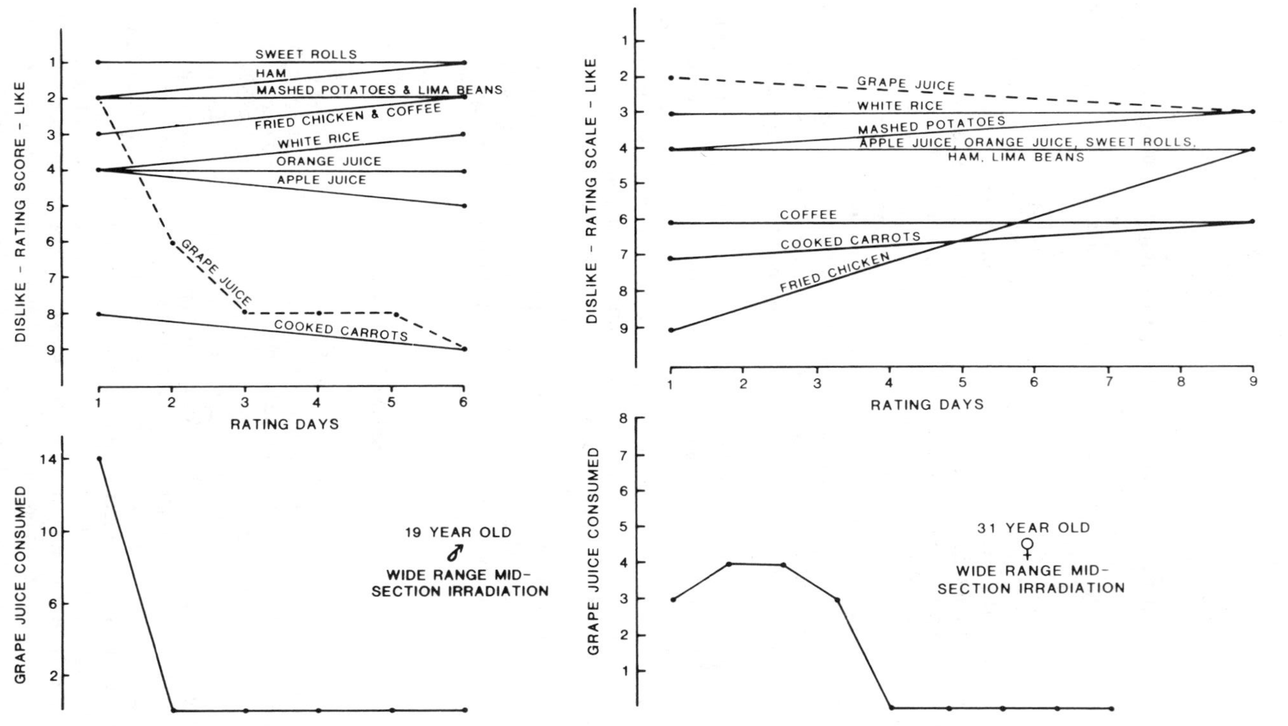

FIGURE 1. (Left) Like-dislike ratings for eleven tastants are plotted as a function of six rating days during the course of radiotherapy for a patient who reported a growing dislike for the grape juice that was daily paired with the radiation treatment. The actual daily consumption of grape juice over the same time period is plotted in the lower portion of the figure. (Right) Similar data for a second patient are shown where the consumption of grape juice decreases to zero by the fourth rating day, but the rating of grape juice was reported as "liked very much" throughout the course of radiotherapy.

ities between the laboratory studies of taste aversion learning and learned taste aversions in more natural settings, we have much yet to learn about the factors controlling this learning in "real life" situations. Dr. Gustavson makes this point quite clearly and calls for conditioned taste-aversion experiments that "include controlled complexity and not limited to the simplicity of investigations using isolated individuals, in isolated cages, where one or two foods are presented serially or concurrently on a daily basis." Similar ideas are expressed in the contributions of Nathan and Bernstein. Data from our own laboratory certainly echo this sentiment.[5] We attempted to demonstrate that a specific taste aversion could be learned by human patients in a radiation therapy clinic. Patients were given a fruit juice prior to abdominal or pelvic irradiation and intake of the juice was recorded prior to subsequent radiotherapy treatments. After an average of six pairings of the juice with irradiation, nine of ten patients refused to drink the juice. During this time we administered a rating scale for eleven common ingestibles (including that of the fruit juice). Examples of the data from two patients are presented in FIGURE 1. In the left panel it can be seen that this patient immediately ceased further drinking of the grape juice and also showed a marked decrease in his rating of the preference for that substance. The patient in the right panel, however, also ceased drinking the grape juice, but she never lowered her rating for it. One could conclude two things from this study. Taste aversion is easy to condition in human patients with partial body irradiation as the US. What the patient "does" in demonstrating an aversion is more important than the patient's "attitude" toward the substance.

In a subsequent study[5] similar to that of Dr. Logue, we observed the eating habits of 56 patients by daily interviews throughout the course of radiotherapy. To our surprise, we found only four cases of a reported taste aversion, i.e., an aversion to a substance ingested close in time to when the therapy was administered. The discrepancy between the results from the contrived experiment and the behavior of the patients in a more natural setting are interesting and lead to several hypotheses for future research.

These results and the findings reported in this session regarding taste-aversion learning in natural settings point to many variables that would be worth studying in more detail in the laboratory setting. Five examples of these are presented in some detail below. Others could have been selected.

Variability

We have numerous examples in these chapters where there were failures to demonstrate learned taste aversions in situations that would seem likely to produce them. In many of the animal studies reported in the literature, we see average aversion scores reported, but little emphasis has been placed on the variability.[3] In the use of chemical aversion treatments of alcoholic patients there is tremendous variability in effectiveness (as cited by Peter Nathan). Some cancer patients show evidence of learned taste aversions in radiotherapy situations, but many show no signs of aversion in spite of similar disease and treatment conditions.[5] In studying the application of taste-aversion learning to human subjects, the topic of variability becomes quite important. In our laboratory we have observed extensive variability in the longevity of radiation-induced taste aversions in rats.[6] In FIGURE 2, data for recovery from a radiation-induced taste aversion are presented for 128 male rats. Four groups (32 rats per group) were given saccharin-radiation, saccharin-sham, water-radiation, or water-sham treatments. The conditioned group shows a gradual recovery over a period of

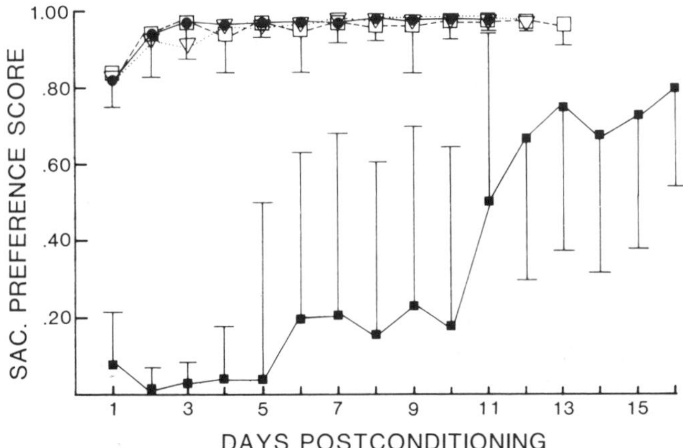

FIGURE 2. Daily median saccharin preference scores for all groups in Experiment 1. Semi-inter-quartile ranges are presented for the group receiving saccharin-radiation (dark squares) and the group receiving saccharin-sham exposure (open squares). The groups receiving water radiation (open triangles) and water-sham exposure (dark circles) are also plotted.

15 days. However, the variability among these rats was quite large. Recovery curves for the 32 individual animals are seen in FIGURE 3. We tried to place them in meaningful categories based on their speed of recovery. On one extreme a large group recovered by the end of four days, but at the other extreme six of the animals showed no signs of recovery even after 15 days. These differences could result from different sensitivities to saccharin or irradiation, different abilities to form association, or other factors. It seems that other studies of the variability among laboratory animals would be helpful in understanding the factors that control such associations in taste-aversion learning in both animals and humans in natural settings.

Selection of Dependent Variables

In this session we see a variety of measures used to determine the occurrence and the magnitude of the learned taste aversion and we seem to make the assumption that they all are valid measures. In the human studies the information is mainly derived from interviews, questionnaires, and observations. The frequency, strength, and generalization of the aversion are inferred from these sources. In addition, we have the luxury of being able to question the human subject about the origin of the aversion. In Nathan's observations, the prime dependent variable is the abstinence rate during the initial post treatment year.

The dependent variables used in the animal studies have also been quite varied.[3] Short-term single bottle and 24-hour two bottle (or pan) tests are the most frequent measures. Even in the well controlled animal studies, it is not clear that all of these dependent variables measure the same thing. Spector *et al.*[6] took six dependent measures following a saccharin-radiation pairing and found that several of these measures were not correlated at all. They measured consumption from a single-bottle of saccharin for a 10-minute period 24 hours after the conditioning. In addition, they gave the animal a 24-hour two bottle preference test for 16 days post irradiation. This allowed

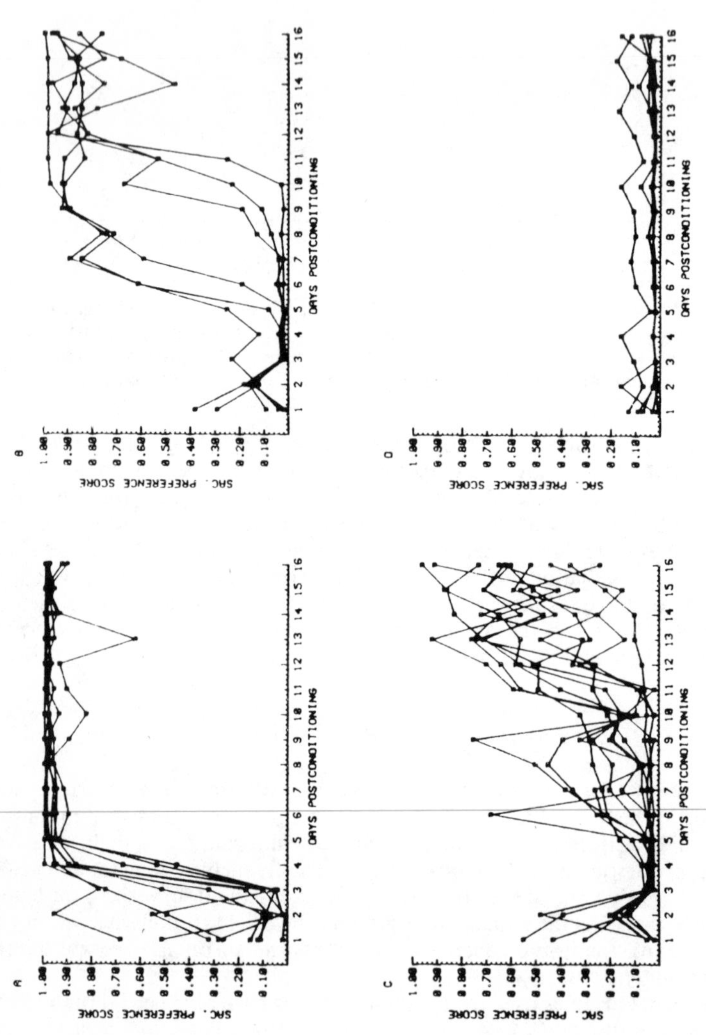

FIGURE 3. Daily saccharin preference scores for individual animals in the saccharin-radiation group are plotted. (Panel A) Rats completely recovered by day 5 postconditioning. (Panel B) Rats completely recovered by day 12 postconditioning. (Panel C) Rats showing a gradual recovery over the 16 postconditioning days. (Panel D) Rats showing little signs of recovery.

TABLE 1. Correlations between Dependent Measures Used with the Saccharin-Radiation Group in Experiment 1[6]

	A	B	C	D	E
B	.09	—	—	—	—
C	−.13	.96	—	—	—
D	.28	.38	.31	—	—
E	.30	.42	.34	.99	—
F	.19	.15	.11	.47	.49

(A) Conditioning day saccharin consumption, (B) 10-min single-bottle test saccharin consumption, (C) Ratio score, (D) Day 1 postconditioning saccharin consumption (in the two-bottle test), (E) Day 1 postconditioning saccharin preference score, and (F) Day 16 area score.

for the measurement of the 24-hour saccharin consumption and the preference score on the first day after conditioning. By integrating the area under the 16-day extinction curve, they could calculate "an area score" that allowed for quantification of the recovery from the aversion. The correlations between these measurements are shown in Table 1. Probably the most important finding from this study is that there is no prediction from the short-term, single-bottle aversion test to the length of time the aversion might last. It is also noteworthy that, except where the numerator (i.e., saccharin consumption) was correlated with the overall ratio, the correlations among the various measures were marginal to low. This suggests that these "standard" measures of taste aversions may be measuring different aspects of the same phenomenon or even perhaps different phenomena.

Longevity of the Aversion

Probably the most important dependent variable for the application of taste-aversion learning to the "natural setting" (animal or human) is how long the aversion lasts. This is most clearly stated in Nathan's paper, but is obviously as important in Gustavson's animal work and Bernstein's work with cancer patients. If the therapy or the disease is instrumental in conditioning food aversions it is only important if it has a lasting and meaningful influence on the dietary habits of the cancer patient.[4,5] In most of the animal studies, little attention has been paid to the longevity of the aversion.[3]

Natural Setting

In the natural setting, there is often little control of the temporal relation between the ingestible and the aversive event. With the cancer patient, for example, many experiences with the radiation may occur without any ingestible being present. It is also quite likely that foods are ingested at many other times than those near enough to the radiation to result in conditioning. Although there are some studies with animal models that have tested the effects of prolonged CS experience or prolonged US experience prior to conditioning,[1,2] much more work is needed in this area. In our laboratory we have seen that postconditioning CS experience has a profound effect on the extinction of a taste aversion.[7] As Gustavson and Bernstein point out, we need animal model studies that involve a variety of ingestibles to more nearly simulate the human condition. In addition, Bernstein's hint that the distinctive taste of ice cream (or other foods) may serve as a "scapegoat," needs to be thoroughly investigated.

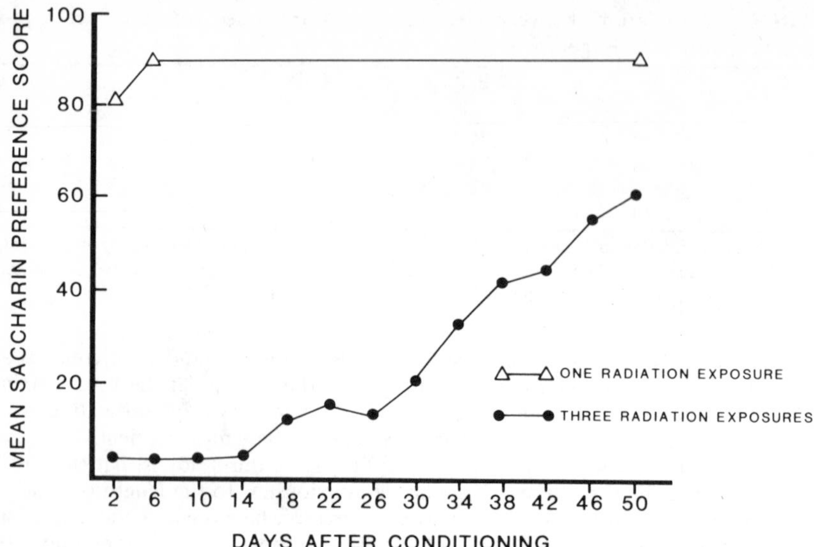

FIGURE 4. Recovery from radiation-induced conditioned taste aversion is seen where mean saccharin preference score is plotted as a function of test days in the postconditioning period. Rats with only one saccharin-radiation pairing (open triangles) showed little initial aversion and recovery by six days. The data point for this group at fifty days is theoretical. The group that received three saccharin-radiation pairings (closed circles) were not recovered to normal saccharin preference even after fifty days.

Multiple Conditioning Trials

More emphasis also needs to be placed in the animal research on multiple conditioning trials. In the applications of taste-aversion learning we need to know more about the effects of repeated CS-US pairings. Cancer patients, for example, may take numerous radiation treatments. There is some evidence that repeated CS-US pairings can result in strong learned taste aversions in spite of extensive familiarity with the CS.[5] In our laboratory we showed that if a rat had 10 days of experience with saccharin-flavored water, one saccharin-radiation pairing resulted in little taste aversion toward the saccharin. However, if the rat received three pairings of the saccharin and radiation, a profound and much longer lasting aversion resulted. This is illustrated in FIGURE 4.

The phenomenon of taste aversion learning can be observed in many applied settings. These aversions occur naturally as humans eat and experience aversive conditions. There is strong evidence that loss of appetite associated with disease may have a significant learning component. Finally, the phenomenon has the potential as a therapeutic technique for treating conditions that involve unwanted ingestion of food and drink. This session presents excellent examples of the application of principles derived from basic research.

REFERENCES

1. BATSON, J. C. & P. J. BEST. 1979. Drug-preexposure effects in flavor aversion learning: As-

sociative interference by conditioned environmental stimuli. J. Exp. Psychol.: Anim. Behav. **5**: 273–283.
2. Elkins, R. L. 1973. Attenuation of drug-induced bait-shyness to a palatable solution as an increasing function of its availability prior to conditioning. Behav. Biol **9**: 221–226.
3. Riley, A. L. & C. M. Clark. 1977. Conditioned taste aversions: A bibliography. *In* Learning Mechanisms in Food Selection. L. M. Barker, M. R. Best & M. Domjan, Eds.: 593–616. Baylor University Press. Waco, TX.
4. Smith, J. C. & J. T. Blumsack. 1981. Learned taste aversion as a factor in cancer therapy. Cancer Treatment Reports **65**: 37–42.
5. Smith, J. C., J. T. Blumsack, F. S. Bilek, A. C. Spector, G. R. Hollander, & D. L. Baker. 1984. Radiation-induced taste aversion as a factor in cancer therapy. Cancer Treatment Reports **68**: 1219–1227.
6. Spector, A. C., J. C. Smith & G. R. Hollander. 1981. A comparison of dependent measures used to quantify radiation-induced taste aversion. Physiol. Behav. **27**: 887–901.
7. Spector, A. C., J. C. Smith & G. R. Hollander. 1983. The effect of postconditioning CS experience on recovery from radiation-induced taste aversion. Physiol. Behav. **30**: 647–649.

Conditioned Food Aversion Learning in Humans[a]

A. W. LOGUE

Department of Psychology
State University of New York at Stony Brook
Stony Brook, New York 11794

The purpose of this article is to describe how conditioned food aversions are acquired by humans. Examination of this topic will aid assessments of the generality of the laws of learning by allowing comparisons between food aversion learning in humans and other species. Second, it will provide information regarding the usefulness of a conditioned food aversion paradigm for treating eating and drinking disorders, particularly alcoholism. Third, it will give some indication as to whether conditioned food aversions are responsible for many of our food aversions. Finally, it will provide information regarding the likelihood that humans' taste aversions will be formed to particular foods, information that may be helpful, for example, in preventing anorexia caused by cancer chemotherapy (cf. Bernstein[1]).

Experiments on conditioned food aversion learning (taste aversion learning) in humans have so far been limited to determining whether taste aversions could or could not be acquired. For example, Bernstein[1,2] has shown that chemotherapy can function as the unconditioned stimulus (US) in taste aversion learning. Several researchers have shown that taste aversions to alcoholic beverages can be acquired by some alcoholics.[3,4] Because ethical considerations prohibit extensive experimentation on taste aversion learning in humans, it has been necessary to rely largely on retrospective questionnaire and interview studies of naturally occurring taste aversions such as those studies by Garb and Stunkard[5] and Logue.[4,6] The majority of the data reviewed in the present article will therefore consist of information collected in these retrospective types of studies. Some of the data, although based on Logue's[4,6] samples, have not been previously reported.

FREQUENCY OF AVERSIONS

The frequency with which naturally acquired taste aversions are reported is almost certainly affected by the conditions under which the subject is asked to report these aversions, by characteristics of the subject, and by characteristics of the aversions. For example, the description of the type of aversions for which the experimenter is looking may affect how many aversions are reported. Very young and very old sub-

[a] Supported by the Department of Psychology, Harvard University, by U.S. Public Health Services Biomedical Research Support Grant 5 S07 RR07067-11 to the State University of New York at Stony Brook, by two State University of New York Research Foundation University Awards to A. W. Logue, by National Institute of Mental Health Grant 1 R03 MH36311-01 to the State University of New York at Stony Brook, and by a grant from the National Science Foundation.

jects may have difficulty recalling or reporting aversions; aversions acquired at less than two years of age are unlikely to be recalled.[7] Therefore comparing frequency of reported aversions across studies is difficult unless the conditions of data collection are constant. The reported frequency of naturally occurring taste aversions can only approximate the actual frequency of these aversions.

In Garb and Stunkard's[5] study, 38% of their 696 subjects reported taste aversions. Garb and Stunkard's youngest subjects were six years of age, and their oldest subjects were over 60. In contrast, Logue, Ophir, and Strauss,[6] working with 517 college students, found that 65% of the subjects reported taste aversions, despite Logue *et al.*'s use of strict criteria for inclusion of a reported aversion in their study. When the data for the college-student age subjects in Garb and Stunkard's study are examined separately, still only about 25% of the subjects reported any aversions. Perhaps the relatively great specificity of Garb and Stunkard's description of a taste aversion in their questionnaire was influential in decreasing the number of reported taste aversions in their study.

Logue, Logue, and Strauss[4] studied naturally occurring taste aversions in humans with eating and drinking disorders. They used the same questionnaire and the same methodology as were used in Logue *et al.*'s[6] study with college students. Therefore the frequencies of the aversions reported in these two studies can be compared. Logue *et al.*[4] found that the 102 hospitalized alcoholics studied reported fewer aversions than did subjects in the original Logue *et al.*[6] study; only 36% of the hospitalized alcoholics reported any taste aversions. However, 63% of a sample of 16 college student heavy drinkers reported taste aversions, comparable to the subjects in Logue *et al.*'s original study with college students. Since there was some overlap in the amount of alcohol consumed by the hospitalized alcoholics and by the college student heavy drinkers, and since there were no differences within these two groups as a function of alcohol consumption, the low frequency with which aversions were reported by the hospitalized alcoholics was apparently due to some difference, other than consumption of alcohol, between them and the college student heavy drinkers. For example, perhaps the hospitalized alcoholics recalled and/or reported fewer aversions because of the effects of their many medical problems in addition to alcoholism.

One other sample was studied by Logue *et al.*:[4] 19 anorexic/bulimic women. A total of 58% of these subjects reported taste aversions, comparable to Logue *et al.*'s[6] original college student sample.

In many samples, over half of the subjects report having acquired at least one taste aversion, even when most of the subjects in the sample have not yet reached the age of 30. Given that reporting a taste aversion requires, first, understanding the experimenter's instructions, second, recall of the taste aversion (keeping in mind that recall may be impossible for aversions acquired at very young ages, or for any aversions acquired with mild illness), and, third, willingness to report the taste aversion, most people may acquire at least a couple of taste aversions during their lifetimes.

Logue *et al.*'s[4,6] studies also found that most of the reported aversions were strong. The mean preference rating of the food to which the aversion was acquired decreased 2.3 points ($SE = 0.1$, $N = 415$) between before and after the aversion formed for the college students, and 2.5 points ($SE = 0.1$, $N = 50$) for the hospitalized alcoholics, in each case on a scale ranging from 1 to 5 (hated it to loved it).

LONG-DELAY LEARNING

Humans can acquire taste aversions with very long delays between the conditioned

TABLE 1. Sensory Modalities to which Aversions Formed

Modality	College Students	Hospitalized Alcoholics
Taste	83%	81%
Smell	51%	46%
Texture	32%	21%
Appearance	26%	19%
Sound	5%	4%
(*N*)	(410)	(48)

stimulus (the CS, consumption of the food) and the US (illness). Garb and Stunkard's[5] subjects reported delays of up to six hours between the CS and the US. Logue *et al.*'s[6] college students reported delays of up to three hours for 91% of the aversions. Another 8% of the aversions were reported as having been acquired with CS-US delays ranging between three and seven hours. One subject reported an even greater CS-US delay: 72 hours. Long-delay learning is also frequently observed with rats.[12]

PREDOMINANCE OF TASTES AS THE AVERSIVE STIMULI

For most species tastes appear to be either easily associated with illness or to potentiate aversions formed to other stimuli when tastes are paired with those stimuli prior to illness.[8-13] For this reason conditioned food aversion learning is usually called taste aversion learning. Tastes also appear to be easily associated with illness by humans. Humans more easily learn to avoid consuming a beverage with illness as the US than with shock as the US.[14] The majority of Garb and Stunkard's[5] subjects reported acquiring their aversions to the taste of a food. Logue *et al.*[4,6] asked college students and hospitalized alcoholics what aspects of the subsequently aversive food became aversive when they acquired naturally occurring taste aversions. Both groups of subjects reported that the taste became aversive for approximately 80% of the aversions (TABLE 1). The next most frequently reported aspect of the food to become aversive for these subjects was the related sensory modality, smell (about 50% of the aversions). The college students and the hospitalized alcoholics reported similar percentages of aversions to the different stimulus modalities.

PREDOMINANCE OF FORWARD CONDITIONING

Previous experiments on taste aversion learning in rats, and, in fact, most experiments on classical conditioning, have found that learning is better when the CS precedes the US.[12,15] This is known as forward conditioning. Consistent with these findings, Logue *et al.*,[4,6] in their studies of naturally occurring taste aversions in college students, alcoholics, college-student heavy drinkers, and anorexic/bulimic women, found virtually no reported instances of aversions in which the US had preceded the CS. In fact, only 7 out of 238 aversions examined were reported as involving backward conditioning. These data therefore suggest that it may be difficult for humans to acquire taste aversions with backward conditioning. They may help to explain why some therapists, who give their patients alcoholic beverages to drink only after making them ill, have had difficulty in inducing taste aversions to alcoholic beverages in a large percentage of their subjects (see, for example, Wiens, Montague, Manaugh & English[16]).

STRENGTH OF ILLNESS

In Logue *et al.*'s[4,6] studies subjects were asked to rate the intensity of the illnesses that resulted in their taste aversions, as well as to state the total number of times in their lives that they had been intensely nauseated. TABLE 2 shows these data for each of the separate populations that Logue *et al.* studied. The hospitalized alcoholics' ratings of the US and those of the anorexic/bulimic women were significantly greater than those of the original college student sample ($t(267) = 2.01$, $0.02 < p < .05$ and $t(237) = 2.92$, $0.002 < p < 0.01$, respectively). These two groups, the hospitalized alcoholics and the anorexic/bulimic women, both consisted of subjects who were likely to have vomited frequently. TABLE 2 shows that these two groups of subjects did indeed report having been intensely nauseated more times in their lives than did the other subjects. However, while the difference between the original college student sample and the hospitalized alcoholics was significant ($t(585) = -6.33$, $p < .002$), the difference between the original college student sample and the anorexic/bulimic women was not ($t(502) = -0.76$, $0.2 < p < 0.5$). Since US familiarity decreases the tendency to form a taste aversion,[12] it is not surprising that the taste aversions acquired by the hospitalized alcoholics were reported as having been formed following stronger illness than in the original college student sample.

GENERALIZATION OF AVERSIONS

All species appear to generalize their taste aversions to foods that taste qualitatively similar.[13] This includes humans who acquire their taste aversions under natural conditions. Logue *et al.*[6] found that their college student subjects reported generalization for about one-third of their aversions. For example, an aversion to chili generalized to Sloppy Joes, an aversion to fried chicken generalized to other greasy, fried foods, an aversion to chocolate chip cookies generalized to anything made of chocolate, and an aversion to Southern Comfort generalized to most strong-smelling and strong-tasting liquors.

TABLE 2. Strength of Illness and Number of Times Nauseated

Sample	Strength of Illness[a]	No. Times Nauseated
College students	4.0(0.1)(221)	34(14)(487)
Hospitalized alcoholics	4.4(0.2)(48)	642(200)(100)
College student heavy drinkers	3.9(0.4)(11)	21(9)(16)
Anorexic/bulimic women	4.7(0.1)(18)	91(34)(17)

Note: Mean (SE) (*N*) is shown.
[a] Illness was rated from 1 (weak nausea) to 5 (extremely strong nausea).

TABLE 3. Percentage of Aversions that Generalized to Other Foods and Drinks

Sample	Percentage (*N*)
College students	29%(403)
Hospitalized alcoholics	10%(49)
College student heavy drinkers	0%(11)
College student nondrinkers	64%(11)
Anorexic/bulimic women	39%(18)

There are some human subjects, however, who do not report generalization of their naturally occurring aversions. Logue *et al.*[4] found that both hospitalized alcoholics and college student heavy drinkers reported virtually no generalization of their aversions. Only 10% of the aversions were reported by the hospitalized alcoholics as having ever generalized, while none of the aversions reported by the college student heavy drinkers generalized. On the other hand, 64% of the aversions of a sample of college student nondrinkers generalized (TABLE 3). The data from these latter subjects were collected at the same time as the data collected from the high consumers of alcohol. Note that the lack of generalization shown by the hospitalized alcoholics and the college student heavy drinkers applied to taste aversions to all foods and drinks, not just to taste aversions to alcoholic beverages.

The lack of generalization shown by these subjects may be related to their indulging in another behavior: excessive drinking. Excessive drinking frequently causes gastrointestinal illness and therefore should result in frequent aversions to alcohol. Indeed, approximately one-fourth of the aversions reported in Logue *et al.*'s[6] original study with college students were to alcoholic beverages. Perhaps part of the reason that some people drink excessively is that these people do not generalize any acquired alcoholic beverages aversions to other alcoholic beverages, thus enabling them to continue drinking. This hypothesis is consistent with previous evidence indicating that alcoholics treated using a taste aversion paradigm will sometimes simply switch to drinking another alcoholic beverage that has not been paired with illness.[17,18]

A recently completed study of food preferences by Logue and Smith[19] showed that in college student populations foods of correlated preference are not necessarily the foods between which aversions tend to generalize. For example, the correlations obtained between the preferences for soda and salt, and candy and salt, were .39 ($N = 302$, $p < .001$) and .35 ($N = 301$, $p < .001$), respectively. However, no aversions to salty foods in the original Logue *et al.*[6] study were reported as having generalized to sweet foods or vice versa, only salty foods to salty foods and sweet foods to sweet foods. Thus, taste aversions tend to generalize to foods that taste qualitatively similar rather than to foods of highly correlated preference.

HYPOTHESES ABOUT THE ORIGINS OF THE ILLNESSES

Taste aversions are frequently acquired by human subjects even though they are convinced that the food to which they have formed the aversion did not make them ill. For example, children ranging from 2 to 18 years of age in Bernstein's[1,20] experiments frequently formed aversions to foods that they consumed prior to chemotherapy even though most of the children knew that their illnesses had been caused by the chemotherapy. In Logue *et al.*'s studies with college students and hospitalized alocholics,[4,6] about 60% of the taste-aversion illnesses were attributed by the subjects to the food that became aversive. However, for about 40% of the aversions the subjects either did not know what caused their illness or they attributed it to another food that did not become aversive or to nonfood-related origins. The responses of the college students and those of the hospitalized alcoholics were similar (TABLE 4). In many cases, pairing of illness and consumption of a food appears sufficient to result in a taste aversion, independent of the cause of the illness.

PREFERENCE AND FAMILIARITY

Rats acquire taste aversions more easily to foods that are less familiar and less preferred.[21,22] Similarly, humans report that their naturally occurring taste aversions are more likely to have occurred to foods that were less familiar and less preferred than other foods eaten at the same time or between that time and the onset of illness. Logue *et al.*[4,6] obtained these results with both their college student and their hospitalized alcoholics samples (TABLE 5). Likewise, approximately 45% of the aversions reported to Garb and Stunkard[5] were to foods that the subjects rated as novel and 53% were to foods that the subjects rated as neutral or nonpreferred.

FOODS TO WHICH AVERSIONS ARE NATURALLY ACQUIRED

More and Less Likely Aversive Foods

The probability is not constant that any given food will become aversive when it precedes illness under natural conditions. Aversions are acquired to some foods much more easily than to others. For example, in Logue *et al.*'s[4,6] studies, a substantial number of aversions were acquired to alcoholic beverages. Such aversions constituted approximately 26% of the 415 aversions reported by the college students,[6] and approximately 30% of the 50 aversions reported by the hospitalized alcoholics[4] (this difference is not significant, χ^2 (1) = 0.22, $0.5 < p < 0.7$). Although the hospitalized alcoholics may have been less likely to acquire a taste aversion than the college students, when they did acquire a taste aversion they were as likely as the college students to report that it had been formed to an alcoholic beverage.

TABLE 4. Origin of Illness Reported for the College Students' Aversions and the Hospitalized Alcoholics' Aversions

Origin of Illness	College Students (N = 405)	Hospitalized Alcoholics (N = 50)
From food that became aversive	57%	64%
Do not know	22%	28%
Not from a food	20%	6%
From another food	1%	2%

TABLE 5. Preference and Familiarity of Foods that Became Aversive, and of Other Foods Eaten at the Same Time or Between the Subsequently Aversive Food and Illness, but Which Did not Become Aversive

	Preference M(SE) (*N*)		Familiarity M(SE) (*N*)	
	College Students	Hospitalized Alcoholics	College Students	Hospitalized Alcoholics
Foods eaten at the same time				
Subsequently aversive food	3.5(0.1)(73)	3.6(0.2)(21)	2.8(0.2)(73)	3.1((0.3)(21)
Food eaten at same time	4.3(0.1)(73)	4.2(0.2)(21)	4.3(0.1)(73)	4.2(0.3)(21)
	$t(72) = -4.88^a$	$t(20) = -3.12^a$	$t(72) = -6.99^a$	$t(20) = -2.60^a$
Foods eaten between subsequently aversive food and illness				
Subsequently aversive food	3.7(0.1)(44)	3.9(0.3)(13)	2.8(0.2)(44)	3.2(0.5)(13)
Food eaten between	4.4(0.1)(44)	4.3(0.3)(13)	4.1(0.2)(44)	4.3(0.3)(13)
	$t(43) = -4.76^a$	$t(12) = -0.92$	$t(43) = -4.82^a$	$t(12) = -1.69$

Note: Preference was rated from 1 (hated it) to 5 (loved it). Familiarity was rated from 1 (never ate it before) to 5 (often ate it before).

[a] $p < .05$.

On the other hand, another common food, bread, was reported as becoming aversive only once. This is so even when all of Logue *et al.*'s[4,6] previous samples are examined, a total of 653 subjects reporting a total of 495 aversions. Further, the bread that was reported as becoming aversive was not ordinary bread, but fruit bread with butter. Since bread is eaten so frequently, it is difficult to believe that bread is virtually never followed by illness. Apparently bread is simply unlikely to become aversive when accompanied by illness.

Another food class to which taste aversions were frequently reported by the subjects in Logue *et al.*'s[4,6] studies was shellfish. Out of 37 aversions to fish, and out of 483 total aversions, 23 aversions to shellfish were reported by the 637 subjects in the original college student, hospitalized alcoholic, and anorexic/bulimic samples. Aversions were more likely to be acquired to shellfish than to other kinds of fish, and aversions to shellfish represented approximately 5% of the total aversions.

A final example concerns the difference in the number of aversions reported to hot dogs and hamburgers. Using the same samples as for shellfish, 12 aversions were reported to hot dogs, while only 5 were reported to hamburgers. A total of 57 aversions were reported to various kinds of meat. Therefore aversions were reported to hot dogs more than twice as often as to hamburgers, hot dog aversions represented approximately 21% of all aversions to meats, and approximately 1 aversion out of every 40 aversions reported to any sort of food was to hot dogs.

Factors Influencing the Tendency of Various Foods to Become Aversive

Not all of the differential tendencies of various foods to become aversive are consistent with an explanation based on differences in prior preference and familiarity of those foods. For example, in Logue *et al.*'s original study with college students,[6] three aversions were reported to hamburgers and 11 to hot dogs. However, there were no significant differences between the preferences for hamburgers and hot dogs prior to the aversions forming ($M = 3.3$, $SE = 0.5$ and $M = 3.6$, $SE = 0.3$, respectively) or between the familiarity of hamburgers and hot dogs prior to the aversions forming ($M = 4.3$, $SE = 0.5$, and $M = 3.9$, $SE = 0.5$, respectively). There are other highly preferred foods that are eaten frequently but to which aversions frequently form. For example, chicken and turkey together were rated a mean preference of 7.8 in the Logue and Smith[19] study ($SE = 0.1$, $N = 303$; scale ranging from 1, dislike extremely, to 9, like extremely), higher than the rating for bread ($M = 7.5$, $SE = 0.1$, $N = 303$), and chicken and turkey are consumed frequently. Yet in the original Logue *et al.* study with college students,[6] 12 out of 415 aversions were reported to either chicken or turkey.

Another factor that could have been influential in the greater tendency of hot dogs to become aversive as compared with hamburgers is the relatively worse reputation of hot dogs. Stories abound concerning offensive hot dog ingredients. One written-questionnaire respondent who had acquired an aversion to hot dogs quite freely expressed his negative opinion of hot dog contents when he was asked whether he would ever consume hot dogs again. Hamburgers are just as likely to spoil as hot dogs, so that it seems unlikely that people are actually made ill more frequently by hot dogs than by hamburgers. Perhaps cultural opinions concerning hot dogs, for example, increase the likelihood that aversions will be formed to them when their consumption is followed by illness, even though the hot dogs have previously been eaten frequently and are highly preferred. In this sense, the particular food to which an aversion is formed may be based on a subject's experience, while the formation of the aversion to the taste of a food is probably not (TABLE 4 and Logue[12]).

TABLE 6. Preference for Foods and Drinks Studied in Logue and Smith[19] Compared with the Number of Aversions Reported to Those Foods and Drinks in Logue *et al.*[6]

Number of Aversions	Preference: Low (rank <19)	Preference: Medium (rank 19–37)	Preference: High (rank >37)
Low (rank <19)	Middle Eastern food Squash Black pepper Coffee Carbonated beverages Salt Tea Yogurt Chili pepper Creamed foods	Butter and margarine Cereal Japanese food Soda French food Spices not including salt and pepper	Bread Salads Bananas Corn
Medium (rank 19–37)	Organ meats Mayonnaise Hot dogs Fish not including shell-fish	Sweet alcoholic beverages Nuts and Seeds Sugar products, candy Mexican food Milk Breads and cereals	Hamburgers Fresh fruit Potatoes Chicken and turkey Chinese food Citrus fruit Cheese
High (rank >37)	Reconstituted meats Beer Hard liquor Cooked or processed fruit	Meat Fish Wine Alcoholic beverages Shellfish Eggs Flour products not including breads and cereals	Dairy products Green vegetables Italian food Noncitrus fruits Vegetables Fruit Vegetables except potatoes

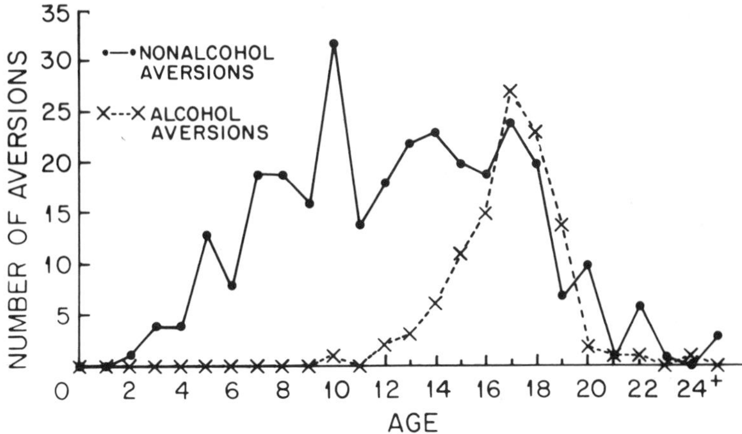

FIGURE 1. Number of aversions to alcoholic beverages and to other foods and drinks as a function of age for the college students studied by Logue *et al.*[6]

The relative reputation of a food may also have been influential in the relatively large numbers of aversions that were reported to shellfish. While some of the 23 aversions to shellfish may have involved contaminated shellfish or allergies to shellfish, it seems unlikely that all of them would have, particularly since they represented 62% of the total aversions to fish. The reputation of shellfish is that it frequently causes illness. Perhaps, in some cases, when a subject has consumed several foods including one reputed to cause illness, and then that subject becomes ill, there is a greater tendency to acquire an aversion to the food with the bad reputation.

TABLE 6 shows the mean preferences for all of the 55 foods and food groups investigated by Logue and Smith,[19] divided according to whether they ranked in the lower, middle, or upper third of the preferences for all of the items. These foods and food groups are also divided according to whether they ranked in the bottom, middle, or upper third of the number of aversions reported to them in Logue *et al.*'s study with college students.[6]

The foods that ranked high in terms of preference tended to be bland rather than spicy and/or strong tasting. For example, bread and dairy products ranked high in preference, whereas black pepper and beer ranked low. The foods to which many aversions were reported tended to be foods which are reputed to frequently cause illness, including allergic reactions. For example dairy products (which can cause unpleasant abdominal reactions in those who are lactose intolerant, a majority of all ethnic groups with the exception of Western Europeans), eggs, and liquor were ranked high in number of reported aversions, while corn, soda, and salt were ranked low. Both preference for and number of aversions reported to all of the spices included in Logue and Smith's study were low. It is impossible to say definitively whether certain foods ranked highly in terms of number of aversions reported to them because they actually make people ill more often than do other foods, or whether illness is just attributed to them more often and so aversions form to them more often, or a mixture of these two factors. In any case, it is clear that there are some foods that ranked high in preference even though they also ranked high in the number of aversions reported to them.

One final factor, opportunity, is responsible for aversions forming more often to certain foods than to others. In the extreme case, a subject cannot form an aversion

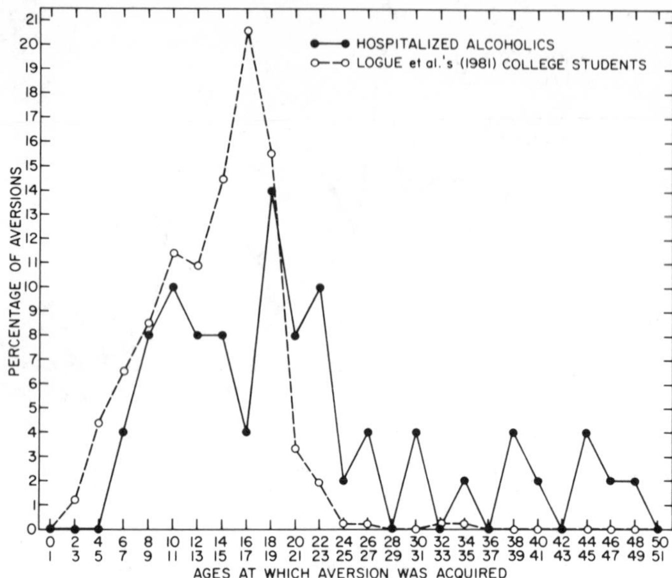

FIGURE 2. The percentage of aversions acquired at different ages by the hospitalized alcoholics[4] and by the college students.[6]

to a food if the subject has never seen or heard of the food before. For example, in TABLE 6, Middle Eastern food may possibly have ranked low in terms of number of aversions reported to it because few college students have ever eaten Middle Eastern food. Although lack of familiarity with a food may increase the probability of an aversion forming to that food, total lack of experience with a food completely removes any chances of aversions being formed to it.

The best example of the effect of opportunity on the formation of taste aversions to specific foods concerns the acquisition of aversions to alcoholic beverages reported in both Logue *et al.*'s[6] original study with college students and in Logue *et al.*'s[4] study with hospitalized alcoholics. FIGURE 1 shows the ages at which aversions were formed to alcoholic beverages and to other foods and drinks by the college students. While the nonalcohol aversions show a slow rise in frequency as a function of age and then a slow decrease in frequency as the upper limit of the ages of the subjects in the study

TABLE 7. Acquisition of Alcoholics' Aversions at Different Ages

Age at Acquisition	No. of Alcohol Aversions	No. of Other Aversions	Percentage to Alcohol
<13	0	14	0
13–17	3	4	43
18–19	4	3	57
20–24	6	3	67
>24	2	10	17
Total	15	35	30

is approached, the alcohol aversions show a sharp peak around the age of 17. The youngest age at which an aversion to an alcoholic beverage was reported was age 10. Prior to the age of 10, children do not customarily have access to alcohol. As they experiment with it in later years, however, they have a large tendency to form aversions to it, usually because of overdrinking. One-fourth of the aversions reported by Logue *et al.*'s college student sample was to alcoholic beverages.[6]

Similar results were obtained with Logue *et al.*'s[4] sample of hospitalized alcoholics. They, like the college student sample, tended to form aversions to alcoholic beverages more frequently in the teen years than at other ages, even though their mean age at the time of the study was 45 years (FIGURE 2 and TABLE 7).

CONCLUSION

Conditioned food aversion learning in humans appears very similar to that in other species. As in other species, aversions can be acquired with long CS-US delays, the aversion most often forms to the taste of the food, the CS usually precedes the US, aversions frequently generalize to foods that taste qualitatively similar, and aversions are more likely to be formed to less preferred, less familiar foods. Aversions are frequently strong. They can be acquired even though the subject is convinced that the food did not cause the subject's illness.

In addition, taste aversion learning appears to occur frequently in humans under natural conditions. The data suggest that, on the average, each of us acquires at least one taste aversion during our lifetime starting at about 2–3 years of age. This number is undoubtedly an underestimate, as reporting conditioned food aversions in a retrospective questionnaire/interview study requires recall of events that may have occurred decades earlier. In fact, it would be impossible to recall any aversions acquired prior to the ages of 2–3 years as events occurring prior to those ages are virtually never recalled. Since aversions are more likely to be formed to novel foods, and infants and toddlers frequently consume novel foods and are frequently ill, aversions are probably acquired prior to the age of 2–3 years. It is also possible that an aversion could be acquired to a particular food following mild illness at any age, and the subject might then be unable to describe how the subject's aversion to that particular food arose. Therefore it appears likely that each of us actually acquires at least several taste aversions during our lifetimes and that taste aversion learning may be responsible for some food aversions of apparently unknown origin.

Several factors appear to be responsible for determining to which foods aversions are acquired. As described above, aversions are more likely to be formed to less preferred, less familiar foods, although aversions are acquired fairly frequently to some foods that are also highly preferred. However, if a food is never eaten, obviously no aversions can be formed to it. Aversions are also more likely to be formed to foods that are reputed to cause illness frequently. For some foods this tendency may reflect a tendency to attribute illness to some foods rather than others, and for other foods it may reflect an actual increased tendency of those foods to make people ill. To what extent each of these possibilities is influential is not clear at present.

Taste aversions appear to be acquired similarly by college students, hospitalized alcoholics, college student heavy drinkers, and anorexic/bulimic women. Hospitalized alcoholics report fewer aversions, hospitalized alcoholics and college student heavy drinkers report less extensive generalization of aversions, and hospitalized alcoholics and anorexic/bulimic women report stronger illness. However in all other respects acquisition of taste aversions by these different groups is similar. Heavy drinkers do acquire taste aversions to alcoholic beverages under natural conditions, just as the other groups of subjects do. However, an aversion of a heavy drinker to an alcoholic beverage is less likely to be reported as generalizing to other alcoholic beverages than are the aversions reported by subjects in other populations. It appears possible to use a taste aversion paradigm to treat alcoholism, but it may be necessary to use strong illness and to pair many different alcoholic beverages with illness in order to achieve low consumption of all alcoholic beverages.

In summary, taste aversion learning appears to occur similarly in humans and other species, and to be a useful paradigm for understanding food aversions and for treating eating and drinking disorders.

ACKNOWLEDGMENTS

Much of the research reported in this article was collected with the help of several students, notably K. Logue, I. Ophir, M. Smith, and K. Strauss. I also thank H. Rachlin, M. Rodriguez, and M. Smith for their comments on a previous version of this chapter.

REFERENCES

1. Bernstein, I. L. 1978. Learned taste aversions in children receiving chemotherapy. Science **200**: 1302–1303.
2. Bernstein, I. L. & M. M. Webster. 1980. Learned taste aversions in humans. Physiol. Behav. **25**: 363–366.
3. Boland, F. J., C. S. Mellor & S. Revusky. 1978. Chemical aversion treatment of alcoholism: Lithium as the aversive agent. Behav. Res. Ther. **16**: 401–409.
4. Logue, A. W., K. R. Logue & K. E. Strauss. 1983. The acquisition of taste aversions in humans with eating and drinking disorders. Behav. Res. Ther. **21**: 275–289.
5. Garb, J. L. & A. J. Stunkard. 1974. Taste aversions in man. Am. J. Psychiat. **131**: 1204–1207.
6. Logue, A. W., I. Ophir & K. E. Strauss. 1981. The acquisition of taste aversions in humans. Behav. Res. Ther. **19**: 319–333.
7. Campbell, B. A. & X. Coulter. 1976. Neural and psychological processes underlying the development of learning and memory. *In* Habituation. T. J. Tighe & R. N. Leaton, Eds.: 129–157. Erlbaum. Hillsdale, NJ.
8. Durlach, P. J. & R. A. Rescorla. 1980. Potentiation rather than overshadowing in flavor-aversion learning: An analysis in terms of within-compound associations. J. Exp. Psychol.: Anim. Behav. Proc. **6**: 175–187.
9. Palmerino, C. C., K. W. Rusiniak & J. Garcia. 1980. Flavor-illness aversions: The peculiar roles of odor and taste in memory for poison. Science **208**: 753–755.
10. Gustavson, C. R. 1977. Comparative and field aspects of learned food aversions. *In* Learning Mechanisms in Food Selection. L. M. Barker, M. R. Best & M. Domjan, Eds.: 23–42. Baylor University Press. Waco, TX.
11. Lett, B. T. 1980. Taste potentiates color-sickness associations in pigeons and quail. Anim. Learn. Behav. **8**: 193–198.
12. Logue, A. W. 1979. Taste aversion and the generality of the laws of learning. Psychol. Bull. **86**: 276–296.
13. Logue, A. W. In press. A comparison of taste aversion learning in humans and other species: Evolutionary pressures in common. *In* Evolution and Learning. R. Bolles & M. Beecher, Eds. Erlbaum. Hillsdale, NJ.
14. Lamon, S., G. T. Wilson & R. C. Leaf. 1977. Human classical aversion conditioning: Nausea versus electric shock in the reduction of target beverage consumption. Behav. Res. Ther. **15**: 313–320.

15. Mackintosh, N. J. 1974. The Psychology of Animal Learning. Academic Press. New York.
16. Wiens, A. N., J. R. Montague, T. S. Manaugh & C. J. English. 1976. Pharmacological aversive counterconditioning to alcohol in a private hospital: One-year follow-up. J. Stud. Alcohol **37**: 1320–1324.
17. Mellor, C. S. & H. P. White. 1978. Taste aversions to alcoholic beverages conditioned by motion sickness. Am. J. Psychiat. **135**: 125–126.
18. Quinn, J. & R. Henbest. 1967. Partial failure of generalization in alcoholism following aversion therapy. Q. J. Stud. Alcohol **28**: 70–75.
19. Logue, A. W. & M. E. Smith. (Manuscript submitted for publication.) Predictors of food preferences in humans.
20. Bernstein, I. L., M. M. Webster & I. D. Bernstein. 1982. Food aversions in children receiving chemotherapy for cancer. Cancer **50**: 2961–2963.
21. Etscorn, F. 1973. Effects of a preferred vs a nonpreferred CS in the establishment of a taste aversion. Physiol. Psychol. **1**: 5–6.
22. Kalat, J. W. 1974. Taste salience depends on novelty, not concentration, in taste-aversion learning in the rat. J. Comp. Physiol. Psychol. **86**: 47–50.

Conditioned Food Aversions and Satiety Signals

PAUL J. KULKOSKY

Center for Psychology and Mental Health
University of Southern Colorado
Pueblo, Colorado 81001

Satiety is a word with nearly antithetical definitions. Most listed meanings of satiety refer to a sad state of gratification to excess or glutting characterized by feelings of disgust and surfeit.[1] A favorable sense of satiety as full satisfaction of need was revived by modern experimentalists.[2] An uncommon term, nimiety, can be selected to refer exclusively to the clearly adverse state resulting from consumption in gross excess of optimal capacity. The distinction of nimiety from satiety eliminates ambiguous usage of satiety and completes the hedonic continuum in feeding: hunger–satiety –nimiety.

The identification of physiological events that trigger satiety and act to terminate a meal is a major goal in recent study of food intake.[3–7] Satiety signals are important in understanding how organisms limit meal size and prevent the acute distress and discomfort of nimiety. The therapeutic manipulation of these stimuli may provide a potential control of the chronic distress and discomfort of intake-related disorders such as obesity. A lively controversy has developed over the use of the conditioned food aversion paradigm as a critical test to verify that a stimulus specifically functions as a satiety signal, rather than as a nonspecific stimulant of distress or toxicosis.[8,9]

Shakespeare's first use of the word satiety refers to "When the Blood is made dull with the Act of Sport,"[1] and presages the conclusion of modern experiments that demonstrate the blood of satiated animals contains a factor that acts to limit meal size.[10] The search for the identity of the blood-borne satiety factor(s) has been guided by the adoption of stringent criteria for verification of candidate satiety factors.[4,11–14] Many putative satiety factors have now been hypothesized, but none has yet satisfied all criteria proposed for validation of an authentic endogenous stimulus of satiation.[13,14]

A humoral satiety signal for feeding must exhibit the following properties: (1) generation endogenously as a prompt and short-acting consequence of food intake, (2) reduction of meal size after exogenous administration that produces circulating levels within the range produced endogenously by food, (3) specific inhibition of food ingestion in a manner that elicits the normal behavioral sequence and self-report of satiety, and (4) support, as an unconditioned stimulus, of dose- and repletion-dependent conditioning of satiety. The conditioned food aversion paradigm has often been used as a method to meet parts of the third and fourth criteria, to verify that a satiety factor inhibits feeding specifically, and not merely as a toxic side effect of production of aversive interoceptive stimuli such as nausea or gut pain. In a conditioned food aversion paradigm, consumption of a novel substance is paired with administration of treatment, and subsequent consumption of that substance is measured. This test, referred to as an experimental analog of "bait shyness," has been widely applied as an index of interoceptor-stimulating toxicity of treatments.[15,16] It is expected that an authentic satiety signal would not be an effective unconditioned stimulus in the conditioned food aversion design, when administered within the low range of doses that specifically reduce food intake.[4,12] Implicit in this expectation is the distinction between satiety and nimiety; that satiety is satisfying, and not identical with the nausea and distress of overeating.

A satiety effect may not be discriminated from an effect of toxicosis simply by changes in food intake, because both effects result in reduced food intake. Rather, an analysis of the behaviors accompanying the meal must show a decline of feeding rate only at the latter part of the meal to be consistent with a satiety effect.[11] Toxins, bitter tastes, and psychoactive drugs affect the initial as well as final feeding rate, and accompanying behaviors do not resemble the typical behavioral sequence seen after normal meal termination.[17] These findings gain importance from the recognition that conditioned aversion tests are not conclusive evidence of toxicosis.[18–22] These considerations led to the combined use of conditioned food aversion tests and meal-pattern analysis to evaluate the specificity of putative satiety signals.

Self-selected food is the natural adequate stimulus for satiety. The experimental literature on food as a reward for hungry subjects is enormous, but that food also serves as the stimulus for nimiety is rarely studied. Nevertheless, the natural stimulus for satiety can also readily condition food aversion, as Tolman noted: "Thus it is well-known that over-indulgence may often induce a permanent distaste for a previously favorite food."[23] The signals elicited by food shift from rewarding to punishing consequences if their intensity is increased. The point where satiety is replaced by nimiety is set by the maximal capacity to digest, store, and utilize food.[24,25] The intensity or dose of a putative circulating satiety factor must be carefully evaluated in relation to endogenous, food-stimulated values to predict its effect as a rewarding event of satiety, as a punishing stimulus of nimiety or toxicosis, or as a physiological novelty. Further, the preferences and aversions conditioned by varying doses of satiety factors have been clearly shown to be dependent on the repletion state of subjects.[4,26,27]

Cholecystokinin (CCK), a gut-brain neuropeptide and hormone,[28] was one of the first circulating factors extensively tested with the conditioned food aversion paradigm as a toxicity test. The original report[12] of CCK's feeding inhibition effect in rats included data from a one-bottle, 10-minute saccharin drinking session. Prior saccharin-paired injection of LiCl induced a conditioned aversion to saccharin in that experiment, but paired injection of NaCl, cholecystokinin, or its octapeptide did not alter saccharin consumption. Single doses of CCK and LiCl were tested, although the CCK dose (40 U/kg) was 67 times higher than the threshold dose required to decrease food intake in fasted rats.

A second experiment[29] examined the effect of repeated saccharin-injection pairings, again using a one-bottle design, but with apomorphine as control. Across seven saccharin drinking sessions, only prior paired injections of apomorphine induced an aversion to saccharin, CCK or its octapeptide (at 40 U/kg) were ineffective. These demonstrations drew sharp methodological criticism.[30,31] A clear aversion to flavors previously paired with a dose of 40 U/kg of CCK was shown in a two-bottle preference test by thirsty rats.[30] Preference tests have long been recognized as providing more sensitive indices of conditioned taste aversion than single-stimulus tests.[32]

The effectiveness of CCK as an unconditioned stimulus in the conditioned food aversion paradigm may therefore depend on the specific testing design employed. We demonstrated[9] that a single pairing of 2 μg/kg of octapeptide of CCK with consumption of a novel saccharin solution in thirsty rats results in a slight and transitory decrease of subsequent saccharin preference. The results of six extinction tests are depicted in FIGURE 1. In the context of extinction, only the LiCl-injected rats showed a consis-

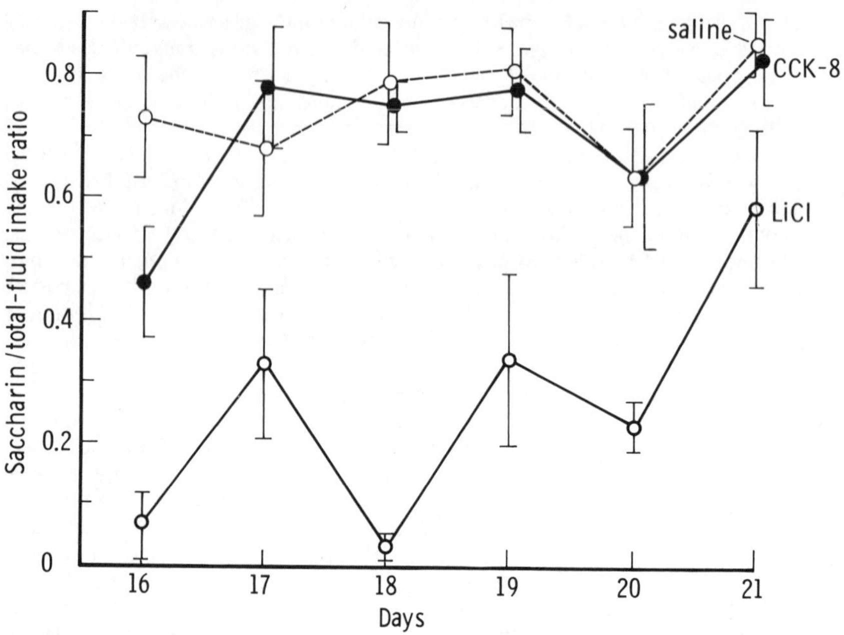

FIGURE 1. Mean (± standard error, SE) saccharin/total fluid intake ratio on six 30-min extinction tests. On day 13 rats received 30-min access to novel 0.125% Na saccharin. Saline (12 ml/kg), CCK-8 (2 μg/kg), or LiCi (12 ml/kg, 0.15 M) was injected i.p. immediately afterwards. Rats received 30-min access to water alone on days 14–15, and two-bottle choice of saccharin and water on days 16–21. (From Smith *et al.*[9] With permission of Haer Institute for Electrophysiological Research.)

tent aversion to associated saccharin. Saline- and CCK-injected means differed on the first extinction test day only. The doses of CCK and LiCl used had been shown to suppress equivalently food intake of hungry rats, but they were not equally effective in altering saccharin preference.

However, the sudden injection of a high dose of hormone after completion of a feeding or drinking session may constitute a sufficiently novel stimulus to elicit neophobic avoidance. Alternatively, the injected hormone may summate with endogenous secretion to produce an aversive signal of over-consumption or nimiety. A more appropriate test of the potential aversive properties of a putative satiety factor would be performed during a feeding session shortened by exogenous administration of that factor, when endogenous satiety signals are diminished. When exogenous CCK has been paired with a taste during a session that permitted feeding, shortened meals but no aversion to associated tastes have been observed. In the first example,[33] sham-feeding rats equipped with open gastric fistulae were injected with NaCl, LiCl, 20% pure CCK, or its octapeptide (1.5 μg/kg) and then given access to a saccharine liquid diet. While LiCl, CCK, and its octapeptide each suppressed sham-feeding, only LiCl-injected rats avoided consumption of the flavored food in a single-stimulus extinction test. In the second example[34] of this effect of testing design, water-deprived rats were allowed food and almond-flavored water during a 30-minute session. Access to almond was preceded by injections of vehicle, 2 μg/kg CCK octapeptide, or LiCl. Both CCK and LiCl equally suppressed the drinking-associated feeding that occurs under these conditions. LiCl, but not CCK, also suppressed almond solution intake. On a subsequent two-bottle test of almond solution and water, only the LiCl-injected rats avoided almond consumption.

These experiments show the importance of design in assessing cholecystokinin in a food aversion test of toxicity. When CCK is associated with tastes under free-feeding conditions, shortened meals but no conditioned aversion to associated tastes is demonstrated. When tested under trace conditioning procedures in drinking tests, CCK can support avoidance conditioning at high doses, although this result has not always been observed.[35] This design specificity in CCK's conditioning ability shows that CCK can condition taste aversions at high doses only if its administration produces a surprise, a physiological novelty—an inappropriately large rise of circulating levels after self-selected consumption, which may function as a signal of nimiety.

This conclusion is supported by the results of single-stimulus conditioned food aversion tests performed in rabbits[36] and pigs[37] with doses of CCK and its structural analogs that effectively inhibit feeding in these species. Food-deprived rabbits did not avoid consumption of flavored feed previously paired with an injection of 40 U/kg of CCK, 100 U/kg of CCK octapeptide, 2 μg/kg of caerulein (a CCK-like peptide), or saline, but pairing of novel flavor with LiCl led to total avoidance of the flavored feed on second presentation. Food-deprived pigs did not avoid consumption of flavored feed previously paired with an injection of 40 U/kg of CCK or CCK-8, 2 μg/kg of caerulein, or saline, but pairing of novel flavor with apomorphine injection induced a strong aversion to the flavored feed.

In summary, CCK-like peptides are typically ineffective unconditioned stimuli in conditioned food aversion designs. Aversions can be demonstrated with high doses of CCK, if administered after completion of a consummatory session, but when CCK acts to decrease a meal, no aversion is observed.

Subsequent to the presentation of cholecystokinin as a candidate satiety signal, many circulating factors have been hypothesized and tested as satiety signals. Bombesin (BBS) is another peptide found in both gut and brain tissues.[38] Bombesin was clearly demonstrated to inhibit specifically the food intake of fasted rats after exogenous administration.[39] Feeding inhibition by BBS was restricted to the latter part of the meal; water intake was not affected by doses that inhibited feeding; the normal behavioral sequence of satiety was observed after a BBS-shortened meal; and the injected rats did not exhibit hypothermia or unusual behaviors. This thorough report was criticized because it omitted a conditioned taste aversion test of the aversive properties of bombesin.[40,41]

Although it can be argued that the conditioned taste aversion, feeding inhibition, and behavioral observations are not foolproof tests of nausea or toxicosis, and that satiety's older definitions have clearly aversive connotations, a sensitive conditioned taste aversion test was performed to evaluate the aversive properties of injected bombesin.[42] Doses of bombesin (4 μg/kg) and LiCl (12 ml/kg, 0.15 M) were chosen that had equivalently suppressed feeding in fasted rats. Water-deprived rats received injections of these doses or equivolumetric saline after 30-minute access to novel saccharin solution. Results from the subsequent two-bottle extinction test are shown in FIGURE 2. LiCl injection conditioned a profound and long-lasting aversion to saccharin, but BBS- or saline-injected rats equally preferred saccharin. A similar saccharin preference design yielded comparable results and support of the conclusion that 4 μg/kg of bombesin effectively reduces feeding but is a relatively ineffective unconditioned stimulus in averting saccharin selection.[35]

However, it has also been shown in rats that three pairings of consumption of

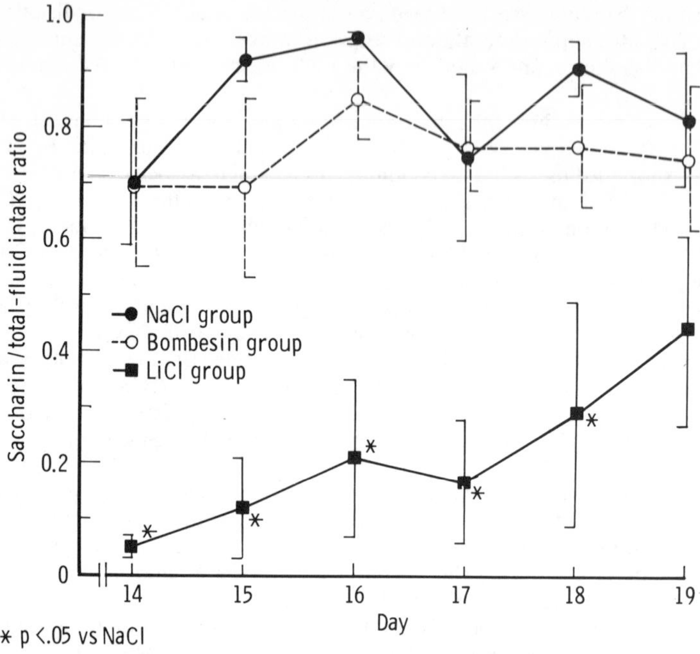

FIGURE 2. Mean (±SE) saccharin/total fluid intake ratio on six 30-min extinction tests. Saline (12 ml/kg), bombesin (4 μg/kg), or LiCl (12 ml/kg, 0.15 M) was injected i.p. immediately following novel saccharin access on day 11. (From Kulkosky *et al.*[42] With permission of Ankho International Inc.)

flavored water and injection of 16 μg/kg bombesin led to a significant decline in flavored-water preference.[43] The dose of BBS chosen in this study is 16 times the threshold dose for feeding inhibition in rats and this dose nonspecifically inhibits both food and water consumption.[44] The demonstration that repeated conditioning trials with a massive dose of a peptide gradually causes a slight preference shift for an associated flavor may indicate that bombesin can condition an aversion to associated cues, as does food, when administered in gross excess of normal levels. Indeed, it has been proposed that it is criterial that a satiety signal act as food in that very high doses (or intakes) can condition repletion-independent food aversions.[4]

The conclusion that bombesin's feeding inhibition effect may be dissociated from its ability to condition taste aversions is further strengthened by results of a study of a bombesin-like peptide, litorin (LIT).[44] Litorin is a peptide that closely resembles bombesin in its structure and physiological actions, and these peptides have been extensively compared.[45] LIT and BBS appear to activate the same receptors that have been identified in mammals.[46] In accord with their structural and physiological similarities, both LIT and BBS decrease food intake of fasted rats after injection, as depicted in FIGURE 3. The initial test of specificity of action of a satiety signal for feeding is to determine its effect on drinking in water-deprived subjects.[47] The results of this test applied to LIT and BBS are shown in FIGURE 4. Both LIT and BBS can reduce water intake, but only at doses that are considerably higher than required to reduce food intake. Thus both peptides are relatively specific inhibitors of food intake. However, several toxins have been shown to induce conditional taste aversion or decrease

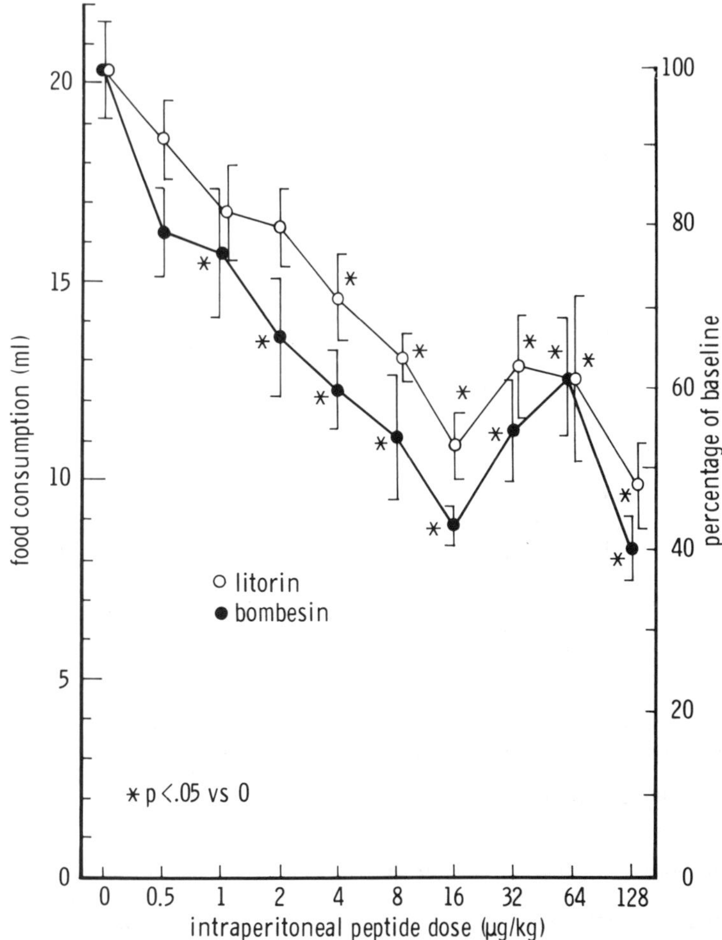

FIGURE 3. Mean (±SE) liquid diet consumption as a function of dose of litorin and bombesin. Rats were deprived of food for 18 hr prior to 30-min access to 25% liquid food. Food presentation was preceded by i.p. injection of saline, bombesin, or litorin. (From Kulkosky & Gibbs.[44] With permission of Pergamon Press, Ltd.)

feeding in food-deprived rats at lower doses than required to decrease drinking in water-deprived rats.[48–50] One study demonstrated that a two-bottle conditioned taste aversion test is a more sensitive measure of the toxicity of physostigmine than a one-bottle test, a consummatory drinking test, or human observations of rat behavior.[51]

As further tests of the specificity of litorin's action, both behavioral observations and a two-bottle conditioned taste aversion test were conducted with LIT, NaCl, and LiCl as unconditioned stimuli. Litorin was tested at a dose that reduced food intake, but not water intake, 8 µg/kg. As in the test of bombesin's aversive properties, a dose of LiCl was chosen that equivalently reduced both food intake and observed feeding behavior of fasted rats. Both LIT and LiCl injection prior to a meal decreased food consumption to a similar degree relative to saline, as depicted in FIGURE 5.

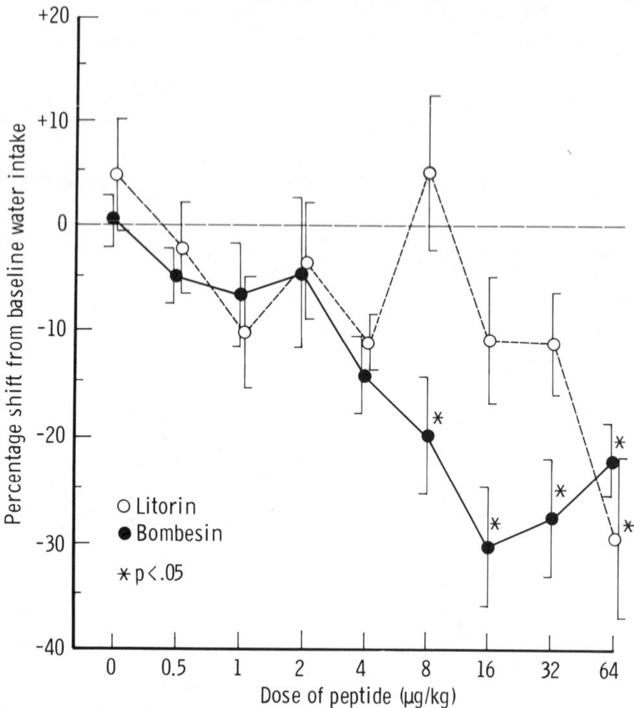

FIGURE 4. Mean (±SE) percentage shift from baseline water intake as a function of dose of litorin and bombesin. Rats were deprived of water for 18 hr prior to 30-min access to water. Water presentation was preceded by i.p. injection of saline, bombesin, or litorin. (From Kulkosky & Gibbs.[44] With permission of Pergamon Press, Ltd.)

Behavioral observations of injected rats were made systematically during this feeding test. Observations were made at one-minute, tone-cued intervals. The categories of behavior and the reliabilities of this time-sampling method have been described.[17,52] Percentage of total observations of behavior made during a 30-minute interval in several categories of behavior of the injected rats is show in FIGURE 6. The results show that LIT and LiCl nearly identically suppressed observed feeding behavior. However, neither LiCl- nor LIT-injected rats differed significantly from saline-injected rats in any other category of behavior. Differences were found in the effects of LiCl and LIT on resting and standing behaviors, but these data reveal the difficulty in distinguishing either treatment from control when behaviors are summarized across a 30-minute interval.

Behavioral observations were further analyzed into five-minute blocks to evaluate initial feeding rate. The resulting meal-related behavioral patterns are shown for NaCl, litorin, and LiCl in FIGURES 7, 8, and 9, respectively.

A striking feature of these observational data is the few significant differences of meal-related behaviors after injections of saline or equi-anorexic doses of litorin and LiCl. LiCl-injected rats differed from both NaCl- and LIT-injected rats in observed feeding behavior only in the first five-minute block. LiCl-injected rats also exhibited less resting than NaCl-or LIT-injected rats in the third five-minute block. Fi-

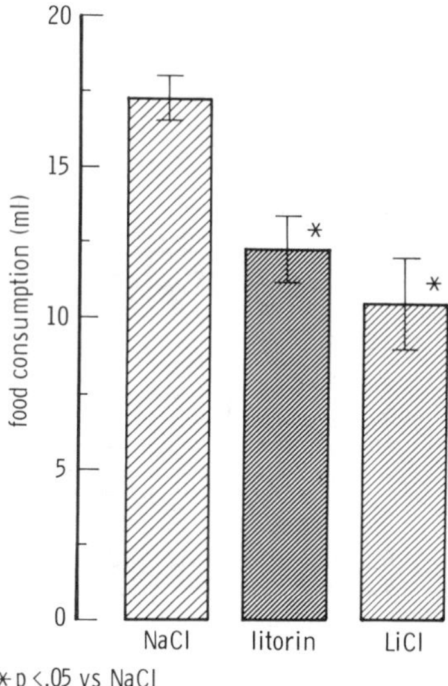

FIGURE 5. Mean (±SE) liquid diet consumption after i.p. injections of saline (8 ml/kg), litorin (8 μg/kg), and LiCl (8 ml/kg, 0.15 M). Rats were deprived of food for 18 hr prior to 30-min access to 25% liquid food. (From Kulkosky & Gibbs.[44] With permission of Pergamon Press, Ltd.)

nally, LiCl-injected rats showed more standing behavior than NaCl-injected rats in the first five-minute block. No other significant difference among treatment means was found in any category, across the five-minute blocks of the 30-minute observation period. Further, treatment-blind human observers could not reliably discriminate these injection groups on the basis of unrecorded casual observations. These findings strengthen the suggestions that a battery of sensitive tests of specificity be applied to any candidate satiety signal. Accordingly, a two-bottle conditioned saccharin aversion test was conducted with the above doses of litorin, LiCl, and NaCl as unconditioned stimuli. The basic design was the same as employed in tests of CCK-8 and BBS: naive, water-deprived rats received one-bottle access to novel 0.125% saccharin for 30 minutes, immediately followed by intraperitoneal injection of LIT, LiCl, or NaCl solutions. On seven succeeding days, a choice of saccharin and water was offered for 30 minutes. The saccharin preferences of LIT-, LiCl-, or NaCl-injected rats across extinction trials are shown in FIGURE 10. These data demonstrate an enormous difference among the treatments. LiCl injection served to condition a near-total and extinction-resistant aversion to paired saccharin, but neither equi-anorexic litorin nor saline was effective in averting saccharin choice.

In conclusion, BBS-like peptides are typically ineffective unconditioned stimuli in conditioned food aversion tests. Aversions can only be produced with a nonspecific high dose of BBS that is repeatedly paired with flavor.

The results of tests of litorin's specific food-reduction effect are compatible with, but do not prove, the hypothesis that endogenous bombesin-like peptide receptors may play a physiological role in induction of satiety. Nevertheless, the following have been argued: these tests of specificity can be shown to provide relatively insensitive indices of the effects of some toxins;[18-22] feeding reduction is the most sensitive index of toxicosis;[53] and mild discomfort and incipient nausea are actually a part of satiety.[34]

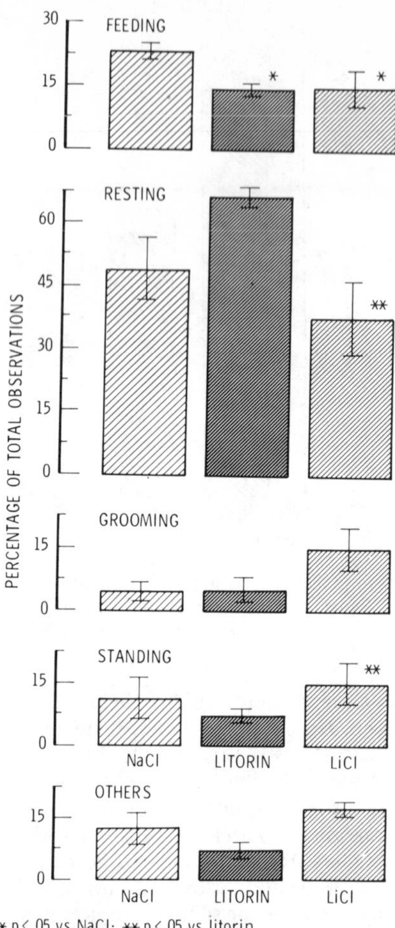

FIGURE 6. Mean (±SE) percentage of total observations of behavior made in the categories of feeding, resting, grooming, standing, and all other categories combined ("others") during the 30-min feeding test described in FIGURE 5. (From Kulkosky & Gibbs.[44] With permission of Pergamon Press, Ltd.)

Each of these criticisms gives pause to the use of simple behavioral observations of animals alone to verify that a stimulus functions as an agent of satiation. The effects in humans of administered candidate satiety signal have attracted considerable attention, not only because of the clear potential therapeutic applications to eating disorders and obesity, but also because human self-report of satiety or sickness may help resolve some of the above criticisms. "Satiety" does refer to a subjective feeling of fullness,[54] and such interoceptive perception is directly accessible via human self-report. However, these data must be evaluated in light of the well-known variable relation between interoceptive stimulation, behavioral change, and human self-report.[55] Both CCK and BBS have been administered experimentally to humans who made self-reports of gut feelings and satiety. A conclusion from these experiments with CCK is that

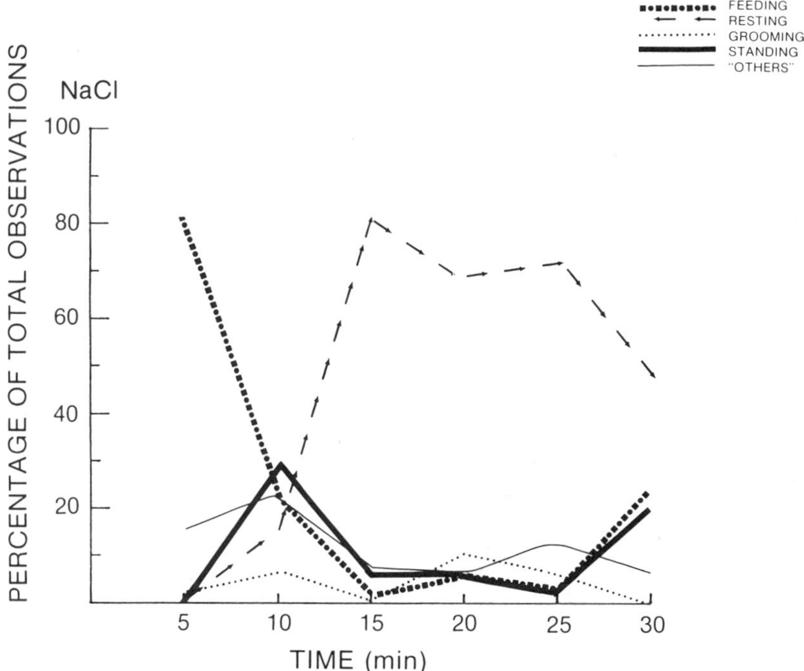

FIGURE 7. Mean percentage of total observations of behavior made in the categories of behavior described in FIGURE 6 for rats receiving saline, across 5-min observation intervals.

when injected at specific doses that reduce human feeding, CCK-like peptides elicit the self-report of satiety, not illness.[56-61] However, many doses of CCK and BBS can elicit reports of cramping, nausea, and other discomfort in humans, as was long known from CCK's use in clinical diagnosis. Caerulein, a CCK-like peptide, reliably elicits vomiting in dogs at certain doses beyond the threshold for feeding inhibition in rats.[62] Bombesin has been administered to humans, with feeding reduction but no correlated reports of sickness observed.[63] A report that concluded BBS may have a physiological role in humans also reported nausea and other side effects as a frequent minor consequence of some doses of BBS injected in humans.[64]

A conclusion possible from the studies of human responses to CCK, caerulein, and BBS administration is that CCK-like peptides and bombesin reduce feeding in man and elicit increments of self-report of both satiety and nausea, although increases of self-reported satiety do not correlate with increases in self-rated nausea. In light of individual variation in response to peptides, this finding could favor the suggestion that satiety signals elicited by food may become aversive, or nimiety signals, if their intensity increases as food intake increases.

Many other food-modulated blood-borne factors have been tested for specificity of satiety action in conditioned food aversion designs. Factors suggested as satiety factors and simultaneously tested as unconditioned stimuli include insulin,[65] glucagon,[66-68] starch,[4,11,26,27] prolactin and estrogen,[69] glucose, arginine, and ammonium ion,[70] glucose and fat,[71,72] calcitonin,[73-75] somatostatin,[76] neurotensin,[77] and corticotropin releasing factor.[78] In these studies, a conditioned aversion to cues associated

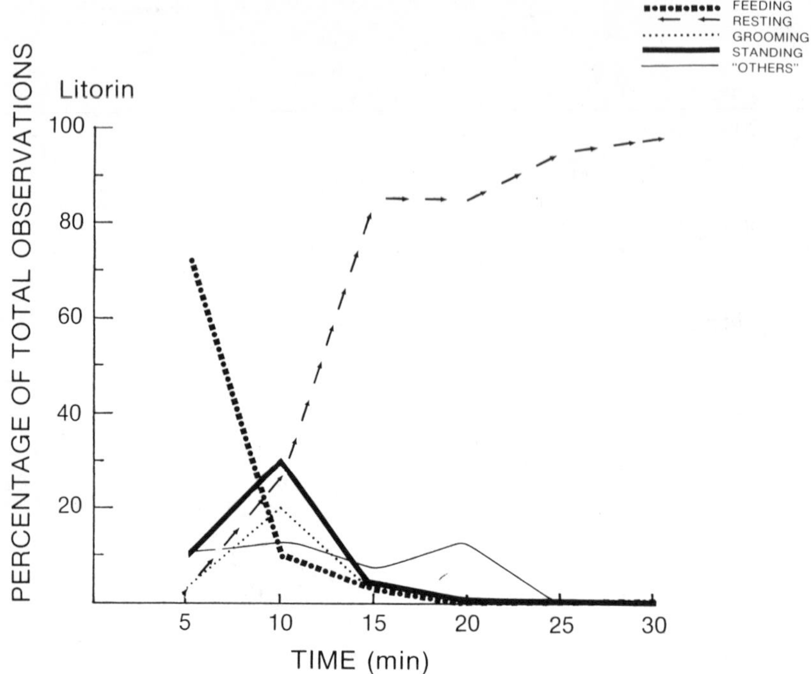

FIGURE 8. Mean percentage of total observations of behavior for rats receiving litorin, across 5-min observation intervals.

with anorexic doses of a factor is not accepted as consistent with a specific satiety action. It has been shown, however, that moderate amounts of food condition aversions as well as preferences that are dependent on repletion state of subjects, and food conditions repletion-independent aversions in overdose.[4] Thus, testing design should evaluate the effects of moderately signal-reduced consumption, and not just the effects of surprisingly high signal strength after self-selected consumption.

Further, it is not entirely clear that satiety's conditioning effects do not reflect the traditional aversive connotations of the term. Experiments assessing the conditioning properties of satiation procedures have often found that cues associated with consumption by hungry subjects are preferred to cues associated with consumption after satiation.[66,79,80] Satiety also produces a well-documented specific short-term aversion to oronasal cues called alliesthesia.[81]

The typical evaluation of circulating satiety factors has been criticized with the argument that feeding reduction may be a more sensitive measure of toxicosis than either behavioral observations or conditioned taste aversion tests.[53] Feeding and drinking reductions, however, have been clearly shown to provide relatively insensitive measures of treatments such as amphetamine,[50] rotational stimulation,[82] cyclophosphamide,[49] and physostigmine,[51] compared to taste aversion measures. Further, increases of non-nutritive feeding or pica have been shown to provide very sensitive indices of toxin administration.[49,82] Pica tests, and other, novel methods of behavioral analysis,[8,83–94] if validated in the context of feeding, may well be applied as parts of

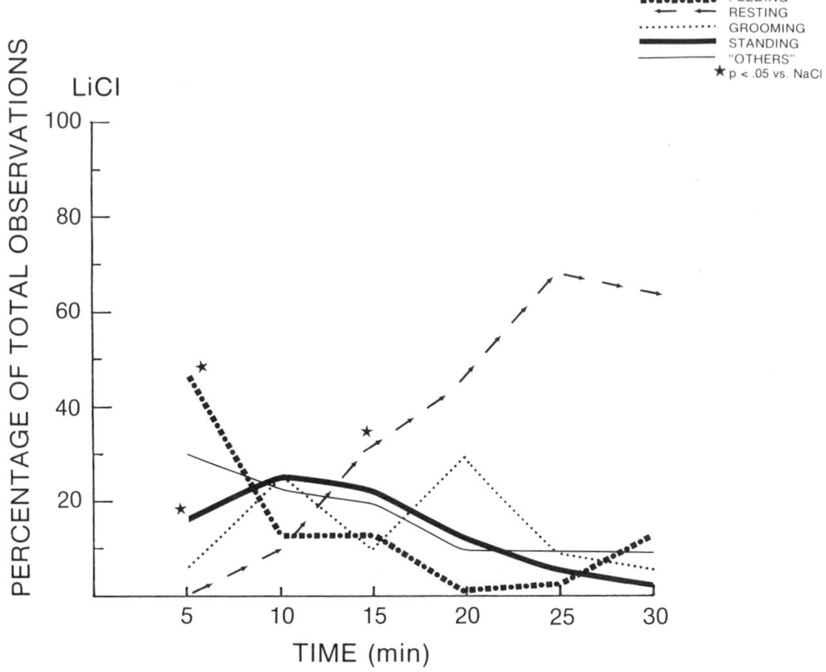

FIGURE 9. Mean percentage of total observations of behavior for rats receiving LiCl, across 5-min observation intervals.

a comprehensive battery of tests of specificity of action. These tests include multiple, systematic behavioral observations, human self-report when available, and demonstration of repletion-dependent conditioned preference and aversion, including a sensitive conditioned taste aversion test to verify that only high, suprathreshold doses condition repletion-independent aversions, just as food does only in excess. The conditioned food aversion test, although well-presented and verified as a test of toxicity,[51,95] has also clearly been shown to provide insensitive measure of certain toxins.[18–22] Clearly, no single test can be shown to provide a foolproof index of all toxicoses. A combination of tests of toxicity must be used to verify that a factor may be involved in satiety and to make the surprisingly subtle distinction between satiation and toxicosis.

Evidence suggests a final common pathway, the vagus nerve, in both satiety elicited by CCK injection and in the production of conditioned aversion to substances like $CuSO_4$, which produce gastrointestinal irritation.[9,96] In early experiments, we observed that total subdiaphragmatic vagotomy eliminated acquisition, but not retention of conditioned taste aversions, and appeared to reduce CCK's satiety effect in rats.[5,97] It is now clear that the feeding inhibition effect of CCK-like peptides depends upon intact gastric vagi,[98–101] and other satiety signals are vagus-independent.[102–105] Similarly, several circulating toxins induce conditioned aversion in vagotomized rats.[22,106,107] Also, intact vagi are required for elicitation of vomiting to some gut-applied stimuli,[108] and for the maintenance of normal meal size.[109] It is tempting to speculate a spectrum of food-contingent signals acting via the vagus, with low and moderate levels

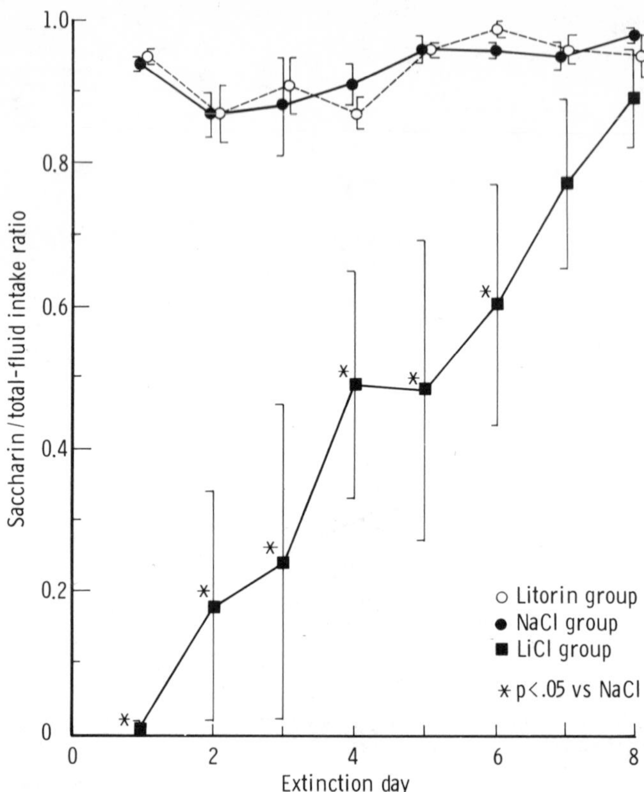

FIGURE 10. Mean (±SE) saccharin/total fluid intake ratio on eight 30-min extinction tests. Saline (8 ml/kg), litorin (8 μg/kg) or LiCl (8 ml/kg, 0.15 M) was injected i.p. immediately following novel saccharin access on day 8 of adaptation to an 18 hr water deprivation schedule. (From Kulkosky & Gibbs.[44] With permission of Pergamon Press, Ltd.)

of food intake and vagal activity effecting hunger reduction and satiety, while higher levels cause nausea and nimiety, and ultimately, vomiting.[34] Qualitative hedonic shifts from hunger to nimiety are correlated with quantitative changes in food intake and associated vagal activity. This consideration, taken together with the recognition that satiety signals act additively and independently to reduce feeding,[110,111] strengthens the foregoing cautions about interpretation of the effects of high doses of a putative satiety factor in any test of aversiveness.

Understanding of the satiety signals that act to limit normal food intake and other caloric intakes, such as ethanol,[112] is hoped to lead to therapeutic advances in treatment of intake-related disorders such as obesity and alcoholism. Administration and non-invasive modulation of these signals at appropriate times and intensities may provide new tools to deal effectively with these pervasive disorders. It is important that candidate satiety signals undergo multiple, rigorous testing according to the established criteria. A sensitive food aversion paradigm can be one, critical part of this screening procedure, when the appropriateness of dose and administration procedure is fully taken into consideration.

ACKNOWLEDGMENT

The author thanks G. P. Smith, J. Gibbs, and S. C. Woods for their many contributions to, and support of this research, and R. F. DeKesthler for his assistance.

REFERENCES

1. Murray, J. A. H., H. Bradley, W. A. Craigie & C. T. Onions, Eds. 1961. Oxford English Dictionary **9**: 118. Oxford University Press. London.
2. Burchfield, R. W., Ed. 1982. Supplement to the Oxford English Dictionary. **3**: 1494. Oxford University Press. London.
3. Smith, G. P. & J. Gibbs. 1979. Postprandial satiety. Prog. Psychobiol. Physiol. Psychol. **8**: 179–242.
4. Booth, D. A. 1981. The physiology of appetite. Br. Med. Bull. **37**: 135–140.
5. Woods, S. C., D. B. West, L. J. Stein, L. D. McKay, E. C. Lotter, S. G. Porte, N. J. Kenney & D. Porte Jr. 1981. Peptides and the control of meal size. Diabetologia **20**: 305–313.
6. Houpt, K. A. 1982. Gastrointestinal factors in hunger and satiety. Neurosci. Biobehav. Rev. **6**: 145–164.
7. Smith, G. P. 1982. Satiety and the problem of motivation. *In* The Physiological Mechanisms of Motivation. D. W. Pfaff, Ed.: 133–143. Springer-Verlag. New York.
8. Deutsch, J. A. 1982. Controversies in food intake regulation. *In* The Neural Basis of Feeding and Reward. B. G. Hoebel & D. Novin, Eds.: 137–148. Haer Institute. Brunswick, Maine.
9. Smith, G. P., J. Gibbs & P. J. Kulkosky. 1982. Relationships between brain-gut peptides and neurons in the control of food intake. *In* The Neural Basis of Feeding and Reward. B. G. Hoebel & D. Novin, Eds.: 149–165. Haer Institute. Brunswick, Maine.
10. Davis, J. D., C. S. Campbell, R. J. Gallagher & M. A. Zurakov. 1971. Disappearance of a humoral satiety factor during food deprivation. J. Comp. Physiol. Psychol. **75**: 476–482.
11. Booth, D. A. 1972. Conditioned satiety in the rat. J. Comp. Physiol. Psychol. **81**: 457–471.
12. Gibbs, J., R. C. Young & G. P. Smith. 1973. Cholecystokinin decreases food intake in rats. J. Comp. Physiol. Psychol. **84**: 488–495.
13. Smith, G. P. 1983. The role of the gut in the control of food intake. Viewpoints Digest. Dis. **15**: 1–4.
14. Smith, G. P. 1983. The place of gut peptides in the treatment of obesity. *In* Biochemical Pharmacology of Obesity. P. B. Curtis-Prior, Ed.: 407–419. Elsevier. New York.
15. Garcia, J., D. J. Kimeldorf & E. L. Hunt 1961. The use of ionizing radiation as a motivating stimulus. Psychol. Rev. **68**: 383–395.
16. Garcia, J., F. R. Ervin & R. A. Koelling. 1967. Bait-shyness: A test for toxicity with N=2. Psychon. Sci. **7**: 245–246.
17. Antin, J., J. Gibbs, J. Holt, R. C. Young & G. P. Smith. 1975. Cholecystokinin elicits the complete behavioral sequence of satiety in rats. J. Comp. Physiol. Psychol. **89**: 784–790.
18. Nachman, M. & P. L. Hartley. 1975. Role of illness in producing learned taste aversions in rats: A comparison of several rodenticides. J. Comp. Physiol. Psychol. **89**: 1010–1018.
19. Ionescu, E. & O. Buresova. 1977. Failure to elicit conditioned taste aversion by severe poisoning. Pharmac. Biochem. Behav. **6**: 251–254.
20. Gamzu, E. 1977. The multifaceted nature of taste-aversion-inducing agents: Is there a single common factor? *In* Learning Mechanisms in Food Selection. L. M. Barker, M. R. Best & M. Domjan, Eds.: 477–509. Baylor University Press. Waco, TX.
21. Goudie, A. J. 1979. Aversive stimulus properties of drugs. Neuropharmac. **18**: 971–979.
22. Ashe, J. H. & M. Nachman. 1980. Neural Mechanisms in taste aversion learning. Prog. Psychobiol. Physiol. Psychol. **9**: 233–262.

23. Tolman, E. C. 1967. Purposive Behavior in Animals and Men. Appleton-Century-Crofts. New York.
24. Adolph, E. F. 1980. Intakes are limited; Satieties. Appetite **1**: 337–342.
25. Adolph, E. F. 1981. Regulations of intakes: clearances. Am. J. Physiol. **240**: R356–R363.
26. Booth, D. A. 1980. Conditioned reactions in motivation. *In* Analysis of Motivational Processes. F. M. Toates & T. R. Halliday, Eds.: 77–102. Academic Press. New York.
27. Booth, D. A. 1982. Normal control of omnivore intake by taste and smell. *In* Determination of Behaviour by Chemical Stimuli. J. E. Steiner & J. R. Ganchrow, Eds.: 233–243. IRL. London.
28. Dockray, G. J. & R. A. Gregory. 1980. Relations between neuropeptides and gut hormones. Proc. R. Soc. Lond. Ser. B **210**: 151–164.
29. Holt, J., J. Antin, J. Gibbs, R. C. Young & G. P. Smith. 1974. Cholecystokinin does not produce bait shyness in rats. Physiol. Behav. **12**: 497–498.
30. Deutsch, J. A. & W. T. Hardy. 1977. Cholecystokinin produces bait shyness in rats. Nature **266**: 196.
31. Gibbs, J. & G. P. Smith. 1977. Reply. Nature **266**: 196.
32. Grote, F. W., Jr & R. T. Brown. 1971. Conditioned taste aversions: Two-stimulus tests are more sensitive than one-stimulus tests. Behav. Res. Meth. Instru. **3**: 311–312.
33. Kraly, F. S., W. J. Carty, S. Resnick & G. P. Smith. 1978. Effect of cholecystokinin on meal size and intermeal interval in the sham-feeding rat. J. Comp. Physiol. Psychol. **92**: 697–707.
34. Kulkosky, P. J. 1980. Reduction of drinking-associated feeding by C-terminal octapeptide of cholecystokinin-pancreozymin. Behav. Neural Biol. **29**: 111–116.
35. West, D. B., R. H. Williams, D. J. Braget & S. C. Woods. 1982. Bombesin reduces food intake of normal and hypothalamically obese rats and lowers body weight when given chronically. Peptides **3**: 61–67.
36. Houpt, T. R., S. M. Anika & N. C. Wolff. 1978. Satiety effects of cholecystokinin and caerulein in rabbits. Am. J. Physiol. **235**: R23–R28.
37. Anika, S. M., T. R. Houpt & K. A. Houpt. 1981. Cholecystokinin and satiety in pigs. Am. J. Physiol. **240**: R310–R318.
38. Melchiorri, P. 1980. Bombesin-like peptides activity in the gastrointestinal tract of mammals and birds. *In* Gastrointestinal Hormones. G. B. Jerzy Glass, Ed.: 717–725. Raven Press. New York.
39. Gibbs, J., D. J. Fauser, E. A. Rowe, B. J. Rolls, E. T. Rolls & S. P. Maddison. 1979. Bombesin suppresses feeding in rats. Nature **282**: 208–210.
40. Deutsch, J. A. 1980. Bombesin—satiety or malaise? Nature **285**: 591.
41. Gibbs, J. & G. P. Smith. 1980. Reply. Nature **285** :591.
42. Kulkosky, P. J., L. Gray, J. Gibbs & G. P. Smith. 1981. Feeding and selection of saccharin after injections of bombesin, LiCl, and NaCl. Peptides **2**: 61–64.
43. Deutsch, J. A. & S. L. Parsons. 1981. Bombesin produces taste aversion in rats. Behav. Neural Biol. **31**: 110–113.
44. Kulkosky, P. J. & J. Gibbs. 1982. Litorin suppresses food intake in rats. Life Sci. **31**: 685–692.
45. Endean, R., V. Erspamer, G. Falconieri Erspamer, G. Improta, P. Melchiorri, L. Negri & N. Sopranzi. 1975. Parallel bioassay of bombesin and litorin, a bombesin-like peptide from the skin of *Litoria aurea*. Br. J. Pharmac. **55**: 213–219.
46. Jensen, R. T., T. Moody, C. Pert, J. E. Rivier & J. D. Gardner. 1978. Interaction of bombesin and litorin with specific membrane receptors on pancreatic acinar cells. Proc. Natl. Acad. Sci. USA **75**: 6139–6143.
47. Mueller, K. & S. Hsiao. 1977. Specificity of cholecystokinin satiety effect: Reduction of food but not water intake. Pharmac. Biochem. Behav. **6**: 643–646.
48. Adams, P. M. 1973. The effects of cholinolytic drugs and cholinesterase blockade on deprivation based activity and appetitive behavior. Neuropharmac. **12**: 825–833.
49. Mitchell, D., C. Wells, N. Hoch, K. Lind, S. C. Woods & L. K. Mitchell. 1976. Poison induced pica in rats. Physiol. Behav. **17**: 691–697.

50. Stolerman, I. P. & G. D. D'Mello. 1978. Amphetamine-induced hypodipsia and its implications for conditioned taste aversion in rats. Pharmac. Biochem. Behav. **8**: 333–338.
51. Parker, L. A., S. Hutchison & A. L. Riley. 1982. Conditioned flavor aversions: A toxicity test of the anticholinesterase agent, physostigmine. Neurobehav. Toxicol. Teratol. **4**: 93–98.
52. Gibbs, J., L. Gray, C. F. Martin, W. T. Lhamon & J. A. Stuckey. 1980. Quantitative behavioral analysis of neuropeptides which suppress food intake. Soc. Neurosci. Abst. **6**: 530.
53. Deutsch, J.A . & M. F. Gonzalez. 1978. Food intake reduction: Satiation or aversion? Behav. Biol. **24**: 317–326.
54. Grossman, M. I. 1960. Satiety signals. Am. J. Clin. Nutr. **8**: 562–568.
55. Razran, G. 1961. The observable unconscious and the inferable conscious in current Soviet psychophysiology: Interoceptive conditioning, semantic conditioning, and the orienting reflex. Psychol. Rev. **68**: 81–147.
56. Sturdevant, R. A. L. & H. Goetz. 1976. Cholecystokinin both stimulates and inhibits human food intake. Nature **261**: 713–715.
57. Stacher, G., H. Bauer & H. Steinringer. 1979. Cholecystokinin decreases appetite and activation evoked by stimuli arising from the preparation of a meal in man. Physiol. Behav. **23**: 325–331.
58. Kissileff, H. R., F. X. Pi-Sunyer, J. Thornton & G. P. Smith. 1981. C-terminal octapeptide of cholecystokinin decreases food intake in man. Am. J. Clin. Nutr. **34**: 154–160.
59. Pi-Sunyer, X., H. R. Kissileff, J. Thornton & G. P. Smith. 1982. C-terminal octapeptide of cholecystokinin decreases food intake in obese men. Physiol. Behav. **29**: 627–630.
60. Stacher, G., H. Steinringer, G. Schmierer, C. Schneider & S. Winklehner. 1982. Cholecystokinin octapeptide decreases intake of solid food in man. Peptides **3**: 133–136.
61. Stacher, G., H. Steinringer, G. Schmierer, C. Schneider & S. Winklehner. 1982. Ceruletide decreases food intake in non-obese men. Peptides **3**: 607–612.
62. Nakamura, N., S. Shiozaki, Y. Koyama, T. Kojima & H. Marumo. 1975. Pharmacological studies of caerulein. II. The possibility of mediation through the central nervous system. Jap. J. Pharmac. **25**: 241–250.
63. Muurahainen, N. E., H. R. Kissileff, J. Thornton & F. X. Pi-Sunyer. 1983. Bombesin: Another peptide that inhibits feeding in man. Soc. Neurosci. Abst. **9**: 183.
64. Basso, N., E. Lezoche & V. Speranza. 1979. Studies with bombesin in man. Wld. J. Surg. **3**: 579–585.
65. Lovett, D., P. Goodchild & D. A. Booth. 1968. Depression of intake of nutrient by association of its odor with effects of insulin. Psychon. Sci. **11**: 27–28.
66. Revusky, S. & J. Garcia. 1970. Learned associations over long delays. Psychol. Learn. Motiv. **4**: 1–84.
67. Martin, J. R. & D. Novin.1977. Decreased feeding in rats following hepatic-portal infusion of glucagon. Physiol. Behav. **19**: 461–466.
68. Geary, N. & G. P. Smith. 1982. Pancreatic glucagon and postprandial satiety in the rat. Physiol. Behav. **28**: 313–322.
69. King, J. M. & V. C. Cox. 1976. Effects of ergocornine and CI-628 on food intake and taste preferences. Physiol. Behav. **16**: 111–113.
70. Martin, G. M. & L. H. Storlien. 1976. Anorexia and conditioned taste aversions in the rat. Learn. Motiv. **7**: 274–282.
71. Koopmans, H. S. & C. A. Maggio. 1978. The effects of specified chemical meals on food intake. Am. J. Clin. Nutr. **31**: S267–S272.
72. Koopmans, H. S. 1981. Peptides as satiety agents: The behavioural evaluation of their effects on food intake. *In* Gut Hormones. 2nd edit. S. R. Bloom & J. M. Polak, Eds.: 464–470. Churchill Livingstone. New York.
73. Perlow, M. J., W. J. Freed, J. S. Carman & R. J. Wyatt. 1980. Calcitonin reduces feeding in man, monkey and rat. Pharmac. Biochem. Behav. **12**: 609–612.
74. Deutsch, J. A. 1981. Calcitonin: Aversive effects in rats? Science **211**: 733–734.

75. Freed, W. J., L. A. Bing & R. J. Wyatt. 1981. Calcitonin: Aversive effects in rats? Science **211**: 734.
76. Lotter, E. C., R. Krinsky, J. M. McKay, C. M. Treneer, D. Porte, Jr. & S. C. Woods. 1981. Somatostatin decreases food intake of rats and baboons. J. Comp. Physiol. Psychol. **95**: 278–287.
77. Luttinger, D., R. A. King, D. Sheppard, J. Strupp, C. B. Nemeroff & A. J. Prange, Jr. 1982. The effect of neurotensin on food consumption in the rat. Eur. J. Pharmac. **81**: 499–503.
78. Gosnell, B. A., J. E. Morley & A. S. Levine. 1983. A comparison of the effects of corticotropin releasing factor and sauvagine on food intake. Pharmac. Biochem. Behav. **19**: 771–775.
79. Revusky, S. H. 1967. Hunger level during food consumption: Effects on subsequent preference. Psychon. Sci. **7**: 109–110.
80. Kurtz, K. H. & R. G. Jarka. 1968. Position preference based on differential food privation. J. Comp. Physiol. Psychol. **66**: 518–521.
81. Cabanac, M. 1979. Sensory pleasure. Q. Rev. Bio. **54**: 1–29.
82. Mitchell, D., M. L. Krusemark & E. Hafner. 1977. Pica: A species relevant behavioral assay of motion sickness in the rat. Physiol. Behav. **18**: 125–130.
83. Kornblith, C. L., G. N. Ervin & R. A. King. 1978. Hypothalamic and locus coeruleus self-stimulation are decreased by cholecystokinin. Physiol. Behav. **21**: 1037–1041.
84. Blundell, J. E., E. Tombros, P. J. Rogers & C. J. Latham. 1980. Behavioural analysis of feeding: Implications for the pharmacological manipulation of food intake in animals and man. Prog. Neuro-Psychopharmac. **4**: 319–326.
85. Booth, D. A. 1981. How should questions about satiation be asked? Appetite **2**: 237–244.
86. VanderWeele, D. A., J. A. Granja & D. A. Deems. 1982. Discomfort or satiety; The spontaneous meal pattern may serve as a predictor. *In* The Neural Basis of Feeding and Reward. B. G. Hoebel & D. Novin, Eds.: 167–173. Haer Institute. Brunswick, Maine.
87. Hsiao, S. & R. Spencer. 1983. Analysis of licking responses in rats: Effects of cholecystokinin and bombesin. Behav. Neurosci. **97**: 234–245.
88. Van Vort, W. & G. P. Smith. 1983. The relationships between the positive reinforcing and satiating effects of a meal in the rat. Physiol. Behav. **30**: 279–284.
89. Mansbach, R. S. & D. N. Lorenz. 1983. Cholecystokinin (CCK-8) elicits prandial sleep in rats. Physiol. Behav. **30**: 179–183.
90. Baldwin, B. A., T. R. Cooper & R. F. Parrott. 1983. Intravenous cholecystokinin octapeptide in pigs reduces operant responding for food, water, sucrose solution or radiant heat. Physiol. Behav. **30**: 399–403.
91. Swerdlow, N. R., C. Van Der Kooy, G. F. Koob & J. R. Wenger. 1983. Cholecystokinin produces conditioned place-aversions, not place-preferences, in food-deprived rats: Evidence against involvement in satiety. Life Sci. **32**: 2087–2093.
92. Crawley, J. N. 1983. Divergent effects of cholecystokinin, bombesin, and lithium on rat exploratory behaviors. Peptides **4**: 405–410.
93. Billington, C. J., A. S. Levine & J. E. Morley. 1983. Are peptides truly satiety agents? A method of testing for neurohumoral satiety effects. Am. J. Physiol. **245**: R920–R926.
94. Ettenberg, A. & G. F. Koob. 1984. Different effects of cholecystokinin and satiety on lateral hypothalamic self-stimulation. Physiol. Behav. **32**: 127–130.
95. Yokel, R. A. & C. D. Ogzewalla. 1981. Effects of plant ingestion in rats determined by the conditioned taste aversion procedure. Toxicon. **19**: 223–232.
96. Coil, J. D., R. C. Rogers, J. Garcia & D. Novin. 1978. Conditioned taste aversions: Vagal and circulatory mediation of the toxic unconditioned stimulus. Behav. Biol. **24**: 509–519.
97. Kulkosky, P. J., E. C. Lotter, D. L. Hjeresen & S. C. Woods. 1974. Elimination of conditioned taste aversions by prior vagotomy. Prog. Ann. Meet. West. Psychol. Soc. **54**: 107.
98. Kulkosky, P. J., C. Breckenridge, R. Krinsky & S. C. Woods. 1976. Satiety elicited by the C-terminal octapeptide of cholecystokinin-pancreozymin in normal and VMH-lesioned rats. Behav. Biol. **18**: 227–234.

99. SMITH, G. P., C. JEROME, B. J. CUSHIN, R. ETERNO & K. J. SIMANSKY. 1981. Abdominal vagotomy blocks the satiety effect of cholecystokinin in the rat. Science **213**: 1036–1037.
100. LORENZ, D. N. & S. A. GOLDMAN. 1982. Vagal mediation of the cholecystokinin satiety effect in rats. Physiol. Behav. **29**: 599–604.
101. SMITH, G. P., C. JEROME, P. KULKOSKY & K. J. SIMANSKY. 1984. Ceruletide acts in the abdomen, not in the brain, to produce satiety. Peptides. (In press.)
102. KRALY, F. S. & J. GIBBS. 1980. Vagotomy fails to block the satiating effect of food in the stomach. Physiol. Behav. **24**: 1007–1010.
103. SMITH, G. P., C. JEROME & J. GIBBS. 1981. Abdominal vagotomy does not block the satiety effect of bombesin in the rat. Peptides **2**: 409–411.
104. MORLEY, J. E., A. S. LEVINE, J. KNEIP & M. GRACE. 1982. The effect of vagotomy on the satiety effects of neuropeptides and naloxone. Life Sci. **30**: 1943–1947.
105. GIBBS, J. & G. P. SMITH. 1982. Gut peptides and food in the gut produce similar satiety effects. Peptides **3**: 553–557.
106. MARTIN, J. R., F. Y. CHENG & D. NOVIN. 1978. Acquisition of learned taste aversion following bilateral subdiaphragmatic vagotomy in rats. Physiol. Behav. **21**: 13–17.
107. KIEFER, S. W., R. J. CABRAL, K. W. RUSINIAK & J. GARCIA. 1980. Ethanol-induced flavor aversions in rats with subdiaphragmatic vagotomies. Behav. Neural Biol. **29**: 246–254.
108. BORISON, H. L. & S. C. WANG. 1953. Physiology and pharmacology of vomiting. Pharmac. Rev. **5**: 193–230.
109. SNOWDON, C. T. & A. N. EPSTEIN. 1970. Oral and intragastric feeding in vagotomized rats. J. Comp. Physiol. Psychol. **71**: 59–67.
110. GIBBS, J., P. J. KULKOSKY & G. P. SMITH. 1981. Effects of peripheral and central bombesin on feeding behavior of rats. Peptides Suppl. 2: 179–183.
111. STEIN, L. J. & S. C. WOODS. 1981. Cholecystokinin and bombesin act independently to decrease food intake in the rat. Peptides **2**: 431–436.
112. KULKOSKY, P. J. 1984. Effect of cholecystokinin octapeptide on ethanol intake in the rat. Alcohol **1**: 125–128.

Predation Control Using Conditioned Food Aversion Methodology: Theory, Practice, and Implications

CARL R. GUSTAVSON[a]

Department of Psychology
North Dakota State University
and
Department of Neuroscience
Division of Psychiatry and Behavioral Science
School of Medicine
University of North Dakota

JOAN C. GUSTAVSON

Department of Neuroscience
Division of Psychiatry and Behavioral Science
School of Medicine
University of North Dakota
Fargo, North Dakota 58102

Since 1972 we have been conducting basic theoretical research on behavior in the applied context using conditioned taste aversion for controlling wildlife damage to human resources. Because of the applied context, this research has often been conducted in circumstances, and has used species, exotic to the psychological laboratory.[1] Our purpose in this paper is to organize the unusual variations presented in this research and to examine these findings as a whole. We report several single case observations that lead us to suggest conditioned taste aversions are expressed differently in the context of social and ecological diversity than in the restricted setting of the laboratory.

In our research we have usually assumed that: (1) our animals are hungry; (2) when animals are hungry food selection is best thought of as having two sequential consummatory components, attack and consumption; and (3) the attack phase is guilded by visual, auditory, and olfactory senses, where as consumption is guilded by taste. We have presumed, but have usually attempted to empirically verify, the parameters for establishing conditioned taste aversion in the laboratory rat would also apply to a diverse number of species.[2-4]

EXPERIMENTAL DIVERSITY

In TABLE 1, the studies were categorized as to the following characteristics: (1) the mobility of the subjects, i.e. whether or not the study was conducted in a captive or

[a] Address correspondence to C. R. G., Department of Psychiatry and Behavioral Science, Rm. 303 Administration Annex, University of Texas Medical Branch, Galveston, TX 77550.

free-ranging environment and (2) the social context of the study (free-ranging subjects were part of a rigid social organization, a feeding affiliate, a seasonal family grouping, or free-ranging individuals; captive subjects lived in social groups, pairs, or as isolated individuals). The type, dose, concentration in food, or route of administration of toxins used in these studies also varied considerably. This information is not included in the table because these variations were always designed to prevent the flavor of the food from being changed. While the organization of TABLE 1 is a post hoc survey of the literature, several broad conclusions seem appropriate.

Apparently taxonomic variables predict little concerning the acquisition of conditioned taste aversions. In fact, a diverse number of vertebrates seem to avoid consuming foods that have in the past been toxic, whether the animals live as isolated individuals or in groups and/or are maintained in captivity or exposed to the food-illness contingency while ranging in their typical habitat. Similarly, irrespective of the diverse food characteristics, taste aversions seem to be eventually learned.

From the information in the table we conclude conditioned taste aversion is a very robust phenomenon, the gross characteristics of which can be observed under a remarkable variety of circumstances. The phenomenon appears so robust that we should find remarkable those instances where a food illness contingency appears to be present and the subjects fail to avoid that food. Under these circumstances the presence of the food illness contingency should be seriously examined.[4–13]

We point this out because confusion seems to exist in the applied literature as to the different effects produced by different aversive stimuli in food avoidance learning. Repellents, conditioned repellents, and poison were paired with food consumption or approach for rats in a variety of environments. Peripheral pain experienced while approaching a food terminated the approach and seemed to inhibit future approach in the area in which the treatment was applied. Neither food consumption nor approach was suppressed in familiar surroundings. Foods paired with poisons prevented consumption regardless of the environment. Consumption of the adulterated food was prevented by repellents only when the repellent was present. Neither the approach nor the consumption was affected when the repellent was absent. This experiment emphasized the importance of maintaining a distinction among peripherally based avoidance conditioning, internally based taste aversion conditioning, and repellents for both practical and theoretical reasons.[14]

ECOLOGICAL CONTEXT

In spite of the broad taxonomic generality and robustness, we do not intend to suggest that ecological variables have no influence on conditioned taste aversion acquisition or expression. Over the past ten years a variety of observations have led us to believe that in order to understand conditioned taste aversions occurring in natural habitats (including human environments), we must understand the context in which the food-illness contingency is presented and the encounter with the averted food is made. What follows are the details of some of these observations.

Captive Subjects

When six captive dingos (*Canis familiaris dingo*) were, on two occasions, simultaneously fed six minced lamb baits that had been treated with Thiabendazole (Merck) the social order of the group prevented one animal from gaining access to the treated

TABLE 1. Conditioned Taste Aversion Studies in Wildlife Management: Experimental Diversity and Results

Mobility	Social Context	Species	Experimental Results	Reference
Free Ranging	Organized			
	Coteries	Prairie dog	Aversion to wheat/oats in feeders	22
	Flocks	Blackbirds	Aversion to sunflower seed baits and seeds in growing heads	23
	Troops	Baboons	Aversion to growing maize	24
	Packs	Wolves	Aversion to beef baits and cattle	21
	Feeding affiliate	Racoons	Aversion to dead and live chicken	19
		Coyotes	Aversion to various camp foods: Animals left area	20
	Seasonal family groups	Coyotes	Aversion to sheep baits, dead sheep, and sheep: Animals left area	16
		Coyotes	Aversion to sheep baits and sheep	25
		Coyotes	Aversion to sheep	26
		Coyotes	Aversion to sheep and turkeys	27
		Coyotes	Aversion to sheep hide/dog food bait	18
	Individuals	Crows	Aversion to colored eggs	28
Captive	Social group	Dingoes	Aversion to minced lamb	15
		N. G. dog	Aversion to minced lamb	15
		Blackbird	Aversion to toxic sunflower seeds and seeds growing in heads in enclosed field	29

	Cape dog	No aversion indicated	**
	Pheasants	Aversion to sprouting corn planted in treated soil	30
	Budgies and finches	Aversion to food adhering to toxin-painted perches	30
Paired	Wolves	Aversion to sheep	16
	N. G. dogs	Aversion to minced lamb	15
Isolates	Dingoes	Aversion to minced lamb	15
	N. G. dogs	Aversion to minced lamb	15
	Wolves	Aversion to chicken franks, canned spaghetti, dog food, and turkey soup	31
	Coyotes	Aversion to rabbits and chickens	16
	Owls	Aversion to chicks/continued kills	18
	Ferrets	Aversion to canned food and mice/continued killing mice	32
	Hawks	Aversion to colored/flavored mice	33
	Bears	Aversion to marshmallows	18
	Magpies	Aversion to rabbit meat	18
	Rats	Aversion to chocolate cookies paired with LiCl/ avoidance of cookies paired with shock or repellents	14
	Coyotes	Aversion to dog food, hamburger, rabbits and sheep	34

meat. During the testing situation this low ranking male dingo, now unharassed by his lamb-diverted cage mates, consumed his fill of the untreated lamb meat.[15]

We conducted an experiment using two wolves (*Canis lupus*),[16] Thomas and Sissy. Sissy had suffered a serious nutritional deficit as a young pup that left her vision impaired by cataracts. As a result she always assumed a subordinate and following role to her brother Thomas. When these animals were presented lithium chloride–laced sheep baits, Thomas immediately seized and consumed one and one-half baits leaving Sissy with half of one bait. When presented with a live sheep several days later, Thomas led the attack, but quickly ceased upon biting the sheep. Sissy having a weak aversion persisted alone for several minutes before giving up. Once again the intraspecific interactions of the two wolves determined the magnitude of the individually acquired taste aversion. In addition, a striking interspecific reaction was observed; the classically docile sheep began attacking the wolves. The wolves were confused by this large, mobile, and unpalatable aggressor and initiated attempts to evaluate the sheep's social status by engaging in play solicitation.

In a dramatic and unique circumstance we failed to establish a conditioned taste aversion to Thiabendazole-laced lamb baits. Two groups of Cape hunting dogs (*Lycaon pictus*), each group made up of three individuals, were being introduced together for display at the Taronga Zoo in Sydney, Australia. Typically these animals have extremely rigid dominance relationships marked by intense aggression when these relationships are disrupted. Zoo personnel were attempting to soothe domestic strife during the introduction process by administering multiple daily injections of barbiturates. We attempted to establish conditioned taste aversions in these six animals by presenting them with six Thiabenzadole-laced sheep baits for three days. The animals were typically lethargic throughout the day, but introduction of the meat baits produced intense fighting and frenzied and rapid feeding. Neither the time required to consume the baits nor the number of baits consumed by individuals in the group changed over the treatment and test days. Whether this failure to reduce consumption was produced by the effect of the tranquilizer or simply the frenzied atmosphere is impossible to determine. But the failure to produce an aversion using a methodology and an illness agent that have worked with dingos, New Guinea wild dogs (*Canis familiaris hallstromi*), and wolves, suggests that frenzied competition, which may be typical for this species,[17] for specific food items may override the impact of conditioned taste aversion.

Free-ranging Subjects

On a national wildlife refuge in eastern Washington,[3,18] interspecific competition between magpies (*Pica pica*) and coyotes (*Canis latrans*) as a function of bait structure was observed. The study was undertaken to examine the target specificity of baits placed in the field to produce conditioned taste aversion in coyotes. Initially, balls of dog food were placed at 14 specific stations about the refuge. These stations were checked daily and missing baits were replaced. Both coyotes and magpies visited the bait stations and consumed baits shortly after the study began. However, within three days magpies began following our vehicles around the refuge and descended on baits upon our departure. Thus, these simple ground meat baits were not available for coyote consumption late in the day. Examination for tracks at bait stations suggested that coyotes seldom visited. At this point in the study we wrapped and sealed all dog food baits in pieces of fresh sheep hide. For several days, as the baits were placed, magpies would descend upon each bait station as we drove away. However, the magpies could not break through the tough hide and after five days they stopped following our vehicles. Coyotes again visited the stations and consumed the baits.

This refuge study continued for an additional two years as weather permitted. During both years, hide-wrapped baits containing lithium chloride were placed daily at stations on one half of the refuge. Hide-wrapped baits without lithium chloride were placed daily at stations on the other half of the refuge. During the first year, daily bait consumption decreased in the treatment area compared to the control area, suggesting that conditioned taste aversions had been established to the hide-wrapped baits. These aversions appeared to remain stable during the winter and spring of the next year when baits were not present. Bait consumption in the treatment area remained suppressed when baits were reintroduced.

Of special interest in this situation are several observations concerning mother-offspring interactions. In this area of eastern Washington coyote pups are born in the late spring and remain with their mothers in loose family affiliations until the next breeding season in the early winter. Based on sightings, estimates of the number of coyotes using the refuge exceeded 90 animals. The number of newborn pups in the treatment area should have exceeded 80. However, during the second year bait consumption in the treatment area averaged .39 per day compared to 2.15 per day for the control area. In addition, there were numerous occasions during the second year when baits at stations were found to be intact, but with both adult and pup coyote tracks evident at the feeding stations. In contrast, whenever tracks of adults and/or pups were present at a control feeding station baits were always missing. Coyote mothers apparently can inform their offspring as to the wholesomeness of food items. The methods by which this tuition is supplied have not been established. However, Galaf[35] suggest some possible mechanisms of socially communicated information about feeding.

An experiment with free ranging raccoons (*Procyon lotor*)[19] provides a contrast to the above observation. Conditioned taste aversions were established in a free-ranging raccoon population by making dead chickens laced with lithium chloride available. The durability of these aversions was tested by simultaneously making available live tethered chickens and dry dog food over a period of eight months. During this eight month period kits were born to the females in the population. As the kits became older, they would visit the testing site, staying back in the trees while their mothers fed on the dog food. During eight months of testing, the adults never killed or consumed the chickens. When the young raccoons first approached the feeder box with their mother, both mothers and kits began consuming dog food. Movements by the tethered chickens attracted the attention and elicited investigations by the kits. The kits killed the chickens and readily began eating them. Within an hour, several of the adults (the kits' mothers first) were also eating the chickens, in spite of eight months of absolute avoidance. The adults returned to killing and eating live chickens when they were presented. Apparently, adult raccoons may take advantage of an inquisitive nature in youth.

Resource Distribution

In addition to assessing conditioned taste aversions by measures of food consumption, four field investigations also evaluated animals' movement patterns. Data from two investigations suggested that the conditioned taste aversions not only changed food selection by the free-ranging animals, but also moved them away from the area in which the averted food was found. Two of the studies showed no indication of animals leaving the area. Moreover, the details of these investigations suggest a solution to these superficially contradictory findings.

One study[16] involved coyotes preying on sheep on a ranch in eastern Washington, which was isolated in a small river valley surrounded by many miles of wheat. In the wheat fields, large, easily captured prey were not abundant. Small rodents were both adundant and equally available on both the ranch and in the wheat fields. Apparently these coyotes were utilizing the sheep on the ranch for large, easily captured meals. However, once aversions were established to sheep the coyotes had no reason to selectively visit the ranch in search of mice, which were just as plentiful in the wheat fields. In another experiment,[20] a group of coyotes had been fed dog food by National Park Personnel for many years. When these personnel moved from the area and the supply of free food disappeared, the coyotes began scavenging a nearby campground. The new park personnel, concerned about camper safety, made available to the scavenging coyotes a wide variety of camping type foods laced with lithium chloride. After several encounters with these different foods, coyote stopped visiting the campground. Apparently these coyotes found eating the more traditional coyote diet preferable to eating easily obtained tainted camp fare. Since the traditional diet was unavailable on the campgrounds the visits ended.

Records of coyote sightings throughout the two years of the refuge study,[3,18] described above, indicate that not only did the coyotes remain in the treatment area, but the population may have increased by as much as 85%. Finally in a fourth experiment,[21] cowhide-wrapped ground beef baits treated with lithium chloride were placed in prime wolf habitat in northeastern Minneosta to protect a small cattle operation from predation by four separate packs of wolves. Each pack had at least one radio-collared member. Aerial tracking of these wolves indicated that the wolves remained in the area even after bait consumption had dropped dramatically.

On the refuge, we imposed a new food on an already established population and an aversion to this new food source did not alter the desirability of the habitat. The northern Minnesota wolf packs were responsible for very little cattle damage (6–12 annually). The pairing of conditioned taste aversions with this trivial and almost accidental food resource apparently did not detract from life in this food-saturated environment. Whether or not free-ranging predators remain in an area following establishment of a food aversion seems to depend upon the relationship of that food to other food resources in the environment and therefore the motives of the animals for frequenting a specific place.

Using this information, we once attempted to drive garbage-can scavenging bears from Mount Rainer National Park campgrounds. All garbage cans in the campgrounds were sprayed several times a day with a strong "minty" flavored lithium chloride solution in hopes that by establishing conditioned taste aversions to the artificially flavored garbage, we would drive the bears away. However, after several days of treatment the bears came upon a solution to the problem that we had not anticipated. Foods being prepared by the campers were not "minty" and the bears began directly intimidating people preparing or eating meals. The study was immediately terminated. The garbage containers were cleaned and the bears were trapped and removed to the high country.

IMPLICATIONS

The collective experience of 12 years of attempting to use conditioned taste aversions in wildlife management contexts suggests that the social organization and ecological context in which conditioned taste aversions are established can affect the rate at which individuals within a population acquire conditioned taste aversions and the way in which the aversion is expressed.

Our information indicates that variations in the results of conditioned taste aversions are not only a function of the parameters traditionally manipulated in psychology laboratories (delay of illness, flavor intensity, novelty or familiarity, illness intensity, and type of drug used to induce illness) but also a function of the complex interaction of these variables along with other variables that are seldom varied in the laboratory setting. Such complexity usually falls under the topic of ecology. We suggest that it is time to expand investigations of conditioned taste aversions to studies that include controlled complexity and not to limit investigations to the simplicity of using isolated individuals, in isolated cages, where one or two foods are presented serially or concurrently on a daily basis. The kind of variability (social organization, mobility, food placement, ease of acquisition, abundance, varied toxicities, competition with consumers of different species, and other complexities of the natural habitats) represented in our studies by accident or opportunism should be brought into the laboratory where the variables can be present at the same time and varied individually and by combination. Such an approach may be expensive and require the development of new technologies to easily identify individuals living in social groups and to monitor complex environments, but such an approach may be especially timely considering that a variety of researchers are attempting to use current knowledge of conditioned taste aversions to bring about desired change in human and animal consumptive behaviors or to explain phenomena occurring in human or veterinary medical settings. In this way we hope to avoid some of the difficulties experienced in other behavioral research areas where isolated animal subjects in simple environmental surroundings have been used to formulate broad theories of behavior, including pathology, only to be met with frustation and insurmountable difficulty.

REFERENCES

1. Riley, A. L. & L. L. Baril. 1976. Conditioned taste aversions: A bibliography. Animal Learning Behav. **4**: 15–135.
2. Gustavson, C. R., L. R. Brett, J. Garcia & D. J. Kelly. 1979. A working model and experimental solutions to the control of predatory behavior. *In* Behavior of Captive Wild Animals. H. Markowitz & V. Stevens, Eds. Nelson-Hall. Chicago, IL.
3. Gustavson, C. R. 1977. Comparative and field aspects of learned food aversions. *In* Learning Mechanisms in Food Selection. L. M. Barker, M. Best & M. Domjan, Eds.: 23–43. Baylor University Press. Waco, TX.
4. Gustavson, C. R. & L. K. Nicolaus. 1981. Taste aversion conditioning in wolves, coyotes and other canids: Retrospect and prospect. Paper presented at the First International Captive Wolf Research Conference. Flint, MI.
5. Burns, R. J. 1977. Conditioned prey aversion and transfer of avoidance to offspring in coyotes. Unpublished manuscript. U.S. Fish and Wildlife Service. Wildlife Research Center. Denver, CO.
6. Burns, R. J. 1980. Evaluation of conditioned predation aversion for controlling coyote predation. J. Wildlife Mgmt. **44**: 938–942.
7. Burns, R. J. & G. E. Connolly. 1980. Lithium chloride did not influence prey killing in coyotes. Proceedings Ninth Vertebrate Pest Conference. 200–203. Fresno, CA.
8. Conover, M. R., J. G. Francik & D. E. Miller. 1977. An experimental evaluation of using taste aversion to control sheep loss due to coyote predation. J. Wildlife Mgmt. **44**: 775–779.
9. Lehner, P. N. & S. W. Horn. 1975. Effectiveness of physiological aversive agents in suppressing predation on rabbits and domestic sheep by coyotes. U.S. Fish and Wildlife Service Research contract. Wildlife Research Center. Denver, CO.
10. Lehner, P. N. & S. W. Horn. 1977. Final research report. U.S. Fish and Wildlife Service. Denver, CO.

11. ELLINS, S. R. & G. C. MARTIN. 1981. Olfactory discrimination of lithium chloride by the coyote (*Canis latrans*). Behav. Neural Biol. **31**: 214–224.
12. WEDDINGTON, W. W. 1982. Psychogenic nausea and vomiting associated with termination of cancer chemotherapy. Psychother. Psychosom. **37**: 129–136.
13. WEDDINGTON, W. W., K. A. BLINDT & S. G. MCCRACKEN. 1983. Relaxation training for anticipatory nausea associated with chemotherapy. Psychosomatics **24**(3): 281–283.
14. GUSTAVSON, C. R. & J. C. GUSTAVSON. 1982. Food avoidance in rats: The differential effects of shock, illness and repellents. Appetite: J. Intake Res. **3**: 335–340.
15. GUSTAVSON, C. R., J. C. GUSTAVSON & G. A. HOLZER. 1983. Thiabendazole-based taste aversions in dingoes *Canis familiaris dingo*) and New Guinea wild dogs (*Canis familiaris hallstromi*). App. Animal Ethol. **10**: 385–388.
16. GUSTAVSON, C. R., D. J. KELLY, M. SWEENEY & J. GARCIA. 1976. Prey-lithium aversions I: Coyotes and wolves. Behav. Biol. **17**: 61–72.
17. DRICKAMER, L. C. & S. H. VESSEY. 1982. Animal Behavior: Concepts, processes, and methods. 312–388. Willard Grand Press. Boston, MA.
18. GUSTAVSON, C. R., D. J. KELLY, M. SWEENEY & G. THOMAS. 1976. Bait density and seasonal effects on learned food aversions in free ranging coyotes, with notes on several wild species. Unpublished manuscript. Washington Game Department. Olympia, WA.
19. NICOLAUS, L. K., T. E. HOFFMAN & C. R. GUSTAVSON. 1982. Taste aversion conditioning in free ranging raccoons (*Procyon lotor*). Northwest Sci. **56**: 165–169.
20. CORNELL, D. & J. E. CORNLEY. 1979. Aversive conditioning of campground coyotes in Joshua Tree National Monument. Wildl. Soc. Bull. **7**: 129–131.
21. GUSTAVSON, C. R. 1982/83. An evaluation of taste aversion control of wolf (*Canis lupus*) predation in northern Minnesota. App. Animal Ethol. **9**: 63–71.
22. HOLZER, G. A. & C. R. GUSTAVSON. 1980. Manipulation of wheat and oat preference in black-tailed prairie dogs: A field demonstration using Methiocarb as a taste aversion agent. Prairie Naturalist **12**(3&4): 114–118.
23. GUSTAVSON, C. R. 1981. The establishment of methylcarbamate based conditioned food aversions in rodents and avians. Research report to Union Carbide Company, Inc. Research Triangle, NC.
24. FORTHMAN-QUICK, D. L. 1982. Controlling crop-raiding baboons with conditioned taste aversion. Paper presented at IX Congress of the International Primate Society. Atlanta, GA.
25. GUSTAVSON, C. R., J. R. JOWEY & D. N. MILLIGAN. 1982. A 3-year evaluation of taste aversion coyote control in Saskatchewan. J. Range Mgmt. **35**(1): 57–59.
26. ELLINS, S. R., S. M. CATALANO & S. A. SCHECHINGER. 1977. Conditioned taste aversion: A field application to coyote predation on sheep. Behav. Biol. **20**: 91–95.
27. ELLINS, S. R. & S. M. CATALANO. 1980. Field application of the conditioned taste aversion paradigm to the control of coyote predation on sheep and turkeys. Behav. Neural Biol. **29**: 532–536.
28. NICOLAUS, L. K., J. F. CASSEL, R. B. CARLSON & C. R. GUSTAVSON. 1983. Taste aversion conditioning of crows to control predation on eggs. Science **220**: 212–214.
29. GUSTAVSON, C. R., G. A. HOLZER, J. C. GUSTAVSON & D. L. VAKOCH. 1982. An evaluation of phenol-methylcarbamates as taste aversion producing agents in caged blackbirds. Appl. Animal Ethol. **8**: 551–559.
30. GUSTAVSON, C. R. 1982. UC 27867 research report #2. Research report to Union Carbide Company, Inc. Research Triangle, NC.
31. ZIEGER, J. M., C. R. GUSTAVSON, G. A. HOLZER & D. GRUBER. 1982/83. Anthelmintic-based taste aversions in wolves (*Canis lupus*). App. Animal Ethol. **9**: 373–377.
32. RUSINIAK, K. W., C. R. GUSTAVSON, W. G. HANKINS & J. GARCIA. 1976. Prey-lithium aversions II: Laboratory rats and ferrets. Behav. Biol. **17**: 73–85.
33. BRETT, L. P., W. G. HANKINS & J. GARCIA. 1976. Prey-lithium averisons III: Buteo hawks. Behav. Biol. **17**: 87–89.
34. GUSTAVSON, C. R., J. GARCIA, W. G. HANKINS & K. W. RUSINIAK. 1974. Coyote predation control by aversive conditioning. Science **184**: 581–583.
35. GALEF, G., JR. 1985. Direct and indirect behavioral pathways to the social transmission of food avoidance. Ann. N.Y. Sci. (This volume.)

Aversion Therapy in the Treatment of Alcoholism: Success and Failure

PETER E. NATHAN

Department of Psychology
Rutgers, The State University
New Brunswick, New Jersey

A very wide range of behavioral treatment methods have been tried out on alcoholic patients (see Nathan and Niaura[1] for an overview of these efforts). For more than 30 years following the initial use of a behavioral approach to alcoholism in 1929[2] however, the treatment of the alcoholic by behavioral means was largely confined to the aversive conditioning therapies. Almost all of this treatment was by means either of electric shock or nausea-inducing drugs to induce aversion. Although two other aversion-induction stimuli—succinylcholine chloride dehydrate, a drug that induces total apneic (respiratory) paralysis,[3] and aversive images, said to induce aversion by imaginal means[4]—have also been employed, electrical and chemical aversion conditioning with nausea-inducing drugs have been the choice of those who treat alcoholism by aversive techniques. Recent research by Revusky and his colleagues[5] suggests that lithium carbonate may be a safer and more effective aversive agent for chemical aversion conditioning, though additional studies of efficacy and safety are necessary before the drug can be routinely substituted for emetine, the drug now used most widely for this purpose.

ELECTRICAL AVERSION

More than 50 years ago, Soviet physician N. V. Kantorovich paired the sight, smell, and taste of a variety of alcoholic beverages with repeated electric shock[2] to treat 20 alcoholic patients. Follow-up of this dramatic new treatment lasted from three weeks to 20 months and revealed that 70% of the patients had remained abstinent. These were extremely encouraging data, especially since Kantorovich, unlike many alcoholism researchers who came from him, followed a matched group of 10 alcoholics provided "standard treatment," which included either hypnotic suggestion or medication. The control group returned to abusive drinking within a few days of their release from the hospital.

Despite the positive nature of Kantorovich's findings, it was not until the 1960s that electrical aversion was reintroduced as a primary behavioral treatment for alcoholism. By contrast, emetine-aversion conditioning was put to routine use in a few specialized alcoholism treatment facilities beginning in the 1930s (see below).

The resurgence of interest in electrical aversion to treat alcoholism and several other behavioral disorders was a consequence, in part, of theoretical papers by Eysenck[6] and Rachman.[7] Rachman's influential paper observed that nausea-inducing drugs are difficult to administer reliably, cause unpleasantness for both patient and therapist, and generate "aggressiveness and hostility on the part of the patient." Contrasting these negative features of chemical aversion with electrical aversion, Rachman went on to note that (1) the long history of aversive conditioning with animals and humans guaranteed better research on therapeutic outcome, (2) the nature of the electrical stimulus permits its reliable and accurate administration, and (3) electrical stimulation also enables use of portable apparatus for delivery of shock to humans, another decided plus. These views, along with similar conclusions by others in favor of electrical aversion, accounted at least in part for the primacy of electric shock as an aversive stimulus in the 1960s and early 1970s.

Shortly after Eysenck's and Rachman's papers appeared (in 1960 and 1961), McGuire and Vallance[8] reported on their initial attempts to treat alcoholism by electrical aversion. They provided straightforward aversive (classical) conditioning to both alcoholics and patients with other behavioral disorders (the latter included a fetishist, an obsessional ruminator, a heavy smoker, and a victim of writer's cramp), concluding that alcoholism responded less well than heavy smoking or fetishism to this treatment method.

One of the most extensive series of electrical aversion studies was conducted shortly thereafter by Blake at the Crichton Royal Hospital, Scotland.[9,10] A more sophisticated application of behavioral principles than McGuire and Vallance's project, Blake's treatment approach combined training in progressive relaxation with electrical aversion conditioning. This broader attack on behaviors associated with chronic alcoholism anticipated similar present day approaches to this disorder. By defining alcoholism as "the result of a learned habit of uncontrollable drinking which is used by the individual in an effort to reduce a disturbance in psychological homeostasis," Blake[9] made clear his acceptance of the anxiety reduction hypothesis of alcoholism etiology[11] in its virtual entirety. He justified his choice of seemingly incompatible treatment methods by noting that electrical aversion is less than a permanent solution to alcoholism in that the maladaptive behavior it confronts (abusive drinking) is itself the consequence of behaviors (heightened fear and anxiety) with which it does not deal directly. As a result, electrical aversion must be employed in conjunction with training in relaxation to confront the fear and anxiety Blake felt was at the center of alcoholism.

In Blake's initial report,[9] the treatment of a single group of 37 alcoholics was described. Subjects were in their middle 40s, had been drawn from higher socioeconomic classes, and suffered from what seems to have been only moderate alcoholism. By DSM-III criteria,[12] some of them would clearly have been diagnosed as suffering from alcohol abuse rather than alcohol dependence. All subjects received relaxation training (which averaged about 12 sessions); "motivational arousal" (designed to increase subjects' motivation for treatment by forcing them to dwell repeatedly on the consequences of their alcohol abuse); and aversion conditioning (lasting about 15 sessions, in which electric shock was begun when a sip of alcohol was taken and terminated when it was spit out—technically, this method constituted aversion relief).

Follow-up data were gathered when subjects returned to the hospital at intervals of 1, 3, 6, 9, and 12 months. At the six- and twelve-month marks, about half the subjects identified at follow-up had remained abstinent. An additional follow-up of the same patients[10] described a comparison of a newly treated group of 25 alcoholic subjects with the original 37 aversion-relaxation subjects. Matched with the original 37 for age, sex, socioeconomic status, chronicity of alcoholism, previous hospitalizations, concurrent psychiatric diagnosis, and intelligence, the 25 new subjects received electrical aversion (aversion relief) therapy alone. Twelve-month follow-up data for both groups show that alcoholics receiving both relaxation training and aversion therapy were more apt to be judged either abstinent or improved than those given electrical aversion therapy alone. However, since Blake did not deal with "time in treatment," the reliability of the follow-up data, or the comparability of his two subject groups in his report, and since he failed to employ an untreated control group for comparative purposes, we believe that his results, although they encourage a multimodal treatment model, must nonetheless be viewed with caution.

In a 1966 study designed to establish the overall efficacy of an aversion relief paradigm similar to Blake's, MacCulloch, Feldman, Orford, and MacCulloch[13] applied the "technique of anticipatory avoidance learning" to a group of four alcoholics. They had previously used this procedure successfully with homosexual subjects. These alcoholic subjects, it is clear, were not as highly motivated for treatment, were more seriously impaired, and were of lower socioeconomic status than Blake's—all factors that by themselves militated against positive outcome. MacCulloch and his colleagues described the alcohol-related stimuli used in their method as follows:

> Subjects are presented with a range of photographs of beer and "spirits," the sight of an actual bottle of alcohol (stoppered), the sight of an open bottle of alcohol, and alcohol in a glass. We also used a tape recording which consists of a repeated invitation to have a drink of . . . the patient's preferred choice. (pp. 187–188)[13]

Slides of orange squash were counterposed as relief stimuli. The complete battery of alcohol-related and nonalcohol-related stimuli was shown randomly to each subject; when an alcohol-related stimulus was presented, it was followed eight seconds later by a shock unless switched off by the subject, at which point the aversion relief stimulus would appear. This treatment design was thought to promote an increase in the reinforcement value of nonalcohol-related stimuli and a concomitant decrease in the reinforcement value of alcohol-related stimuli within the context of a combined operant-classical conditioning paradigm.

In reporting their essentially negative findings (all four subjects returned to drinking within relatively short periods of time) the authors of the study observed that three of the four had consistently failed to avoid shock during conditioning by refusing to switch off alcohol-related stimuli (in other words, they failed in large part to permit themselves to be conditioned). The authors observed further that the unknown role of biochemical factors in alcoholism might have played a role in determining these negative results in view of the method's apparent success with homosexuals. Finally, they felt that social factors implicit in the maintenance of uncontrolled drinking may have been stronger maintainers of that behavior than similar factors in the environments of homosexuals.

The late 1960s and early 1970s signaled the advent of more sophisticated treatment research by behavior therapists. What this meant to those studying electrical aversion was that control groups began to be employed, more subjects were chosen for each study, better measures of outcome were used, and electrical aversion was more often embedded in more comprehensive treatment packages than before. Among studies completed from this more advanced research perspective were those by Vogler and his colleagues,[14,15] who reported encouraging short-term abstinence data but disproportionate losses of subjects from electrical aversion treatment groups. Miller and his coworkers[16] failed to identify differences in consumption between experimental and control subjects on Miller's "taste test." And Hedberg and Campbell,[17] comparing four separate behavioral treatment approaches (behavioral family counseling, systematic desensitization, covert sensitization, and electrical aversion), reported that electrical aversion, unlike the other three treatments, had absolutely no impact on drinking by alcoholic subjects.

Subsequently, Vogler and his colleagues reported on two additional studies involving electrical aversion. Their investigation of the efficacy of four multifaceted treatment packages, one of which included electrical aversion, with alcoholics[18] and problem drinkers,[19] yielded equivocal results: The short-term positive changes in drinking rate that were observed could not be attributed to any single component of the treatment package, including electrical aversion.

One of the most convincing demonstrations of the ineffectiveness of electrical aversion as a treatment for alcoholism was the 1975 study by Wilson and Nathan,[20] who directly tested the widespread presumption that electrical aversion conditioning establishes conditioned aversion to ethanol. After a very large number of aversion conditioning trials extending over several days, alcoholics were permitted to drink *ad libitum* in a laboratory setting that neither encouraged nor discouraged drinking. Subjects drank with undiminished enthusiasm in this environment, just as they had during a comparable pretreatment *ad libitum* period; Wilson and his coworkers concluded that conditioned aversion had not been established by the aversion conditioning procedure.

Wilson concluded a comprehensive 1978 review of the electrical aversion literature[21] by noting that ". . . the evidence on the efficacy of electrical aversion conditioning is overwhelmingly negative. Its use as a treatment modality with alcoholics should be discontinued." We agree with this view of the data on the efficacy of electrical aversion.

Continuing his discussion beyond this point, Wilson went on to question the continued use of electrical aversion on two other bases, conceptual and ethical. By conceptual, Wilson referred to the assumption, naive so far as Wilson was concerned, that electrical aversion ought to be the treatment of choice for alcoholism because it suppresses the excessive drinking that defines the disorder; this approach to alcoholism treatment, so far as Wilson was concerned, unfortunately fails to attend to the diverse antecedent, mediational, and consequent variables (interpersonal, socioeconomic, and psychological) that play crucial roles in the disorder. Wilson's ethical concerns about electrical aversion referred to the essential impossibility of obtaining truly informed consent to its use by many of the individuals to whom it has customarily been offered. Some of these persons are coerced into treatment, effectively removing all possibility of freely given consent. Moreover, even those who are not coerced cannot be expected to weigh for themselves the conflicting data on the efficacy of electrical aversion, necessary before truly informed consent to a therapeutic procedure is possible.

CHEMICAL AVERSION

In the 1940s and 1950s, Voegtlin, Lemere, and their colleagues at the Shadel Hospital in Seattle published a series of reports describing the productive use of chemical aversion to treat alcoholism. With the exception of a recent series of publications by Wiens, Neubuerger, and their colleagues reviewed below, additional reports on chemical aversion have been conspicuously absent from the literature. This surprising lack of interest in a treatment as efficacious as chemical aversion with nausea-inducing drugs derived in large part from much stronger, long-lived interest among behavioral clinicians in electric shock as a stimulus for conditioning aversion to ethanol. As noted above, however, despite its attractiveness on both theoretical and traditional grounds, electric shock is not effective as an aversive stimulus for the development of a conditioned aversion to ethanol.

In partial explanation for the apparent success of emetine aversion and the failure of electrical aversion to establish conditioned aversion to ethanol, Wilson and Davison[22] and Garcia and his colleagues[23] have suggested that nausea is "biologically appropriate" to alcohol while electric shock is not: Many people have experienced nausea after drinking, few have experienced electric shock. For this reason alcoholics are more likely to develop and maintain an association between alcohol and nausea than between alcohol and shock.

The actual procedures followed at the Shadel Hospital were described in detail by Voegtlin in 1940[24] and Lemere and Voegtlin in 1950.[25] In brief, patients were hospitalized for approximately 10 days; the five treatment sessions were spaced on alternate days. Treatment sessions were held in rooms specially designed to minimize distractions and maximize visibility of a large array of alcoholic beverages. An emetine-pilocarpine-ephedrine mixture was administered intravenously, producing nausea within two to eight minutes. Immediately prior to initial signs of nausea, the patient was given a drink of his/her favorite alcoholic beverage to smell, then to taste. Additional drinks were provided over a 30–60 minute period, as nausea, vomiting, sweating, increased respiration, and other consequences of the three-drug mixture were experienced.

"Booster" reconditioning sessions were offered to all aversive conditioning patients at any time they felt the urge to drink or, routinely, six and 12 months after inpatient treatment. With some variation (administration of drugs is no longer by infusion; reconditioning sessions are more frequent; several additional components of treatment are offered), a similar aversive conditioning treatment sequence continues to be followed at the Shadel Hospital (now the several Shick-Shadel Hospitals), as well as at the several Raleigh Hills Hospitals, which also offer chemical aversion as the cornerstone of their alcoholism treatment efforts.

Results of the first 13 years of treatment at the Shadel Hospital were based on follow-up of 4,096 of 4,468 patients treated, a most impressive follow-up rate of 92%. Forty-four percent of these patients had remained totally abstinent for from two to 13 years while another 7% had relapsed and been successfully retreated. Of the 4,096 patients followed-up, 60% had been abstinent for one year, 51% for two years, 38% for five years, and 23% for 10 years.

These outcome data are remarkably similar to those reported more recently by other facilities offering chemical aversion treatment. Following seven years of emetine conditioning treatment at the Washingtonian Hospital in Boston, Thimann, in 1949,[26] reported a total success rate of 51% of patients who could be located for follow-up, a figure identical to that of Lemere and Voegtlin's. Similarly, Wiens and his colleagues, in 1976,[27] reported that 63% of 261 alcoholic patients treated by emetine conditioning at the Raleigh Hills Hospital in Portland were abstinent after a year, results strikingly comparable to the one-year figure of 60% cited by Lemere and Voegtlin. The figure reported by Wiens and his coworkers is even more impressive since the Portland group considered patients who could not be located for follow-up to be treatment failures. Notable, as well, is the fact that the Raleigh Hills treatment program was a multifaceted one that included a range of individual, group, and behavioral treatment components along with the aversive conditioning that was at the heart of the program.

Wiens and his colleagues updated their 1976 report in 1983, confirming the earlier outcome figures and identifying demographic and treatment variables predictive of outcome in the Raleigh Hills emetine conditioning program.[28] Of the 835 patients admitted to the hospital in 1978 and 1979, 711 completed treatment and could be located for a one-year follow-up. Sixty-three percent of this group was abstinent at the one-year mark, a figure identical to Wiens' 1976 report. As interesting are data linking outcome to demographic and treatment factors. For example, Wiens and his colleagues[28] found that while only 2% of the 1978 patients who achieved abstinence did not return to the hospital for "booster" reconditioning and only 4% of the successful patients came back only once for reconditioning, 59% of the patients who were treated successfully according to this criterion came back for all six scheduled "booster" sessions. In fact, the correlation between number of "booster" sessions and average length of sobriety for the 1978 patients was .70 ($p < .001$); for the 1979 patients it was .67 ($p < .001$).

The same report[28] indicates that older male patients were more successfully treated than younger male patients; but that age did not predict treatment outcome for women. Married male patients were more likely to meet the one-year abstinence criterion than their unmarried male counterparts whereas marital status was unrelated to treatment outcome in women. Educational level, occupational status (employed or unemployed) and type (white- versus blue-collar), and history of prior treatment for alcoholism did not predict outcome.

A series of outcome studies of patients treated at another Raleigh Hills hospital have recently been reported by Neubuerger and his colleagues.[29-31] The Raleigh Hills Hospital in Fair Oaks, California, utilizes a treatment program very similar to that employed at the Portland, Oregon, Raleigh Hills Hospital at which Wiens and his colleagues worked.

Surveying 1,263 patients treated during the years 1976–1979 inclusive at the Fair Oaks Raleigh Hills Hospital, Neubuerger and his co-workers report an overall abstinence rate at the one-year mark of 52%, more than ten percentage points lower than the rate at which the Portland Raleigh Hills patients met the same criterion. Possible explanations for the difference include a larger percentage of younger, unemployed, unmarried, and less well-educated patients in the Fair Oaks sample, since these variables negatively influenced outcome in either the Portland or Fair Oaks samples, or both.

Why do these outcome data appear to be so much better than those from other approaches to alcoholism and, this being so, why hasn't a rush to establish chemical aversion facilities followed their publication? The answer to the first question also responds to the second. It is that alcoholics undergoing chemical aversion treatment now, as in the 1940s, enter treatment with better prognoses than those who enter most other kinds of treatment.[25,28,31]

To begin with, patients entering chemical aversion programs (which are costly) must have substantial private financial resources, health insurance, or another source of third-party reimbursement; both of the first two funding sources would require patients to be either recently or still employed. Recent or current employment, in turn, suggests that the individual retains a modicum of ability to function adequately in the world. Further, many of these patients also differ markedly in educational and socioeconomic level from alcoholics treated elsewhere, additional indications of their superior treatment potential. Finally, patients who complete a chemical aversion treatment sequence must be highly motivated to change their drinking behavior, since the treatment is both expensive and extremely unpleasant. It is a given, of course, that positive treatment motivation is one of the most important predictors of successful treatment.

Do these data mean that chemical aversion, its outcome data so encouraging, is not as promising a treatment for alcoholism as it might seem? Probably not, since few treatment approaches have yielded outcomes as positive. Instead, one must recognize that a largely homogeneous group of well-motivated, relatively well-educated, largely intact alcoholics have benefitted from chemical aversion. To assume that patients widely disparate from this group would also benefit is to go farther beyond these data than we are prepared to go.

Chemical aversion is not the only therapeutic modality available to patients at the

Shick-Shadel and Raleigh Hills facilities. Indeed, rehabilitation and personal counseling, family therapy, behavior therapy and biofeedback, and access to local Alcoholics Anonymous groups, all provided in a supportive atmosphere, are regular components of the therapy package offered at these facilities. This being so, one might ask just how significant chemical aversion *per se* is to the treatment provided at these hospitals.

Research demonstrating that pairing chemically induced nausea with alcohol produces a reliable aversion to alcohol in humans has only recently been reported;[5,32] research linking the strength of an alcohol aversion to treatment outcome, currently in progress,[33] has not yet been reported. However, inpatient facilities offering a treatment package excluding chemical aversion have not reported outcomes as positive as those with chemical aversion included. On the other hand, Burt[34] interviewed 34 patients who had relapsed an average of 18 months after completing the Shadel program; only five of them reported nausea or fear before their first drink. Further, Voegtlin[35] acknowledged that some of his patients did not develop alcohol aversions despite vomiting during the conditioning process. Finally, Wilson[21] concludes that conditioning is a cognitive process, not one which works automatically without the patient's knowledge or consent.

We conclude that chemical aversion can be effective in the context of a carefully orchestrated treatment program accompanied by adjunctive counseling and attention to social support systems and followed by booster sessions. What seems most important, as a consequence, is consideration of ways to reduce the cost and increase the availability of a treatment approach with demonstrated utility.

REFERENCES

1. Nathan, P. E. & R. S. Niaura. 1985. Behavioral assessment and treatment of alcoholism. *In* Diagnosis and Treatment of Alcoholism. J. H. Mendelson & N. K. Mello, Eds. 2nd edit. McGraw-Hill. New York.
2. Kantorovich, N. V. 1930. An attempt at associative-reflex therapy in alcoholism (1929). Psychol. Abstr. **4**: 493.
3. Sanderson, R. E., D. Campbell & S. G. Laverty. 1963. An investigation of a new aversive conditioning treatment for alcoholism. Q. J. Stud. Alcoh. **24**: 261–275.
4. Elkins, R. L. 1980. Covert sensitization treatment of alcoholism: contributions of successful conditioning to subsequent abstinence maintenance. Addict. Behav. **5**: 67–89.
5. Boland, F. J., C. S. Mellor & S. Revusky. 1978. Chemical aversion treatment of alcoholism: lithium as the aversive agent. Behav. Res. Ther. **16**: 401–409.
6. Eysenck, H. J., Ed. 1960. Behavior Therapy and the Neuroses. Pergamon Press. London.
7. Rachman, S. 1961. Sexual disorders and behavior therapy. Am. J. Psychiat. **118**: 235–240.
8. McGuire, R. J. & M. Vallance. 1964. Aversion therapy by electric shock, a simple technique. Brit. Med. J. **1**: 151–152.
9. Blake, B. G. 1965. The application of behavior therapy to the treatment of alcoholism. Behav. Res. Ther. **3**: 75–85.
10. Blake, B. G. 1967. A follow-up of alcoholics treated by behavior therapy. Behav. Res. Ther. **5**: 89–94.
11. Cappell, H. & C. P. Herman. 1972. Alcohol and tension reduction: A review. Q. J. Stud. Alcoh. **33**: 33–64.
12. American Psychiatric Association. 1980. Diagnostic and Statistical Manual of Mental Disorders. 3rd edit. American Psychiatric Association. Washington, DC.
13. MacCulloch, M. J., M. P. Feldman, J. F. Orford & M. L. MacCulloch. 1966. Anticipatory avoidance learning in the treatment of alcoholism: A record of therapeutic failure. Behav. Res. Ther. **4**: 187–196.

14. Vogler, R. E., S. E. Lunde, G. R. Johnson & P. L. Martin. 1970. Electrical aversion conditioning with chronic alcoholics. J. Consult. Clin. Psychol. **34**: 302–307.
15. Vogler, R. E., S. E. Lunde & P. L. Martin. 1971. Electrical aversion conditioning with chronic alcoholics: Follow-up and suggestions for research. J. Consult. Clin. Psychol. **36**: 450.
16. Miller, P. M. & M. Hersen. 1972. Quantitative changes in alcohol consumption as a function of electrical aversive conditioning. J. Clin. Psychol. **28**: 590–593.
17. Hedberg, A. G. & L. Campbell. 1974. A comparison of four behavioral treatments of alcoholism. J. Behav. Ther. Exper. Psychiat. **5**: 251–256.
18. Vogler, R. E., J. V. Compton & T. A. Weissbach. 1975, Integrated behavior change techniques for alcoholics. J. Consult. Clin. Psychol. **43**: 233–243.
19. Vogler, R. E., T. A. Weissbach, J. V. Compton & G. T. Martin. 1977. Integrated behavior change techniques for problem drinkers in the community. J. Consult. Clin. Psychol. **45**: 267–279.
20. Wilson, G. T. & P. E. Nathan. 1975. The aversive control of excessive drinking by chronic alcoholics in the laboratory setting. J. Appl. Behav. Anal. **8**: 13–26.
21. Wilson, G. T. 1978. Booze, beliefs, and behavior: Cognitive processes in alcohol use and abuse. *In* Alcoholism: New Directions in Behavioral Research and Treatment. P. E. Nathan & G. A. Marlatt, Eds. Plenum Press. New York.
22. Wilson, G. T. & G. C. Davison. 1969. Aversion techniques in behavior therapy: Some theoretical and metatheoretical considerations. J. Consult. Clin. Psychol. **33**: 327–329.
23. Garcia, J., W. G. Hankins & K. W. Rusiniak. 1974. Behavioral regulation of the milieu interne in man and rat. Science **185**: 824–831.
24. Voegtlin, W. L. 1940. The treatment of alcoholism by establishing a conditioned reflex. Am. J. Med Sci. **199**: 802–809.
25. Lemere, F. & W. L. Voegtlin. 1950. An evaluation of the aversion treatment of alcoholism. Q. J. Stud. Alcoh. **11**: 199–204.
26. Thimann, J. 1949. Conditioned reflex treatment of alcoholism. II. The risk of its application, its indications, contraindications and psychotherapeutic aspects. New Eng. J. Med. **241**: 408–410.
27. Wiens, A. N., J. R. Montague, T. S. Manaugh & C. J. English. 1976. Pharmacological aversive counterconditioning to alcohol in a private hospital: One year follow-up. J. Stud. Alcoh. **37**: 1320–1324.
28. Wiens, A. N. & C. E. Menustik. 1983. Treatment outcome and patient characteristics in an aversion therapy program for alcoholism. Am. Psychol. **38**: 1089–1096.
29. Neubuerger, O. W., J. D. Matarazzo, R. E. Schmitz & H. H. Pratt. 1980. One year follow-up of total abstinence in chronic alcoholic patients following emetic counterconditioning. Alcoh.: Clin. Exp. Res. **4**: 306–312.
30. Neubuerger, O. W., N. Hasha, J. D. Matarazzo, R. E. Schmitz & H. H. Pratt. 1981. Behavioral-chemical treatment of alcoholism: An outcome replication. J. Stud. Alcoh. **42**: 806–810.
31. Neubuerger, O. W., S. I. Miller, R. E. Schmitz, J. D. Matarazzo, H. H. Pratt & N. Hasha. 1982. Replicable abstinence rates in an alcoholism treatment program. J. Am. Med. Assoc. **248**: 960–963.
32. Cannon, D. S. & T. B. Baker. 1981. Emetic and electric shock alcohol aversion therapy: Assessment of conditioning. J. Consult. Clin. Psychol. **49**: 20–33.
33. Cannon, D. S. & T. Baker. 1981. Proposal to evaluate alcohol aversion therapy. Advanced Health Systems, Inc. Irvine, CA.
34. Burt, D. W. 1974. Characteristics of the relapse situation of alcoholics treated with aversive conditioning. Behav. Res. Ther. **12**: 121–123.
35. Voegtlin, W. L. Conditioned reflex therapy of chronic alcoholism: Ten years experience with the method. Rocky Mt. Med. J. **44**: 807–812.

Learned Food Aversions in the Progression of Cancer and Its Treatment[a]

ILENE L. BERNSTEIN

Department of Psychology
University of Washington
Seattle, Washington 98195

Patients suffering from cancer are exposed to a variety of experiences that can provide the basis for the development of learned aversions, particularly learned aversions to foods. Prominent among these experiences are the severe nausea and vomiting that commonly accompany chemotherapy and radiotherapy.[1] Since drug and radiation treatments are well established as effective unconditioned stimuli in the acquisition of learned taste aversions, foods eaten before such treatments are potential targets for the development of learned aversions.[2,3] Drug side effects are also involved in the phenomenon of conditioned or anticipatory nausea and vomiting.[4-6] This is a form of classical conditioning that occurs in some patients when stimuli associated with repeated drug treatments come to elicit these symptoms before the drugs are actually administered.

Another source of learned aversions is the disease process itself. Animal studies indicate that the aversive physiological consequences of tumor growth may become associated with specific diets, leading to the development of learned aversions to those diets.[7,8] Such aversions have been shown to lead to depressions in food intake and body weight.

The studies discussed in this paper examine the learned food aversions that arise both as a result of antineoplastic drug therapy and as a result of neoplastic disease. Chemotherapy-induced aversions have largely been studied in humans in a clinical setting, although an animal model of chemotherapy-induced aversions has played a role in the development of intervention strategies. Tumor-induced aversions have been examined in animal experiments using rats implanted with experimental tumors. In describing this work I will present the evidence on which I base the conclusion that learned food aversions arise in patients and in animals with cancer and that these aversions contribute to the appetite problems associated with this disease. I will also outline the direction of our current and future work.

DRUG-INDUCED LEARNED FOOD AVERSIONS

Learned Taste Aversions in Patients Receiving Chemotherapy

Our studies in this area were stimulated by the dramatic and compelling nature

[a] Supported by grant R01-CA26419 from the National Cancer Institute, Department of Health, Education, and Welfare.

of taste aversion learning in animals. We suspected that humans exposed to pairings of foods and GI toxicity in the course of cancer treatments would develop aversions to those foods. Interview studies[9] suggested that humans often develop profound distastes for foods that were coincidentally associated with gastrointestinal (GI) discomfort. The clinical setting provided an opportunity to examine taste aversion learning in humans experimentally. It was important to determine whether learned food aversions were an inadvertent side effect of cancer chemotherapy and whether ways could be devised to prevent them.

The first study in this series examined learned taste aversions in pediatric cancer patients receiving chemotherapy.[10] We asked whether children receiving drugs that were associated with nausea and vomiting would acquire aversions to a novel food consumed before their drug treatments. We used a novel food as our target stimulus because novel foods are apparently much more susceptible to aversion conditioning than are familiar foods.[11] The "novel food" target in this study was "Mapletoff" ice cream, chosen because children, even anxious and "nondeprived" children, are generally willing to eat ice cream. The novelty was introduced by using unusual flavorings.

Subjects were outpatients, between the ages of two and 16 years, being treated at the Children's Orthopedic Hospital and Medical Center Hematology Clinic in Seattle. Patients scheduled to receive GI toxic chemotherapy were randomly assigned to one of two groups: the Experimental Group, which consumed Mapletoff ice cream shortly before their scheduled drug treatment, or the Drug Control Group, which received similar drug treatments but no exposure to the ice cream. A Taste Control Group composed of patients who either received chemotherapy not associated with GI symptoms (vincristine) or no drug treatment was also included. Patients in this group consumed the same ice cream as the Experimental Group. Approximately two to four weeks later, patients were tested for the development of aversions by being offered a choice between eating Mapletoff ice cream or playing with a game.

Only 21 percent (3/14) of the patients in the Experimental Group chose Mapletoff ice cream during the test session compared to 67 percent (8/12) and 73 percent (11/15) in the two Control Groups. The proportion of subjects selecting ice cream in the Experimental Group was significantly lower than in the combined Control Groups ($p < .01$) suggesting that children will avoid eating a food that has previously been associated with GI toxic chemotherapy.

To evaluate the flavor specificity of these aversions, we offered experimental and control patients a choice between two ice cream flavors: Mapletoff (the flavor previously paired with GI toxic therapy in the experimental condition) and Hawaiian Delight (orange-pineapple). We asked the patients to taste both ice cream flavors, indicate which they preferred, and eat as much of each as they wished. Flavor preference and amount consumed were recorded. Preference for Mapletoff ice cream, whether measured by the amount consumed or the patients' stated preference, was significantly lower in the Experimental Group than in the Control Groups. Thus, aversions appear to be specific to the particular ice cream flavor presented during conditioning.

Although the observation of taste aversion learning in human subjects was not particularly unexpected, there are some interesting features of these results. First, the aversions were acquired in a single conditioning trial even though lengthy delays were likely to have occurred between the tasting of the ice cream and the onset of aversive symptoms. (Symptoms may begin a few minutes to a few hours after drug administration.) Second, many of the patients had received a large number of prior drug treatments. Furthermore, most of the patients were old enough to understand that the cause of their symptoms of nausea and vomiting was their drug therapy and not Mapletoff ice cream. Because factors such as these would be expected to reduce aversion conditioning, the demonstration of significant aversions suggests that humans are relatively susceptible to taste aversion learning.

These studies were subsequently extended to an adult patient population[12] where we found that adults, like children, can acquire learned taste aversions in a single trial. Apparently the cognitive development of adults does not override this conditioning.

Animal Models of Drug-induced Aversions

Since taste aversion studies in the rat originally pointed us to the existence of drug-induced aversions in humans, it seemed particularly appropriate to turn to animal models of these aversions to learn more about the mechanisms involved and to develop intervention strategies.

The vast majority of previous taste aversion studies have employed deprived subjects and novel, flavored solutions. Therefore, our first task was to modify the aversion conditioning paradigm so that it would more closely model the clinical situation. It is obvious that a number of important differences exist between the eating habits of laboratory rats and human patients. Laboratory rats are typically reared on a single, complete food (i.e., commercial laboratory chow). Humans in our society, on the other hand, have a dazzling variety of foods available to them throughout life although the foods they actually consume from day to day are considerably more restricted. In order to provide a target food that was not totally novel, but also was not as familiar as laboratory chow,[13] we exposed rats to a single, complete diet (AIN meal; ICN, Cleveland, OH) for five days before subjecting them to a course of drug (cyclophosphamide) treatments: four i.p. injections of either cyclophosphamide or physiological saline spaced three days apart. The cyclophosphamide dosage used was 20 mg/kg of body weight, which is in the low range of dosages in clinical use. AIN diet was continuously available *ad lib* throughout the 12 days. A 24-hr two food preference test, which offered rats a choice between AIN and a novel diet of comparable palatability, was used to evaluate food aversion learning. Preference scores were calculated for each animal by dividing the amount of AIN diet consumed by total food intake during the test. Drug-treated animals displayed significantly lower preferences than saline-treated controls for the AIN target diet, a strong indication that the drug-treated animals developed learned aversions to the AIN diet. These findings are interesting because the animals were not deprived, and in fact had received five days of "safe" pre-exposure to the AIN diet prior to the first drug treatment. Furthermore the diet was present continuously during the 17-day experiment—i.e. exposure was not linked temporally to the drug treatments in any narrow sense.

Since this treatment model was capable of producing significant diet aversions, we tested a variety of intervention methods for reducing or eliminating the aversions. We rated the success of these interventions by the degree to which they reduced aversions to the AIN diet. The approaches evaluated were: (1) depriving animals of food for six hours before and after each drug treatment; (2) introducing a novel flavor in the animals' water around the time of each treatment; (3) exposing animals to a combination of food deprivation and novelly flavored water; and (4) replacing the animals' standard AIN diet with a novel food on treatment days. As can be seen in FIGURE 1, only the introduction of a novel diet on treatment days was effective in preventing diet aversions. In spite of the fact that the animals in the Novel Diet group consumed very little of the novel food (and therefore would appear to be similar to the Deprivation group), aversions to the AIN diet were completely eliminated. Food deprivation and novel liquid interference stimuli did not reliably reduce the magnitude of AIN

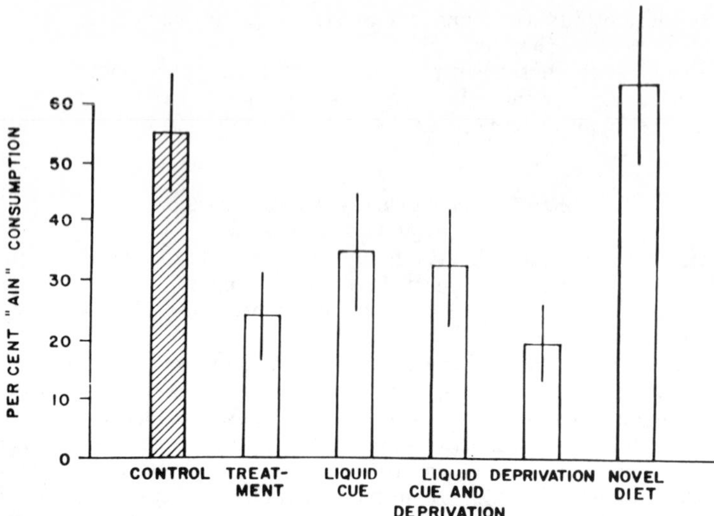

FIGURE 1. Average preference (± SE) for AIN meal in the 24-hour two-food choice test [AIN meal vs. chocolate chow (a novel diet)]. (Reprinted with permission from Bernstein *et al.*[13] Copyright 1980 by the American Psychological Association.)

aversions. The lack of interference by flavored solutions was not due to a failure of these solutions to become conditioned aversive stimuli since strong aversions were acquired to the liquid flavor cues as well as to the target diet. These results suggest that exposure to a novel food interference stimulus might be effective in preventing or reducing learned food aversions to standard diet items in cancer patients receiving chemotherapy. These findings also suggest that asymmetries exist between the potency of foods and drinks as targets in aversion conditioning.[14]

While documenting chemotherapy-induced food aversions in the clinic (using questionnaires described in the next section) as well as food aversions that spontaneously arose in healthy University of Washington undergraduates, we were intrigued to note that a substantial proportion of aversions appeared to be directed at foods that were protein sources (e.g. fish, eggs, meat). Aversions to carbohydrate sources appeared far less frequently. This observation, although interesting and potentially important, is difficult to evaluate critically using survey methods. To date the experimental literature on taste aversions does not provide much information on this topic. Although numerous animal studies have looked at the novelty and intensity of the CS as determinants of conditioning strength, the issue of the salience of specific macronutrients has been largely neglected.

Determining whether protein sources are more likely targets for conditioned aversions than are other macronutrients is of practical as well as theoretical interest. Although examination of this question is complicated by difficulties in equating certain features of these nutrients, such as their flavor intensity and postingestive consequences, it is possible that these features contribute to the salience of proteins as targets in aversion conditioning. We addressed this question by allowing rats to self-select from separate protein and carbohydrate macronutrient sources during a sequence of cyclophosphamide injections. We found that significant aversions developed to the protein but not the carbohydrate source in three studies that varied the composition of both protein and carbohydrate diets. These results suggest that animals on a dietary self-selection regimen are more likely to develop conditioned aversions to the protein source than the carbohydrate source. A final study in this series examined the generality of the above findings by determining whether aversions would selectively arise to protein but not carbohydrate when nutrients were conditioned in a single trial, using a meal feeding paradigm. Proteins again proved to be more salient targets for aversions than carbohydrates. These findings suggest that the tendency to associate proteins with drug-induced illness more readily than carbohydrates is not limited to a self-selection regimen.[15] Although the specific properties of proteins that contribute to their associability in a taste aversion paradigm have yet to be identified, two possibilities are differences in postingestive and/or taste properties of proteins and carbohydrates.

These findings could lead one to speculate that the propensity to avoid proteins rather than carbohydrates has some adaptive value, particularly if potential sources of toxicosis in the natural diet of rat or human are more likely to be proteins. Our results also imply that the nutritional consequences of learned food aversions, particularly those arising in cancer patients, may involve dietary quality rather than total energy intake.

Learned Aversions to Familiar Foods

We now ask whether aversions affect patients' preference for familiar foods in their routine diets, and not just novel target foods.[16] This study used diet inventories or questionnaires to assess changes in food preferences and food choices as a result of GI toxic chemotherapy. Pediatric patients completed diet inventories during an initial treatment session and again at a subsequent evaluation session that occurred at least a week later. These forms were completed at the same time that some subjects were participating in the previously described "ice cream" study. Children (with the help of their parents) listed their favorite foods, foods they were reluctant to eat, and typical breakfast, lunch, and dinner menus. During the initial session, they also indicated specific food items they had consumed in the four to five hour period before coming to the clinic. Patients receiving GI toxic chemotherapy composed the Experimental Group and the specific foods they had eaten before their drug therapy were considered the targets for the formation of aversions. To assess aversions the two questionnaires from each patient were compared and scored by a rater blind to the group membership of subjects; an aversion was scored when a specific food eaten before therapy was no longer preferred, became actively disliked, or was no longer listed in usual menus. We determined the number of patients whose inventories showed at least one such aversion. Patients receiving vincristine or no drug provided a Control Group that allowed us to compare inventory changes in the Experimental Group to a comparable patient population not currently receiving GI toxic therapy. Control Group changes from Session 1 to Session 2 provided an estimate of the rate such changes occur due to chance, forgetting, or some other factor.

A multiple regression analysis showed that the number of food items consumed before therapy made the greatest contribution to the variance in incidence of aversions. However, when we controlled for the number of "pretherapy items" in the analysis, and classified patients in the Experimental Group with regard to whether they had consumed Mapletoff ice cream before treatment (Group 1) or not (Group 2), an interesting finding emerged. We found that GI toxic drug treatment was significantly associated with the incidence of aversions in Group 2, where nausea symptoms were experienced without ice cream exposure (TABLE 1). In contrast, the incidence of aversions in Group 1 was intermediate between controls (Group 3) and Group 2 and did not differ significantly from either. Thus Group 1 patients exposed to a novel taste

TABLE 1. Aversions to Food in the Diet

	Number of Patients Showing Aversions
Group 1	
GI toxic drugs/ice cream	14/25 (56%)
Group 2	
GI toxic drugs/no ice cream	16/23 (70%)
Group 3	
Controls	11/31 (36%)

Difference between two proportions: Groups 1 and 2 (combined) versus Group 3 = $p < 0.02$. (After Bernstein *et al.*[16])

(Mapletoff ice cream) before treatments did not show a significantly higher incidence of aversions than controls. Since patients scheduled for GI toxic therapy were randomly assigned to Groups 1 and 2 the observation that drug treatment was significantly associated with the formation of diet aversions only in the group not exposed to ice cream suggests that the ice cream may have blocked the development of aversions to foods in the diet. It should be noted that this study was not designed to examine interference effects; but was rather a serendipitous outcome of looking at diet aversions in the same patients that had been in the "ice cream study." The findings are suggestive of an interference effect that clearly needs to be examined further. However, these observations are consistent with some of the results of our animal studies; namely that a novel food presented in association with toxic drug treatment can interfere with aversions to a target food. Perhaps deliberate exposure in the clinic to novel, "scapegoat" tastes prior to chemotherapy treatments would protect normal diet items from becoming the targets for learned food aversions.

The prevalence of aversions to familiar diet items in our pediatric population is somewhat surprising in view of the emphasis placed on stimulus novelty in the taste aversion literature. Possible explanations of our findings include the following: (1)

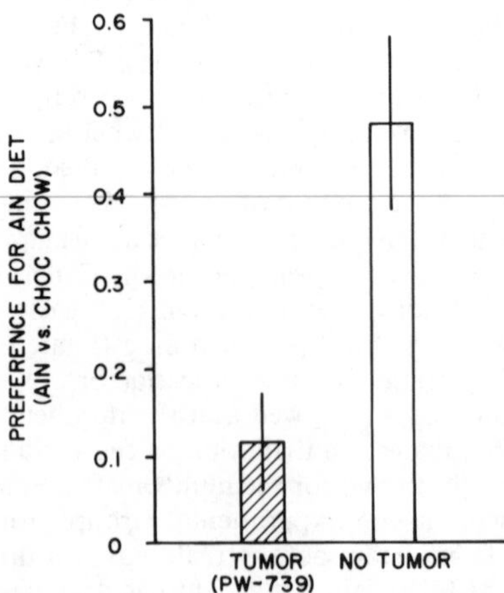

FIGURE 2. Average preference (± SE) for AIN meal in the 24-hour two-food choice test [AIN meal versus chocolate chow (a novel diet)]. Average total consumption: tumor, 18.3 g; control, 17.4 g. (Reprinted with permission from Bernstein & Sigmundi.[7] Copyright 1980 by the AAAS.)

Foods appear to be far more potent stimuli for taste aversion conditioning than are flavored solutions, and conclusions based largely on studies using flavored solutions may not apply. (2) Repeated trials increase the likelihood of aversions to familiar foods.[17] If children tend to consume particular foods repeatedly for breakfast or lunch, when they receive multiple chemotherapy treatments, then one or more of those foods may receive multiple conditioning trials. (3) Familiar foods may taste "novel" to cancer patients since cancer and cancer therapy can induce changes in taste bud function.[18,19]

TUMOR-INDUCED LEARNED FOOD AVERSIONS

In the course of developing an animal model for drug-induced food aversions we began to ask questions regarding the causes of tumor anorexia, i.e., the decline in food intake that frequently accompanies tumor growth. We speculated that aversions could arise in response to the association of a diet with the aversive physiological effects of the tumor itself. Thus, tumor-induced appetite loss could result, at least in part, from the development of learned aversions, with the US being some chronic symptom of tumor growth rather than the acute effects of a drug injection.[7]

To investigate this hypothesis, we implanted transplantable, polyoma virus-induced sarcomas (PW-739) subcutaneously in the flanks of syngeneic Wistar-Furth rats. Control animals received an incision and suture but no tumors. The growth of this tumor is associated with significant depressions in food intake and body weight that typically begin approximately five to six weeks after the tumor is implanted. To determine whether learned aversions would also develop, tumor-bearing and control animals were exposed to a distinctive target diet (AIN meal) for ten days. At the end of the diet exposure period the food intake of tumor-bearing animals had declined significantly below that of controls. Aversions were assessed as previously described.

Mean AIN preference scores are depicted in FIGURE 2. Tumor-bearing animals exhibited conspicuously lower preferences than controls for the AIN diet, the diet that had been available during recent tumor growth. Furthermore, when an alternate diet was available during the preference test, we saw striking elevations of 24-hr food intake in tumor-bearing animals but not in controls. These findings indicate that tumor-bearing animals had developed a pronounced aversion to the AIN target diet by the day of the preference test.

In additional studies, aversions were shown to be specific to the particular diet available during tumor growth, thus excluding the possibility that our original findings were a nonspecific effect of tumor growth on taste preference. We have concluded that tumor-induced aversions are based on learning, that is, the association of a specific food with some symptom(s) of tumor growth. We are currently seeking answers to three questions: (1) What is the overall contribution of learned food aversions to tumor anorexia? (2) How general are tumor-induced aversions? and (3) What are the physiological mechanisms responsible for the development of tumor-induced aversions?

ASSESSING THE CONTRIBUTION OF LEARNED FOOD AVERSIONS TO ANOREXIA

Continuous LiCl Infusions: Conditioned Effects on Food Intake and Preference

Since there is clear evidence that learned food aversions arise in tumor-bearing animals, an important question is whether the preference shifts that characterize "learned aversions" can actually lead to hypophagia and weight loss. In this regard it is necessary to distinguish between depressions in food intake that are the direct result of tumor-induced physiological changes and those that are secondary to the development of learned aversions. We began these investigations by modeling the effects of a tumor in undiseased animals.[20] We used osmotic minipumps (Alza, Palo Alto, CA), which are small, implantable capsules, to infuse a concentrated solution of lithium chloride (LiCl) over a seven day period. This provided a controlled chemical simulation of the presumed chronic US exposure experienced by tumor-bearing animals. To separate learned from direct effects, we compared the response to LiCl infusions of animals consuming their familiar maintenance diet to those consuming a novel diet. As noted earlier, familiar tastes are relatively resistant to the development of learned food aversions whereas novel tastes rapidly become the target of such aversions.[11] Thus, even though drug infusions were the same in both groups, the likelihood of forming strong aversions was quite different, because the group with a novel diet had a more salient target. Differences in food intake would be a reflection of greater learned aversions in the novel food group.

Rats were assigned either to Novel diet groups (which were given *ad lib* access to C-21, a novel diet in place of their usual diet) or to Familiar diet groups (which received their usual brand of commercial laboratory chow). The next day, an osmotic minipump was implanted in the peritoneal cavity of each subject. We gave half the animals in each diet condition (Drug-Novel and Drug-Familiar groups) minipumps containing a saturated aqueous solution of LiCl. The pumps deliver a relatively constant i.p. infusion of solution (one μl per hour) for approximately seven days. Control animals (Control-Novel and Control-Familiar groups) received nonfunctional pumps. Animals had free access to their assigned diet for six days of LiCl infusion. Food intake was measured daily. On Day 7 we tested for the presence of aversions in a 24-hour two-food preference test. The two foods provided in the test were the target diet, (either ground laboratory chow for familiar diet groups or C-21 for novel diet groups) and AIN meal (a diet novel to both groups).

Food intake over the drug infusion period can be seen in FIGURE 3. Striking differences between Novel and Familiar drug-treated animals are evident, with chronic drug infusions lowering food intake substantially in animals consuming a novel food while those consuming familiar laboratory chow are only slightly different from controls. Furthermore, significant food aversions developed in animals with a novel diet-drug association but not in animals with a familiar diet-drug association.

Two factors were likely to contribute to the decline of food intake associated with minipump infusions. One factor, the direct or unconditioned effect of drug-induced malaise on appetite, presumably afflicts novel and familiar groups equally. On the other hand, the conditioned effect would be based on a diet-illness association. As expected, the novel diet proved much more susceptible to conditioned effects. Since diet aversions arose in the novel but not the familiar diet group the considerable difference in appetite suppression between animals on familiar and novel diets may largely be attributed to the contribution of learned food aversions.

A second study confirmed that it was novelty of the C-21 diet and not some intrinsic difference between the C-21 and the laboratory chow that was responsible for differences in intake suppression. In this study, novel and familiar groups consumed the same diet (C-21) during the infusion period but differed in their prior experience with it. Significant anorexia appeared in animals unfamiliar with the diet but not in those familiar with it, which supports the hypothesis that differential intakes were not due to nutritional or taste properties of the diets but to novelty and differential aversion conditioning.

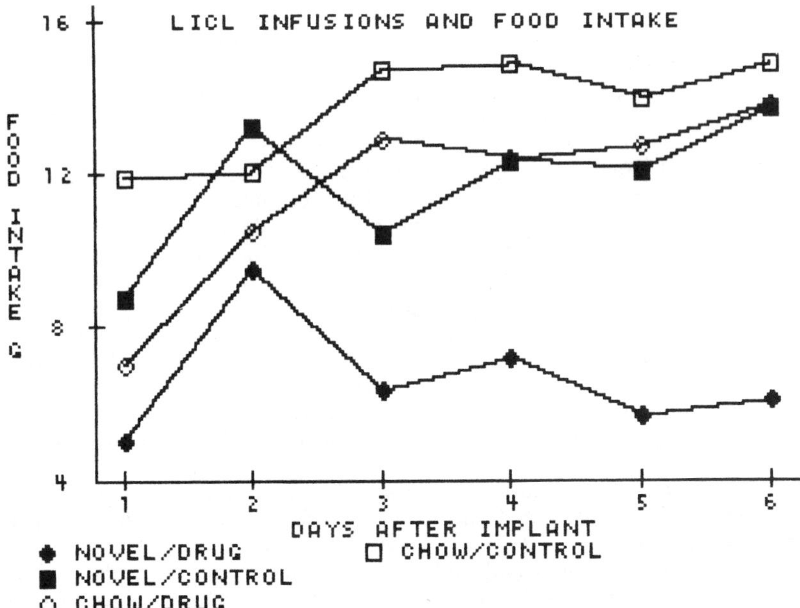

FIGURE 3. Mean daily food intake during LiCl infusions (drug) or no infusions (control). Groups were consuming either C-21 diet (novel) or familiar Wayne lab chow (chow).

Diet Novelty and Tumor Anorexia

The striking effects of diet novelty on food intake in the previous study led us to examine whether parallel effects would be found in tumor-bearing animals. Similar findings would provide strong evidence that learned aversions play a major role in tumor anorexia. Specifically, the hypothesis that tumors suppress appetite directly would not predict a differential effect of diet novelty on severity of appetite depression; whereas the hypothesis that learned aversions contribute substantially to tumor-induced anorexia would predict that animals eating a familiar diet would display less intake depression than those eating a novel diet. When we compared the food intake and preferences of tumor-bearing rats consuming a novel diet to those of rats consuming a familiar diet, we found that animals that consumed familiar laboratory chow did not develop aversions to it and had relatively mild transient anorexia. In contrast, tumor-bearing animals consuming a novel diet (C-21) developed strong aversions to that diet and displayed severe anorexia.[21] These results are consistent with the hypothesis that differential food aversion conditioning led to the striking differences in severity of anorexia seen in tumor-bearing animals consuming familiar and novel diets.

Another prediction from our hypothesis that learned food aversions can make a substantial contribution to anorexia is that frequent changes in diet should attenuate anorexia either by preventing the formation of learned aversions or by repeatedly replacing aversive foods with new ones. In a test of this prediction we fed one group of tumor-bearing animals a variety of diets while maintaining a second group on a single diet. Two control groups were exposed to the comparable diet exposure. Three of the diets were commercially available dog or cat foods; the remaining three were semisynthetic rodent diets. Animals assigned to the Varied Diet groups participated in initial preference testing, during which each diet was paired with every other diet for a 24 hr period. Preference ratios for these diets over the numerous preference tests were averaged and ranked providing an estimate of relative preference for these diets. In ascending order of palatability the six diets were Safeway Puppy Chow; Friskies Cat Food; Blue Mountain Dog Food; Soy meal diet; AIN meal; and C-21. The diet that was preferred relative to all others (C-21) was used as the single diet offered to the animals in the Same Diet groups. Animals in the Varied Diet group received each diet for three days. The diets were presented in ascending order of palatability. At the end of 18 days a preference test was run to evaluate the development of aversions to C-21, which was the single food source of the Same Diet groups and the last food presented to the Varied Diet groups.

Food intake in both tumor-bearing groups declined during the first few days of observation. However, the tumor-bearing animals receiving a different diet every three days showed average food intakes that were often more than twice what was eaten by the tumor-bearing group with access to the same (initially highly preferred) food (FIGURE 4). Although both tumor groups had significantly lower food intakes than their respective control groups, food intake in the Varied/Tumor group was significantly higher than in the C-21/Tumor group.

The results of the preference test indicated that the rats in the Same Diet-Tumor Group had significant aversion to C-21 relative to their controls. In the Varied Diet-Tumor Group preference for C-21 was lower than in the Varied Diet-Control group, but the differences were not significant. Thus, providing a continually varying menu to tumor-bearing animals significantly elevated their food intake over the amount consumed when a single food was present. This supports the notion that the prevention of learned food aversions, or the presentation of non-aversive foods, can attenuate anorexia in tumor-bearing animals.

Contribution of Learned Food Aversions to Anorexia Syndromes

Although the studies presented in this section had the specific focus of assessing the contribution of learned food aversions to tumor anorexia, there is a more general focus to these studies as well. The general issue is that the symptoms of hypophagia and weight loss, which can be produced by any of a number of experimental treatments, may to a lesser or greater extent be the product of specific learned aversions acquired via the association of treatment symptoms with a specific diet. This suggests that some of the anorexia syndromes that result from brain lesions or other surgical modifications may actually be, partly or wholly, based on learned food aversions. For example, renewed interest in the role of the vagus nerve has been generated by reports that subdiaphragmatic vagotomy produces hypophagia and weight loss in normal rats[22,23] and can reverse the hyperphagia and obesity of rats with ventromedial hypothalamic lesions.[24] Vagotomy can also produce symptoms of nausea and discomfort, symptoms that are highly effective USs in food aversion conditioning. We recently asked whether some of the depression in food intake observed in rats with vagotomy could be due to the development of aversions to the foods eaten after surgery.[26] Significant aversions developed to a novel diet consumed after surgery, but not to familiar laboratory chow. Likewise, hypophagia was more long lasting and severe in animals with a novel diet. We concluded that learned food aversions can contribute to the appetite and weight loss exhibited by vagotomized animals and that the magnitude of this contribution depends on procedural details such as diet exposure and recovery time, which are often unspecified. Similarly, intestinal bypass surgery in rats apparently produces strong conditioned taste aversions to a novel solution presented

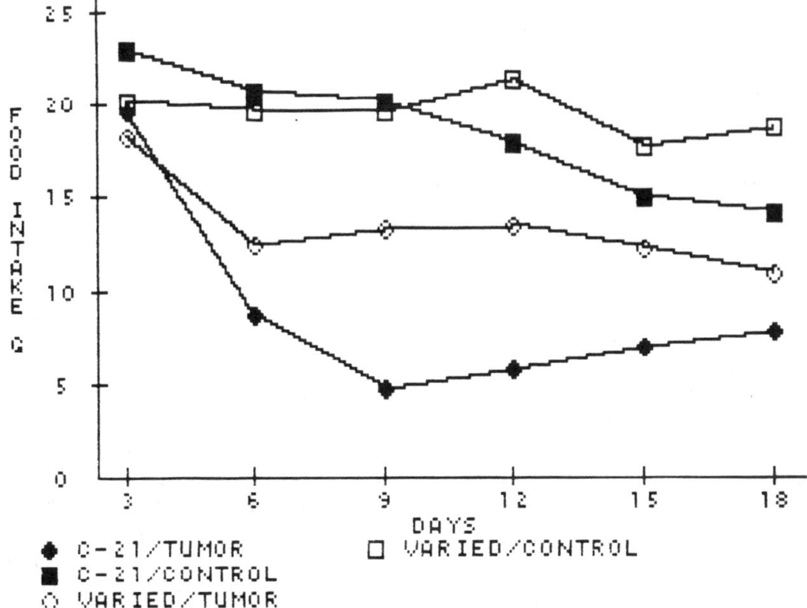

FIGURE 4. Mean daily food intake in three-day blocks for tumor-bearing and control animals. Animals received either C-21 throughout the 18-day period or a succession of diets (Varied) presented for three days each. For the varied group each three-day block represents a different diet. Diets are described in the text.

after surgery.[27] These few studies provide clear evidence supporting the idea that learned food aversions can contribute to anorexia. However, because experimenters typically do not test for learned aversions when their treatments reduce food intake we do not yet have a clear picture of the actual contribution of learned aversions to the total "anorexia" picture.

ASSESSING THE GENERALITY OF TUMOR-INDUCED AVERSIONS

Other experimental tumors besides the PW-739 have been used in recent years to study the physiological bases of tumor-induced anorexia. These include the Walker 256 carcinosarcoma[28,29] and a Leydig cell tumor (LTW(m)).[30] Although growth of all three transplantable tumors is associated with significant declines of food intake and body weight, the mechanisms by which they induce anorexia may be different. The Walker tumor is a rapidly growing tumor that constitutes a substantial proportion (30%) of the animal's body weight at the time significant declines in food intake become apparent.[28,31] The LTW(m) tumor, on the other hand, produces symptoms of appetite loss when the tumor itself weighs less than a gram.[30] The PW-739 tumor is intermediate in its growth rate and effects on food intake and body weight. We were interested in examining the effects of the Walker 256 and LTW(m) tumors on food intake and diet preference and comparing their effects to those of PW-739 tumors.

TABLE 2. Preference Test Scores:[a] Leydig-LTW(m) Tumors

AIN Target	
Tumor	0.13 (±.05)
Control	0.40 (±.08)
C-21 Target	
Tumor	0.14 (±.08)
Control	0.69 (±.07)

[a] Preference test scores = grams of target diet consumed divided by total food consumption during the test.

In studies patterned after our original work,[8] animals were implanted with either LTW(m) or Walker tumors and exposed to target diets. We measured food intake daily and administered a preference test after anorexia was evident. Significant declines in food intake were seen with LTW(m) tumors at 17 days post-implant and with Walker tumor at four weeks post-implant. Results of the preference tests can be seen in TABLES 2 and 3. Animals with LTW(m) tumors, like those with PW-739 tumors, developed strong aversions to the specific diet they had been eating after tumor implant. On the other hand, animals with Walker tumors did not develop diet aversions, displaying instead preferences for the target diet that were indistinguishable from those of healthy controls.

Thus although both tumors produced clear declines in food intake, their effects on target diet preference were different. These results suggest that learned food aversions contribute to anorexia in animals with LTW(m) but not Walker tumors. Such findings emphasize that there are multiple factors contributing to the decline in food intake accompanying tumor growth and that "tumor anorexia" is not a unitary phenomenon with a single cause. It is likely that the clinical picture is at least as heterogeneous.

The presence of learned aversions in animals with certain tumors indicates that physiological consequences of tumor growth can act as USs in aversion conditioning. The finding that the induction of food aversions is not common to all experimental rat tumors indicates that illness and tumor growth per se are not sufficient conditions for the development of aversions. This suggests that tumor-induced aversions are caused by specific physiological changes, not merely by general malaise, and that these changes may prove identifiable.

ASSESSING THE PHYSIOLOGICAL BASIS OF TUMOR-INDUCED AVERSIONS

In considering potential candidates for the physiological USs responsible for tumor-

TABLE 3. Preference Test Scores:[a] Walker 256 Tumor

AIN Target	
Tumor	0.01 (±.01)
Control	0.07 (±.03)
C-21 Target	
Tumor	0.81 (±.03)
Control	0.78 (±.03)

[a] Preference test scores = grams of target diet consumed divided by total food consumption during the test.

induced aversions, two categories of stimuli come to mind. One is substances secreted abnormally or in unusually large amounts by the tumor; it is possible that such substances could have toxic effects that would act as USs in food aversion conditioning. The other possibility is that the tumor-bearing animals' striking similarity to animals on nutrient-deficient diets[32] may be more than coincidental. That is, the tumor may actually produce a state of nutrient deficiency in the host organism by its excessive and preferential utilization of some essential nutrient(s).[33] Both the toxin and nutrient deficiency hypotheses are attractive and, at this point, we cannot favor one over the other. In fact, given the heterogeneity evident in experimental tumors it remains possible that both types of mechanisms are triggering tumor-induced aversions and the one involved may depend on the specific tumor being studied.

One approach to defining the physiological mechanisms responsible for tumor-induced aversions is to identify the neural circuitry mediating the effect. Early efforts to assess the involvement of particular brain regions in tumor anorexia were directed at effects of lesions in the lateral or ventromedial areas of the hypothalamus because of the overwhelming evidence implicating the hypothalamus in the regulation of feeding behavior. These lesions did not prevent or attenuate the appearance of tumor-induced anorexia, and the apparently independent effects of lesions and tumor manipulations on food intake strongly suggested that they are unlikely to involve the same control mechanisms.[34,35] A region of the brain that has received considerable recent attention for its presumed role in taste aversion learning and regulation of food intake is the area postrema (AP).[36-38] Located in the brain stem, the area postrema has also been identified as the chemoreceptor trigger zone for nausea and emesis.[39] Lesioning of the area postrema and the nearby caudal medial nucleus of the solitary tract (AP/cmNTS) is a potentially useful technique for us in our search for the physiological US for tumor-induced food aversions. If the AP is involved in detection of a blood-borne US produced by the tumor, then animals with lesions in this region might be expected to show attenuation or elimination of tumor-induced aversions as well as milder anorexia.[40] However, since AP lesions are themselves associated with substantial reductions in food intake and body weight, effects of a tumor would necessarily be superimposed on the AP syndrome.

In the following experiment thermal lesions were produced in the AP/cmNTS.[41] Half the animals were given AP lesions, the other half were sham operated. Six weeks were allowed for recovery from the acute effects of the lesions. Half the animals with AP lesions and half the sham-operated animals were then implanted with Leydig LTW(m) tumors. Two weeks elapsed after tumor implant before animals were exposed to AIN meal as their sole diet for eight days with intake measured daily. On the ninth day they received a two hour preference test in which they chose between AIN and C-21.

Mean body weights of AP-lesioned animals at the time of tumor implant was approximately 230 g as compared to the weights of unlesioned controls, which were 320 g. The weight differences were statistically significant and reflect the substantial weight loss associated with lesions of the AP. However, sufficient time elapsed between lesioning and tumor implant to allow for stabilization of weights at a new lower level.

Average food intake over the diet exposure period: AP-Tumor = 14.9g; AP-Control = 16.0g; Sham-Tumor = 11.5g; and Sham-Control = 19.9g. It is evident that AP-Control animals eat less than Sham-Control animals, although intake is not different if expressed relative to the animals' body weights. Effects of tumor implant on food intake are dramatically different in lesioned and unlesioned animals. Sham-operated animals develop tumor anorexia as manifested by food intake which declines to levels that are half those seen in controls, a finding consistent with the numerous studies we have already reported. In contrast, AP-lesioned animals show little or no tumor anorexia. A repeated measures analysis of variance yielded a significant main

TABLE 4. Area Postrema Lesions and Tumor-induced Food Aversions

Groups	Preference for AIN[a] (±SE)
AP-tumor	.67 (±.08)
AP-control	.81 (±.09)
Sham-tumor	.02 (±.00)
Sham-control	.92 (±.04)

[a] Preference for AIN = grams of AIN consumed divided by total food consumption during the test.

effect of tumor and a significant interaction. Planned comparisons indicated that food intake of the Sham-Tumor group is significantly lower than the Sham-Control group and the AP-Tumor group. The AP-Tumor group is not significantly different from the AP-Control group. Tumor growth was also associated with considerably less weight loss in AP-lesioned animals than in sham-operated animals. Although AP lesions themselves lead to hypophagia and weight loss, the pattern of results does not suggest that lesion effects obscured the appearance of tumor-induced symptoms. Rather we found that AP-Tumor animals consumed significantly more food and lost significantly less weight than Sham-Tumor animals.

We observed complementary effects of AP lesions on tumor-induced food aversions. As can be seen in TABLE 4 significant severe aversions were evident in Sham-Tumor animals but not in AP-Tumor animals. Thus, the area postrema appears to be involved in the development and/or expression of LTW(m) tumor-induced anorexia, weight loss, and food aversions since its destruction prevents or postpones the appearance of the symptoms that generally follow implant. These findings are important because they suggest that detection by the area postrema of some blood-borne chemical may be involved in the aversions and anorexia produced by the LTW(m) tumor. They also provide another line of evidence for a direct relationship between aversions and anorexia in this tumor model. It remains to be determined whether the role of the area postrema in tumor anorexia is largely due its detection of chemical unconditioned stimuli in aversion conditioning or whether direct effects on the regulation of food intake and body weight are involved. This is an interesting question because of the apparently multiple functions of area postrema in regulation of food intake and body weight as well as food aversion learning.

SUMMARY AND CONCLUSIONS

The studies included in this chapter examine the learned food aversions that develop as a result of cancer and cancer treatment. Clinical studies have shown that cancer patients can develop learned aversions to a novel ice cream flavor when it is consumed before drug treatments that produce nausea and vomiting. They also provided evidence that patients can acquire aversions to food in their usual diets when these foods are eaten before similar drug treatments. Observations in the clinic, supported by complementary studies with animal models, suggest that learned aversions are more likely to arise to protein foods than to other nutrient sources and that the presentation of a novel food in association with drug treatments may act as a "scapegoat" in blocking the development of aversions to foods in the normal diet.

Laboratory studies using transplantable tumors in rats have shown that tumor growth can be associated with the development of strong aversions to the available diet. These aversions are specific to the diet eaten during tumor growth and they appear to play a causal role in the development of tumor-induced anorexia. The food aversions apparent in animals with certain experimental tumors point to physiological consequences of tumor growth that act as unconditioned stimuli in taste aversion conditioning. The identification of these changes and development of methods for correcting them are the current goals of our research in this area.

ACKNOWLEDGMENTS

The collaboration of M.M. Webster, C.M. Treneer, L.E. Goehler, and Dr. D.P. Fenner in various aspects of this research is gratefully acknowledged.

REFERENCES

1. Lazslo, J. 1983. Nausea and vomiting as major complications of cancer chemotherapy. Drugs **25** (Suppl. 1): 1–6.
2. Garcia, J., W. G. Hankins & K. W. Rusiniak. 1974. Behavioral regulation of the milieu interne in man and rat. Science **185**: 824–831.
3. Riley, A. L. & C. M. Clarke. 1977. Conditioned taste aversions: A bibliography. *In* Learning Mechanisms in Food Selection, L. M. Barker, M. R. Best & M. Domjan, Eds. Baylor University Press. Waco, TX.
4. Nesse, R. M., T. Carli, G. C. Curtis & P. D. Kleinman. 1980. Pretreatment nausea in cancer chemotherapy: A conditioned response? Psychosom. Med. **42**(1): 33–36.
5. Morrow, G. R. & C. Morrell 1982. Behavioral treatment for the anticipatory nausea and vomiting induced by cancer chemotherapy. N. Engl. J. Med. **307**(24): 1476–1480.
6. Redd, W. H. & G. V. Andresen. Conditioned aversion in cancer patients. Behav. Therapist **4**(2): 3–4.
7. Bernstein, I. L. & R. A. Sigmundi. 1980. Tumor anorexia: A learned food aversion? Science **209**: 416–418.
8. Bernstein I. L. & D. P. Fenner. 1983. Learned food aversions: Heterogeneity of animal models of tumor-induced anorexia. Appetite **4**: 79–86.
9. Garb, J. L. & A. J. Stunkard. 1974. Taste aversions in man. Am. J. Psychiatry **131**: 1204–1207.
10. Bernstein, I. L. 1978. Learned taste aversions in children receiving chemotherapy. Science **200**: 1302–1303.
11. Revusky, S. H. & E. W. Bedarf. 1967. Association of illness with prior ingestion of novel foods. Science **155**: 219–220.
12. Bernstein, I. L. & M. M. Webster. 1980. Learned taste aversions in humans. Physiol. Behav. **25**: 363–366.
13. Bernstein, I. L., M. V. Vitiello & R. A. Sigmundi. 1980. Effects of interference stimuli on the acquisition of learned aversions to food in the rat. J. Comp. Physiol. Psychol. **94**: 921–931.
14. Bernstein, I. L., L. E. Goehler & M. E. Bouton. 1983. Relative potency of foods and drinks as targets in aversion conditioning. Behav. Neural Biol. **37**: 134–148.
15. Bernstein, I. L., L. E. Goehler & D. P. Fenner. 1984. Learned aversions to proteins in rats on a dietary self-selection regimen. Behav. Neurosci. **6**: 1065–1072.
16. Bernstein, I. L., M. M. Webster & I. D. Bernstein. 1982. Food aversions in children receiving chemotherapy for cancer. Cancer **50**: 2961–2963.
17. Elkins, R. L. 1974. Conditioned flavor aversions to familiar tap water in rats: An adjustment with implications for aversion therapy treatment of alcoholism and obesity. J. Abn. Psychol. **83**(4): 411–417.
18. Conger, A. D. 1973. Loss and recovery of taste acuity in patients irradiated to the oral cavity. Rad. Res **53**: 338–347.

19. DEWYS, W. D. 1974. Abnormalities of taste as a remote effect of a neoplasm. Ann. N.Y. Acad. Sci. **230**: 426–434.
20. BERNSTEIN, I. L. & L. E. GOEHLER. 1983. Chronic lithium chloride infusions: Conditioned suppression of food intake and preference. Behav. Neurosci. **97**: 290–298.
21. BERNSTEIN, I. L., C. M. TRENEER, L. E. GOEHLER & E. MUROWCHICK. 1985. Tumor growth in rats: conditioned suppression of food intake and preference. Behav. Neurosci. (In press.)
22. NOVIN, D. 1976. Visceral mechanisms in the control of food intake. *In* Hunger: Basic Mechanisms and Clinical Implications. D. Novin, W. Wyrwicka & G. Bray, Eds. Raven Press. New York.
23. OPSAHL, C. A. & T. L. POWLEY. 1977. Body weight and gastric acid secretion in rats with subdiaphragmatic vagotomy and lateral hypothalamic lesions. J. Comp. Physiol. Psychol. **226**: 25–33.
24. POWLEY, T. L. & C. A. OPSAHL. 1974. Ventromedial hypothalamic obesity abolished by subdiaphragmatic vagotomy. Am. J. Physiol. **226**: 25–33.
25. KENNEDY T. 1974. The vagus and the consequences of vagotomy. Med. Clinics N. Am. **58**: 1231–1246.
26. BERNSTEIN, I. L. & L. E. GOEHLER. 1983. Vagotomy produces learned food aversions in the rat. Behav. Neurosci. **97**: 585–594.
27. SCLAFANI, A. & H. S. KOOPMANS. 1981. Intestinal bypass surgery produces conditioned taste aversion in rats. Int. J. Obesity **5**: 497–500.
28. MORRISON, S. D. 1973. Control of food intake during growth of a Walker 256 carcinosarcoma. Cancer Res. **33**: 526–528.
29. KRAUSE, R., J. H. JAMES, V. ZIPARO & J. E. FISCHER. 1979. Brain tryptophan and the neoplastic anorexia-cachexia syndrome. Cancer **44**: 1003–1008.
30. MORDES, J. P. & A. A. ROSSINI. 1981. Tumor-induced anorexia in the Wistar rat. Science **213**: 565–567.
31. MORRISON, S. D. 1976. Control of food intake in cancer cachexia: A challenge and a tool. Physiol. Behav. **17**: 705–714.
32. ROZIN, P. & J. W. KALAT. 1971. Specific hungers and poison avoidance as adaptive specializations of learning. Psychol. Rev. **78**: 459–486.
33. LAWSON, D. H., A. RICHMOND & D. RUDMAN. 1982. Metabolic approaches to cancer cachexia. Annu Rev. Nutr. **2**: 277–301.
34. BAILLIE, P., F. K. MILLAR & A. W. PRATT. 1965. Food and water intakes and Walker tumor growth in rats with hypothalamic lesions. Am. J. Physiol. **209**: 293–300.
35. LIEBELT, R. A., A. G. LIEBELT & H. M. JOHNSTON. 1971. Lipid mobilization and food intake in experimentally obese mice bearing transplanted tumors. Proc. Soc. Exp. Biol. **138**: 482–490.
36. BERGER, B. D., C. D. WISE & J. STEIN. 1973. Area postrema damage and bait shyness. J. Comp. Physiol. Psychol. **82**: 475–479.
37. COIL, J. D. & R. NORGREN. 1981. Taste aversions conditioned with intravenous copper sulfate: Attenuation by ablation of the area postrema. Brain Res. **212**: 425–433.
38. HYDE, T. M. & R. R. MISELIS. 1983. Effects of area postrema/caudal medial nucleus of solitary tract lesions on food intake and body weight. Am. J. Physiol. **244**: R577–R587.
39. BORISON, H. L. & S. C. WANG. 1953. Physiology and pharmacology of vomiting. Pharmacol. Rev. **5**: 193–230.
40. BERNSTEIN, I. L., C. M. TRENEER & J. N. KOTT. 1985. Area postrema mediates tumor effects on body weight, food intake and learned aversions. (Submitted for publication.)
41. MCGLONE, J. J., S. RITTER & K. W. KELLEY. 1980. The antiaggressive effect of lithium is abolished by area postrema lesion. Physiol. Behav. **24**: 1095–1100.

PART VI. CONDITIONED FOOD AVERSIONS: A BIBLIOGRAPHY

Conditioned Food Aversions: A Bibliography

ANTHONY L. RILEY AND DIANE L. TUCK

Psychopharmacology Laboratory
Department of Psychology
The American University
Washington, D.C. 20016

As evidenced from the breadth of topics covered in the present collection of chapters, it is clear that the area of conditioned food aversions has grown immensely since the early findings of John Garcia and his colleagues that x-irradiated rats would avoid consumption of flavored solutions that had been present during the irradiation episode. What began as an interesting biological response with clear implications for traditional models of learning has now become a broad research area in and of itself. Not only is attention being focused on understanding the associative, biological, physiological and pharmacological bases of food aversion learning, but the phenomenon itself has recently become an applied research tool in pharmacology, toxicology, predation control, and clinical treatment.

This growing interest in conditioned food aversions has been reflected in the number of articles published over the past 30 years. While over 600 papers had been published on taste aversion learning as of 1977, this number now stands at 1,373. The present bibliography is an attempt to update our earlier reports (see Riley & Baril, 1976 and Riley & Clarke, 1977) and brings the literature from 1955 to 1985 into a workable list.

In determining what topics are relevant for inclusion, some degree of arbitrariness is certain. The present list is no exception. Only articles directly related to conditioned food aversions are included. By this restriction, a number of interesting and important related topics have been excluded, e.g., conditioned preferences, mimicry, neophobia, and unconditioned drug effects. These topics are listed only if they are examined in relation to conditioned food aversions. Also, although every attempt was made to include every food aversion article, some are certain to be missed. We apologize in advance for these oversights.

In compiling the bibliography, references were obtained from individual journals in the areas of psychology, physiology, pharmacology, and animal behavior and from computer searches from *Medline* and *Psychological Abstracts*. References were also obtained from the bibliographies of individual articles. A final source of references was provided by individual researchers in the field of conditioned food aversions who freely contributed both preprints and reprints of their work.

Abelson, J. S., Pierrel-Sorrentino, R., & Blough, P. M. Some conditions for the rapid extinction of a learned taste aversion. *Bulletin of the Psychonomic Society,* 1977, **9**: 51–52.

Adams, C. D. Post-conditioning devaluation of an instrumental reinforcer has no effect on extinction performance. *Quarterly Journal of Experimental Psychology,* 1980, **32**: 447–458.

Adams, C. D. Variations in the sensitivity of instrumental responding to reinforcer devaluation. *Quarterly Journal of Experimental Psychology*, 1982, **34B**: 77–98.

ADAMS, C. D., & DICKINSON, A. Instrumental responding following reinforcer devaluation. *Quarterly Journal of Experimental Psychology,* 1981, **33B**: 109–121.

ADER, R. "Strain" differences in illness-induced taste aversion. *Bulletin of the Psychonomic Society*, 1973, **1**: 253–254.

ADER, R. Effects of early experiences on shock- and illness-induced passive avoidance behaviors. *Developmental Psychobiology*, 1973, **6**: 547–555.

ADER, R. Letter to the editor. *Psychosomatic Medicine*, 1974, **36**: 183–184.

ADER, R. Conditioned adrenocortical steroid elevations in the rat. *Journal of Comparative and Physiological Psychology,* 1976, **90**: 1156–1163.

ADER, R. A note on the role of olfaction in taste aversion learning. *Bulletin of the Psychonomic Society*, 1977, **10**: 402–404.

ADER, R. Conditioned taste aversions and immunopharmacology. *Annals of The New York Academy of Sciences,* 1985, **443**: 293–307.

ADER, R. Conditioned immunopharmacologic effects in animals: Implications for a conditioning model of pharmacotherapy. In L. White, B. Tursky and G. Schwartz (Eds.), *Placebo: Clinical phenomena and new insights.* New York: Guilford Press, in press.

ADER, R., & COHEN, N. Behaviorally conditioned immunosuppression. *Psychosomatic Medicine.* 1975, **37**: 333–340.

ADER, R., & COHEN, N. Conditioned immunopharmacologic effects. In R. Ader (Ed.), *Psychoneuroimmunology*. New York: Academic Press, 1981.

ADER, R., & COHEN, N. Behaviorally conditioned immunosuppression and murine systemic lupus erythematosus. *Science*, 1982, **215**: 1534–1536.

ADER, R., & COHEN, N., & BOVBJERG, D. Conditioned suppression of humoral immunity in the rat. *Journal of Comparative and Physiological Psychology,* 1982, **96**: 517–521.

ADER, R., COHEN, N., & BOVBJERG, D. Immunoregulation by behavioral conditioning. *Trends in Pharmacological Sciences*, 1983, **4**: 78–80.

ADER, R., COHEN, N., & GROTA, L. J. Adrenal involvement in conditioned immunosuppression. *International Journal of Immunopharmacology,* 1979, **1**: 141–145.

ADER, R., GROTA, L. J., & BUCKLAND, R. Effects of adrenalectomy on taste aversion learning. *Physiological Psychology*, 1978, **6**: 359–361.

ADER, R., & PECK, J. H. Early learning and retention of a conditioned taste aversion. *Developmental Psychobiology*, 1977, **10**: 213–218.

AGGLETON, J. P., PETRIDES, M., & IVERSEN, S. D. Differential effects of amygdaloid lesions on conditioned taste aversion learning by rats. *Physiology & Behavior*, 1981, **27**: 397–400.

AHLERS, R. H., & BEST, P. J. Novelty vs temporal contiguity in taste aversions. *Psychonomic Science,* 1971, **25**: 34–36.

AHLERS, R. H., & BEST, P. J. Retrograde amnesia for discriminated taste aversions: A memory deficit. *Journal of Comparative and Physiological Psychology*, 1972, **79**: 371–376.

ALEKSANYAN, Z. A., BURESOVA, O., & BURES, J. Modification of unit responses to gustatory stimuli by conditioned taste aversion in rats. *Physiology & Behavior*, 1976, **17**: 173–179.

ALEKSANYAN, Z. A., BURESOVA, O., BURES, J., & VASSILEVSKI, N. N. Modification of hypothalamic unit activity by conditioned taste aversion and instrumental control of blood pressure. *Activitas Nervosa Superior*, 1977, **19**: 59–60.

AMIT, Z., LEVITAN, D. E., BROWN, Z. W., & ROGAN, F. Possible involvement of central factors in the mediation of conditioned taste aversion. *Neuropharmacology*, 1977, **16**: 121–124.

AMIT, Z., & SUTHERLAND, E. A. The relevance of recent animal studies for the development of treatment procedures for alcoholics. *Drug and Alcohol Dependence*, 1975, **1**: 3.

ANANT, S. S. A note on the treatment of alcoholics by a verbal aversion technique. *Canadian Psychologist*, 1967, **8**: 12–22.

ANANT, S. S. Treatment of alcoholics and drug addicts by verbal aversion techniques. *The International Journal of the Addictions,* 1968, **3**: 381–388.

ANDERSON, C. E., TILSON, H. A., & MITCHELL, C. L. Conditioned taste aversion following acutely administered acrylamide. *Neurobehavioral Toxicology and Teratology*, 1982, **4**: 497–499.

ANDREWS, E. A., & BRAVEMAN, N. S. The combined effects of dosage level and interstimulus interval on the formation of one-trial poison-based aversions in rats. *Animal Learning & Behavior,* 1975, **3**: 287–289.

ANIKA, S. M., HOUPT, T. R., & HOUPT, K. A. Cholecystokinin and satiety in pigs. *American Journal of Physiology*, 1981, **240**: R310–R318.

ARAVICH, P. F., & SCLAFANI, A. Dietary preference behavior in rats fed bitter tasting quinine and sucrose octa acetate adulterated diets. *Physiology & Behavior*, 1980, **25**: 157–160.

ARCHER, T., COTIC, T., & JARBE, T. U. C. Attenuation of the context effect and lack of unconditioned stimulus-preexposure effect in taste-aversion learning following treatment with DSP4, the selective nonradrenaline neurotoxin. *Behavioral and Neural Biology*, 1982, **35**: 159–173.

ARCHER, T., MOHAMMED, A. K., & JARBE, T. U. C. Latent inhibition following systemic DSP4: Effects due to presence and absence of contextual cues in taste-aversion learning. *Behavioral and Neural Biology*, 1983, **38**: 287–306.

ARCHER, T., & SJODEN, P-O. Positive correlation between pre- and postconditioning saccharin intake in taste-aversion learning. *Animal Learning & Behavior*, 1979, **7**: 144–148.

ARCHER, T., & SJODEN, P-O. Neophobia in taste-aversion conditioning: Individual differences and effects of contextual changes. *Physiological Psychology*, 1979, **7**: 364–369.

ARCHER, T., & SJODEN, P-O. Context-dependent taste-aversion learning with a familiar conditioning context. *Psychological Psychology*, 1980, **8**: 40–46.

ARCHER, T., & SJODEN, P-O. Environment-dependent taste-aversion extinction: A question of stimulus novelty at conditioning. *Psychological Psychology*, 1981, **9**: 102–108.

ARCHER, T., & SJODEN, P-O. Higher-order conditioning and sensory preconditioning of a taste aversion with an exteroceptive CS1. *Quarterly Journal of Experimental Psychology,* 1982, **34B**: 1–17.

ARCHER, T., SJODEN, P-O., & CARTER, N. Control of taste-aversion extinction by exteroceptive cues. *Behavioral and Neural Biology,* 1979, **25**: 217–226.

ARCHER, T., SJODEN, P-O, & NILSSON, L-G. Contextual control of taste-aversion conditioning and extinction. In P. Balsam and A. Tomie (Eds.), *Context and learning*. Hillsdale, N.J.: Lawrence Erlbaum Associates, 1985.

ARCHER, T., SJODEN, P-O., NILSSON, L-G., & CARTER, N. Role of exteroceptive background context in taste-aversion conditioning and extinction. *Animal Learning & Behavior,* 1979, **7**: 17–22.

ARCHER, T., SJODEN, P-O., NILSSON, L-G., & CARTER, N. Exteroceptive context in taste-aversion conditioning and extinction: Odour, cage, and bottle stimuli. *Quarterly Journal of Experimental Psychology,* 1980, **32**: 197–214.

ARTHUR, J. B. Taste aversion learning is impaired by interpolated amygdaloid stimulation but not by posttraining amygdaloid stimulation. *Behavioral Biology,* 1975, **13**: 369–376.

ASHE, J. H., & NACHMAN, M. Neural mechanisms in taste aversion learning. In J. Sprague and A. Epstein (Eds.), *Progress in psychobiology and physiological psychology* (*vol. 9*). New York: Academic Press, 1980.

ASHEM, B., & DONNER, L. Covert sensitization with alcoholics: A controlled replication. *Behaviour Research and Therapy*, 1968, **6**: 7–12.

BABINE, A. M., & SMOTHERMAN, W. P. Uterine position and conditioned taste aversion. *Behavioral Neuroscience*, 1984, **96**: 461–466.

BAKER, L. J., BAKER, T. B., & KESNER, R. P. Taste aversion learning in young and adult rats. *Journal of Comparative and Physiological Psychology*, 1977, **91**: 1168–1178.

BAKER, T. B., & CANNON, D. S. Taste aversion therapy with alcoholics: Techniques and evidence of a conditional response. *Behaviour Research and Therapy*, 1979, **17**: 229–242.

BAKER, T. B., & CANNON, D. S. Alcohol and taste-mediated learning. *Addictive Behaviors*, 1982, **7**: 221–230.

BAKER, T. B., CANNON, D. S., STEPHENSON, G., & DROUBAY, E. Procedures for taste aversion therapy for alcoholics. *American Journal of Psychiatry*, 1978, **135**: 1439.

BALAGURA, S., BROPHY, J., & DEVENPORT, L. D. Modification of learned aversion to LiCl and NaCl by multiple experiences with LiCl. *Journal of Comparative and Physiological Psychology,* 1972, **81**: 212–219.

BALAGURA, S., RALPH, T., & GOLD, R. Effect of electrical brain stimulation of diencephalic and mesencephalic structures on the generalized NaCl aversion after LiCl poisoning. *Physiologist,* 1972, **15**: 77.

BALAGURA, S., & SMITH, D. F. Role of lithium and environmental stimuli on generalized learned aversion to NaCl in the rat. *American Journal of Physiology*, 1970, **219**: 1231–1234.

BALCOM, F. W., COLEMAN, W. R., & NORMAN, J. L. Taste aversion learning and long-term retention in juvenile rats. *Psychological Reports*, 1981, **49**: 266.

BALSTER, R. L., & BORZELLECA, J. F. Behavioral toxicity of trihalomethane contaminants of drinking water in mice. *Environmental Health Perspectives*, 1982, **46**: 127–136.

BANERJEE, U., & DAS, P. Amnesic effects of electroshock and anoxia on conditioned taste aversion learning in rats. *Behavioural Processes*, 1977, **2**: 175–186.

BANERJEE, U., & DAS, P. Conditioned taste aversion by lithium and saline: A methodological evaluation. *Chemical Senses*, 1980, **5**: 175–183.

BARKER, L. M. CS duration, amount and concentration effects in conditioning taste aversions. *Learning and Motivation*, 1976, **7**: 265–273.

BARKER, L. M., BEST, M. R., & DOMJAN, M. (Eds.). *Learning mechanisms in food selection.* Waco, Texas: Baylor University Press, 1977.

BARKER, L. M., & JOHNS, T. Effect of ethanol preexposure on ethanol-induced conditioned taste aversion. *Journal of Studies on Alcohol*, 1978, **39**: 39–46.

BARKER, L. M., & SMITH, J. C. A comparison of taste aversions induced by radiation and lithium chloride in CS-US and US-CS paradigms. *Journal of Comparative and Physiological Psychology*, 1974, **87**: 644–654.

BARKER, L. M., SMITH, J. C., & SUAREZ, E. M. "Sickness" and the backward conditioning of taste aversions. In L. Barker, M. Best and M. Domjan (Eds.), *Learning mechanisms in food selection*. Waco, Texas: Baylor University Press, 1977.

BARKER, L. M., SUAREZ, E. M., & GRAY, D. Backward conditioning of taste aversions in rats using cyclophosphamide as the US. *Physiological Psychology*, 1974, **2**: 117–119.

BARNETT, S. A., COWAN, P. E., RADFORD, G. G., & PRAKASH, I. Peripheral anosmia and the discrimination of poisoned food by *Rattus rattus L. Behavioral Biology*, 1975, **13**: 183–190.

BARRETT, T. J., & SACHS, L. B. Test of the classical conditioning explanation of covert sensitization. *Psychological Reports*, 1974, **34**: 1312–1314.

BATSON, J. D. Effects of repeated lithium injections on temperature, activity, and flavor conditioning in rats. *Animal Learning & Behavior*, 1983, **11**: 199–204.

BATSON, J. D., & BEST, P. J. Drug-preexposure effects in flavor-aversion learning: Associative interference by conditioned environmental stimuli. *Journal of Experimental Psychology: Animal Behavior Processes*, 1979, **5**: 273–283.

BATSON, J. D., & BEST, M. R. Single-element assessment of conditioned inhibition. *Bulletin of the Psychonomic Society*, 1981, **18**: 328–330.

BATSON, J. D., & BEST, M. R. Lithium-mediated disruptions of latent inhibition: Overshadowing by the unconditioned stimulus in flavor conditioning. *Learning and Motivation,* 1982, **13**: 167–184.

BAUERMEISTER, J. J., & SCHAEFFER, R. W. Relations between preconditioned rate of solution ingestion and rate of post-irradiation intake. *Psychology & Behavior*, 1969, **4**: 1019–1021.

BAUM, M., FOIDART, D. S., & LAPOINTE, A. Rapid extinction of a conditioned taste aversion following unreinforced intraperitoneal injection of the fluid CS. *Physiology & Behavior,* 1974, **12**: 871–873.

BEALER, S. L. Intensity coding in the transient portion of the rat chorda tympani response. *Journal of Comparative and Physiological Psychology*, 1978, **92**: 185–195.

BEKOFF, M. Reply to C. Gustavson, D. Kelly, & J. Garcia. *Science,* 1975, **187**: 1096.

BELKNAP, J K., BELKNAP, N. D., BERG, J. H., & COLEMAN, R. Preabsorptive vs. postabsorptive control of ethanol intake in C57BL&6J and DBA&2J mice. *Behavior and Genetics,* 1977, **7**: 413–425.

BELKNAP, J. K., COLEMAN, R. R., & FOSTER, K. Alcohol consumption and sensory threshold differences between C57BL&6J and DBA&2J mice. *Physiological Psychology*, 1978, **6**: 71–74.

BERG, D., & BAENNINGER, R. Predation: Separation of aggressive and hunger motivation by conditioned aversion. *Journal of Comparative and Physiological Psychology*, 1974, **86**: 601–606.

BERGER, B. D. Conditioning of food aversions by injections of psychoactive drugs. *Journal of Comparative and Physiological Psychology*, 1972, **81**: 21–26.

BERGER, B. D., WISE, C. D., & STEIN, L. Area postrema damage and bait shyness. *Journal of Comparative and Physiological Psychology,* 1973, **82**: 475–479.

Berk, A. M., & Miller, R. R. LiCl-induced aversions to audiovisual cues as a function of response measure and CS-US interval. *Behavioral Biology*, 1978, **24**: 185–208.

Berman, R. F., & Cannon, D. S. The effect of prior ethanol experience on ethanol-induced saccharin aversions. *Physiology & Behavior*, 1974, **12**: 1041–1044.

Bermudez-Rattoni, F., Rusiniak, K. W., & Garcia, J. Flavor-illness aversions: Potentiation of odor by taste is disrupted by application of novocaine into amygdala. *Behavioral and Neural Biology*, 1983, **37**: 61–75.

Bernstein, I. L. Learned taste aversions in children receiving chemotherapy. *Science*, 1978, **200**: 1302–1303.

Bernstein, I. L. Physiological and psychological mechanisms of cancer anorexia. *Cancer Research*, 1982, **42**: 7152–7172.

Bernstein, I. L. Learned food aversions in the progression of cancer and its treatment. *Annals of The New York Academy of Sciences*, 1985, **443**: 365–380.

Bernstein, I. L., & Bernstein, I. D. Learned food aversions and cancer anorexia. *Cancer Treatment Reports*, 1981, **65**: 37–42.

Bernstein, I. L., & Fenner, D. P. Learned food aversions: Heterogeneity of animal models of tumor-induced anorexia. *Appetite: Journal for Intake Research*, 1983, **4**: 79–86.

Bernstein, I. L., & Goehler, L. E. Chronic lithium chloride infusions: Conditioned suppression of food intake and preference. *Behavioral Neuroscience*, 1983, **97**: 290–298.

Bernstein, I. L., & Goehler, L. E. Vagotomy produces learned food aversions in the rat. *Behavioral Neuroscience*, 1983, **97**: 585–594.

Bernstein, I. L., Goehler, L. E., & Bouton, M. E. Relative potency of foods and drinks as targets in aversion conditioning. *Behavioral and Neural Biology*, 1983, **37**: 134–148.

Bernstein, I. L. & Sigmundi, R. A. Tumor anorexia: A learned food aversion? *Science*, 1980, **209**: 416–418.

Bernstein, I. L., Vitiello, M. V., & Sigmundi, R. A. Effects of tumor growth on taste-aversion learning produced by antitumor drugs in the rat. *Physiological Psychology*, 1980, **8**: 51–55.

Bernstein, I. L., Vitiello, M. V., & Sigmundi, R. A. Effects of interference stimuli on the acquisition of learned aversions to foods in the rat. *Journal of Comparative and Physiological Psychology*, 1980, **94**: 921–931.

Bernstein, I. L., Wallace, M. J., Bernstein, I. D., Bleyer, W. A., Chard, R. L., & Hartmann, J R. Learned food aversions as a consequence of cancer treatment. In J. van Eys, M. Seelig and B. Nichols (Eds.), *Nutrition and cancer.* New York: Spectrum Publications, 1979.

Bernstein, I. L., & Webster, M. M. Learned taste aversions in humans. *Physiology & Behavior*, 1980, **25**: 363–366.

Bernstein, I. L., Webster, M. M., & Bernstein, I. D. Food aversions in children receiving chemotherapy for cancer. *Cancer*, 1982, **50**: 2961–2963.

Berridge, K., Grill, H. J., & Norgren, R. Relation of consummatory responses and preabsorptive insulin release to palatability and learned taste aversions. *Journal of Comparative and Physiological Psychology*, 1981, **95**: 363–382.

Best, M. R. Conditioned and latent inhibition in taste-aversion learning: Clarifying the role of learned safety. *Journal of Experimental Psychology: Animal Behavior Processes*, 1975, **104**: 97–113.

Best, M. R., & Barker, L. M. The nature of "learned safety" and its role in the delay of reinforcement gradient. In L. Barker, M. Best and M. Domjan (Eds.), *Learning mechanisms in food selection.* Waco, Texas: Baylor University Press, 1977.

Best, M. R., & Batson, J. D. Enhancing the expression of flavor neophobia: Some effects of the ingestion-illness contingency. *Journal of Experimental Psychology: Animal Behavior Processes*, 1977, **3**: 132–143.

Best, M. R., & Domjan, M. Associative and nonassociative sources of interference with the acquisition of a flavor aversion. In M. Commons, R. Herrnstein and A. Wagner (Eds.), *Quantiatative analyses of behavior (vol. 2): Acquisition.* Cambridge: Ballinger, in press.

Best, M. R., & Domjan, M. Characteristics of the lithium-mediated proximal US-preexposure effect in flavor-aversion conditioning. *Animal Learning & Behavior*, 1979, **7**: 433–440.

Best, M. R., Domjan, M., & Haskins, W. L. Long-term retention of flavor familiarization: Effects of number and amount of prior exposures. *Behavioral Biology*, 1978, **23**: 95–99.

BEST, M. R., & GEMBERLING, G. A. Role of short-term processes in the conditioned stimulus preexposure effect and the delay of learning. *Journal of Experimental Psychology: Animal Behavior Processes*, 1977, **3**: 253–263.

BEST, M. R., GEMBERLING, G. A., & JOHNSON, P. E. Disrupting the conditioned stimulus preexposure effect in flavor-aversion learning: Effects of interoceptive distractor manipulations. *Journal of Experimental Psychology: Animal Behavior Processes*, 1979, **5**: 321–334.

BEST, P. J., BEST, M. R., & AHLERS, R. H. Transfer of discriminated taste aversion to a lever-pressing task. *Psychonomic Science*, 1971, **25**: 281–282.

BEST, P. J., BEST, M. R., & HENGGELER, S. The contribution of environmental non-ingestive cues in conditioning with aversive internal consequences. In L. Barker, M. Best and M. Domjan (Eds.), *Learning mechanisms in food selection.* Waco, Texas: Baylor University Press, 1977.

BEST, P. J., BEST, M. R., & LINDSEY, G. P. The role of cue additivity in salience in taste aversion conditioning. *Learning and Motivation*, 1976, **7**: 254–264.

BEST, P. J., BEST, M. R., & MICKLEY, G. A. Conditioned aversion to distinct environmental stimuli resulting from gastrointestinal distress. *Journal of Comparative and Physiological Psychology*, 1973, **85**: 250–257.

BEST, P. J., & ORR, J., JR. Effects of hippocampal lesions on passive avoidance and taste aversion conditioning. *Physiology & Behavior*, 1973, **10**: 193–196.

BEST, P. J., & ZUCKERMAN, K. Subcortical mediation of learned taste aversion. *Physiology & Behavior*, 1971, **7**: 317–320.

BHARDWAJ, D., & KHAN, J. A. Effect of texture of food on bait-shy behaviour in wild rats (*Rattus rattus*). *Applied Animal Ethology*, 1979, **5**: 361–367.

BIEDERMAN, G. B. The search for the chemistry of memory: Recent trends and the logic of investigation in the role of cholinergic and adrenergic transmitters. In G. Kerkut and J. Phillips (Eds.), *Progress in neurobiology (vol. 2).* New York: Pergamon Press, 1974.

BIEDERMAN, G. B., MILGRAM, N. W., HEIGHINGTON, G. A., STOCKMAN, S. M., & O'NEILL, W. Memory of conditioned food aversion follows a U-shape function in rats. *Quarterly Journal of Experimental Psychology*, 1974, **26**: 610–615.

BITTERMAN, M. E. Flavor aversion studies. *Science*, 1976, **192**: 266–267.

BLAIR, R., & AMIT, Z. Morphine conditioned taste aversion reversed by periaqueductal gray lesions. *Pharmacology, Biochemistry & Behavior*, 1981, **15**: 651–655.

BOLAND, F. J. Saccharin aversions induced by lithium chloride toxicosis in a backward conditioning paradigm. *Animal Learning & Behavior*, 1973, **1**: 3–4.

BOLAND, F. J., MELLOR, C. S., & REVUSKY, S. Chemical aversion treatment of alcoholism: Lithium as the aversive agent. *Behaviour Research and Therapy*, 1978, **16**: 401–409.

BOLAND, F. J., & STERN, M. H. Suppression by lithium of voluntary alcohol intake in the rat: Mechanism of action. *Pharmacology, Biochemistry & Behavior*, 1980, **12**: 239–248.

BOLAS, K. C., BELLINGHAM, W. P., & MARTIN, G. M. Aversive properties of cycloheximide versus memory inhibition in chickens' formation of visually cued food aversions. *Pharmacology, Biochemistry & Behavior*, 1979, **10**: 251–254.

BOLLES, R. C. Associative processes in the formation of conditioned food aversions: An emerging functionalism? *Annals of The New York Academy of Sciences*, 1985, **443**: 1–7.

BOLLES, R. C., RILEY, A. L., & LASKOWSKI, B. A further demonstration of the learned safety effect in food-aversion learning. *Bulletin of the Psychonomic Society*, 1973, **1**: 190–192.

BOND, N. W. Transferred odor aversions in adult rats. *Behavioral and Neural Biology*, 1982, **35**: 417–421.

BOND, N. W. Reciprocal overshadowing in flavour-aversion learning. *Quarterly Journal of Experimental Psychology*, 1983, **35B**: 265–274.

BOND, N. W., & CORFIELD-SUMNER, P. K. Taste aversion learning and schedule-induced polydipsia in the rat. *Animal Learning & Behavior*, 1978, **6**: 413–416.

BOND, N., & DI GUISTO, E. Amount of solution drunk is a factor in the establishment of taste aversion. *Animal Learning & Behavior*, 1975, **3**: 81–84.

BOND, N. W., & DI GUISTO, E. L. One trial higher-order conditioning of a taste aversion. *Australian Journal of Psychology*, 1976, **28**: 53–55.

BOND, N., & HARLAND, W. Higher order conditioning of a taste aversion. *Animal Learning & Behavior*, 1975, **3**: 295–296.

BOND, N., & HARLAND, W. Effect of amount of solution drunk on taste-aversion learning. *Bulletin of the Psychonomic Society,* 1975, **5**: 219–220.

BOND, N. W., & WESTBROOK, R. F. The role of amount consumed in flavor preexposure effects and neophobia. *Animal Learning & Behavior,* 1982, **10**: 511–515.

BOOTH, D. A. Satiety and appetite are conditioned reactions. *Psychosomatic Medicine*, 1977, **39**: 76–81

BOOTH, D. A. The physiology of appetite. *British Medical Bulletin*, 1981, **37**: 135–140.

BOOTH, D. A. Food-conditioned eating preferences and aversions with interoceptive elements: Conditioned appetites and satieties. *Annals of The New York Academy of Sciences,* 1985, **443**: 22–41.

BOOTH, D. A., LOVETT, D., & MCSHERRY, G. M. Postingestive modulation of the sweetness preference gradient in the rat. *Journal of Comparative and Physiological Psychology*, 1972, **78**: 485–512.

BOOTH, D. A., & PILCHER, C. W. T. Behavioural effects of protein synthesis inhibitors: Consolidation blockade or negative reinforcement. In G. Ansell and P. Bradley (Eds.), *Macromolecules and behaviour.* Birmingham, England: MacMillan, 1973.

BOOTH, D. A., PILCHER, C. W. T., D'MELLO, G. D., & STOLERMAN, I. P. Comparative potencies of amphetamine, fenfluramine and related compounds in taste aversion experiments in rats. *British Journal of Pharmacology,* 1977, **61**: 669–677.

BOOTH, D. A., & SIMSON, P. C. Food preferences acquired by association with variations in amino acid nutrition. *Quarterly Journal of Experimental Psychology*, 1971, **23**: 135–145.

BOOTH, D. A., & SIMSON, P. C. Aversion to a cue acquired by its association with effects of an antibiotic in rats. *Journal of Comparative and Physiological Psychology*, 1973, **84**: 319–323.

BOOTH, D. A., & SIMSON, P. C. Taste aversion induced by an histidine-free amino acid load. *Physiological Psychology*, 1974, **2**: 349–351.

BOUTON, M. E. Lack of reinstatement of an extinguished taste aversion. *Animal Learning & Behavior,* 1982. **10**: 233–241.

BOUTON, M. E., & WHITING, M. R. Simultaneous odor-taste and taste-taste compounds in poison-avoidance learning. *Learning and Motivation*, 1982, **13**: 472–494.

BOVBJERG, D., ADER, R., & COHEN, N. Acquisition and extinction of conditioned suppression of a graft-vs-host response. *Journal of Immunology*, 1984, **132**: 111–113.

BOVBJERG, D., ADER, R., & COHEN, N. Behaviorally conditioned suppression of a graft-versus-host response. *Proceedings of the National Academy of Sciences*, 1982, **79**: 583–585.

BRACKBILL, R. M., & BROOKSHIRE, K. H. Conditioned taste aversions as a function of the number of CS-US pairs. *Psychonomic Science*, 1971, **22**: 25–26.

BRACKBILL, R. M., ROSENBUSH, S. N., & BROOKSHIRE, K. H. Acquisition and retention of conditioned taste aversions as a function of the taste quality of the CS. *Learning and Motivation*, 1971, **2**: 341–350.

BRADLEY, R. M., & MISTRETTA, C. M. Intravascular taste in rats as demonstrated by conditioned aversion to sodium saccharin. *Journal of Comparative and Physiological Psychology*, 1971, **75**: 186–189.

BRAUN, J. J. Foundations of residual associative taste salience in rats lacking gustatory neocortex. *Bulletin of the Psychonomic Society*, 1983, **21**: 337.

BRAUN, J. J., KIEFER, S. W., & OUELLET, J. V. Psychic ageusia in rats lacking gustatory neocortex. *Experimental Neurology*, 1981, **72**: 711–716.

BRAUN, J. J., LASITER, P. S., & KIEFER, S. W. The gustatory neocortex of the rat. *Physiological Psychology*, 1982, **10**: 13–45.

BRAUN, J. J., & MCINTOSH, H., JR. Learned taste aversions induced by rotational stimulation. *Physiological Psychology*, 1973, **1**: 301–304.

BRAUN, J. J., & ROSENTHAL, B. Relative salience of saccharin and quinine in long-delay taste aversion learning. *Behavioral Biology*, 1976, **16**: 341–352.

BRAUN, J. J., SLICK, T. B., & LORDEN, J. F. Involvement of gustatory neocortex in the learning of taste aversions. *Physiology & Behavior*, 1972, **9**: 637–641.

BRAUN, J. J., & SNYDER, D. R. Taste aversions and acute methyl mercury poisoning in rats. *Bulletin of the Psychonomic Society*, 1973, **1**: 419–420.

BRAVEMAN, N. S. Poison-based avoidance learning with flavored or colored water in guinea pigs. *Learning and Motivation*, 1974, **5**: 182–194.

BRAVEMAN, N. S. Formation of taste aversions in rats following prior exposure to sickness. *Learning and Motivation*, 1975, **6**: 512–534.

BRAVEMAN, N. S. Relative salience of gustatory and visual cues in the formation of poison-based food aversions by guinea pigs (*Cavia porcellus*). *Behavioral Biology*, 1975, **14**: 189–199.

BRAVEMAN, N. S. Visually guided avoidance of poisonous foods in mammals. In L. Barker, M. Best and M. Domjan (Eds.), *Learning mechanisms in food selection*. Waco, Texas: Baylor University Press, 1977.

BRAVEMAN, N. S. What studies on preexposure to pharmacological agents tell us about the nature of the aversion-inducing treatment. In L. Barker, M. Best and M. Domjan (Eds.), *Learning mechanisms in food selection*. Waco, Texas: Baylor University Press, 1977.

BRAVEMAN, N. S. The role of handling cues in the treatment preexposure effect in taste aversion learning. *Bulletin of the Psychonomic Society*, 1978, **12**: 74–76.

BRAVEMAN, N. S. Preexposure to feeding-related stimuli reduces neophobia. *Animal Learning & Behavior*, 1978, **6**: 417–422.

BRAVEMAN, N. S. The role of blocking and compensatory conditioning in the treatment preexposure effect. *Psychopharmacology*, 1979, **61**:177–189.

BRAVEMAN, N. S. & CRANE, J. Amount consumed and the formation of conditioned taste aversions. *Behavioral Biology*, 1977, **21**: 470–477.

BRAVEMAN, N. S., & JARVIS, P. S. Independence of neophobia and taste aversion learning. *Animal Learning & Behavior*, 1978, **6**: 406–412.

BRETT, L. P., HANKINS, W. G., & GARCIA, J. Prey-lithium aversions. III: Buteo hawks. *Behavioral Biology*, 1976, **17**: 87–98.

BRETT, L. P., & LEVINE, S. The pituitary-adrenal response to "minimized" schedule-induced drinking. *Physiology & Behavior*, 1981, **26**: 153–158.

BROOKSHIRE, K. H. Function of the "onset of illness" in the preference changes of alloxan-diabetic rats. *Journal of Comparative and Physiological Psychology*, 1974, **87**: 1069–1072.

BROOKSHIRE, K. H., & BRACKBILL. R. M. Formation and retention of conditioned taste aversions and UCS habituation. *Bulletin of the Psychonomic Society*, 1976, **7**: 125–128.

BROOKSHIRE, K. H., STEWART, C. N., & BHAGAVAN, H. N. Saccharin aversion in alloxan-diabetic rats. *Journal of Comparative and Physiological Psychology*, 1972, **79**: 385–393.

BROWDER, J. A., UPCHURCH, W. M., & KIRBY, R. H. Preference for drinking deionized water over D_2O in the rat. *Physiological Psychology*, 1974, **2**: 461–463.

BROWER, L. P. Ecological chemistry. *Scientific American*, 1969, **220**: 22–29.

BROWER, L. P., & FINK, L. S. A natural toxic defense system: Cardenolides in butterflies *vs* birds. *Annals of The New York Academy of Sciences*, 1985, **443**: 171–188.

BROWN, R. T. Taste-aversion learning in dead rats: A procedural note. *The Worm Runner's Digest*, 1974, **16**: 105.

BROWN, R. T., STEWART, R. I., & HALL, T. L. Extinction of a taste aversion in the absence of the consummatory response. *Animal Learning & Behavior*, 1976, **4**: 213–216.

BROWN, Z. W., AMIT, Z., SMITH, B., & ROCKMAN, G. E. Differential effects on conditioned taste aversion learning with peripherally and centrally administered acetaldehyde. *Neuropharmacology*, 1978, **17**: 931–935.

BROWN, Z. W., AMIT, Z., SMITH, B., & ROCKMAN, G. Disruption of taste aversion learning by pretreatment with diazepam and morphine. *Pharmacology, Biochemistry & Behavior*, 1979, **10**: 17–20.

BROZEK, G. Electrophysiological analysis of conditioned taste aversion in rats. *Acta Neurobiologiae Experimentalis*, 1982, **42**: 29–41.

BROZEK, G., BURESOVA, O., & BURES, J. Effect of bilateral cortical spreading depression on the hippocampal theta activity induced by oral infusion of aversive gustatory stimulus. *Experimental Neurology*, 1974, **42**: 661–668.

BROZEK, G., BURESOVA, O., & BURES, J. Electrophysiological analysis of retrieval of conditioned taste aversion: Physiological techniques and data processing. *Physiologia Bohemoslovaca*, 1979; **28**: 537–544.

BROZEK, G., BURESOVA O., & BURES, J. Electrophysiological correlates of memory retrieval. In C. Marsan & H. Matthies (Eds.), *Neuronal plasticity and memory formation*. New York: Raven Press, 1982.

BROZEK, G., SIEGFRIED, B., KLIMENKO, V. M., & BURES, J. Lick triggered intracranial stimulation interferes with retrieval of conditioned taste aversion. *Physiology & Behavior,* 1979, **23**: 625–631.

BUCKWALD, N. A., GARCIA, J., FEDER, B. H., & BACH-Y-RITA, G. Ionizing radiation as a perceptual and aversive stimulus. II: Electrophysiological studies. In T. Haley and R. Snider (Eds.), *Response of the nervous system to ionizing radiation.* New York: Little Brown, 1964.

BURES, J. New models and methods in the electrophysiology of learning. *Activitas Nervosa Superior,* 1976, **18**: 51–57.

BURES, J., & BURESOVA, O. Gustatory recognition time in rats with conditioned taste aversion. *Physiologia Bohemoslovaca,* 1976, **25**: 257.

BURES, J., & BURESOVA, O. Physiological mechanisms of conditioned food aversion. In N. Milgram, L. Krames and T. Alloway (Eds.), *Food aversion learning.* New York: Plenum Press, 1977.

BURES, J., & BURESOVA, O. Biological significance and physiological mechanisms of conditioned taste aversion. In T. Oniani (Ed.), *Neurophysiological bases of memory.* Tbilisi, USSR: Metsniereba Publishers, 1979.

BURES, J., & BURESOVA, O. Neurophysiological analysis of conditioned taste aversion. In A. Brazier (Ed.), *Brain mechanisms in memory and learning: From the single neuron to man.* New York: Raven Press, 1979.

BURES, J., & BURESOVA, O. Elementary learning phenomena in food selection. In G. Adam, I. Meszaros, and E. Banyai (Eds.), *Advances in physiological sciences, vol. 17. Brain and behaviour.* Budapest: Pergamon Press, 1981.

BURES, J., & BURESOVA, O. Ethological models in research into the neural mechanisms of short-term memory. *Journal of Physiology,* 1982, **78**: 870–871.

BURESOVA, O. Differential role of the cerebral cortex and subcortical centres in the acquisition and extinction of conditioned taste aversion. *Activitas Nervosa Superior,* 1976, **18**: 118–119.

BURESOVA, O. Neocortico-amygdalar interaction in the conditioned taste aversion in rats. *Activitas Nervosa Superior,* 1978, **20**: 224–230.

BURESOVA, O., ALEKSANYAN, Z. A., & BURES, J. Electrophysiological analysis of retrieval of conditioned taste aversion in rats. Unit activity changes in critical brain regions. *Physiologia Bohemoslovaca,* 1979, **28**: 525–536.

BURESOVA, O., & BURES, J. Cortical and subcortical components of the conditioned saccharin aversion. *Physiology & Behavior,* 1973, **11**: 435–439.

BURESOVA, O., & BURES, J. Cortical and subcortical components of conditioned saccharin aversion in rats. *Acta Neurobiologia Experimentalis,* 1973, **33**: 689–698.

BURESOVA, O., & BURES, J. The mechanisms of conditioned saccharin aversion. In H. Matthies (Ed.), *Neurobiological basis of memory formation.* Berlin: Veb Verlag Volk and Gesundheit, 1974.

BURESOVA, O., & BURES, J. Functional decortication in the CS-US interval decreases efficiency of taste aversion learning. *Behavioral Biology,* 1974, **12**: 357–364.

BURESOVA, O., & BURES, J. The antagonistic influence of anesthesia and functional decortication on conditioned taste aversion. *Activitas Nervosa Superior,* 1975, **17**: 58.

BURESOVA, O., & BURES, J. Functional decortication by cortical spreading depression does not prevent forced extinction of conditioned saccharin aversion in rats. *Journal of Comparative and Physiological Psychology,* 1975, **88**: 47–52.

BURESOVA, O., & BURES, J. Post-ingestion interference with brain function prevents attenuation of neophobia in rats. *Behavioural Brain Research,* 1980, **1**: 299–312.

BURESOVA, O., & BURES, J. The effect of anesthesia on acquisition and extinction of conditioned taste aversion. *Behavioral Biology,* 1977, **20**: 41–50.

BURESOVA, O., & BURES, J. The anterograde effect of ECS on the acquisition, retrieval and extinction of conditioned taste aversion. *Physiology & Behavior,* 1979, **22**: 641–645.

BURESOVA, O., & BURES, J. Extinction of a newly acquired conditioned aversion: Effect of gustatory CS administered under anesthesia. *Behavioral Processes,* 1980, **4**: 329–339.

BURESOVA, O., & BURES, J. Threshold hypothermia disrupting acquisition of conditioned taste aversion and attenuation of neophobia in rats. *Behavioral and Neural Biology,* 1981, **31**: 274–282.

BURESOVA, O., BURES, J., & SKOPKOVA, J. Specificity of the effect of desglycinamide (8-D-Arginine) deaminovasopressin on short-term memory. *Physiologia Bohemoslovaca*, 1983, **32**: 403.

BURESOVA, O., SEMENOV, L., & BURES, J. Electrical stimulation or chemical blockade of vestibular nuclei can serve as the unconditioned stimulus in the conditioned taste aversion paradigm. *Acta Biologica Academical Scientiarum Hungaricae*, 1982, **33**: 139–148.

BURGHARDT, G. M., WILCOXON, H. C., & CZAPLICKI, J. A. Conditioning in garter snakes: Aversion to palatable prey induced by delayed illness. *Animal Learning & Behavior*, 1973, **1**: 317–320.

BURT, G. S., & SMOTHERMAN, W. P. Amygdalectomy-induced deficits in conditioned taste-aversion: Possible pituitary-adrenal involvement. *Physiology & Behavior*, 1980, **24**: 651–655.

BUSKIST, W. F., MILLER, H. L., JR., DUNCAN, P., & FLEMING, D. E. Associative history determines stregnth of taste-aversion conditioning in thiamine-deficient rats. *Physiology & Behavior*, 1980, **25**: 989–992.

BUSKIST, W. F., MILLER, H. L., JR., FLEMING, D. E., & SPARENBORG, S. P. Associative history, not familiarity, determines strength of taste-aversion conditioning in thiamine-deficient rats. *Bulletin of the Psychonomic Society*, 1981, **17**: 104–106.

CAIN, N. W., & BAENNINGER, R. Habituation to illness: Effects of prior experience with the US on the formation of learned taste aversions in rats. *Animal Learning & Behavior*, 1977, **5**: 359–364.

CAIRNIE, A. B. Adverse effects of radioprotector WR2721. *Radiation Research*, 1983, **94**: 221–226.

CAIRNIE, A. B., & LEACH, K. E. Dexamethasone: A potent blocker for radiation-induced taste aversion in rats. *Pharmacology, Biochemistry & Behavior*, 1982, **17**: 305–311.

CAMPBELL, B. A., & ALBERTS, J. R. Ontogeny of long-term memory for learned taste aversions. *Behavioral and Neural Biology*, 1979, **25**: 139–156.

CANNON, D. S., & BAKER, T. B. Emetic and electric shock alcohol aversion therapy: Assessment of conditioning. *Journal of Consulting and Clinical Psychology*, 1981, **49**: 20–33.

CANNON, D. S., BAKER, T. B., & BERMAN, R. F. Taste aversion disruption by drug pretreatment: Dissociative and drug-specific effects. *Pharmacology, Biochemistry & Behavior*, 1977, **6**: 93–100.

CANNON, D., BAKER, T., & WEHL, C. Emetic and electric shock alcohol aversion therapy: Six- and twelve-month follow-up. *Journal of Consulting and Clinical Psychology*, 1981, **49**: 360–368.

CANNON, D. S., BERMAN, R. F., BAKER, T. B., & ATKINSON, C. A. Effect of preconditioning unconditioned stimulus experience on learned taste aversions. *Journal of Experimental Psychology: Animal Behavior Processes*, 1975, **104**: 270–284.

CANNON, D. S., BEST, M. R., BATSON, J. D., & FELDMAN, M. Taste familiarity and apomorphine-induced taste aversion in humans. *Behaviour Research and Therapy*, 1983, **21**: 669–673.

CAPPELL, H., & LEBLANC, A. E. Conditioned aversion to saccharin by single administrations of mescaline and d-amphetamine. *Psychopharmacologia*, 1971, **22**: 352–356.

CAPPELL, H., & LEBLANC, A. E. Aversive conditioning by d-amphetamine. In J. Singh, L. Miller and H. Lal (Eds.), *Drug addiction: Experimental pharmacology*. New York: Futura, 1972.

CAPPELL, H., & LEBLANC, A. E. Punishment of saccharin drinking by amphetamine in rats and its reversal by chlordiazepoxide. *Journal of Comparative and Physiological Psychology*, 1973, **85**: 97–104.

CAPPELL, H., & LEBLANC, A. E. Conditioned aversion by psychoactive drugs: Does it have significance for an understanding of drug dependence? *Addictive Behaviors*, 1975, **1**: 55–64.

CAPPELL, H., & LEBLANC, A. E. Conditioned aversion by amphetamine: Rate of acquisition and loss of the attenuating effects of prior exposure. *Psychopharmacologia*, 1975, **43**: 157–162.

CAPPELL, H., & LEBLANC, A. E. Gustatory avoidance conditioning by drugs of abuse: Relationships to general issues in research on drug dependence. In. N. Milgram, L. Krames and T. Alloway (Eds.), *Food aversion learning*. New York: Plenum Press, 1977.

CAPPELL, H., & LEBLANC, A. E. Parametric investigations of the effects of prior exposure to amphetamine and morphine on conditioned gustatory aversion. *Psychopharmacology*, 1977, **51**: 265–271.

CAPPELL, H., LEBLANC, A. E., & ENDRENYI, L. Effects of chlordiazepoxide and ethanol on the extinction of a conditioned taste aversion. *Physiology & Behavior*, 1972, **9**: 167–169.

CAPPELL, H., LEBLANC, A. E., & ENDRENYI, L. Aversive conditioning by psychoactive drugs: Effects of morphine, alcohol and chlordiazepoxide. *Psychopharmacologia*, 1973, **29**: 239–246.

CAPPELL, H., LEBLANC, A. E., & HERLING, S. Modification of the punishing effect of psychoactive drugs in rats by previous drug experience. *Journal of Comparative and Physiological Psychology*, 1975, **89**: 347–356.

CAPPELL, H., & POULOS, C. X. Associative factors in drug pretreatment effects on gustatory conditioning: Cross-drug effects. *Psychopharmacology*, 1979, **64**: 209–213.

CAPRETTA, P. J. An experimental modification of food preference in chickens. *Journal of Comparative and Physiological Psychology*, 1961, **54**: 238-242.

CAPRETTA, P. J., & MOORE, M. J. Appropriateness of reinforcement to cue in the conditioning of food aversions in chickens (*Gallus gallus*). *Journal of Comparative and Physiological Psychology*, 1970, **72**: 85–89.

CAPRETTA, P. J., MOORE, M. J., & ROSSITER, T. R. Establishment and modification of food and taste preferences: Effects of experience. *The Journal of General Psychology*, 1973, **89**: 27–46.

CAREY, R. J. Acquired aversion to amphetamine solutions. *Pharmacology, Biochemistry & Behavior*, 1973, **1**: 227–229.

CAREY, R. J. Long-term aversion to a saccharin solution induced by repeated amphetamine injections. *Pharmacology, Biochemistry & Behavior*, 1973, **1**: 265–270.

CAREY, R. J. A comparison of the food intake suppression produced by giving amphetamine as an aversion treatment versus as an anorexic treatment. *Psychopharmacology*, 1978, **56**: 45–48.

CAREY, R. J., & GODDALL, E. B. Amphetamine-induced taste aversion: A comparison of d- versus l-amphetamine. *Pharmacology, Biochemistry & Behavior*, 1974, **2**: 325–330.

CAREY, R. J., & GOODALL, E. B. A conditioned taste aversion induced by alpha-methyl-p-tyrosine. *Neuropharmacology*, 1974, **13**: 595–600.

CARROLL, M. E., DINC, H. I., LEVY, C. J., & SMITH, J. C. Demonstrations of neophobia and enhanced neophobia in the albino rat. *Journal of Comparative and Physiological Psychology*, 1975, **89**: 457–467.

CARROLL, M. E., & SMITH, J. C. Time course of radiation-induced taste aversion conditioning. *Physiology & Behavior*, 1974, **13**: 809–812.

CAUTELA, J. R. Treatment of compulsive behavior by covert sensitization. *Psychological Reports*, 1966, **16**: 33–41.

CAUTELA, J. R. Covert sensitization. *Psychological Reports*, 1967, **20**:459–468.

CAUTELA, J. R. Covert reinforcement. *Behavior Therapy*, 1970, **1**: 33–50.

CAZA, P. A., BROWN, L., & SPEAR, N. E. Epinephrine-induced conditioned taste aversion. *Hormones and Behavior*, 1982, **16**: 31–45.

CAZA, P., STEINERT, P. A., & SPEAR, N. E. Comparison of circadian susceptibility to LiCl-induced taste aversion learning between preweanling and adult rats. *Physiology & Behavior*, 1980, **25**: 389–396.

CHAMBERS, K. C. Hormonal influences on sexual dimorphism in the rate of extinction of a conditioned taste aversion in rats. *Journal of Comparative and Physiological Psychology*, 1976, **90**: 851–856.

CHAMBERS, K. C. Progesterone, estradiol, testosterone and dihydrotestosterone: Effects on rate of extinction of a conditioned taste aversion in rats. *Physiology & Behavior*, 1980, **24**: 1061–1065.

CHAMBERS, K. C. Failure of ACTH to prolong extinction of a conditioned taste aversion in the absence of the testes. *Physiology & Behavior*, 1982, **29**: 915–919.

CHAMBERS, K. C. Sexual dimorphisms as an index of hormonal influences on conditioned food aversions. *Annals of The New York Academy of Sciences,* 1985, **443**: 110–125.

CHAMBERS, K. C., & SENGSTAKE, C. B. Sexually dimorphic extinction of a conditioned taste aversion in rats. *Animal Learning & Behavior*, 1976, **4**: 181–185.

CHAMBERS, K. C., & SENGSTAKE, C. B. Pseudo-castration effects of social isolation on extinction of a taste aversion. *Physiology & Behavior*, 1978, **21**: 29–32.

CHAMBERS, K. C., & SENGSTAKE, C. B. Temporal aspects of the dependency of a dimorphic rate of extinction on testosterone. *Physiology & Behavior*, 1979, **22**: 53–56.

CHAMBERS, K. C., SENGSTAKE, C. B., YODER, R. L., & THORNTON, J. E. Sexually dimorphic acquisition of a conditioned taste aversion in rats: Effects of gonadectomy, testoseterone replacement and water deprivation. *Physiology & Behavior,* 1981, **27**: 83–88.

CHANG, J. J., & GELPERIN, A. Rapid taste-aversion learning by an isolated molluscan central nervous system. *Proceedings of the National Academy of Sciences of the United States of America,* 1980, **77**: 6204–6206.

CHEATLE, M. D., & RUDY, J. W. Analysis of second-order odor-aversion conditioning in neonatal rats: Implications for Kamin's blocking effect. *Journal of Experimental Psychology: Animal Behavior Processes,* 1978, **4**: 237–249.

CHEATLE, M. D., & RUDY, J. W. Ontogeny of second-order odor-aversion conditioning in neonatal rats. *Journal of Experimental Psychology: Animal Behavior Processes,* 1979, **5**: 142–151.

CHEN, J-S., & AMSEL, A. Recall (versus recognition) of taste and immunization against aversive taste anticipations based on illness. *Science,* 1980, **209**: 831–833.

CHEN, J-S., DRISCOLL, C., & RILEY, E. Ingestional aversion learning in preweanling rats exposed to alcohol prenatally. *Alcoholism: Clinical & Experimental Research,* 1978, **6**: 138.

CHENY, C. D., & ELDRED, N. L. Lithium-chloride-induced aversions in the opossum (*Didelphais virginiana*). *Physiological Psychology,* 1980, **8**: 383–385.

CHIPKIN, R. E., & ROSECRANS, J. A. Aversiveness of oral methadone in rats. *Psychopharmacology,* 1978, **57**: 303–310.

CHITTY, D. (Ed.), Control of rats and mice (vol 1). Oxford: Clarendon Press, 1954

CHITTY, D. (Ed.), Control of rats and mice (vol 2). Oxford: Clarendon Press, 1954.

CHITTY, D. The study of the brown rat and its control by poison. In D. Chitty (Ed.), *Control of rats and mice (vol 1).* Oxford: Clarendon Press, 1954.

CLARKE, J. C., & WESTBROOK, R. F. Control of polydipsic drinking by a taste aversion procedure. *Pharmacology, Biochemistry & Behavior,* 1978, **9**: 283–286.

CLARKE, J. C., WESTBROOK, R. F., & IRWIN, J. Potentiation instead of overshadowing in the pigeon. *Behavioral and Neural Biology,* 1979, **25**: 18–29.

CLODY, D. E., & VOGEL, J. R. Drug-induced conditioned aversion to mouse-killing in rats. *Pharmacology, Biochemistry & Behavior,* 1973, **1**: 477–481.

COHEN, N., ADER, R., GREEN, N., & BOVBJERG, D. Conditioned suppression of a thymus-independent antibody response. *Psychosomatic Medicine,* 1979, **41**: 487–491.

COIL, J. D., HANKINS, W. G., JENDEN, D. J., & GARCIA, J. The attenuation of a specific cue-to-consequence association by antiemetic agents. *Psychopharmacology,* 1978, **56**: 21–25.

COIL, J. D., & NORGREN, R. Taste aversions conditioned with intravenous copper sulfate: Attenuation by ablation of the area postrema. *Brain Research,* 1982, **212**: 425–433.

COIL, J. D., ROGERS, R. C., GARCIA, J., & NOVIN, D. Conditioned taste aversions: Vagal and circulatory mediation of the toxic unconditioned stimulus. *Behavioral Biology,* 1978, **24**: 509–519.

COLBY, J. J., & SMITH, N. F. The effect of three procedures for eliminating a conditioned taste aversion in the rat. *Learning and Motivation,* 1977, **8**: 404–413.

CONCANNON, J. T., & FREDA, J. Modulation of conditioned taste aversion by sodium pentobarbital. *Pharmacology, Biochemistry & Behavior,* 1980, **13**: 761–764.

CONOVER, M. R., FRANCIK, J. G., & MILLER, D. E. An experimental evaluation of using taste aversion to control sheep loss due to coyote predation. *Journal of Wildlife Management,* 1977, **44**: 775–779.

COOMBES, S., REVUSKY, S., & LETT, B. T. Long-delay taste aversion learning in an unpoisoned rat: Exposure to a poisoned rat as the unconditioned stimulus. *Learning and Motivation,* 1980, **11**: 256–266.

COOPER, A., & CAPRETTA, P. J. Olfactory bulb removal and taste aversion learing in mice. *Bulletin of the Psychonomic Society,* 1976, **7**: 235–236.

COOPER, R. L., MCNAMARA, M. C., & THOMPSON, W. G. Vasopressin and conditioned flavor aversion in aged rats. *Neurobiology of Aging,* 1980, **1**: 53–57.

CORCORAN, M. E. Role of drug novelty and metabolism in the aversive effects of hashish injections in rats. *Life Sciences,* 1973, **12**: 63–72.

CORCORAN, M. E., BOLOTOW, I., AMIT, Z., & MCCAUGHRAN, J. A., JR. Conditioned taste aversions produced by active and inactive cannabinoids. *Pharmacology, Biochemistry & Behavior,* 1974, **2**: 725–728.

CORCORAN, M. E., LEWIS, J., & FIBIGER, H. C. Forebrain noradrenaline and oral self-administration of ethanol by rats. *Behavioural Brain Research*, 1983, **8**: 1–21.

CORFIELD-SUMNER, P. K., & BOND, N. W. Taste aversion learning and schedule-induced alcohol consumption in rats. *Pharmacology, Biochemistry & Behavior*, 1978, **9**: 731–733.

CORNELL, D., & CORNELY, J. E. Aversive conditioning of campground coyotes in Joshua Tree National Monument. *Wildlife Society Bulletin*, 1979, **7**: 129–131.

COUSSENS, W. R. Conditioned taste aversion: Route of drug adminsitration. In J. Singh and H. Lal (Eds.), *Drug addiction: Neurobiology and influences on behavior (vol 3)*. Miami: Symposium Specialists, 1974.

COUSSENS, W. R., CROWDER, W. F., & DAVIS, W. M. Morphine-induced saccharin aversion in alpha-methyltyrosine pretreated rats. *Psychopharmacologia*, 1973, **29**: 151–157.

CRABBE, J. C., RIGTER, H., & KERBUSCH, S. Analysis of behavioural responses to an ACTH analog in CXB:BY recombinant inbred mice. *Behavioural Brain Research*, 1982, **4**: 289–314.

CRAWFORD, D., & BAKER, T. B. Alcohol dependence and taste-mediated learning in the rat. *Pharmacology, Biochemistry & Behaviour*, 1982, **16**: 253–261.

CREIM, J. A., LOVELY, R. H., KAUNE, W. T., & PHILLIPS, R. D. Attempts to produce taste-aversion learning in rats exposed to 60-Hz electric fields. *Bioelectromagnetics*, 1984, **5**: 271–282.

CULLEN, J. W. Modification of salt-seeking behavior in the adrenalectomized rat via gamma-ray irradiation. *Journal of Comparative and Physiological Psychology*, 1969, **68**: 524–529.

CULLEN, J. W. Modification of NaCl appetite in the adrenalectomized rat consequent to extensive LiCl poisoning. *Journal of Comparative and Physiological Psychology*, 1970, **72**: 79–84.

CUNNINGHAM, C. L. Alcohol interacts with flavor during extinction of conditioned taste aversion. *Physiological Psychology*, 1978, **6**: 510–516.

CUNNINGHAM, C. L. Flavor and location aversions produced by ethanol. *Behavioral and Neural Biology*, 1979, **27**: 362–367

CUNNINGHAM, C. L. Spatial aversion conditioning with ethanol. *Pharmacology, Biochemistry & Behavior*, 1981, **14**: 263–264.

CUNNINGHAM, C. L. & LINAKIS, J. G. Paradoxical aversive conditioning with ethanol. *Pharmacology, Biochemistry & Behavior*, 1980, **12**: 337–341.

CZAPLICKI, J. A., BORREBACH, D. E., & WILCOXON, H. C. Stimulus generalization of illness-induced aversion to different intensities of colored water in Japanese quail. *Animal Learning & Behavior*, 1976, **4**: 45–48.

CZAPLICKI, J. A., PORTER, R. H., & WILCOXON, H. C. Olfactory mimicry involving garter snakes and artificial models and mimics. *Behaviour*, 1975, **54**: 60–71.

DACANAY, R. J., MASTROPAOLO, J. P., OLIN, D. A., & RILEY, A. L. Sex differences in taste aversion learning: An analysis of the minimal effective dose. *Neurobehavioral Toxicology and Teratology*, 1984, **6**: 9–11.

DACANAY, R. J., & RILEY, A. L. The UCS preexposure effect in taste aversion learning: Tolerance and blocking are drug specific. *Animal Learning & Behavior*, 1982, **10**: 91–96.

DALRYMPLE, A. J., & GALEF, B. G., JR. Visual discrimination pretraining facilitates subsequent visual-cue-toxicosis conditioning in rats. *Bulletin of the Psychonomic Society*, 1981, **18**: 267–270.

DALY, M., RAUSCHEBERGER, J., & BEHRENDS, P. Food aversion learning in Kangaroo rats: A specialist-generalist comparison. *Animal Learning & Behavior*, 1982, **10**: 314–320.

D'AMATO, M. R., & SAFARJAN, W. R. Differential effects of delay of reinforcement on acquisition of affective and instrumental responses. *Animal Learning & Behavior*, 1981, **9**: 209–215.

DANGUIR, J., & NICOLADIS, S. Impairments of learned aversion acquisition following paradoxical sleep deprivation in the rat. *Physiology & Behavior*, 1976, **17**: 489–492.

DANGUIR, J., & NICOLADIS, S. Lack of reacquisition in learned taste aversions. *Animal Learning & Behavior*, 1977, **5**: 395–397.

DANTZER, R. Conditioned taste aversion as an index of lead toxicity. *Pharmacology, Biochemistry & Behavior*, 1980, **13**: 133–135.

DAS GUPTA, K., & JEFFERSON, J. W. Lithium and "accidentally" induced food aversion. *Journal of Clinical Psychiatry*, 1980, **41**: 10.

DAVIDSON, W. S. Studies of aversive conditioning for alcoholics: A critical review of theory and research methodology. *Psychological Bulletin*, 1974, **81**: 571–581.

DAVIS, J. L. Saccharin aversion acquired during unilateral spreading depression. *Physiological Psychology*, 1975, **3**: 253–254.

DAVIS, J. L., & BURES, J. Disruption of saccharin-aversion learning in rats by cortical spreading depression in the CS-US interval. *Journal of Comparative and Physiological Psychology*, 1972, **80**: 398–402.

DAVIS, J. L., BURESOVA, O., & BURES, J. Cortical spreading depression and conditioned taste aversion: An attempt to resolve a controversy. *Behavioral and Neural Biology*, 1983, **37**: 338–343.

DAVIS, J. L., PICO, R. M., & CHERKIN, A. Dose-dependent and time-dependent action of oxytocin on chick memory. *Brain Research*, 1983, **266**: 355–358.

DAVIS, R. S. Breakthrough on the Honn Ranch. *Defenders of Wildlife International*, in press.

DAVISON, C. S., CORWIN, G., & MCGOWAN, T. Alcohol-induced taste aversion in golden hamsters. *Journal of Studies on Alcohol*, 1976, **37**: 606–610.

DAVISON, C. S., & HOUSE, W. J. Alcohol as the aversive stimulus in conditioned taste aversion. *Bulletin of the Psychonomic Society*, 1975, **6**: 49–50.

DAWLEY, J. M. Generalization of the CS-preexposure effect transfers to taste-aversion learning. *Animal Learning & Behavior*, 1979, **7**: 23–24.

DECASTRO, J. M., & BALAGURA, S. Fornicotomy: Effect on the primary and secondary punishment of mouse killing by LiCl poisoning. *Behavioral Biology*. 1975, **13**: 483–489.

DENEBERG, V. H., HOFMANN, M., GARBANATI, J. A., SHERMAN, G. F., ROSEN, G. D., & YUTZEY, D. A. Handling in infancy, taste aversion, and brain laterality in rats. *Brain Research*, 1980, **200**: 123–133.

DER-KARABETIAN, A., & GORRY, T. Amount of different flavors consumed during the CS-US interval in taste-aversion learning and interference. *Physiological Psychology*, 1974, **2**: 457–460.

DEUTSCH, J. A. Bombesin: Satiety or malaise? *Nature*, 1980, **285**: 592.

DEUTSCH, J. A. Calcitonin: Aversive effects in rats? *Science*, 1981, **211**: 733–734.

DEUTSCH, J. A. Controversies in food intake regulation. In B. Hoebel and D. Novin (Eds.), *The neural basis of feeding and reward*. Brunswick, ME: Haer Institute, 1982.

DEUTSCH, J. A., & CANNIS, J. T. Rapid induction of voluntary alcohol choice in rats. *Behavioral and Neural Biology*, 1980, **30**: 292–298.

DEUTSCH, J. A., DAVIS, J. K., & CAP, M. Conditioned taste aversion: Oral and post ingestional factors. *Behavioral Biology*, 1976, **18**: 545–550.

DEUTSCH, J. A., & EISNER, A. Ethanol self-administration in the rat induced by forced drinking of ethanol. *Behavioral Biology*, 1977, **20**: 81–90.

DEUTSCH, J. A., & GONZALEZ, M. F. Food intake reduction: Satiation or aversion? *Behavioral Biology*, 1978, **24**: 317–326.

DEUTSCH, J. A., & HARDY, W. T. Ethanol tolerance in the rat measured by the untasted intake of alcohol. *Behavioral Biology*, 1976, **17**: 379–389.

DEUTSCH, J. A., & HARDY, W. T. Cholecystokinin produces bait shyness in rats. *Nature*, 1977, **266**: 196.

DEUTSCH, J. A., MOLINA, F., & PUERTO, A. Conditioned taste aversion caused by palatable nontoxic nutrients. *Behavioral Biology*, 1976, **16**: 161–174.

DEUTSCH, J. A., & PARSONS, S. L. Bombesin produces taste aversion in rats. *Behavioral and Neural Biology*, 1981, **31**: 110–113.

DEUTSCH, J. A., PUERTO, A., & WANG, M-L. The pyloric sphincter and differential food preference. *Behavioral Biology*, 1977, **19**: 543–547.

DEUTSCH, J. A., WALTON, N. Y., & THIEL, T. R. The importance of postingestional factors in limiting alcohol consumption in the rat. *Behavioral Biology*, 1978, **22**: 128–131.

DEUTSCH, R. Conditioned hypoglycemia: A mechanism for saccharin-induced sensitivity to insulin in the rat. *Journal of Comparative and Physiological Psychology*, 1974, **86**: 350–358.

DEUTSCH, R. Effects of CS amount on conditioned taste aversion at different CS-US intervals. *Animal Learning & Behavior*, 1978, **6**: 258–260.

DEUTSCH, R. Effects of atropine on conditioned taste aversion. *Pharmacology, Biochemistry & Behavior*, 1978, **8**: 685–694.

DEVENPORT, L. D. Aversion to a palatable saline solution in rats: Interactions of physiology and experience. *Journal of Comparative and Physiological Psychology*, 1973, **83**: 98–105.

DIAMENT, C., & WILSON, G. T. An experimental investigation of the effects of covert sensitization in an analog eating situation. *Behavior Therapy*, 1975, **6**: 499–509.

DICKINSON, A., NICHOLAS, D. J., & ADAMS, C. D. The effect of the instrumental training contingency on susceptibility to reinforcer devaluation. *Quarterly Journal of Experimental Psychology*, 1983, **35B**: 35–51.

DINC, H. I., & SMITH, J. C. Role of the olfactory bulbs in the detection of ionizing radiation by the rat. *Physiology & Behavior*, 1966, **1**: 139–144.

DIVAC, I., GADE, A., & WIKMARK, R. E. G. Taste aversion in rats with lesions in the frontal lobes: No evidence for interoceptive agnosia. *Physiological Psychology*, 1975, **3**: 43–46.

D'MELLO, G. D., GOLDBERG, D. M., GOLDBERG, S. R., & STOLERMAN, I. P. Conditioned taste aversion and operant behaviour in rats: Effects of cocaine and a cocaine analogue (Win 35, 428). *Neuropharmacology*, 1979, **18**: 1009–1010.

D'MELLO, G. D., GOLDBERG, D. M., GOLDBERG, S. R., & STOLERMAN I. P. Conditioned taste aversion and operant behavior in rats: Effects of cocaine, apomorphine and some long-acting derivatives. *Journal of Pharmacology and Experimental Therapeutics*, 1981, **219**: 60–68.

D'MELLO, G. D., & STOLERMAN, I. P. Suppression of fixed-interval responding by flavour-amphetamine pairings in rats. *Pharmacology, Biochemistry & Behavior*, 1978, **9**: 395–398.

D'MELLO, G. D., STOLERMAN, I. P., BOOTH, D. A., & PILCHER, C. W. T. Factors influencing flavour aversions conditioned with amphetamine in rats. *Pharmacology, Biochemistry & Behavior*, 1977, **7**: 185–190.

DOMJAN, M. CS preexposure in taste-aversion learning: Effects of deprivation and preexposure duration. *Learning and Motivation*, 1972, **3**: 389–402.

DOMJAN, M. Role of ingestion in odor-toxicosis learning in the rat. *Journal of Comparative and Physiological Psychology*, 1973, **84**: 507–521.

DOMJAN, M. Poison-induced neophobia in rats: Role of stimulus generalization of conditioned taste aversions. *Animal Learning & Behavior*, 1975, **3**: 205–211.

DOMJAN, M. The nature of the thirst stimulus: A factor in conditioned taste-aversion behavior. *Physiology & Behavior*, 1975, **14**: 809–813.

DOMJAN, M. Attentuation and enhancement of neophobia for edible substances. In L. Barker, M. Best and M. Domjan (Eds.), *Learning mechanisms in food selection*. Waco, Texas: Baylor University Press, 1977.

DOMJAN, M. Effects of proximal unconditioned stimulus preexposure on ingestional aversions learned as a result of taste presentation following drug treatment. *Animal Learning & Behavior*, 1978, **6**: 133–142.

DOMJAN, M. Effects of the intertrial interval on taste-aversion learning in rats. *Physiology & Behavior*, 1980, **25**: 117–125.

DOMJAN, M. Ingestional aversion learning: Unique and general processes. In J. Rosenblatt, R. Hinde, C. Beer and M. Busnel (Eds.), *Advances in the study of behavior* (*vol. 11*). New York: Academic Press, 1980.

DOMJAN, M. Biological constraints on instrumental and classical conditioning: Implications for general process theory. In G. Bower (Ed.), *The psychology of learning and motivation* (*vol. 17*). New York: Academic Press, 1983.

DOMJAN, M. Cue-consequence specificity and long-delay learning revisited. *Annals of The New York Academy of Sciences*, 1985, **443**: 54–66.

DOMJAN, M., & BEST, M. R. Paradoxical effects of proximal unconditioned stimulus preexposure: Interference with and conditioning of a taste aversion. *Journal of Experimental Psychology: Animal Behavior Processes*, 1977, **3**: 310–321.

DOMJAN, M., & BEST, M. R. Interference with ingestional aversion learning produced by preexposure to the unconditioned stimulus: Associative and nonassociative aspects. *Learning and Motivation*, 1980, **11**: 522–537.

DOMJAN, M., & BOWMAN, T. G. Learned safety and the CS-US delay gradient in taste-aversion learning. *Learning and Motivation*, 1974, **5**: 409–423.

DOMJAN, M., FOSTER, K., & GILLAN, D. J. Effects of distribution of the drug unconditioned stimulus on taste-aversion learning. *Physiology & Behavior*, 1979, **23**: 931–938.

DOMJAN, M., & GALEF, B. G., JR. Biological constraints on instrumental and classical conditioning: Retrospect and prospect. *Animal Learning & Behavior*, 1983, **11**: 151–161.

DOMJAN, M., & GEMBERLING, G. A. Effects of expected vs. unexpected proximal US preexposure on taste-aversion learning. *Animal Learning & Behavior,* 1980, **8**: 204–210.

DOMJAN, M., GEMBERLING, G. A., & GILLAN, D. J. Increased drinking stimulated by exposure to lithium-conditioned taste cues: Effects of conditioning trials and drug dose. *Pharmacology, Biochemistry & Behavior,* 1980, **12**: 789–795.

DOMJAN, M., & GILLAN, D. J. Aftereffects of lithium-conditioned stimuli on consummatory behavior. *Journal of Experimental Psychology: Animal Behavior Processes,* 1977, **3**: 322–334.

DOMJAN, M., GILLAN, D. J., & GEMBERLING, G. A. Aftereffects of lithium-conditioned stimuli on consummatory behavior in the presence or absence of the drug. *Journal of Experimental Psychology: Animal Behavior Processes,* 1980, **6**: 49–64.

DOMJAN, M., & GREGG, B. Long-delay backward taste-aversion conditioning with lithium. *Physiology & Behavior,* 1977, **18**: 59–62.

DOMJAN, M., & HANLON, M. J. Poison-avoidance learning to food-related tactile stimuli: Avoidance of texture cues by rats. *Animal Learning & Behavior,* 1982, **10**: 293–300.

DOMJAN, M., & LEVY, C. J. Taste aversions conditioned by the aversiveness of insulin and formalin: Role of CS specificity. *Journal of Experimental Psychology: Animal Behavior Processes,* 1977, **3**: 119–131.

DOMJAN, M., MILLER, V., & GEMBERLING, G. A. Note on aversion learning to the shape of food by monkeys. *Journal of the Experimental Analysis of Behavior,* 1982, **38**: 87–92.

DOMJAN, M., SCHORR, R., & BEST, M. Early environmental influences on conditioned and unconditioned ingestional and locomotor behaviors. *Developmental Psychobiology,* 1977, **10**: 499–506.

DOMJAN, M., & SIEGEL, S. Attenuation of the aversive and analgesic effects of morphine by repeated administration: Different mechanisms. *Physiological Psychology,* 1983, **11**: 155–158.

DOMJAN, M., & WILSON, N. E. Specificity of cue to consequence in aversion learning in the rat. *Psychonomic Science,* 1972, **26**: 143–145.

DOMJAN, M., & WILSON, N. E. Contribution of ingestive behaviors to taste-aversion learning in the rat. *Journal of Comparative and Physiological Psychology,* 1972, **80**: 403–412.

DORRANCE, M., & ROY, L. Aversive conditioning tests of black bears in beeyards. *Proceedings of the Vertebrate Pest Conference,* 1978, **8**: 251–254.

DOURISH, C. T., GREENSHAW, A. J., & BOULTON, A. A. Deuterium substitution enhances the effects of beta-phenylethylamine on spontaneous motor activity in the rat. *Pharmacology, Biochemistry & Behavior,* 1983, **19**: 471–475.

DRAGOIN, W. B. Conditioning and extinction of taste aversions with variations in intensity of the CS and UCS in two strains of rats. *Psychonomic Science,* 1971, **22**: 303–305.

DRAGOIN, W., HUGHES, G., DEVINE, M., & BENTLEY, J. Long-term retention of conditioned taste aversions: Effects of gustatory interference. *Psychological Reports,* 1973, **33**: 511–514.

DRAGOIN, W., MCCLEARY, G. E., & MCCLEARY, P. A comparison of two methods of measuring conditioned taste aversions. *Behavior Research Methods and Instrumentation,* 1971, **3**: 309–310.

DRAY, S. M., & TAYLOR, A. N. ACTH4–10 enhances retention of conditioned taste aversion learning in infant rats. *Behavioral and Neural Biology,* 1982, **35**: 147–158.

DUDEK, B. C. Ethanol-induced conditioned taste aversions in mice that differ in neural sensitivity to ethanol. *Journal of Studies on Alcohol,* 1982, **43**: 129–136.

DUDEK, B. C., & FULLER, J. L. Task-dependent genetic influences on behavioral response of mice (*Mus musculus*) to acetaldehyde. *Journal of Comparative and Physiological Psychology,* 1978, **92**: 749–758.

DUGAS, D. V. X., HER, C., & MAC, L. P. Qualitative discrimination of sweet stimuli: Behavioural study on rats. *Chemical Senses,* 1981, **6**: 143–148.

DURLACH, P. J., & RESCORLA, R. A. Potentiation rather than overshadowing in flavor-aversion learning: An analysis in terms of within-compound associations. *Journal of Experimental Psychology: Animal Behavior Processes,* 1980, **6**: 175–187.

EARLEY, C. J. Taste aversion as a method for assessing the effects of gonadal hormones on behavior. *Israel Journal of Medical Sciences,* 1978, **147**: 24–27.

EARLEY, C. J., & LEONARD, B. E. Androgenic involvement in conditioned taste aversion. *Hormones and Behavior,* 1978, **11**: 1–11.

EARLEY, C. J., & LEONARD, B. E. Effects of prior exposure on conditioned taste aversion in the rat: Androgen- and estrogen-dependent events. *Journal of Comparative and Physiological Psychology*, 1979, **93**: 793–805.

ECKARDT, M. J. Conditioned taste aversion produced by the oral ingestion of ethanol in the rat. *Physiological Psychology*, 1975, **3**: 317–321.

ECKHARDT, M. J. The role of orosensory stimuli from ethanol and blood-alcohol levels in producing conditioned taste aversion in the rat. *Psychopharmacologia*, 1975, **44**: 267–271.

ECKHARDT, M. J. Alcohol-induced conditioned taste aversion in rats: Effects of concentration and prior exposure to alcohol. *Journal of Studies on Alcohol*, 1976, **37**: 334–346.

ECKHARDT, M. J., SKURDAL, A. J., & BROWN, J. S. Conditioned taste aversion produced by low doses of alcohol. *Physiological Psychology*, 1974, **2**: 89–92.

EISNER, T., & GRANT, R. P. Toxicity, odor aversion, and "olfactory aposematism." *Science*, 1981, **213**: 476.

ELKINS, R. L. Attenuation of drug-induced baitshyness to a palatable solution as an increasing function of its availability prior to conditioning. *Behavioral Biology*, 1973, **9**: 221–226.

ELKINS, R. L. Individual differences in baitshyness: Effects of drug dose and measurement technique. *The Psychological Record*, 1973, **23**: 349–358.

ELKINS, R. L. Bait-shyness acquisition and resistance to extinction as functions of US exposure prior to conditioning. *Physiological Psychology*, 1974, **2**: 341–343.

ELKINS, R. L. Conditioned flavor aversions to familiar tap water in rats: An adjustment with implications for aversion therapy treatment of alcoholism and obesity. *Journal of Abnormal Psychology*, 1974, **83**: 411–417.

ELKINS, R. L. Aversion therapy for alcoholism: Chemical, electrical, or verbal imaginary? *The International Journal of the Addictions*, 1975, **10**: 157–209.

ELKINS, R. L. A note on aversion therapy for alcoholism. *Behaviour Research and Therapy*, 1976, **14**: 159–160.

ELKINS, R. L. A therapeutic phoenix: Emergent normal drinking by "failures" in an abstinence-oriented program of verbal aversion therapy for alcoholism. *Scandinavian Journal of Behaviour Therapy*, 1977, **6**: 55.

ELKINS, R. L. Covert sensitization treatment of alcoholism: Contributions of successful conditioning to subsequent abstinence maintenance. *Addictive Behavior*, 1980, **5**: 67–89.

ELKINS, R. L. A reconsideration of the relevance of recent animal studies for development of treatment procedures for alcoholics. *Drug and Alcohol Dependence*, 1980, **5**: 101–113.

ELKINS, R. L. Attenuation of x-ray-induced taste aversions by olfactory-bulb or amygdaloid lesions. *Physiology & Behavior*, 1980, **24**: 515–521.

ELKINS, R. L. Taste-aversion retention: An animal experiment with implications for consummatory-aversion alcoholism treatments. *Behaviour Research and Therapy*, 1984, **22**: 179–186.

ELKINS, R. L., FRASER, J., & HOBBS, S. H. Differential olfactory bulb contributions to baitshyness and place avoidance learning. *Physiology & Behavior*, 1977, **19**: 787–793.

ELKINS, R. L., & HARRISON, W. Rotation-induced taste aversions in strains of rats selectively bred for strong or weak acquisition of drug-induced taste aversions. *Bulletin of the Psychonomic Society*, 1983, **21**: 57–60.

ELKINS, R. L., & HOBBS, S. H. Forgetting, preconditioning CS familiarization and taste aversion learning: An animal experiment with implications for alcoholism treatment. *Behaviour Research and Therapy*, 1979, **17**: 567–573.

ELKINS, R. L., & HOBBS, S. H. Taste aversion proneness: A modulator of conditioned consummatory aversions in rats. *Bulletin of the Psychonomic Society*, 1982, **20**: 257–260.

ELKINS, R. L., & MURDOCK, R. P. The contribution of successful conditioning to abstinence maintenance following covert sensitization (verbal aversion) treatment of alcoholism. *IRCS Medical Science: Psychology and Psychiatry: Social and Occupational Medicine*, 1977, **5**: 167.

ELLINS, S. R., & CATALANO, S. M. Field application of the conditioned taste aversion paradigm to the control of coyote predation on sheep and turkeys. *Behavioral and Neural Biology*, 1980, **29**: 532–536.

ELLINS, S. R., CATALANO, S. M., & SCHECHINGER, S. A. Conditioned taste aversion: A field application to coyote predation on sheep. *Behavioral Biology*, 1977, **20**: 91–95.

ELLINS, S. R., GUSTAVSON, C. R., & GARCIA, J. Conditioned taste aversion in predators: Response to Sterner and Shumake. *Behavioral Biology*, 1978, **24**: 554–556.

Ellins, S. R., & Martin, G. C. Olfactory discrimination of lithium chloride by the coyote (*Canis latrans*). *Behavioral and Neural Biology*, 1981, **31**: 214–224.

Ellins, S. R., Thompson, L., & Swanson, W. E. Effects of novelty and familiarity on illness-induced aversions to food and place cues in coyotes (*Canis latrans*). *Journal of Comparative Psychology*, 1983, **97**: 302–309.

Ellis, M. E., & Kesner, R. P. Physostigmine and norepinephrine: Effects of injection into the amygdala on taste associations. *Physiology & Behavior*, 1981, **27**: 203–209.

Elsmore, T. F., & Fletcher, G. V. Delta-9-tetrahydrocannabinol: Aversive effects in rat at high doses. *Science*, 1972, **175**: 911–912.

Elton, C. Research on rodent control by the bureau of animal population September 1939 to July 1947. In D. Chitty (Ed.), *Control of rats and mice* (*vol I*). Oxford: Clarendon Press, 1954.

Emmerick, J. J., & Snowdon, C. T. Failure to show modification of male golden hamster mating behavior through taste-odor aversion learning. *Journal of Comparative and Physiological Psychology*, 1976, **90**: 857–869.

Engwall, D. B., & Kristal, M. B. Placentophagia in rats is modifiable by taste aversion conditioning. *Physiology & Behavior*, 1977, **18**: 495–502.

Enns, M. P., & Grinker, J. A. Conditioned aversion to sweet and salt in genetically obese and lean Zucker rats. *Chemical Senses*, 1980, **5**: 219–231.

Ervin, G. N., Carter, R. B., Webster, E. L., Moore, S. I., & Cooper, B. R. Evidence that taste aversion learning induced by 1-5-hydroxytryptophan is mediated peripherally. *Pharmacology, Biochemistry & Behavior*, 1984, **20**: 799–802.

Etscorn, F. Effects of a preferred vs a nonpreferred CS in the establishment of a taste aversion. *Physiological Psychology*, 1973, **1**: 5–6.

Etscorn, F. Illness-induced aversion learning in a desert species of rodent (*Acomys cahirinus*). *Physiological Psychology*, 1977, **5**: 336–338.

Etscorn, F. Suppression of feeding but not killing of a prey species in the ringtail cat (*Bassariscus astutus*). *Physiological Psychology*, 1978, **6**: 261–262.

Etscorn, F. Sucrose aversions in mice as a result of injected nicotine or passive tobacco smoke inhalation. *Bulletin of the Psychonomic Society*, 1980, **15**: 54–56.

Etscorn, F., & Miller, R. L. Variations in the strength of conditioned taste-aversion in rats as a function of time of inducement. *Physiological Psychology*, 1975, **3**: 270–272.

Etscorn, F., & Parson, P. Taste aversion in mice using phencyclidine and ketamine as the aversive agents. *Bulletin of the Psychonomic Society*, 1979, **14**: 19–21.

Etscorn, F., & Stephens, R. Establishment of conditioned taste aversions with a 24-hour CS-US interval. *Physiological Psychology*, 1973, **1**: 251–253.

Ettenberg, A., Sgro, S., & White, N. Algebraic summation of the affective properties of a rewarding and an aversive stimulus in the rat. *Physiology & Behavior*, 1982, **28**: 873–877.

Ettenberg, A., van der Kooy, D., Le Moal, M., Koob, G., & Bloom, F. Can aversive properties of (peripherally-injected) vasopressin account for its putative role in memory? *Behavioural Brain Research*, 1983, **7**: 331–350.

Ettenberg, A., & White, N. Pimozide attenuates conditioned taste preferences induced by self-stimulation in rats. *Pharmacology, Biochemistry & Behavior*, 1981, **15**: 915–919.

Farber, P. D., Gorman, J. E., & Reid, L. D. Morphine injections in the taste aversion paradigm. *Physiological Psychology*, 1976, **4**: 365–368.

Farley, J. A., McLaurin, W. A., Scarborough, B. B., & Rawlings, T. D. Pre-irradiation saccharin habituation: A factor in avoidance behavior. *Psychological Reports*, 1964, **14**: 491–496.

Feinberg, A. Effect of treatment-test interval and proferrin on x-irradiation-induced saccharin aversion. *JSAS Catalog of Selected Documents in Psychology*, 1973, **3**: 119–141.

Fenner, D. P., & Bernstein, I. L. Interference in food aversion conditioning by reducing drug dose or conditioning trials. *Behavioral and Neural Biology*, 1984, **40**: 114–118.

Fenwick, S., Mikulka, P. J., & Klein, S. B. The effect of different levels of pre-exposure to sucrose on the acquisition and extinction of a conditioned aversion. *Behavioral Biology*, 1975, **14**: 231–235.

FERNANDEZ, B., & TERNES, J. W. Conditioned aversion to morphine with lithium chloride in morphine-dependent rats. *Bulletin of the Psychonomic Society*, 1975, **5**: 331–332.

FISCHER, G. J., & VAIL, B. J. Preexposure to delta-9-THC blocks THC-induced conditioned taste aversion in the rat. *Behavioral and Neural Biology*, 1980, **30**: 191–196.

FITZGERALD, R. E., & BURTON, M. J. Neophobia and conditioned taste aversion deficits in the rat produced by undercutting temporal cortex. *Physiology & Behavior*, 1983, **30**: 203–206.

FJERDINGSTAD, E. J. Chemical transfer of radiation induced avoidance: A replication. *Scandinavian Journal of Psychology*, 1972, **13**: 145–151.

FLEIGER, D. L., & ZINGLE, H. W. Covert sensitization treatment with alcoholics. *Canadian Counsellor*, 1973, **7**: 269–277.

FOLTIN, R. W., PRESTON, K. L., WAGNER, G. C., & SCHUSTER, C. R. The aversive stimulus properties of repeated infusions of cocaine. *Pharmacology, Biochemistry & Behavior*, 1981, **15**: 71–74.

FOLTIN, R. W., & SCHUSTER, C. R. The effects of dl-cathinone in a gustatory avoidance paradigm. *Pharmacology, Biochemistry & Behavior*, 1981, **14**: 907–909.

FOLTIN, R. W., & SCHUSTER, C. R.The effects of cocaine in a gustatory avoidance paradigm: A procedural analysis. *Pharmacology, Biochemistry & Behavior*, 1982, **16**: 347–352.

FORBES, D. T., & HOLLAND, P. C. Positive and negative patterning after CS preexposure in flavor aversion conditioning. *Animal Learning & Behavior*, 1980, **8**: 595–600.

FORD, K. A., & RILEY, A. L. The effects of LiCl preexposure on amphetamine-induced taste aversions: An assessment of blocking. *Pharmacology, Biochemistry & Behavior*, 1984, **20**: 643–645.

FOREYT, J. P., & HAGEN, R. L. Covert sensitization: Conditioning or suggestions? *Journal of Abnormal Psychology*, 1973, **82**: 17–23.

FOX, R. A. Poison aversion and sexual behavior in the golden hamster. *Psychological Reports*, 1977, **41**: 993–994.

FOX, R. A., & DAUNTON, N. G. Conditioned feeding suppression in rats produced by cross-coupled and simple motions. *Aviation, Space, and Environmental Medicine*, 1982, **53**: 218–220.

FOX, R. A., LAUBER, A. H., DAUNTON, N. G., PHILLIPS, M., & DIAZ, L. Off-vertical rotation produces conditioned taste aversions and suppressed drinking in mice. *Aviation, Space, and Environmental Medicine*, 1984, **55**: 632–635.

FRANCHINA, J. J., & DIETZ, S. Taste aversion following backward conditioning procedures in preweanling and adult rats. *Developmental Psychobiology*, 1981, **14**: 499–505.

FRANCHINA, J. J., DOMATO, G. C., & MCCLEESE, D. Learning and retention of sucrose taste aversion in weanling rats. *Bulletin of the Psychonomic Society*, 1979, **14**: 91–94.

FRANCHINA, J. J., DOMATO, G. C., PATSIOKAS, A. T., & GRIESEMER, H. A. Effects of number of pre-exposures on sucrose taste aversion in weanling rats. *Developmental Psychobiology*, 1980, **13**: 25–31.

FRANCHINA, J. J., & HOROWITZ, S. W. Effects of age and flavor preexposures on taste aversion performance. *Bulletin of the Psychonomic Society*, 1982, **19**: 41–44.

FRANCHINA, J. J., SILBER, S., & MAY, B. Novelty and temporal contiquity in taste aversion learning: Within-subjects conditioning effects. *Bulletin of the Psychonomic Society*, 1981, **18**: 99–102.

FRANK, M. E., NOWLIS, G. H., & PFAFFMANN, C. Specificity of acquired aversions to taste qualities in hamsters and rats. *Journal of Comparative and Physiological Psychology*, 1980, **94**: 932–942.

FRANKO, C. M., & WAGNER, G. C. Gustatory avoidance in rats: Effects of cocaine under a mild water deprivation schedule. *Drug and Alcohol Dependence*, 1983, **11**: 409–413.

FRANKS, C. M. Behavior therapy, the principles of conditioning and the treatment of the alcoholic. *Quarterly Journal of Studies on Alcohol*, 1963, **24**: 511–529.

FRANKS, C. M. Conditioning and conditioned aversion therapies in the treatment of the alcoholic. *International Journal of the Addictions*, 1966, **1**: 61–68.

FREED, W. J., BING, L. A., & WYATT, R. J. Reply to Deutsch. *Science*, 1981, **211**: 734.

FREED, W. J., PERLOW, M. J., & WYATT, R. J. Calcitonin: Inhibitory effect on eating in rats. *Science*, 1979, **206**: 850–852.

FREEDMAN, N. L., & WARD, R. Saccharin aversion produced by reversible functional cortical ablation. *Physiological Psychology*, 1976, **4**: 485–488.

FREEMAN, F. G., MIKULKA, P. J., PHILLIPS, J., MEGARR, M., & MEISEL, L. Generalization of conditioned aversion and limbic lesions in rats. *Behavioral and Neural Biology*, 1978, **24**: 520–526.

FREGLY, M. J. Specificity of the sodium chloride appetite of adrenalectomized rats: Substitution of lithium chloride for sodium chloride. *American Journal of Physiology*, 1958, **195**: 645–653.

FRENK, H., & ROGERS, G. H. The suppressant effects of naloxone on food and water intake in the rat. *Behavioral and Neural Biology*, 1979, **26**: 23–40.

FREY, A. H., & FELD, S. R. Avoidance by rats of illumination with low power nonionizing electromagnetic energy. *Journal of Comparative and Physiological Psychology*, 1975, **89**: 183–188.

FRUMKIN, K. Interaction of LiCl aversion and sodium-specific hunger in the adrenalectomized rat. *Journal of Comparative and Physiological Psychology*, 1971, **75**: 32–40.

FRUMKIN, K. Effects of deprivation schedule on the maintenance of a preoperative salt aversion by adrenalectomized rats. *Physiological Psychology*, 1975, **3**: 101–106.

FRUMKIN, K. Failure of sodium- and calcium-deficient rats to acquire conditioned taste aversions to the object of their specific hunger. *Journal of Comparative and Physiological Psychology*, 1975, **89**: 329–339.

FRUMKIN, K. Differential potency of taste and audiovisual stimuli in the conditioning of morphine withdrawal in rats. *Psychopharmacologia*, 1976, **46**: 245–248.

FUDIM, O. K. Sensory preconditioning of flavors with a formalin-produced sodium need. *Journal of Experimental Psychology: Animal Behavior Processes*, 1978, **4**: 276–285.

FUKUDA, N. An experimental study of conditioned taste aversion: Stimulus discrimination in extinguished process. *Journal of Child Development*, 1980, **16**: 37–43.

GADUSEK, F. J., & KALAT, J. W. Effects of scopolamine on the retention of taste-aversion learning in rats. *Physiological Psychology*, 1975, **3**: 130–132.

GAINES, T. B., & HAYES, W. J., JR. Bait shyness to antu in wild Norway rats. *Public Health Report*, 1952, **63**: 306–311.

GALE, K. Catecholamine-independent behavioral and neurochemical effects of cocaine in rats. In C. Sharp (Ed.), *Nida Monograph*, in press.

GALEF, B. G., JR. Direct and indirect behavior pathways to the social transmission of food avoidance. *Annals of The New York Academy of Sciences*, 1985, **443**: 203–215.

GALEF, B. G., JR., & DALRYMPLE, A. J. Active transmission of poison avoidance among rats? *Behavioral Biology*, 1978, **24**: 265–271.

GALEF, B. G., JR., & DALRYMPLE, A. J. Toxicosis-based aversions to visual cues in rats: A test of the Testa and Ternes hypothesis. *Animal Learning & Behavior*, 1981, **9**: 332–334.

GALEF, B. G., JR., & OSBORNE, B. Novel taste facilitation of the association of visual cues with toxicosis in rats. *Journal of Comparative and Physiological Psychology*, 1978, **92**: 907–916.

GALEF, B. G., JR., WIGMORE, S. W., & KENNETT, D. J. A failure to find socially mediated taste aversion learning in Norway rats (*R. norvegicus*). *Journal of Comparative Psychology*, 1983, **97**: 358–363.

GAMZU, E. The multifaceted nature of taste-aversion inducing agents: Is there a single common factor? In L. Barker, M. Best and M. Domjan (Eds.), *Learning mechanisms in food selection*. Waco, Texas: Baylor University Press, 1977.

GAMZU, E., VINCENT, G., & BOFF, E. A pharmacological perspective of drugs used in establishing conditioned food aversions. *Annals of The New York Academy of Sciences*, 1985, **443**: 231–249.

GARB, J. L., & STUNKARD, A. J. Taste aversions in man. *American Journal of Psychiatry*, 1974, **131**: 1204–1207.

GARCIA, J. The faddy rat and us. *New Scientist and Science Journal*, 1974, **49**: 254–256.

GARCIA, J. Mitchell, Scott, and Mitchell are not supported by their own data. *Animal Learning & Behavior*, 1978, **6**: 116.

GARCIA, J., & BRETT, L. P. Conditioned responses to food odor and taste in rats and wild predators. In M. Kare and O. Maller (Eds.), *The chemical senses and nutrition*. New York: Academic Press, 1977.

GARCIA, J., BUCHWALD, N. A., FEDER, B. H., KOELLING, R. A., & TEDROW, L. F. Ionizing radiation as a perceptual and aversive stimulus. I. Instrumental conditioning studies. In T. Haley and R. Snider (Eds.), *Response of the nervous system to ionizing radiation.* New York: Little Brown, 1964.

GARCIA, J., & ERVIN, F. R. Appetites, aversions, and addictions: A model for visceral memory. In J. Wortis (Ed.), *Recent advances in biological psychiatry.* New York: Plenum Press, 1968.

GARCIA, J., & ERVIN, F. R. Gustatory-visceral and telereceptor-cutaneous conditioning: Adaptation in internal and external milieus. *Communications in Behavioral Biology*, 1968, **1**: 389–415.

GARCIA, J., ERVIN, F. R., & KOELLING. R. A. Learning with prolonged delay of reinforcement. *Psychonomic Science*, 1966, **5**: 121–122.

GARCIA, J., ERVIN, F. R., & KOELLING, R. A. Bait-shyness: A test for toxicity with N=2. *Psychonomic Science*, 1967, **7**: 245–246.

GARCIA, J., ERVIN, F. R., & KOELLING. R. A. Toxicity of serum from irradiated donors. *Nature*, 1967, **213**: 682–683.

GARCIA, J., ERVIN, F. R., YORKE, C. H., & KOELLING, R. A. Conditioning with delayed vitamin injections. *Science*, 1967, **155**: 716–718.

GARCIA, J., FORTHMAN-QUICK, D., & WHITE, B. Conditioned disgust and fear from mollusk to monkey. In D. Alkon and J. Farley (Eds.), *Primary neural substrates of learning and behavioral change.* New York: Cambridge University Press, 1984.

GARCIA, J., GREEN, K. F., & MCGOWAN, B. K. X-ray as an olfactory stimulus. In C. Pffafmann (Ed.), *Olfaction and taste.* New York: Rockefeller University Press, 1969.

GARCIA, J., & HANKINS, W. G. The evolution of bitter and the acquisition of toxiphobia. In D. Denton (Ed.), *Olfaction and taste* (*vol. 5*). New York: Academic Press, 1975.

GARCIA, J., & HANKINS, W. On the origin of food aversion paradigms. In L. Barker, M. Best and M. Domjan (Eds.), *Learning mechanisms in food selection.* Waco Texas: Baylor University Press, 1977.

GARCIA, J., HANKINS, W. G., & COIL, J. D. Koalas, men, and other conditioned gastronomes. In N. Milgram, L. Krames and T. Alloway (Eds.), *Food aversion learning.* New York: Plenum Press, 1977.

GARCIA, J., HANKINS, W. G., ROBINSON, J. H., & VOGT, J. L. Baitshyness: Tests of CS-US mediation. *Physiology & Behavior*, 1972, **8**: 807–810.

GARCIA, J., HANKINS, W. G., & RUSINIAK, K. W. Behavioral regulation of the milieu interne in man and rat. *Science*, 1974, **185**: 824–831.

GARCIA, J., HANKINS, W. G., & RUSINIAK, K. W. Flavor aversion studies. *Science*, 1976, **192**: 265–266.

GARCIA, J., & KIMELDORF, D. J. Temporal relationship within the conditioning of a saccharine aversion through radiation exposure. *Journal of Comparative and Physiological Psychology*, 1957, **50**: 180–183.

GARCIA, J., & KIMELDORF, D. J. The effect of ophthalmectomy upon responses of the rat to radiation and taste stimuli. *Journal of Comparative and Physiological Psychology*, 1958, **51**: 288–291.

GARCIA, J., & KIMELDORF, D. J. Some factors which influence radiation-conditioned behavior of rats. *Radiation Research*, 1960, **12**: 719–727.

GARCIA, J., & KIMELDORF, D. J. Conditioned avoidance behaviour induced by low-dose neutron exposure. *Nature*, 1960, **185**: 261–262.

GARCIA, J., KIMELDORF, D. J., & HUNT, E. L. Conditioned responses to manipulative procedures resulting from exposure to gamma radiation. *Radiation Research*, 1956, **5**: 79–87.

GARCIA, J., KIMELDORF, D. J., & HUNT, E. L. Spatial avoidance behavior in the rat as a result of exposure to ionizing radiation. *British Journal of Radiology*, 1957, **30**: 318–320.

GARCIA, J., KIMELDORF, D. J., & HUNT, E. L. The use of ionizing radiation as a motivating stimulus. *Psychological Review*, 1961, **68**: 383–395.

GARCIA, J., KIMELDORF, D. J., HUNT, E. L., & DAVIES, B. P. Food and water consumption of rats during exposure to gamma-radiation. *Radiation Research*, 1956, **4**: 33–41.

GARCIA, J., KIMELDORF, D. J., & KOELLING, R. A. Conditioned aversion to saccharin resulting from exposure to gamma radiation. *Science*, 1955, **122**: 157–158.

GARCIA, J., & KOELLING, R. A. Relation of cue to consequence in avoidance learning. *Psychonomic Science*, 1966, **4**: 123–124.

GARCIA, J., & KOELLING, R. A. A comparison of aversions induced by x-rays, toxins, and drugs in the rat. *Radiation Research Supplement*, 1967, **7**: 439–450.

GARCIA, J., & KOELLING, R. A. The use of ionizing rays as a mammalian olfactory stimulus. In L. Beidler (Ed.), *Handbook of sensory physiology* (*vol. 4*), *Chemical senses: Olfaction* (*Part I*). New York: Springer-Verlag, 1971.

GARCIA, J., KOVNER, R., & GREEN, K. F. Cue properties vs palatability of flavors in avoidance learning. *Psychonomic Science*, 1970, **20**: 313–314.

GARCIA, J., LASITER, P. S., BERMUDEZ-RATTONI, F., & DEEMS, D. A. A general theory of aversion learning. *Annals of The New York Academy of Sciences*, 1985, **443**: 8–21.

GARCIA, J., MCGOWAN, B. K., ERVIN, F. R., & KOELLING, R. A. Cues: Their relative effectiveness as a function of the reinforcer. *Science*, 1968, **160**: 794–795.

GARCIA, J., MCGOWAN, B. K., & GREEN, K. F. Biological constraints on conditioning. In A. Black and W. Prokasy (Eds.), *Classical conditioning II: Current research and theory.* New York: Appleton-Century-Crofts, 1972.

GARCIA, J., PALMERINO, C. C., RUSINIAK, K. W., & KIEFER, S. W. Taste aversions and the nature of instinct. In J. McGaugh and R. Thompson (Eds.), *The neurobiology of learning and memory.* New York: Plenum Press, 1985.

GARCIA, J., & RUSINIAK, K. W. Visceral feedback and the taste signal. *NATO Conference Series* (*III-Human Factors*) (*vol. 2*): *Biofeedback and behavior.* New York: Plenum Press, 1977.

GARCIA, J., & RUSINIAK, K. W. What the nose learns from the mouth. In D. Muller-Schwarze and R. Silverstein (Eds.), *Chemical signals.* New York: Plenum Press, 1980.

GARCIA, J., RUSINIAK, K. W., & BRETT, L. P. Conditioning food-illness aversion in wild animals: *Caveant canonici.* In H. Davis and H. Hurwitz (Eds.), *Operant-Pavlovian interactions.* New Jersey: Lawrence Erlbaum Associates, 1977.

GARCIA, J., RUSINIAK, K. W., KIEFER, S. W., & BERMUDEZ-RATTONI, F. The neural integration of feeding and drinking habits. In C. Woody (Ed.), *Conditioning.* New York: Plenum Press, 1982.

GARCIA, Y., ROBERTSON, R., & GARCIA, J. X-rays and learned taste aversions: Historical and psychological ramifications. In T. Burish, S. Levy and B. Meyerowitz (Eds.), *Cancer, nutrition and eating behavior: A biobehavioral perspective.* New Jersey: Lawrence Erlbaum Associates, in press.

GASTON, K. E. An illness-induced conditioned aversion in domestic chicks: One-trial learning with a long delay of reinforcement. *Behavioral Biology*, 1977, **20**: 441–453.

GASTON, K. E. Brain mechanisms of conditioned taste aversion learning: A review of the literature. *Physiological Psychology*, 1978, **6**: 340–353.

GASTON, K. E. Interocular transfer of a visually mediated conditioned food aversion in chicks. *Behavioral Biology*, 1978, **24**: 272–278.

GASTON, K. E. Evidence for separate and concurrent avoidance learning in the two hemispheres of the normal chick brain. *Behavioral and Neural Biology*, 1980, **28**: 129–137.

GAY, P. E., LEAF, R. C., & ARBLE, F. B. Inhibitory effects of pre- and posttest drugs on mouse-killing by rats. *Pharmacology, Biochemistry & Behavior*, 1975, **3**: 33–45.

GEARY, N., & SMITH, G. P. Pancreatic glucagon and postprandial satiety in the rat. *Physiology & Behavior*, 1982, **28**: 313–322.

GELPERIN, A. Rapid food-aversion learning by a terrestrial mollusk. *Science*, 1975, **189**: 567–570.

GELPERIN, A., CHANG, J. J., & REINGOLD, S. C. Feeding motor program in *Limax*. I. Neuromuscular correlates and control by chemosensory input. *Journal of Neurobiology*, 1978, **9**: 285–300.

GELPERIN, A., & FORSYTHE, D. Neuroethological studies of learning in mollusks. In J. Fentress (Ed.), *Simpler networks and behavior.* Massachusetts: Sinauer, 1976.

GEMBERLING, G. A., & DOMJAN, M. Selective associations in one-day-old rats: Taste-toxicosis and texture-shock aversion learning. *Journal of Comparative and Physiological Psychology*, 1982, **96**: 105–113.

GEMBERLING, G. A., DOMJAN, M., & AMSEL, A. Aversion learning in 5-day-old rats: Taste-toxicosis and texture-shock associations. *Journal of Comparative and Physiological Psychology*, 1980, **94**: 734–735.

GENOVESE, R. F., & BROWNE, M. P. Sickness-induced learning in chicks. *Behavioral Biology*, 1978, **24**: 68–76.

GIBBS, J., KULKOSKY, P. J., & SMITH, G. P. Effects of peripheral and central bombesin on feeding behavior of rats. *Peptides*, 1981, **2**: 179–183.

GIBBS, J., & SMITH, G. P. Response to Deutsch. *Nature*, 1977, **266**: 196.

GIBBS, J., & SMITH, G. P. Response to Deutsch. *Nature*, 1980, **285**: 592.

GIBBS, J., YOUNG, R. C., & SMITH, G. P. Cholecystokinin decreases food intake in rats. *Journal of Comparative and Physiological Psychology*, 1973, **84**: 488–495.

GILLAN, D. J. Learned suppression of ingestion: Role of discriminative stimuli, ingestive responses, and aversive tastes. *Journal of Experimental Psychology: Animal Behavior Processes*, 1979, **5**: 258–272.

GILLAN, D. J., & DOMJAN, M. Taste-aversion conditioning with expected versus unexpected drug treatment. *Journal of Experimental Psychology: Animal Behavior Processes*, 1977, **3**: 297–309.

GILLETTE, K., & BELLINGHAM, W. P. Loss of within-compound flavour associations: Configural preconditioning. *Experimental Animal Behaviour*, 1982, **1**: 1–17.

GILLETTE, K., BELLINGHAM, W. P., & MARTIN, G. M. Transfer of a taste aversion from food to water under various states of deprivation. *Animal Learning & Behavior*, 1979, **7**: 441–446.

GILLETTE, K., IRWIN, J. D., THOMAS, D. K., & BELLINGHAM, W. P. Transfer of coloured food and water aversions in domestic chicks. *Bird Behaviour*, 1980, **2**: 37–47.

GILLETTE, K., MARTIN, G. M., & BELLINGHAM, W. P. Differential use of food and water cues in the formation of conditioned aversions by domestic chicks (*Gallus gallus*). *Journal of Experimental Psychology: Animal Behavior Processes*, 1980, **6**: 99–111.

GILLETTE, K., THOMAS, D. K., & BELLINGHAM, W. P. A parametric study of flavoured food avoidance in chicks. *Chemical Senses*, 1983, **8**: 41–57.

GLEITMAN, H. Getting animals to understand the experimenter's instructions. *Animal Learning & Behavior*, 1974, **2**: 1–5.

GLOWA, J. R., & BARRETT, J. E. Response suppression by visual stimuli paired with postsession d-amphetamine injections in the pigeon. *Journal of the Experimental Analysis of Behavior*, 1983, **39**: 165–173.

GOETT, J. M., & KAY, E. J. Lithium chloride and delta-9-THC lead to conditioned aversions in the pigeon. *Psychopharmacology*, 1981, **72**: 215–216.

GOLD, R. M., & PROULX, D. M. Bait-shyness acquisition is impaired by VMH lesions that produce obesity. *Journal of Comparative and Physiological Psychology*, 1972, **79**: 201–209.

GOLUS, P., & MCGEE, R. Metrazol produces conditioned taste aversion in rats. *Psychopharmacology*, 1980, **68**: 257–259.

GOLUS, P., MCGEE, R., & KING, M. G. Melatonin and melanocyte-stimulating hormone (MSH) do not produce conditioned taste aversions. *IRCS Medical Science: Biochemistry; Dentistry and Oral Biology; Drug Metabolism and Toxicology; Nervous System; Pharmacology; Psychology and Psychiatry*, 1981, **9**: 437.

GORDON, D. Effects of forebrain ablation on taste aversion in goldfish (*Carassius auratus*). *Experimental Neurology*, 1979, **63**: 356–366.

GORMAN, J. E., DE OBALDIA, R. N., SCOTT, R. C., & REID, L. D. Morphine injections in the taste aversion paradigm: Extent of aversions and readiness to consume sweetened morphine solutions. *Physiological Psychology*, 1978, **6**: 101–109.

GOSNELL, B. A., MORLEY, J. E., & LEVINE, A. S. A comparison of the effects of corticotropin releasing factor and sauvagine on food intake. *Pharmacology, Biochemistry & Behavior*, 1983, **19**: 771–775.

GOUDIE, A. J. Temporal factors in hedonic responses to drugs of abuse. *Experimental Brain Research*, 1978, **32**: 54.

GOUDIE, A. J. Aversive stimulus properties of drugs. *Neuropharmacology*, 1979, **18**: 971–979.

GOUDIE, A. J. Aversive stimulus properties of cocaine following inhibition of hepatic enzymes. *IRCS Medical Sciences: Biochemistry; Metabolism and Toxicology; Pharmacology; Psychology and Psychiatry*, 1980, **8**: 58–59.

GOUDIE, A. J. Conditioned food aversion: An adaptive specialisation of learning? *IRCS Journal of Medical Science*, 1980, **8**: 591–594.

GOUDIE, A. J. Stimulus properties of cocaine/chlordiazepoxide mixtures in rodents. *IRCS Medical*

Sciences: Biochemistry; Drug Metabolism and Toxicology; Nervous System; Pharmacology; Psychology and Psychiatry, 1981, **9**: 663–664.

GOUDIE, A. J. Aversive stimulus properties of drugs: The conditioned taste aversion paradigm. In A. Greenshaw and C. Dourish (Eds.), *Experimental approach in psychopharmacology.* New Jersey: Humana Press, in press.

GOUDIE, A. J., & DEMELLWEEK, C. Naloxone fails to block amphetamine-induced anorexia and conditioned taste aversion. *Journal of Pharmacy and Pharmacology*, 1980, **32**: 653–656.

GOUDIE, A. J., & DICKINS, D. W. Aversive properties of drugs of abuse in rats and their possible relationship to drug abuse in humans. In J. Madden, R. Walker and W. Kenyon (Eds.), *Aspects of alcohol and drug dependence.* London: Pittman Medical, 1980.

GOUDIE, A. J., & DICKINS, D. W. Nitrous oxide-induced conditioned taste aversions in rats: The role of duration of drug exposure and its relation to the taste aversion-self-administration "paradox." *Pharmacology, Biochemistry & Behavior*, 1978, **9**: 587–592.

GOUDIE, A. J., DICKINS, D. W., & THORNTON, E. W. Cocaine-induced conditioned taste aversions in rats. *Pharmacology, Biochemistry & Behavior*, 1978, **8**: 757–761.

GOUDIE, A. J., STOLERMAN, I. P., DEMELLWEEK, C., & D'MELLO, G. D. Does conditioned nausea mediate drug-induced conditioned taste aversion? *Psychopharmacology*, 1982, **78**: 277–281.

GOUDIE, A. J., TAYLOR, M., & ATHERTON, H. Effects of prior drug experience on the establishment of taste aversions in rats. *Pharmacology, Biochemistry & Behavior*, 1975, **3**: 947–952.

GOUDIE, A. J., & THORNTON, E. W. Effects of drug experience on drug induced conditioned taste aversions: Studies with amphetamine and fenfluramine. *Psychopharmacologia*, 1975. **44**: 77–82.

GOUDIE, A. J., & THORNTON, E. W. Role of drug metabolism in the aversive properties of d-amphetamine. *IRCS Medical Sciences: Dentistry and Oral Biology; Drug Metabolism and Toxicology; Nervous System; Pharmacology; Psychology and Psychiatry*, 1977, **5**: 93.

GOUDIE, A. J., THORNTON, E. W., & WHEATLEY, J. Effects of p-chlorophenylalanine on drinking suppressed by punishment. *IRCS Medical Sciences: Neurobiology and Neurophysiology; Pharmacology; Psychology*, 1975, **3**: 265.

GOUDIE, A. J., THORNTON, E. W., & WHEATLEY, J. Attenuation by alpha-methyltyrosine of amphetamine induced conditioned taste aversion in rats. *Psychopharmacologia*, 1975, **45**: 119–123.

GOUDIE, A. J., THORNTON, E. W., & WHEELER, T. J. Drug pretreatment effects in drug induced taste aversions: Effects of dose and duration of pretreatment. *Pharmacology, Biochemistry & Behavior*, 1976, **4**: 629–633.

GREEN, K. F. Aversions to grape juice induced by apomorphine. *Psychonomic Science*, 1969, **17**: 168–169.

GREEN, K. F., & CHURCHILL, P. A. An effect of flavors on strength of conditioned aversions. *Psychonomic Science*, 1970, **21**: 19–20.

GREEN, K. F., & GARCIA, J. Recuperation from illness: Flavor enhancement for rats. *Science*, 1971, **173**: 749–751.

GREEN, K. F., HART, G. L., & HAGEN, H. S. Toxic heat as a UCS in conditioning in internal and external milieus in rats. *Physiology & Behavior*, 1981, **27**: 77–82.

GREEN, K. E., HOLMSTROM, L. S., & WOLLMAN, M. A. Relation of cue to consequence in rats: Effect of recuperation from illness. *Behavioral Biology*, 1974, **10**: 491–503.

GREEN, L., BOUZAS, A., & RACHLIN, H. Test of an electric-shock analog to illness-induced aversion. *Behavioral Biology*, 1972, **7**: 513–518.

GREEN, L., & RACHLIN, H. The effect of rotation on the learning of taste aversions. *Bulletin of the Psychonomic Society*, 1973, **1**: 137–138.

GREEN, L., & RACHLIN, H. Learned taste aversions in rats as a function of delay, speed, and duration of rotation. *Learning and Motivation*, 1976, **7**: 283–289.

GREENSHAW, A. J., & BURESOVA, O. Learned taste aversion to saccharin following intraventricular or intraperitoneal administration of d,l-amphetamine. *Pharmacology, Biochemistry & Behavior*, 1982, **17**: 1129–1133.

GREENSHAW, A. J., & DOURISH, C. T. β-phenylethylamine and d-amphetamine: Differential potency in the conditioned taste aversion paradigm. In A. Boulton, G. Baker, W. Dewhurst and A. Sandler (Eds.), *Neurobiology of the trace amines.* New Jersey: Humana Press, in press.

GREENSHAW, A. J., & DOURISH, C. T. Differential aversive stimulus properties of beta-phenylethylamine, and d-amphetamine. *Psychopharmacology*, 1984, **82**: 189–193.

GREGG, B., KITTREL, E. M. W., DOMJAN, M., & AMSEL, A. Ingestional aversion learning in preweanling rats. *Journal of Comparative and Physiological Psychology*, 1978, **92**: 785–795.

GRILL, H. J. Discussion of physiological mechanisms in conditioned taste aversions. *Annals of The New York Academy of Sciences*, 1985, **443**: 67–88.

GRILL, H. J., & NORGREN, R. The taste reactivity test. I. Mimetic responses to gustatory stimuli in neurologically normal rats. *Brain Research*, 1978, **143**: 263–279.

GRILL, H. J., & NORGREN, R. The taste reactivity test. II. Mimetic responses to gustatory stimuli in chronic thalamic and chronic decerebrate rats. *Brain Research*, 1978, **143**: 281–297.

GRILL, H. J., & NORGREN, R. Chronically decerebrate rats demonstrate satiation but not bait shyness. *Science*, 1978, **201**: 267–269.

GROTE, F. W., JR., & BROWN, R. T. Conditioned taste aversions: Two-stimulus tests are more sensitive than one-stimulus tests. *Behavior Research Methods and Instrumentation*, 1971, **3**: 311–312.

GROTE, F. W., JR., & BROWN, R. T. Rapid learning of passive avoidance by weanling rats: Conditioned taste aversion. *Psychonomic Science*, 1971, **25**: 163–164.

GROTE, F. W., JR., & BROWN, R. T. Deprivation level affects extinction of a conditioned taste aversion. *Learning and Motivation*, 1973, **4**: 314–319.

GRUNBERG, N. E. Specific taste preferences: An alternative explanation for eating changes in cancer patients. In T. Burish, S. Levy, and B. Meyerowitz (Eds.), *Cancer, nutrition and eating behavior: A biobehavioral perspective*. Hillsdale, New Jersey: Lawrence Erlbaum Associates, in press.

GRUPP, L. A. Effects of pimozide on the acquisition, maintenance and extinction of an amphetamine-induced taste aversion. *Psychopharmacologia*, 1977, **53**: 235–242.

GRUPP, L. A., LINESMAN, M. A., & CAPPELL, H. Effects of amygdala lesions on taste aversions produced by amphetamine and LiCl. *Pharmacology, Biochemistry & Behavior*, 1976, **4**: 541–544.

GUANOWSKY, V., MISANIN, J. R., & RICCIO, D. C. Retention of conditioned taste aversion in weanling, adult, and old-age rats. *Behavioral and Neural Biology*, 1983, **37**: 173–178.

GUBERNICK, L. T., & ALBERTS, J. R. A specialization of taste aversion learning during suckling and its weaning-associated transformation. *Developmental Psychobiology*, 1984, **17**: 613–628.

GUSTAVSON, C. R. Taste aversion conditioning of predators. *The Chronicle of the Horse*, 1975, **38**: 12–13.

GUSTAVSON, C. R. Comparative and field aspects of learned food aversions. In L. Barker, M. Best and M. Domjan (Eds.), *Learning mechanisms in food selection*. Waco, Texas: Baylor University Press, 1977.

GUSTAVSON, C. R. An evaluation of taste aversion control of wolf (*Canis lupus*) predation in Northern Minnesota. *Applied Animal Ethology*, 1982, **9**: 63–71.

GUSTAVSON, C. R., BRETT, L. P., GARCIA, J., & KELLY, D. J. A working model and experimental solutions to the control of predatory behavior. In H. Markowitz and V. Stevens (Eds.), *Studies of captive wild animals*. Chicago: Nelson Hall, 1976.

GUSTAVSON, C. R., & GARCIA, J. Aversive conditioning: Pulling a gag on the wily coyote. *Psychology Today*, 1974, **8**: 69–72.

GUSTAVSON, C. R., GARCIA, J., HANKINS, W. G., & RUSINIAK, K. W. Coyote predation control by aversive conditioning. *Science*, 1974, **184**: 581–583.

GUSTAVSON, C. R., & GUSTAVSON, J. C. Spiked lamb dulls coyote appetite. *Defenders of Wildlife International*, 1974, **49**: 293–294.

GUSTAVSON, C. R., & GUSTAVSON, J. C. Food avoidance in rats: The differential effects of shock, illness and repellents. *Appetite: Journal for Intake Research*, 1982, **3**: 335–340.

GUSTAVSON, C. R., & GUSTAVSON, J. C. Control of predation using conditioned food aversion methodology: Theory, practice and implications. *Annals of The New York Academy of Sciences*, 1985, **443**: 348–356.

GUSTAVSON, C. R., GUSTAVSON, J. C., & HOLZER, G. A. Thiabandazole-based taste aversions in dingoes (*Canis familiaris dingo*) and New Guinea wild dogs (*Canis familiaris hallstromi*). *Applied Animal Ethology*, 1983, **10**: 385–388.

GUSTAVSON, C. R., HOLZER, G. A., GUSTAVSON, J. C., & VAKOCH, D. L. An evaluation of phenol methylcarbamates as taste aversion producing agents in caged blackbirds. *Applied Animal Ethology,* 1982, **8**: 551–559.

GUSTAVSON, C. R., JOWSEY, J. R., & MILLIGAN, D. N. A 3-year evaluation of taste aversion coyote control in Saskatchewan. *Journal of Range Management,* 1982, **35**: 57–59.

GUSTAVSON, C. R., KELLY, D. J., SWEENEY, M., & GARCIA, J. Prey-lithium aversions. I. Coyotes and wolves. *Behavioral Biology,* 1976, **17**: 61–72.

HALE, C., & GREEN, L. Effect of initial-pecking consequences on subsequent pecking in young chicks. *Journal of Comparative and Physiological Psychology,* 1979, **93**: 730–735.

HALPERN, B. P., & MAROWITZ, L. A. Taste responses to lick-duration stimuli. *Brain Research,* 1973, **57**: 473–478.

HALPERN, B. P., & TAPPER, D. N. Taste stimuli: Quality coding time. *Science,* 1971, **171**: 1256–1258.

HAMBURGER, J. N., & KUTSCHER, C. L. LiCl-induced selective depression of saccharin drinking in the mouse. *Pharmacology, Biochemistry & Behavior,* 1979, **10**: 651–655.

HAMILTON, L. W., & CAPOBIANCO, S. Consumption of sodium chloride and lithium chloride in normal rats and in rats with septal lesions. *Physiological Psychology,* 1973, **1**: 213–218.

HANKINS, W. G., GARCIA, J., & RUSINIAK, K. W. Dissociation of odor and taste in baitshyness. *Behavioral Biology,* 1973, **8**: 407–419.

HANKINS, W. G., GARCIA, J., & RUSINIAK, K. W. Cortical lesions: Flavor illness and noise-shock conditioning. *Behavioral Biology,* 1974, **10**: 173–181.

HANKINS, W. G., RUSINIAK, K. W., & GARCIA, J. Dissociation of odor and taste in shock-avoidance learning. *Behavioral Biology,* 1976, **18**: 345–358.

HARDY, W. T., & DEUTSCH, J. A. Preference for ethanol in dependent rats. *Behavioral Biology,* 1977, **20**: 482–492.

HARGRAVE, G. E., & BOLLES, R. C. Rat's aversion to flavors following induced illness. *Psychonomic Science,* 1971, **23**: 91–92.

HARLOW, H. F. Effects of radiation on the central nervous system and on behavior: General survey. In T. Haley and R. Snider (Eds.), *Response of the nervous system to ionizing radiation.* New York: Academic Press, 1962.

HARRIMAN, A. E., & KARE, M. R. Preference for sodium chloride over lithium chloride by adrenalectomized rats. *American Journal of Physiology,* 1964, **207**: 941–943.

HARRIMAN, A. E., NANCE, D. M., & MILNER, J. S. Discrimination between equimolar NaCl and LiCl solutions by anosmic, adrenalectomized rats. *Physiology & Behavior,* 1968, **3**: 887–889.

HAROUTUNIAN, V., & RICCIO, D. C. Acquisition of rotation-induced taste aversion as a function of drinking-treatment delay. *Physiological Psychology,* 1975, **3**: 273–277.

HAROUTUNIAN, V., RICCIO, D. C., & GANS, D. P. Suppression of drinking following rotational stimulation as an index of motion sickness in the rat. *Physiological Psychology,* 1976, **4**: 467–472.

HASEGAWA, Y. Recuperation for lithium-induced illness: Flavor enhancement for rats. *Behavioral and Neural Biology,* 1981, **33**: 252–255.

HASEGAWA, Y., & MATSUZAWA, T. Food-aversion conditioning in Japanese monkeys (*Macaca fuscala*): A dissociation of feeding in two separate situations. *Behavioral and Neural Biology,* 1981, **33**: 237–242.

HENNESSY, J. W., & LEVINE, S. STRESS, arousal and the pituitary-adrenal system: A psychoendocrine hypothesis. In J. Sprague and A. Epstein (Eds.), *Progress in psychobiology and physiological psychology, vol. 8.* New York: Academic Press, 1979.

HENNESSY, J. W., SMOTHERMAN, W. P., & LEVINE, S. Conditioned taste aversion and the pituitary-adrenal system. *Behavioral Biology,* 1976, **16**: 413–424.

HENNESSY, J. W., SMOTHERMAN, W. P., & LEVINE, S. Investigations into the nature of the dexamethasone and ACTH effects upon learned taste aversion. *Physiology & Behavior,* 1980, **24**: 645–649.

HOBBS, S. H., CLINGERMAN, H., & ELKINS, R. L. Illness-induced taste aversions in normal and bulbectomized hamsters. *Physiology & Behavior,* 1976, **17**: 235–238.

HOBBS, S. H., & ELKINS, R. L. Baitshyness retention in rats with olfactory-bulb ablations. *Physiological Psychology,* 1976, **4**: 391–394.

HOBBS, S. H., ELKINS, R. L., & PEACOCK, L. J. Taste-aversion conditioning in rats with septal lesions. *Behavioral Biology*, 1974, **11**: 239–245.

HOLLAND, P. C. Acquisition of representation-mediated conditioned food aversions. *Learning and Motivation*, 1981, **12**: 1–18.

HOLLAND, P. C. Representation-mediated overshadowing and potentiation of conditioned aversions. *Journal of Experimental Psychology: Animal Behavior Processes*, 1983, **9**: 1–13.

HOLLAND, P. C., & FORBES, D. T. Effects of compound or element preexposure on compound flavor aversion conditioning. *Animal Learning & Behavior*, 1980, **8**: 199–203.

HOLLAND, P. C., & FORBES, D. T. Representation-mediated extinction of conditioned flavor aversions. *Learning and Motivation*, 1982, **13**: 454–471.

HOLLAND, P. C., & RESCORLA, R. A. The effect of two ways of devaluing the unconditioned stimulus after first- and second-order appetitive conditioning. *Journal of Experimental Psychology: Animal Behavior Processes*, 1975, **1**: 355–363.

HOLLAND, P. C., & STRAUB, J. J. Differential effects of two ways of devaluing the unconditioned stimulus after Pavlovian appetitive conditioning. *Journal of Experimental Psychology: Animal Behavior Processes*, 1979, **5**: 65–78.

HOLMAN, E. W. Some conditions for the dissociation of consummatory and instrumental behavior in rats. *Learning and Motivation*, 1975, **6**: 358–366.

HOLMAN, E. W. The effect of drug habituation before and after taste aversion learning in rats. *Animal Learning & Behavior*, 1976, **4**: 329–332.

HOLT, J., ANTIN, J., GIBBS, J., YOUNG, R. C., & SMITH, G. P. Cholecystokinin does not produce bait shyness in rats. *Physiology & Behavior*, 1974, **12**: 497–498.

HOLZER, G. A. & GUSTAVSON, C. R. Manipulation of wheat and oat preference in black-tailed prairie dogs: A field demonstration using methiocarb as a taste aversion agent. *Prairie Naturalist*, 1980, **12**: 114–118.

HORN, S. W., & LEHNER, P. N. Conditioned avoidance in coyotes: Effects of administering LiCl during selected phases of the predatory sequence. *Bulletin of the Psychonomic Society*, 1981, **7**: 209–212.

HOROWITZ, G. P., & WHITNEY, G. Alcohol-induced conditioned aversion: Genotypic specificity in mice (*Mus musculus*). *Journal of Comparative and Physiological Psychology*, 1975, **89**: 340–346.

HOUPT, K. A., ZAHORIK, D. M., ANIKA, S. M., & HOUPT, T. R. Taste aversion learning in suckling and weanling pigs. *Veterinary Science Communications*, 1979, **3**: 165–169.

HOUPT, T. R., ANIKA, S. M., & WOLFF, N. C. Satiety effects of cholecystokinin and caerulein in rabbits. *American Journal of Physiology*, 1978, **235**: R23–R28.

HOWARD, W. E., MARSH, R. E., & COLE, R. E. Duration of associative memory to toxic bait in deer mice. *Journal of Wildlife Management*, 1977, **41**: 484–486.

HOWARD, W. E., PALMATEER, S. D., & NACHMAN, M. Aversion to strychnine sulfate by Norway rats, roof rats, and pocket gophers. *Toxicology and Applied Pharmacology*, 1968, **12**: 229–241.

HULSE, E., & DEMPSEY, B. Radiation conditioning: A specific aversion to feeding after a single exposure to 50 R. *International Journal of Radiation Biology*, 1964, **8**: 97–99.

HUNT, E. L., CARROLL, H. W., & KIMELDORF, D. J. Humoral mediation of radiation-induced motivation in parabiont rats. *Science*, 1965, **150**: 1747–1748.

HUNT, E. L., CARROLL, H. W., & KIMELDORF, D. J. Effects of dose and of partial-body exposure on conditioning through a radiation-induced humoral factor. *Physiology & Behavior*, 1968, **3**: 809–813.

HUNT, E. L., & KIMELDORF, D. J. The humoral factor in radiation-induced motivation. *Radiation Research*, 1967, **30**: 404–419.

HUNT, T., AMIT, Z., SWITZMAN, L., & SINYOR, D. An aversive naloxone-morphine interaction in rats. *Neuroscience Letters*, 1983, **35**: 311–315.

HUTCHISON, S. L., JR. Taste aversion in albino rats using centrifugal spin as an unconditioned stimulus. *Psychological Reports*, 1973, **33**: 467–470.

HYSON, R. L., SICKEL, J. L., KULKOSKY, P. J., & RILEY, A. L. The insensitivity of schedule-induced polydipsia to conditioned taste aversions: Effect of amount consumed during conditioning. *Animal Learning & Behavior*, 1981, **9**: 281–286.

IDA, M. Acquisition and extinction in long-delay taste aversion learning. *Journal of Child Development*, 1980, **16**: 44–50.

INFURNA, R. N. Daily biorhythmicity influences homing behavior, psychopharmacological responsiveness, learning, and retention of suckling rats. *Journal of Comparative and Physiological Psychology*, 1981, **95**: 896–914.

INFURNA, R. N., & SPEAR, L. P. Developmental changes in amphetamine-induced taste aversions. *Pharmacology, Biochemistry & Behavior*, 1979, **11**: 31–35.

INFURNA, R. N., STEINERT, P. A., FREDA, J. S., & SPEAR, N. E. Sucrose preference and LiCl illness-induced aversion as a function of drug dose and phase of the illumination cycle. *Physiology & Behavior*, 1979, **22**: 955–961.

INFURNA, R. N., STEINERT, P. A., & SPEAR, N. E. Ontogenetic changes in the modulation of taste aversion learning by home environmental cues in rats. *Journal of Comparative and Physiological Psychology*, 1979, **93**: 1097–1108.

INGRAM, D. K. Conditioned taste aversion in genetically obese (OB/OB) mice. *Behaviour Analysis Letters*, 1981, **1**: 199–206.

INGRAM, D. K. Lithium chloride-induced taste aversion in C57BL:6J and DBA:2J mice. *Journal of General Psychology*, 1982, **106**: 233–249.

INGRAM, D. K., & CORFMAN, T. P. Strain-dependent sexual dimorphism in the extinction of conditioned taste aversion in mice. *Animal Learning & Behavior*, 1981, **9**: 101–107.

INGRAM, D. K., & PEACOCK, L. J. Conditioned taste aversion as a function of age in mature male rats. *Experimental Aging Research*, 1980, **6**: 113–123.

IONESCU, E., & BURES, J. Ontogenetic development of conditioned food aversion in chickens. *Behavioural Processes*, 1976, **1**: 233–241.

IONESCU, E., & BURESOVA, O. Failure to elicit conditioned taste aversion by severe poisoning. *Pharmacology, Biochemistry & Behavior*, 1977, **6**: 251–254.

IONESCU, E., & BURESOVA, O. The significance of amygdala for learning and retrieval of the conditioned taste aversion. *Studia Psychologica*, 1977, **19**: 210–211.

IONESCU, E., & BURESOVA, O. Effects of hypothermia on the acquisition of conditioned taste aversion in rats. *Journal of Comparative and Physiological Psychology*, 1977, **91**: 1297–1307.

IONESCU, E., BURESOVA, O., & BURES, J. The significance of gustatory and visual cues for conditioned food aversion in rats and chickens. *Physiologia Bohemoslovaca*, 1975, **24**: 58.

ISLAM, S. Eliciting conditioned taste aversion by cobra venom neurotoxin in rats. *Indian Journal of Physiology and Pharmacology*, 1978, **22**: 368–371.

ISLAM, S. Severe conditioned taste aversion elicited by venom of Russell's viper. *Experientia*, 1979, **35**: 1206–1207.

ISLAM, S. Conditioned taste aversion elicited in anesthetized rats of scorpion venom. *Physiologia Bohemoslovaca*, 1980, **29**: 361–366.

ISLAM, S. Snake neurotoxins and conditioned taste aversion in mice. *International Journal of Neuroscience*, 1980, **11**: 41–43.

ISLAM, S., BURESOVA, O., & BURES, J. Antihistamines fail to prevent acquisition of conditioned taste aversion induced by viper venom. *Biology of Behavior*, 1982, **7**: 101–108.

JACKSON, T. R., & SMITH, J. W. A comparison of two aversion treatment methods for alcoholism. *Journal of Studies on Alcohol*, 1978, **39**: 187–191.

JACOBS, W. J., ZELLNER, D. A., LOLORDO, V. M., & RILEY, A. L. The effect of post-conditioning exposure to morphine on the retention of a morphine-induced conditioned taste aversion. *Pharmacology, Biochemistry & Behavior*, 1981, **14**: 779–785.

JACOBS, W. W., & LABOWS, J. N. Conditioned aversion, bitter taste and the avoidance of natural toxicants in wild guinea pigs. *Physiology & Behavior*, 1979, **22**: 173–178.

JACQUET, Y. F. Conditioned aversion during morphine maintenance in mice and rats. *Physiology & Behavior*, 1973, **11**: 527–541.

JAKINOVICH, W., JR. Stimulation of the gerbil's gustatory receptors by artificial sweeteners. *Brain Research*, 1981, **210**: 69–81.

JAKINOVICH, W., JR. Taste aversion to sugars by the gerbil. *Physiology & Behavior*, 1982, **28**: 1065–1072.

JANCSAR, S. M., & LEONARD, B. E. The effects of antidepressant drugs on conditioned taste aversion learning of the olfactory bulbectomized rat. *Neuropharmacology*, 1981, **20**: 1341–1345.

JANDA, L. H., & RIMM, C. D. Covert sensitization in the treatment of obesity. *Journal of Abnormal Psychology*, 1972, **80**: 37–42.

JESSUP, B. The role of diet in migraine: Conditioned taste aversion. *Headache*, 1978, **18**: 229.

JOHNSON, C., BEATON, R., & HALL, K. Poison-based avoidance learning in nonhuman primates: Use of visual cues. *Physiology & Behavior*, 1975, **14**: 403–407.

JOHNSTON, R. E., & ZAHORIK, D. M. Taste aversions to sexual attractants. *Science*, 1975, **189**: 893–894.

JOHNSTON, R. E., ZAHORIK, D. M., IMMLER, K., & ZAKON, H. Alterations of male sexual behavior by learned aversions to hamster vaginal secretion. *Journal of Comparative and Physiological Psychology*, 1978, **92**: 85–93.

JOLICOEUR, F. B., RONDEAU, D. B., WAYNER, M. J., MINTZ, R. B., & MERKEL, A. D. Barbiturates and alcohol consumption. *Biobehavioral Reviews*, 1977, **1**: 177–196.

JOLICOEUR, F. B., WAYNER, M. J., MERKEL, A. D., RONDEAU, D. B., & MINTZ, R. B. The effects of various barbiturates on LiCl induced taste aversion. *Pharmacology, Biochemistry & Behavior*, 1980, **12**: 613–617.

JOLICOEUR, F. B., WAYNER, M. J., RONDEAU, D. B., & MERKEL, A. D. The effects of phenobarbitol on lithium chloride induced taste aversion. *Pharmacology, Biochemistry & Behavior*, 1978, **9**: 845–847.

JOLICOEUR, F. B., WAYNER, M. J., RONDEAU, D. B., MERKEL, A. D., & BASSANO, D. A. Effects of phenobarbitol on taste aversion induced by x-radiation. *Pharmacology, Biochemistry & Behavior*, 1979, **11**: 709–712.

JONES, L. Taste aversion conditioning and 'T' maze behaviour. *Australian Journal of Psychology*, 1980, **32**: 95–110.

JONES, L., & BELLINGHAM, W. P. Taste aversion conditioning and barpressing: A quality-quantity interaction. *Australian Journal of Psychology*, 1981, **33**: 61–71.

JONES, L., & BELLINGHAM, W. P. Effect of taste aversion conditioning on barpressing: Incentive or response interference. *Australian Journal of Psychology*, 1981, **33**: 247–252.

JONES, L., BELLINGHAM, W. P., & MARTIN. G. M. Avoidance of toxins by the Galah *Cacatua roseicapilla*. *The Emu*, 1978, **78**: 231–233.

KALAT, J. W. Taste-aversion learning in dead rats. *The Worm Runner's Digest*, 1973, **15**: 59–60.

KALAT, J. W. Taste salience depends on novelty, not concentration, in taste-aversion learning in the rat. *Journal of Comparative and Physiological Psychology*, 1974, **86**: 47–50.

KALAT, J. W. Taste-aversion learning in infant guinea pigs. *Developmental Psychobiology*, 1975, **8**: 383–387.

KALAT, J. W. Should taste-aversion learning experiments control duration or volume of drinking on the training day? *Animal Learning & Behavior*, 1976, **4**: 96–98.

KALAT, J. W. Status of "learned safety" or "learned non-correlation" as a mechanism in taste-aversion learning. In L. Barker, M. Best and M. Domjan (Eds.), *Learning mechanisms in food selection*. Waco, Texas: Baylor University Press, 1977.

KALAT, J. W. Biological significance of food aversion learning. In N. Milgram, L. Krames and T. Alloway (Eds.), *Food aversion learning*. New York: Plenum Press, 1977.

KALAT, J. W., & ROZIN, P. "Salience:" A factor which can override temporal contiquity in taste-aversion learning. *Journal of Comparative and Physiological Psychology*, 1970, **71**: 192–197.

KALAT, J. W., & ROZIN, P. Role of interference in taste-aversion learning. *Journal of Comparative and Physiological Psychology*, 1971, **77**: 53–58.

KALAT, J. W., & ROZIN, P. You can lead a rat to poison but you can't make him think. In M. Seligman and J. Hager (Eds.), *Biological boundaries of learning*. New York: Appleton-Century-Crofts, 1972.

KALAT, J. W., & ROZIN, P. "Learned safety" as a mechanism in long-delay taste-aversion learning in rats. *Journal of Comparative and Physiological Psychology*, 1973, **83**: 198–207.

KALLMAN, M. J., LYNCH, M. R., & LANDAUER, M. R. Taste aversions to several halogenated hydrocarbons. *Neurobehavioral Toxicology and Teratology*, 1983, **5**: 23–28.

KANAREK, R. B., ADAMS, K. S., & MAYER, J. Conditioned taste aversion in the Mongolian gerbil (*Meriones unquiculatus*). *Bulletin of the Psychonomic Society*, 1975, **6**: 303–305.

KATZ, E. R. Conditioned aversion to chemotherapy. *Psychosomatics*, 1982, **23**: 650–651.

KAY, E. J. Aversive effects of repeated injections of THC in rats. *Psychological Reports*, 1975, **37**: 1051–1054.

KEMBLE, E. D., & NAGEL, J. A. Failure to form a learned taste aversion in rats with amygdaloid lesions. *Bulletin of the Psychonomic Society*, 1973, **2**: 155–156.

KEMBLE, E. D., STUDELSKA, D. R., & SCHMIDT, M. K. Effects of central amygdaloid nucleus lesions on ingestion, taste reactivity, exploration and taste aversion. *Physiology & Behavior*, 1979, **22**: 789–793.

KENDLER, K., HENNESSY, J. W., SMOTHERMAN, W. P., & LEVINE, S. An ACTH effect on recovery from conditioned taste aversion. *Behavioral Biology*, 1976, **17**: 225–229.

KENNEY, N. J., MOE, K. E., & SKOOG, K. M. The antidipsogenic action of peripheral prostaglandin E2. *Pharmacology, Biochemistry & Behavior*, 1981, **15**: 263–269.

KESNER, R. P., & BERMAN, R. F. Effects of midbrain reticular formation, hippocampal, and lateral hypothalmic stimulation upon recovery from neophobia and taste aversion learning. *Physiology & Behavior*, 1977, **18**: 763–768.

KESNER, R. P., BERMAN, R. F., BURTON, B., & HANKINS. W. G. Effects of electrical stimulation of amygdala upon neophobia and taste aversion. *Behavioral Biology*, 1975, **13**: 349–358.

KESNER, R. P., HARDY, J. D., & CALDER, L. D. Phencyclidine and behavior: I. Sensory-motor function, activity level, taste aversion and water intake. *Pharmacology, Biochemistry & Behavior*, 1981, **15**: 7–13.

KEYMER, A., CROMPTON, D. W., & SAHAKIAN, B. J. Parasite-induced learned taste aversion involving nippostrongylus in rats. *Parasitology*, 1983, **86**: 455–460.

KIEFER, S. W. Two-bottle discrimination of equimolar NaCl and LiCl solutions by rats. *Physiological Psychology*, 1978, **6**: 191–198.

KIEFER, S. W. Neural mediation of conditioned food aversions. *Annals of The New York Academy of Sciences*, 1985, **443**: 100–109.

KIEFER, S. W., & BRAUN, J. J. Absence of differential associative responses to novel and familiar taste stimuli in rats lacking gustatory neocortex. *Journal of Comparative and Physiological Psychology*, 1977, **91**: 498–507.

KIEFER, S. W., & BRAUN, J. J. Acquisition of taste avoidance habits in rats lacking gustatory neocortex. *Physiological Psychology*, 1979, **7**: 245–250.

KIEFER, S. W., CABRAL, R. J., RUSINIAK, K. W., & GARCIA, J. Ethanol-induced flavor aversions in rats with subdiaphragmatic vagotomies. *Behavioral and Neural Biology*, 1980, **29**: 246–254.

KIEFER, S. W., LEACH, L. R., & BRAUN, J. J. Taste agnosia following gustatory neocortex ablation: Dissociation from odor and generality across taste qualities. *Behavioral Neuroscience*, 1984, **98**: 590–608.

KIEFER, S. W., PHILLIPS, J. A., & BRAUN, J. J. Preexposure to conditioned and unconditioned stimuli in taste-aversion learning. *Bulletin of the Psychonomic Society*, 1977, **10**: 226–228.

KIEFER, S. W., RUSINIAK, K. W., & GARCIA, J. Flavor-illness aversions: Gustatory neocortex ablations disrupt taste but not taste-potentiated odor cues. *Journal of Comparative and Physiological Psychology*, 1982, **96**: 540–548.

KIEFER, S. W., RUSINIAK, K. W., GARCIA, J., & COIL, J. D. Vagotomy facilitates extinction of conditioned taste aversions in rats. *Journal of Comparative and Physiological Psychology*, 1981, **95**: 114–122.

KIMBLE, D. P., BREMILLER, R., SCHROEDER, L., & SMOTHERMAN, W. P. Hippocampal lesions slow extinction of a conditioned taste aversion in rats. *Physiology & Behavior*, 1979, **23**: 217–222.

KIMELDORF, D. J. Radiation-conditioned behavior. In T. Haley and R. Snider (Eds.), *Response of the nervous system to ionizing radiation*. New York: Academic Press, 1962.

KIMELDORF, D. J., GARCIA, J., & RUBADEAU, D. O. Radiation-induced conditioned avoidance behavior in rats, mice, and cats. *Radiation Research*, 1960, **12**: 710–718.

KIMELDORF, D. J., & HUNT, E. L. Conditioned behavior and the radiation stimulus. In T. Haley and R. Snider (Eds.), *Response of the nervous system to ionizing radiation.* Boston: Little Brown, 1964.

KING, J. M., & COX, V. C. Effects of ergocornine and CI-628 on food intake and taste preferences. *Physiology & Behavior*, 1976, **16**: 111–113.

KLEIN, S. B., BARTER, M. J., MURPHY, A. L., & RICHARDSON, J. H. Aversion to low doses of mercuric chloride in rats. *Physiological Psychology*, 1974, **2**: 397–400.

KLEIN, S. B., DOMATO, G. C., HALLSTEAD, C., STEPHENS, I., & MIKULKA, P. J. Acquisition of a conditioned aversion as a function of age and measurement technique. *Physiological Psychology*, 1975, **3**: 379–384.

KLEIN, S. B., MIKULKA, P. J., DOMATO, G. C., & HALLSTEAD, C. Retention of internal experiences in juvenile and adult rats. *Physiological Psychology*, 1976, **5**: 63–66.

KLEIN, S. B., MIKULKA, P. J., & HAMEL, K. Influence of sucrose preexposure on acquisition of a conditioned aversion. *Behavioral Biology*, 1976, **16**: 99–104.

KLEIN, S. B., MIKULKA, P. J., ROCHELLE, F. P., & BLAIR, V. Postconditioning CS-alone exposure as a source of interference in a taste aversion paradigm. *Physiological Psychology*, 1978, **6**: 255–260.

KLING, J. W. Demonstration experiments in learned taste aversions. *Teaching of Psychology*, 1981, **8**: 166–169.

KLUNDER, C. S., & O'BOYLE, M. Suppression of predatory behaviors in laboratory mice following lithium chloride injections or electric shock. *Animal Learning & Behavior*, 1979, **7**: 13–16.

KOLB, B., NONNEMAN, A. J., & ABPLANALP, P. Studies on the neural mechanisms of baitshyness in rats. *Bulletin of the Psychonomic Society*, 1977, **10**: 389–392.

KOOPMANS, H. S. Peptides as satiety agents: The behavioural evaluation of their effects on food intake. In S. Bloom and J. Polak (Eds.), *Gut hormones*. New York: Churchill Livingstone, 1981.

KOOPMANS, H. S. A stomach hormone that inhibits food intake. *Journal of the Autonomic Nervous System*, 1983, **9**: 157–171.

KOOPMANS, H. S., & MAGGIO, C. A. The effects of specified chemical meals on food intake. *American Journal of Clinical Nutrition*, 1978, **31**: 267–272.

KRAL, P. A. Interpolation of electroconvulsive shock during CS-US interval as an impediment to the conditioning of taste aversion. *Psychonomic Science*, 1970, **19**: 36–37.

KRAL, P. A. Electroconvulsive shock during taste-illness interval: Evidence for induced dissociation. *Physiology & Behavior*, 1971, **7**: 667–670.

KRAL, P. A. ECS between tasting and illness: Effects of current parameters on a taste aversion. *Physiology & Behavior*, 1971, **7**: 779–782.

KRAL, P. A. Effects of scopolamine injection during CS-US interval on conditioning. *Psychological Reports*, 1971, **28**: 690.

KRAL, P. A. Localized ECS impedes taste aversion learning. *Behavioral Biology*, 1972, **7**: 761–765.

KRAL, P. A., & BEGGERLY, H. D. Electroconvulsive shock impedes association formation: Conditioned taste aversion paradigm. *Physiology & Behavior*, 1973, **10**: 145–147.

KRAL, P. A., & ST. OMER, V. V. Beta-adrenergic receptor involvement in the mediation of learned taste aversions. *Psychopharmacologia*, 1972, **26**: 79–83.

KRALY, F. S., CARTY, W. J., RESNICK, S., & SMITH, G. P. Effect of cholecystokinin on meal size and intermeal in the sham-feeding rat. *Journal of Comparative and Physiological Psychology*, 1978, **92**: 697–707.

KRAMER, T. H., SCLAFANI, A., KINDYA, K., & PEZNER, M. Conditioned taste aversion in lean and obese rats with ventromedial hypothalamic knife cuts. *Behavioral Neuroscience*, 1983, **97**: 110–119.

KRAMES, L., MILGRAM, N. W., & CHRISTIE, D. P. Predatory aggression: Differential suppression of killing and feeding. *Behavioral Biology*, 1973, **9**: 641–647.

KRANE, R. V. Toxiphobia conditioning with exteroceptive cues. *Animal Learning & Behavior*, 1980, **8**: 513–523.

KRANE, R. V., & ROBERTSON, D. P. Trace decay and the priming of short-term memory in long-delay taste aversion learning: Disruptive effects of novel exteroceptive stimulation. *Learning and Motivation*, 1982, **13**: 434–453.

KRANE, R. V., SINNAMON, H. M., & THOMAS, G. J. Conditioned taste aversions and neophobia in rats with hippocampal lesions. *Journal of Comparative and Physiological Psychology*, 1976, **90**: 680–693.

KRANE, R. V., & WAGNER, A. R. Taste aversion learning with a delayed shock US: Implications for the "generality of the laws of learning." *Journal of Comparative and Physiological Psychology*, 1975, **88**: 882–889.

KRATZ, C. M., & LEVITSKY, D. A. The role of a noxious taste in determining food intake in the rat. *Physiology & Behavior*, 1980, **24**: 1027–1030.

KRESEL, J. J., & BAROFSKY, I. Conditioned saccharin aversion development following administration of hypotensive agents. *Physiology & Behavior*, 1979, **23**: 733–736.

KRISTAL, M. B., STEUER, M. A., NISHITA, J. K., & PETERS, L. C. Neophobia and water intake after repeated pairings of novel flavors with toxicosis. *Physiology & Behavior*, 1980, **24**: 979–982.

KUCHARSKI, D., & SPEAR, N. E. Potentiation of a conditioned taste aversion in preweanling and adult rats. *Behavioral and Neural Biology,* 1984, **40**: 44–57.

KUCHARSKI, D., & SPEAR, N. E. Potentiation and overshadowing in preweaning and adult rats. *Journal of Experimental Psychology: Animal Behavior Processes,* in press.

KULKOSKY, P. J. Reduction of drinking-associated feeding by C-terminal octapeptide of cholecystokinin-pancreozymin. *Behavioral and Neural Biology,* 1980, **29**: 111–116.

KULKOSKY, P. J. Conditioned food aversions and satiety signals. *Annals of the New York Academy of Sciences,* 1985, **443**: 330–347.

KULKOSKY, P. J., & GIBBS, J. Litorin suppresses food intake in rats. *Life Sciences,* 1982, **31**: 685–692.

KULKOSKY, P. J., GRAY, L., GIBBS, J., & SMITH, G. P. Feeding and selection of saccharin after injections of bombesin, LiCl, and NaCl. *Peptides,* 1981, **2**: 61–64.

KULKOSKY, P. J., RILEY, A. L., WOODS, S. C., & KRINSKY, R. Interaction of brain stimulation and conditioned taste aversion: Osmotically induced drinking. *Physiological Psychology,* 1975, **3**: 297–299.

KULKOSKY, P. J., SICKEL, J. L., & RILEY, A. L. Total avoidance of saccharin consumption by rats after repeatedly paired injections of ethanol or LiCl. *Pharmacology, Biochemistry & Behavior,* 1980, **13**: 77–80.

KULKOSKY, P. J., ZELLNER, D. A., HYSON, R. L., & RILEY, A. L. Ethanol consunption of rats in individual, group, and colonial housing conditions. *Physiological Psychology,* 1980, **8**: 56–60.

KUMAR, R., PRATT, J. A., & STOLERMAN, I. P. Characteristics of conditioned taste aversion produced by nicotine in rats. *British Journal of Pharmacology,* 1983, **79**: 245–253.

KURZ, E. M., & LEVITSKY, D. A. Novelty of contextual cues in taste aversion learning. *Animal Learning & Behavior,* 1982, **10**: 229–232.

KUSNECOV, A. W., SIVYER, M., KING, M. G., HUSBAND, A. J., CRIPPS, A. W., & CLANCY, R. L. Behaviorally conditioned suppression of the immune response by antilymphocyte serum. *Journal of Immunology,* 1983, **130**: 2117–2120.

KUTSCHER, C. L., & WRIGHT, W. A. Unconditioned taste aversion to quinine induced by injections of NaCl and LiCl: Dissociation of aversion from cellular dehydration. *Physiology & Behavior,* 1977, **18**: 87–94.

KUTSCHER, C. L., WRIGHT, W. A., & LISCH, M. NaCl and LiCl efficacy in the induction of aversion for quinine and saccharin solutions immediately following injection. *Pharmacology, Biochemistry & Behavior,* 1977, **6**: 567–569.

KUTSCHER, C. L., & YAMAMOTO, B. K. Altered saccharin preference during chronic dietary administration of lead in adult rats. *Neurobehavioral Toxicology,* 1979, **1**: 259–262.

KUTSCHER, C. L., YAMAMOTO, B. K., & HAMBURGER, J. N. Increased and decreased preference for saccharin immediately following injections of various agents. *Physiology & Behavior,* 1979, **23**: 461–464.

LAMON, S., WILSON, G. T., & LEAF, R. C. Human classical aversion conditioning: Nausea versus electric shock in the reduction of target beverage consumption. *Behaviour Research and Therapy,* 1977, **15**: 313–320.

LANDAUER, M. R., LYNCH, M. R., BALSTER, R. L., & KALLMAN, M. J. Trichloromethane-induced taste aversions in mice. *Neurobehavioral Toxicology and Teratology,* 1982, **4**: 305–309.

LANDAUER, M. R., TOMLINSON, W. T., BALSTER, R. L., & MACPHAIL, R. C. Some effects of the formamidine pesticide chlordimeform on the behavior of mice. *Neurotoxicology,* 1984, **5**: 91–100.

LANGHANS, W., & SCHARRER, E. Changes in food intake and meal patterns following injection of D-mannoheptulose in rats. *Behavioral and Neural Biology,* 1983, **38**: 269–286.

LANGHANS, W., WIESENREITER, F., & SCHARRER, E. Plasma metabolites and food intake reduction following heparinoid injection in rats. *Physiology & Behavior,* 1983, **30**: 113–119.

LANGLEY, W. Failure of food-aversion conditioning to suppress predatory attack of the grasshopper mouse, *Onychomys leucogaster. Behavioral and Neural Biology,* 1981, **33**: 317–333.

LANGLEY, W. M., & KNAPP, K. Importance of olfaction to suppression of attack response through conditioned taste aversion in the grasshopper mouse. *Behavioral and Neural Biology,* 1982, **36**: 368–378.

LASITER, P. S. Cortical substrates of taste aversion learning: Direct amygdalocortical projections to the gustatory neocortex do not mediate conditioned taste aversion learning. *Physiological Psychology*, 1982, **10**: 377–383.

LASITER, P. S. Gastrointestinal reactivity in rats lacking anterior insular neocortex. *Behavioral and Neural Biology*, 1983, **39**: 149–154.

LASITER, P. S., & BRAUN, J. J. Shock facilitation of taste aversion learning. *Behavioral and Neural Biology*, 1981, **32**: 277–281.

LASITER, P. S., & GLANZMAN, D. L. Cortical substates of taste aversion learning: Dorsal prepiriform (insular) lesions disrupt taste aversion learning. *Journal of Comparative and Physiological Psychology*, 1982, **96**: 376–392.

LAVIN, M. J. The establishment of flavor-flavor associations using a sensory preconditioning training procedure. *Learning and Motivation*, 1976, **7**: 173–183.

LAVIN, M. J., FREISE, B., & COOMBES, S. Transferred flavor aversions in adult rats. *Behavioral and Neural Biology*, 1980, **28**: 15–33.

LEANDER, J. D., & GAU, B. A. Flavor aversions rapidly produced by inorganic lead and triethyltin. *Neurotoxicology*, 1980, **1**: 635–642.

LEBLANC, A. E., & CAPPELL, H. Attenuation of punishing effects of morphine and amphetamine by chronic prior treatment. *Journal of Comparative and Physiological Psychology*, 1974, **87**: 691–698.

LEBLANC, A. E., & CAPPELL, H. Antagonism of morphine-induced aversive conditioning by naloxone. *Pharmacology, Biochemistry & Behavior*, 1975, **3**: 185–188.

LEBLANC, A. E., POULOS, C. X., & CAPPELL, H. Tolerance as a behavioral phenomenon: Evidence from two experimental paradigms. In N. Krasnegor (Ed.), *Behavioral tolerance: Research and treatment implications. NIDA Research Monograph (vol. 18).* Rockville, Maryland: DHEW Publications, 1978.

LEHR, P. P., & NACHMAN, M. Lateralization of learned taste aversion by cortical spreading depression. *Physiology & Behavior*, 1973, **10**: 79–83.

LE MAGNEN, J., MARFAING-JALLAT, P., & MICELI, D. A bioassay of ethanol-dependence in rats. *Pharmacology, Biochemistry & Behavior*, 1980, **12**: 701–704.

LE MAGNEN, J., MARFAING-JALLAT, P., MICELI, D., & DEVOS, M. Pain modulating and reward systems: A single brain mechanism? *Pharmacology, Biochemistry & Behavior*, 1980, **12**: 729–733.

LEMERE, F., & VOEGTLIN, W. L. An evaluation of the aversion treatment of alcoholism. *Quarterly Journal of the Studies on Alcohol*, 1950, **11**: 199–204.

LEPIANE, F. G., & PHILLIPS, A. G. Differential effects of electrical stimulation of amygdala, caudate-putamen or substantia nigra pars compacta on taste aversion and passive avoidance in rats. *Physiology & Behavior*, 1978, **21**: 979–985.

LESHEM, M. Suppression of feeding by naloxone in rat: A dose-response comparison of anorexia and conditioned taste aversion suggesting a specific anorexic effect. *Psychopharmacology*, 1984, **82**: 127–130.

LESTER, D., NACHMAN, M., & LE MAGNEN, J. Aversive conditioning by ethanol in the rat. *Journal of Studies on Alcohol*, 1970, **31**: 578–586.

LETT, B. T. Taste potentiates color-sickness associations in pigeons and quail. *Animal Learning & Behavior*, 1980, **8**: 193–198.

LETT, B. T. Pavlovian drug-sickness pairings result in the conditioning of an antisickness response. *Behavioral Neuroscience*, 1983, **97**: 779–784.

LETT, B. T. Taste potentiation in poison avoidance learning. In M. Commons, R. Herrnstein and A. Wagner (Eds.), *Quantitative analyses of behavior (vol. 3), Acquisition.* Cambridge, Mass.: Ballinger, in press.

LETT, B. T. The painlike effect of gallamine and naloxone differs from sickness induced by lithium. *Behavioral Neuroscience*, 1985, **99**: 145–150.

LETT, B. T., & HARLEY, C. W. Stimulation of laternal hypothalamus during sickness attenuates learned flavor aversions. *Physiology & Behavior*, 1974, **12**: 79–83.

LEVAN, H., & MOOS, W. An effect of DMSO on post-irradiation saccharin avoidance in mice. *Experientia*, 1967, **23**: 276–277.

LEVAN, H., & MOOS, W. Possible effects of radiation produced hydrogen peroxide on post-irradiation aversion in mice. *Experientia*, 1967, **23**: 749–751.

LEVAN, H., MOOS, W., & HEBRON, D. Direct and indirect effect of x-irradiation on conditioned avoidance behavior. *Medicina Experimentalis*, 1968, **18**: 161–168.

LEVAN, H., MOOS, W., & MASON, H. Attenuation of transferability of radiation-induced behavior by dimethyl sulfoxide in mice. *Journal of Biological Psychology*, 1970, **12**: 41–44.

LEVINE, S., SMOTHERMAN, W. P., & HENNESSY, J. W. Pituitary-adrenal hormones and learned taste aversion. In L. Miller, C. Sandman and A. Kastin (Eds.), *Neuropeptide influences on the brain and behavior.* New York: Raven Press, 1977.

LEVINE, T. E. Conditioned aversion following ingestion of methylmercury in rats and mice. *Behavioral Biology*, 1978, **22**: 489–496.

LEVY, C. J., CARROLL, M. E., SMITH, J. C., & HOFER, K. G. Antihistamines block radiation-induced taste aversions. *Science*, 1974, **186**: 1044–1046.

LEVY, C. J., CARROLL, M. E., SMITH, J. C., & HOFER, K. G. Reply to Sessions. *Science*, 1975, **190**: 403.

LEVY, C. K., ERVIN, F. R., & GARCIA, J. Effect of serum from irradiated rats on gastrointestinal function. *Nature*, 1970, **225**: 463–464.

LIEBLING, D. S., EISNER, J. D., GIBBS, J., & SMITH, G. P. Intestinal satiety in rats. *Journal of Comparative and Physiological Psychology*, 1975, **89**: 955–965.

LIGON, J. D., & MARTIN, D. J. Pinon seed assessment by the pinon jay, *Gymnorhinus cyanocephalus. Animal Behaviour*, 1974, **22**: 421–429.

LINAKIS, J. G., & CUNNINGHAM, C. L. Effects of concentration of ethanol injected intraperitoneally on taste aversion, body temperature, and activity. *Psychopharmacology*, 1979, **64**: 61–65.

LINDBERG, M. A., BEGGS, A. L., CHEZIK, D. D., & RAY, D. Flavor-toxicosis associations: Tests of three hypothesis of long delay learning. *Physiology & Behavior*, 1982, **29**: 439–442.

LINDSEY, G. P., & BEST, P. J. Overshadowing of the less salient of two novel fluids in a taste-aversion paradigm. *Physiological Psychology*, 1973, **1**: 13–15.

LITTLE, E. E. Conditioned aversion to amino acid flavors in the catfish (*Ictalurus punctatus*). *Physiology & Behavior*, 1977, **19**: 743–747.

LITTLE, L. M., & CURRAN, J. P. Covert sensitization: A clinical procedure in need of some explanations. *Psychological Bulletin*, 1978, **85**: 513–531.

LIU, W. F., HU, N. W., & BEATON, J. M. Behavioral toxicological assessment of oral pralidoxime methanesulphonate in the rat. *Neurobehavioral Toxicology and Teratology*, in press.

LOGUE, A. W. Taste aversion and the generality of the laws of learning. *Psychological Bulletin*, 1979, **86**: 276–296.

LOGUE, A. W. Visual cues for illness-induced aversions in the pigeon. *Behavioral and Neural Biology*, 1980, **28**: 372–377.

LOGUE, A. W. Conditioned food aversion learning in humans. *Annals of The New York Academy of Sciences*, 1985, **443**: 316–329.

LOGUE, A. W. A comparison of taste aversion learning in humans and other species: Evolutionary pressures in common. In R. Bolles and M. Beecher (Eds.), *Evolution and Learning*, Hillsdale, New Jersey: Lawrence Erlbaum Associates, in press.

LOGUE, A. W., LOGUE, K. R., & STRAUSS, K. E. The acquisition of taste aversions in humans with eating and drinking disorders. *Behaviour Research and Therapy*, 1983, **21**: 275–289.

LOGUE, A. W., OPHIR, I., & STRAUSS, K. E. The acquisition of taste aversions in humans. *Behaviour Research and Therapy*, 1981, **19**: 319–333.

LORDEN, J. F. Effects of lesions of the gustatory neocortex on taste aversion learning in the rat. *Journal of Comparative and Physiological Psychology*, 1976, **90**: 665–679.

LORDEN, J. F. Alteration of the characteristics of learned taste aversion by manipulation of serotonin levels in the rat. *Pharmacology, Biochemistry & Behavior*, 1978, **8**: 13–18.

LORDEN, J. F., CALLAHAN, M., & DAWSON, R., JR. Effects of forebrain serotonin depletion on fenfluramine-induced taste aversions. *Physiological Psychology*, 1979, **7**: 97–101.

LORDEN, J. F., CALLAHAN, M., & DAWSON, R., JR. Depletion of central catecholamines alters amphetamine- and fenfluramine-induced taste aversions in the rat. *Journal of Comparative and Physiological Psychology*, 1980, **94**: 99–114.

LORDEN, J. F., KENFIELD, M., & BRAUN, J. J. Response suppression to odors paired with toxicosis. *Learning and Motivation*, 1970, **1**: 391–400.

LORDEN, J. F., & MARGULES, D. L. Enhancement of conditioned taste aversions by lesions of the midbrain raphe nuclei that deplete serotonin. *Physiological Psychology*, 1977, **5**: 273–279.

LORDEN, J. F., & NUNN, W. B. Effects of central and peripheral pretreatment with fluoxetine in gustatory conditioning. *Pharmacology, Biochemistry & Behavior,* 1982, **17**: 435–444.

LORDEN, J. F., & OLTMANS, G. A. Alteration of the characteristics of learned taste aversion by manipulation of serotonin levels in the rat. *Pharmacology, Biochemistry & Behavior,* 1978, **8**: 13–18.

LOTTER, E. C., KRINSKY, R., MCKAY, J. M., TRENEER, C. M., PORTE, D., JR., & WOODS, S. C. Somatostatin decreases food intake of rats and baboons. *Journal of Comparative and Physiological Psychology,* 1981, **95**: 278–287.

LOULLIS, C. C., WAYNER, M. J., & JOLICOEUR, F. B. Thalamic taste nuclei lesions and taste aversion. *Physiology & Behavior,* 1978, **20**: 653–655.

LOVETT, D., & BOOTH, D. A. Four effects of exogenous insulin on food intake. *Quarterly Journal of Experimental Psychology,* 1970, **22**: 406–419.

LOVETT, D., GOODCHILD, P., & BOOTH, D. A. Depression of intake of nutrient by association of its odor with effects of insulin. *Psychonomic Science,* 1968, **11**: 27–28.

LOWE, W. C., & O'BOYLE, M. Suppression of cricket killing and eating in laboratory mice following lithium chloride injections. *Physiology & Behavior,* 1976, **17**: 427–430.

LUNDE, G. E., & VOGLER, R. E. Generalization of results in studies of aversion conditioning with alcoholics. *Behavioural Research and Therapy,* 1970, **8**: 313–314.

LUONGO, A. F. Stimulus selection in discriminative taste-aversion learning in the rat. *Animal Learning & Behavior,* 1976, **4**: 225–230.

LUTTINGER, D., KING, R. A., SHEPPARD, D., STRUPP, J., NEMEROFF, C. B., & PRANGE, A. J., JR. The effect of neurotensin on food consumption in the rat. *European Journal of Pharmacology,* 1982, **81**: 499–503.

LYNCH, M. R., PORTER, J. H., & ROSECRANS, J. A. Latent inhibition in the aversion to oral methadone. *Pharmacology, Biochemistry & Behavior,* 1984, **20**: 467–472.

MACKAY, B. Conditioned food aversion produced by toxicosis in Atlantic cod. *Behavioral Biology,* 1974, **12**: 347–355.

MACKAY, B. Visual and flavor cues in toxicosis conditioning of codfish. *Behavioral Biology,* 1977, **19**: 87–97.

MACPHAIL, R. C. Studies on the flavor aversions induced by trialkyltin compounds. *Neurobehavioral Toxicology and Teratology,* 1982, **4**: 225–230.

MACPHAIL, R. C., & ELSMORE, T. F. Ethanol-induced flavor aversions in mice: A behavior-genetics analysis. *Neurotoxicology,* 1980, **1**: 625–634.

MACPHAIL, R. C., & LEANDER, J. D. Flavor aversions induced by chlordimeform. *Neurobehavioral Toxicology,* 1980, **2**: 363–365.

MAGGIO, C. A., & KOOPMANS, H. S. Food intake after intragastric meals of short-, medium-, or long-chain triglyceride. *Physiology & Behavior,* 1982, **28**: 921–926.

MALONE, P. E., & COX, V. C. Development of taste aversions to individual components of a compound gustatory stimulus. *Communications in Behavioral Biology,* 1971, **6**: 341–344.

MANNING, F. J., & JACKSON, M. C., JR. Enduring effects of morphine pellets revealed by conditioned taste aversion. *Psychopharmacology,* 1977, **51**: 279–283.

MARFAING-JALLAT, P., & LE MAGNEN, J. Ethanol-induced taste aversion in ethanol-dependent and normal rats. *Behavioral and Neural Biology,* 1979, **26**: 106–114.

MARGULIES, D. L. Beta-adrenergic receptors in the hypothalamus for learned and unlearned taste aversions. *Journal of Comparative and Physiological Psychology,* 1970, **73**: 13–21.

MARTIN, G. M. Examination of factors which might disrupt a learned association between pentobarbital and LiCl. *Learning and Motivation,* 1982, **13**: 185–199.

MARTIN, G. M. Effect of pairings of pentobarbital with lithium chloride on the capacity of pentobarbital to maintain a conditioned aversion. *Behavioral and Neural Biology,* 1983, **39**: 145–148.

MARTIN, G. M. Disruption of chickens' color aversions when training and test mediums are different. *Animal Learning & Behavior,* 1984, **12**: 79–88.

MARTIN, G. M., & BELLINGHAM, W. P. Learning of visual food aversions by chickens (*Gallus gallus*) over long delays. *Behavioral and Neural Biology,* 1979, **25**: 58–68.

MARTIN, G. M., BELLINGHAM, W. P., & STORLIEN, L. H. Effects of varied color experience on chickens' formation of color and texture aversions. *Physiology & Behavior,* 1977, **18**: 415–420.

MARTIN, G. M., & STORLIEN, L. H. Anorexia and conditioned taste aversions in the rat. *Learning and Motivation,* 1976, **7**: 274–282.

MARTIN, G. M., & TIMMINS, W. K. Taste-sickness associations in young rats over varying delays, stimulus, and test conditions. *Animal Learning & Behavior*, 1980, **8**: 529–533.

MARTIN, J. C. Spatial avoidance in a paradigm in which ionizing irradiation precedes spatial confinement. *Radiation Research*, 1966, **27**: 284–289.

MARTIN, J. C. Saccharin preference and aversion as a function of irradiation and supplier in the albino rat. *Psychonomic Science*, 1968, **13**: 251–252.

MARTIN, J. C., & ELLINWOOD, E. H., JR. Conditioned aversion to a preferred solution following metamphetamine injections. *Psychopharmacologia*, 1973, **29**: 253–261.

MARTIN, J. C., & ELLINWOOD, E. H., JR. Conditioned aversion in spatial paradigms following metamphetamine injection. *Psychopharmacologia*, 1974, **36**: 323–335.

MARTIN, J. R. Coeliactomy: Differential toxiphobia conditioning with apomorphine and copper sulfate. *Pharmacology, Biochemistry & Behavior*, 1979, **11**: 331–334.

MARTIN, J. R., CHENG, F. Y., & NOVIN, D. Acquisition of learned taste aversion following bilateral subdiaphragmatic vagotomy in rats. *Physiology & Behavior*, 1978, **21**: 13–17.

MARTIN, J. R., & NOVIN, D. Decreased feeding in rats following hepatic-portal infusion of glucagon. *Physiology & Behavior*, 1977, **19**: 461–466.

MARTIN, L. T., & ALBERTS, J. R. Taste aversions to mother's milk: The age-related role of nursing in acquisition and expression of a learned association. *Journal of Comparative and Physiological Psychology*, 1979, **93**: 430–445.

MARTIN, L. T., & LAWRENCE, C. D. The importance of odor and texture cues in food aversion learning. *Behavioral and Neural Biology*, 1979, **27**: 503–515.

MARTIN, R. L., & HAMMOND, G. R. Lateral hypothalamic electrode implantation disrupts lithium-chloride-based generalized aversion to sodium chloride by enhancing sodium appetite. *Physiological Psychology*, 1983, **11**: 63–72.

MARTINEZ, J. L., JR., & RIGTER, H. Assessment of retention capacities in old rats. *Behavioral and Neural Biology*, 1983, **39**: 181–191.

MARUNIAK, J. A., MASON, J. R., & KOSTELC, J. G. Conditioned aversions to an intravascular odorant. *Physiology & Behavior*, 1983, **30**: 617–620.

MASON, J. R., RABIN, M. D., & STEVENS, D. A. Conditioned taste aversions: Skin secretions used for defense by tiger salamanders, *Ambystoma tigrinum*. *Copeia*, 1982, **3**: 667–671.

MASON, J. R., & REIDINGER, R. F. Observational learning of food aversions in red-winged blackbirds (*Agelaius phoeniceus*). *The Auk*, 1982, **99**: 548–554.

MASON, J. R., & REIDINGER, R. F., JR. Conspecific individual recognition between starlings after toxicant-induced sickness. *Animal Learning & Behavior*, 1983, **11**: 332–336.

MASON, J. R., & REIDINGER, R. F., JR. Importance of color for methiocarb-induced food aversions in red-winged blackbirds. *Journal of Wildlife Management*, 1983, **47**: 383–393.

MASON, J. R., & REIDINGER, R. F., JR. Generalization of and effects of pre-exposure on color-avoidance learning by red-winged blackbirds (*Agelaius phoeniceus*). *The Auk*, 1983, **100**: 461–468.

MASON, J. R., & SILVER, W. L. Trigeminally mediated odor aversions in starling. *Brain Research*, 1983, **269**: 196–199.

MASON, S. T., & FIBIGER, H. C. Noradrenaline and extinction of conditioned taste aversion in the rat. *Behavioral and Neural Biology*, 1979, **25**: 206–216.

MASON, S. T., & IVERSEN, S. D. Reward, attention and the dorsal noradrenergic bundle. *Brain Research*, 1978, **150**: 135–148.

MASSEY, O. T., & CALHOUN, W. H. Stimulus generalization according to palatability in lithium-chloride-induced taste aversions. *Bulletin of the Psychonomic Society*, 1977, **10**: 92–94.

MATSUZAWA, T., & HASEGAWA, Y. Food-aversion conditioning in Japanese monkeys (*Macacca fuscata*): Suppression of key-pressing. *Behavioral and Neural Biology*, 1982, **36**: 298–303.

MATSUZAWA, T., & HASEGAWA, Y. Food aversion learning in Japanese monkeys (*Macaca fuscata*): A strategy to avoid a noxious food. *Folica Primatologica*, 1983, **40**: 247–255.

MATSUZAWA, T., HASEGAWA, Y., GOTOH, S., & WADA, K. One-trial long-lasting food aversion learning in wild Japanese monkeys (*Macaca fuscata*). *Behavioral and Neural Biology*, 1983, **39**: 155–159.

MCCOY, D. F., NALLAN, G. B., & PACE, G. M. Some effects of rotation and centrifugally produced high gravitiy on taste aversion in rats. *Bulletin of the Psychonomic Society*, 1980, **16**: 255–257.

McFarland, D. J. Stimulus relevance and homeostasis. In R. Hinde and J. Stevenson-Hinde (Eds.), *Constraints on Learning*. London: Academic Press, 1973.

McFarland, D. J., Kostas, J., & Drew, Wm. G. Dorsal hippocampal lesions: Effects of preconditioning CS exposure on flavor aversion. *Behavioral Biology*, 1978, **22**: 398–404.

McGlone, J. J., Ritter, S., & Kelley, K. W. The antiaggressive effect of lithium is abolished by area postrema lesion. *Physiology & Behavior*, 1980, **24**: 1095–1100.

McGowan, B. K., Garcia, J., Ervin, F. R., & Schwartz, J. Effects of septal lesions on bait-shyness in the rat. *Physiology & Behavior*, 1969, **4**: 907–909.

McGowan, B. K., Hankins, W. G., & Garcia, J. Limbic lesions and control of the internal and external environment. *Behavioral Biology*, 1972, **7**: 841–852.

McIntosh, S. M., & Tarpy, R. M. Retention of latent inhibition in a taste-aversion paradigm. *Bulletin of the Psychonomic Society*, 1977, **9**: 411–412.

McLaurin, W. A. Postirradiation saccharin avoidance in rats as a function of the interval between ingestion and exposure. *Journal of Comparative and Physiological Psychology*, 1964, **57**: 316–317.

McLaurin, W. A., Farley, J. A., & Scarborough, B. B. Inhibitory effect of preirradiation saccharin habituation on conditioned avoidance behavior. *Radiation Research*, 1963, **18**: 473–478.

McLaruin, W. A., Farley, J. A., Scarborough, B. B., & Rawlings, T. D. Post-irradiation saccharin avoidance with non-coincident stimuli. *Psychological Reports*, 1964, **14**: 507–512.

McLaurin, W. A., & Scarborough, B. B. Extension of the interstimulus interval in saccharin avoidance conditioning. *Radiation Research*, 1963, **20**: 317–324.

McLaurin, W. A., Scarborough, B. B., & Farley, J. A. Delay of postirradiation test fluids: A factor in saccharin avoidance behavior. *Radiation Research*, 1964, **22**: 45–52.

McManus, F. E., & Wyers, E. J. Olfaction and selective association in the earthworm, *Lumbricus terrestris*. *Behavioral and Neural Biology*, 1979, **25**: 39–57.

Meliza, L. L., Leung, P. M., & Rogers, Q. R. Effect of anterior prepyriform and medial amygdaloid lesions on acquisition of taste-avoidance and response to dietary amino acid imbalance. *Physiology & Behavior*, 1981, **26**: 1031–1035.

Mellor, C. S., & White, H. P. Taste aversions to alcoholic beverages conditioned by motion sickness. *American Journal of Psychiatry*, 1978, **135**: 125–126.

Miceli, D., Marfaing-Jallat, P., & Le Magnen, J. Non-specific enhancement of ethanol-induced taste of aversion by naloxone. *Pharmacology, Biochemistry & Behavior*, 1979, **11**: 391–394.

Miceli, D., Marfaing-Jallat, P., & Le Magnen, J. Ethanol aversion induced by parenterally administered ethanol acting both as CS and UCS. *Physiological Psychology*, 1980, **8**: 433–436.

Middleton, A. Rural rat control. In D. Chitty (Ed), *Control of rats and mice* (*vol 2*). Oxford: Clarendon Press, 1954.

Mikulka, P. J., Freeman, F. G., & Lidstrom, P. The effect of training technique and amygdala lesions on the acquisition and retention of a taste aversion. *Behavioral Biology*, 1977, **19**: 509–517.

Mikulka, P. J., & Klein, S. B. The effect of CS familiarization and extinction procedure on the resistance to extinction of a taste aversion. *Behavioral Biology*, 1977, **19**: 518–522.

Mikulka, P., & Klein, S. Resistance to extinction of a taste aversion: Effects of level of training and procedures used in acquisition and extinction. *American Journal of Psychology*, 1980, **93**: 631–641.

Mikulka, P. J., Krone, P. D., Rapisardi, P. L., & Kirby, R. H. Discrimination between deionized water and D_2O in a runway using olfaction in the rat. *Physiological Psychology*, 1975, **3**: 92–94.

Mikulka, P. J., Leard, B., & Klein, S. B. Illness-alone exposure as a source of interference with the acquisition and retention of a taste aversion. *Journal of Experimental Psychology: Animal Behavior Processes*, 1977, **3**: 189–201.

Mikulka, P. J., Pitts, E., & Philput, C. Overshadowing not potentiation in taste aversion conditioning. *Bulletin of the Psychonomic Society*, 1982, **20**: 101–104.

Mikulka, P., Vaughn, P., & Hughes, J. Lithium chloride-produced prey aversion in the toad (*Bufo americanus*). *Behavioral and Neural Biology*, 1981, **33**: 220–229.

Milgram, N. W., Krames, L., & Alloway, T. M. (Eds.). *Food aversion learning*. New York:

Plenum Press, 1977.

MILGRAM, N. W., CAUDARELLA, M., & KRAMES, L. Suppression of interspecific aggression using toxic reinforcers. In N. Milgram, L. Krames and T. Alloway (Eds.), *Food aversion learning*. New York: Plenum Press, 1977.

MILLARD, W. J. Lithium chloride-induced avoidance of a conspecific odor: Effect of prior exposure to the conditional stimulus. *Behavioral and Neural Biology*, 1982, **34**: 404–410.

MILLER, C. R., ELKINS, R. L., FRASER, J., PEACOCK, L. J., & HOBBS, S. H. Taste aversion and passive avoidance in rats with hippocampal lesions. *Physiological Psychology*, 1975, **3**: 123–126.

MILLER, C. R., ELKINS, R. L., & PEACOCK, L. J. Disruption of a radiation-induced preference shift by hippocampal lesions. *Physiology & Behavior*, 1971, **6**: 283–285.

MILLER, D. B., & MILLER, L. L. Bupropion, d-amphetamine, and amitriptyline-induced conditioned taste aversion in rats: Dose effects. *Pharmacology, Biochemistry & Behavior*, 1983, **18**: 737–740.

MILLER, R. R., & HOLZMAN, A. D. Neophobias and conditioned taste aversions in rats following exposure to novel flavors. *Animal Learning & Behavior*, 1981, **9**: 89–100.

MILLER, R. R., & HOLZMAN, A. D. Neophobia: Generality and function. *Behavioral and Neural Biology*, 1981, **33**: 17–44.

MILLER, V. Selective aversion learning in the rat. *Learning and Motivation*, in press.

MILLER, V., & DOMJAN, M. Specificity of cue to consequence in aversion learning in the rat: Control for US-induced differential orientations. *Animal Learning & Behavior*, 1981, **9**: 339–345.

MILLER, V., & DOMJAN, M. Selective sensitization induced by lithium malaise and footshock in rats. *Behavioral and Neural Biology*, 1981, **31**: 42–55.

MILLNER, J. R., & PALFAI, T. Metrazol impairs conditioned aversion produced by LiCl: A time dependent effect. *Pharmacology, Biochemistry & Behavior*, 1975, **3**: 201–204.

MINEKA, S., SELIGMAN, M. E. P., HETRICK, M., & ZUELZER, K. Poisoning and conditioned drinking. *Journal of Comparative and Physiological Psychology*, 1972, **79**: 377–383.

MISANIN, J. R., GUANOWSKY, V., & RICCIO, D. C. The effect of CS-preexposure on conditioned taste aversion in young and adult rats. *Physiology & Behavior*, 1983, **30**: 859–862.

MITCHELL, D. Reply to Revusky. *Animal Learning & Behavior*, 1977, **5**: 321–322.

MITCHELL, D. The psychological vs. the ethological rat: Two views of the poison avoidance behavior of the rat compared. *Animal Learning & Behavior*, 1978, **6**: 121–124.

MITCHELL, D., KIRSCHBAUM, E. H., & PERRY, R. L. Effects of neophobia and habituation on the poison-induced avoidance of exteroceptive stimuli in the rat. *Journal of Experimental Psychology: Animal Behavior Processes*, 1975, **104**: 47–55.

MITCHELL, D., LAYCOCK, J. D., & STEPHENS, W. F. Motion sickness-induced pica in the rat. *The American Journal of Clinical Nutrition*, 1977, **30**: 147–150.

MITCHELL, D., PARKER, L. F., & JOHNSON, R. Absence of a generalization decrement in the poison-induced avoidance of interoceptive stimuli in the rat. *Physiological Psychology*, 1976, **4**: 121–123.

MITCHELL, D., SCOTT, D. W., & MITCHELL, L. K. Attenuated and enhanced neophobia in the taste-aversion "delay of reinforcement" effect. *Animal Learning & Behavior*, 1977, **5**: 99–102.

MITCHELL, D., WINTER, W., & MOFFITT, T. Cross-modality contrast: Exteroceptive context habituation enhances taste neophobia and conditioned taste aversions. *Animal Learning & Behavior*, 1980, **8**: 524–528.

MITCHELL, D., WINTER, W., & MORISAKI, C. M. Conditioned taste aversions accompanied by geophagia: Evidence for the occurrence of "psychological" factors in the etiology of pica. *Psychosomatic Medicine*, 1977, **39**: 402–412.

MIYAGAWA, M. Conditioned taste aversion induced by inhalation exposure to methyl bromide in rats. *Toxicology Letters*, 1982, **10**: 411–416.

MIYAGAWA, M., HONMA, T., SATO, M., & HASEGAWA, H. Conditioned taste aversion induced by toluene administration in rats. *Neurobehavioral Toxicology and Teratology*, 1984, **6**: 33–37.

MONAHAN, J.C., & HENTON, W. W. Microwave absorption and taste aversion as a function of 915 MHz radiation. In D. Hazzard (Ed.), *Symposium on biological effects and measurement of radio frequency: Microwaves*. Rockville, Md: DHEW, 1977.

MONROE, B., & BARKER, L. M. A contingency analysis of taste aversion conditioning. *Animal Learning & Behavior*, 1979, **7**: 141–143.

MOORE, M. J., & CAPRETTA, P. J. Changes in colored or flavored food preferences in chickens as a function of shock. *Psychonomic Science*, 1968, **12**: 195–196.

MORRIS, D. D., & SMITH, J. C. X-ray-conditioned saccharin aversion induced during the immediate post exposure period. *Radiation Research*, 1964, **21**: 513–519.

MORRISON, G. R., & COLLYER, R. Taste-mediated conditioned aversion to an exteroceptive stimulus following LiCl poisoning. *Journal of Comparative and Physiological Psychology*, 1974, **86**: 51–55.

MORRISON, G. R., & JESSUP, A. Does saccharin have a dual taste for the rat? In J. Weiffenbach (Ed.), *Taste and development*. Bethesda: DHEW, 1977.

MOUNTJOY, P. T., & ROBERTS, A. E. Radiation produced avoidance to morphine. *Psychonomic Science*, 1967, **9**: 427–428.

MURPHY, L. R., & BROWN, T. S. Hippocampal lesions and learned taste aversion. *Physiological Psychology*, 1974, **2**: 60–64.

MYERS, R. H., & DE CASTRO, J. M. Learned aversion to intracerebral carbachol. *Physiology & Behavior*, 1977, **19**: 467–472.

NACHMAN, M. Learned aversion to the taste of lithium chloride and generalization to other salts. *Journal of Comparative and Physiological Psychology*, 1963, **56**: 343–349.

NACHMAN, M. Taste preferences for lithium chloride by adrenalectomized rats. *American Journal of Physiology*, 1963, **205**: 219–221.

NACHMAN, M. Learned taste and temperature aversions due to lithium chloride sickness after temporal delays. *Journal of Comparative and Physiological Psychology* 1970, **73**: 22–30.

NACHMAN, M. Limited effects of electroconvulsive shock on memory of taste stimulation. *Journal of Comparative and Physiological Psychology*, 1970, **73**: 31–37.

NACHMAN, M., & ASHE, J. H. Learned taste aversions in rats as a function of dosage, concentrations and route of administration of LiCl. *Physiology & Behavior*, 1973, **10**: 73–78.

NACHMAN, M., & ASHE, J. H. Effects of basolateral amygdala lesions on neophobia, learned taste aversions, and sodium appetite in rats. *Journal of Comparative and Physiological Psychology*, 1974, **87**: 622–643.

NACHMAN, M., & COLE, L. P. Role of taste in specific hungers. In L. Beidler (Ed.), *Handbook of sensory physiology (vol 4): Chemical senses (Part 2): Taste.* New York: Springer-Verlag, 1971.

NACHMAN, M., & HARTLEY, P. L. Role of illness in producing learned taste aversions in rats: A comparison of several rodenticides. *Journal of Comparative and Physiological Psychology*, 1975, **89**: 1010–1018.

NACHMAN, M., & JONES, D. R. Learned taste aversions over long delays in rats: The role of learned safety. *Journal of Comparative and Physiological Psychology*, 1974, **86**: 949–956.

NACHMAN, M., LESTER, D., & LE MAGNEN, J. Alcohol aversion in the rat: Behavioral assessment of noxious drug effects. *Science*, 1970, **168**: 1244–1246.

NACHMAN, M., RAUSCHENBERGER, J., & ASHE, J. H. Stimulus characteristics in food aversion learning. In N. Milgram, L. Krames and T. Alloway (Eds.), *Food aversion learning*. New York: Plenum Press, 1977.

NACHMAN, M., RAUSCHENBERGER, J., & ASHE, J. H. Studies of learned aversions using non-gustatory stimuli. In L. Barker, M. Best and M. Domjan (Eds.), *Learning mechanisms in food selection*. Waco, Texas: Baylor University Press, 1977.

NAKAJIMA, S. Conditioned aversion of water produced by cycloheximide injection. *Physiological Psychology*, 1974, **2**: 484–486.

NATHAN, B. A., & VOGEL, J. R. Taste aversions induced by d-amphetamine: Dose-response relationship. *Bulletin of the Psychonomic Society*, 1975, **6**: 287–288.

NATHAN, P. E. Aversion therapy in the treatment of alcoholism: Success and failure. *Annals of The New York Academy of Sciences*, 1985, **443**: 357–364.

NEUBERGER, O. W., HASHA, N., MATARAZZO, J. D., SCHMITZ, R. E., & PRATT, H. H. Behavioral-chemical treatment of alcoholism: An outcome replication. *Journal of Studies on Alcohol*, 1981, **42**: 806–810.

NEUBERGER, O. W., MATARAZZO, J. D., SCHMITZ, R. E., & PRATT, H. H. One year follow-up of total abstinence in chronic alcoholic patients following emetic counterconditioning. *Alcoholism: Clinical and Experimental Research*, 1980, **4**: 306–312.

NEUBERGER, O. W., MILLER, S. I., SCHMITZ, R. E., MATARAZZO, J. D., PRATT, H. H., & HASHA, N. Replicable abstinence rates in an alcoholism treatment program. *Journal of the American Medical Association*, 1982, **248**: 960–963.

NICOLAUS, L. K., CASSEL, J. F., CARLSON, R. B., & GUSTAVSON, C. R. Taste-aversion conditioning of crows to control predation on eggs. *Science*, 1983, **220**: 212–214.

NICOLAUS, L. K., HOFFMAN, T. E., & GUSTAVSON, C. R. Taste aversion conditioning in free ranging raccoons (*Procyon lotor*). *Northwest Science*, 1982, **56**: 165–169.

NONNEMAN, A. J., & CURTIS, S. D. Strength of conditioning determines the effects of septohippocampal lesions on taste aversion learning. *Physiological Psychology*, 1978, **6**: 249–254.

NOWLIS, G. H. Conditioned stimulus intensity and acquired alimentary aversions in the rat. *Journal of Comparative and Physiological Psychology*, 1974, **86**: 1173–1184.

NOWLIS, G. H., FRANK, M. E., & PFAFFMANN, C. Specificity of acquired aversions to taste qualities in hamsters and rats. *Journal of Comparative and Physiological Psychology*, 1980, **94**: 932–942.

O'BOYLE, M., LOONEY, T. A., & COHEN, P. S. Suppression and recovery of mouse killing in rats following immediate lithium-chloride injections. *Bulletin of the Psychonomic Society*, 1973, **1**: 250–252.

OMURA, K., TAKAGI, S. F., & HARADA, O. On the mechanism of the repellant action of narmycin to rats. *Gunma Journal of Medical Sciences*, 1961, **10**: 217–227.

OPITZ, K. Effect of fenfluramine on alcohol and saccharin consumption in the rat. *South African Medical Journal*, 1972, **46**: 742–744.

OSSENKOPP, K-P. Taste aversions conditioned with gamma radiation: Attenuation by area postrema lesions in rats. *Behavioural Brain Research*, 1983, **7**: 297–305.

OSSENKOPP, K-P. Area postrema lesions in rats enhance the magnitude of body rotation-induced conditioned taste aversions. *Behavioral and Neural Biology*, 1983, **38**: 82–96.

OSSENKOPP, K-P., & FRISKEN, N. L. Defecation as an index of motion sickness in the rat. *Physiological Psychology*, 1982, **10**: 355–360.

OSTROWSKI, N. L., FOLEY, T. L., LIND, M. D., & REID, L. D. Naloxone reduces fluid intake: Effect of water and food deprivation. *Pharmacology, Biochemistry & Behavior*, 1980, **12**: 431–435.

OVERALL, J. E., BROWN, W. L., & LOGIE, L. C. Instrumental behaviour of albino rats in response to incident x-radiation. *British Journal of Radiology*, 1959, **32**: 411–414.

PAGER, J., & ROYET, J. P. Some effects of conditioned aversion on food intake and olfactory bulb electrical responses in the rat. *Journal of Comparative and Physiological Psychology*, 1976, **90**: 67–77.

PAIN, J. F., & BOOTH, D. A. Toxiphobia for odors. *Psychonomic Science*, 1968, **10**: 363–364.

PALMERINO, C. C., RUSINIAK, K. W., & GARCIA, J. Flavor-illness aversions: The peculiar roles of odor and taste in memory for poision. *Science*, 1980, **208**: 753–755.

PANHUBER, H. Effect of odor quality and intensity on conditioned odor aversion learning in the rat. *Physiology & Behavior*, 1982, **28**: 149–154.

PANKSEPP, J., POLLACK, A., MEEKER, R. B., & SULLIVAN, A. C. (–)-hydroxycitrate and conditioned aversions. *Pharmacology, Biochemistry & Behavior*, 1977, **6**: 683–687.

PARKER, H. B., & SMITH, R. E. Flavor- vs. tone-cued shock avoidance. *Animal Learning & Behavior*, 1981, **9**: 335–338.

PARKER, L. A. Conditioned suppression of drinking: A measure of the CR elicited by a lithium-conditioned flavor. *Learning and Motivation*, 1980, **11**: 538–559.

PARKER, L. A. Nonconsummatory and consummatory behavioral CRs elicited by lithium- and amphetamine-paired flavors. *Learning and Motivation*, 1982, **13**: 281–303.

PARKER, L. A., HUTCHISON, S., & RILEY, A. L. Conditioned flavor aversions: A toxicity test of the anticholinesterase agent, physostigmine. *Neurobehavioral Toxicology and Teratology*, 1982, **4**: 93–98.

PARKER, L. A., & REVUSKY, S. Failure of Sprague-Dawley rats to transfer taste-aversions or preferences by, odor-marking the spout. *Behavioral Biology*, 1975, **15**: 383–387.

PARKER, L. A., & REVUSKY, S. Generalized conditioned flavor aversions: Effects of toxicosis training with one flavor on the preference for different novel flavors. *Animal Learning & Behavior*, 1982, **10**: 505–510.

PARKER, L., FAILOR, A., & WEIDMAN, K. Conditioned preferences in the rat with an unnatural need state: Morphine withdrawal. *Journal of Comparative and Physiological Psychology*, 1973, **82**: 294–300.

PARKER, L. F., & RADOW, B. L. Morphine-like physical dependence: A pharmacological method for drug assessment using the rat. *Pharmacology, Biochemistry & Behavior*, 1974, **2**: 613–618.

PARKER, L. F., & RADOW, B. L. Effects of parachlorophenylalanine on ethanol self-selection in the rat. *Pharmacology, Biochemistry & Behavior*, 1976, **4**: 535–540.

PASSOF, P. C., MARSH, R. E., & HOWARD, W. E. Alpha-naphthylthiourea as a conditioning repellant for protecting conifer seed. In W. Johnson (Ed.), *Proceedings sixth vertebrate pest conference*. Anaheim, California, 1974.

PEACOCK, L. J., & WATSON, J. A. Radiation-induced aversion to alcohol. *Science*, 1964, **143**: 1462–1463.

PEARLMAN, C. A. Interference with taste familiarization by several drugs in rats. *Behavioral Biology*, 1978, **24**: 307–316.

PECK, J. H., & ADER, R. Illness-induced taste aversion under states of deprivation and satiation. *Animal Learning & Behavior*, 1974, **2**: 6–8.

PELCHAT, M. L., GRILL, H. J., ROZIN, P., & JACOBS, J. Quality of acquired responses to tastes by *Rattus norvegicus* depends on type of associated discomfort. *Journal of Comparative Psychology*, 1983, **97**: 140–153.

PELCHAT, M. L., & ROZIN, P. The special role os nausea in the acquisition of food dislikes by humans. *Appetite: Journal for Intake Research*, 1982 **3**: 341–351.

PERLOW, M. J., FREED, W. J., CARMAN, J. S., & WYATT, R. J. Calcitonin reduces feeding in man, monkey and rat. *Pharmacology, Biochemistry & Behavior*, 1980, **12**: 609–612.

PERRY, N. W., JR. Avoidance conditioning of NaCl with x-irradiation of the rat. *Radiation Research*, 1963, **20**: 471–476.

PERSINGER, M. A., & FISS, T. B. Mesenteric mast cell degranulation is not essential for conditioned taste aversion. *Pharmacology, Biochemistry & Behavior*, 1978, **9**: 725–730.

PETERS, R. H. Learned aversions to copulatory behaviors in male rats. *Behavioral Neuroscience*, 1983, **97**: 140–145.

PETERS, R. H., & REICH, M. J. Effects of ventromedial hypothalamic lesions on conditioned sucrose aversions in rats. *Journal of Comparative and Physiological Psychology*, 1973, **84**: 502–506.

PETTIJOHN, T. F. Conditioned olfactory aversion in the male Mongolian gerbil. *Physiological Psychology*, 1979, **7**: 299–302.

PETTIJOHN, T. F., & JAMORA, C. M. Learned aversion to soiled bedding in male Mongolian gerbils. *Physiology & Behavior*, 1980, **24**: 1031–1034.

PHILLIPS, A. G., & LEPIANE, F. G. Electrical stimulation of the amygdala as a conditioned stimulus in a bait-shyness paradigm. *Science*, 1978, **201**: 536–538.

PHILLIPS, A. G., & LEPIANE, F. G. Disruption of conditioned taste aversion in the rat by stimulation of amygdala: A conditioning effect, not amnesia. *Journal of Comparative and Physiological Psychology*, 1980, **94**: 664–674.

PHILLIPS, A. G., & MCDONALD, A. C. Conditioned aversion to brain-stimulation reward: Effects of electrode placement and prior experience. *Brain Research*, 1979, **170**: 523–531.

PILCHER, C. W. T., & JONES, S. M. Social crowding enhances aversiveness of naloxone in rats. *Pharmacology, Biochemistry & Behavior*, 1981, **14**: 299–303.

PILCHER, C. W. T., JONES, S. M., & STOLERMAN, I. P. Possible GABA involvement in the mediation of narcotic antagonist-induced aversions. In E. Way (Ed.), *Endogenous and exogenous opiate agonists and antagonists*. Oxford: Pergamon, 1979.

PILCHER, C. W. T., JONES, S. M., & BROWNE, J. Rhythmic nature of naloxone-induce aversions and nociception in rats. *Life Sciences*, 1982, **31**: 1249–1252.

PILCHER, C. W. T., & STOLERMAN, I. P. Recent approaches to assessing opiate dependence in rats. In H. Kosterlitz (Ed.), *Opiates and endogenous opioid peptides*. Amsterdam: Elsevier North Holland Press, 1976.

PILCHER, C. W. T., & STOLERMAN, I. P. Conditioned flavor aversions for assessing precipitated morphine abstinence in rats. *Pharmacology, Biochemistry & Behavior*, 1976, **4**: 159–163.

PILCHER, C. W., STOLERMAN, I. P., & D'MELLO, G. D. Aversive effects of narcotic antagonists in rats. In J. van Ree and L. Terenius (Eds.), *Characteristics and function of opioids*. Amsterdam: Elsevier North Holland Press, 1978.

POLING, A., CLEARY, J., & MONAGHAN, M. Burying by rats in response to aversive and nonaversive stimuli. *Journal of the Experimental Analysis of Behavior*, 1981, **35**: 31–44.

POLLOCK, J. D., & ROWLAND, N. Peripherally administered serotonin decreases food intake in rats. *Pharmacology, Biochemistry & Behavior*, 1981, **15**: 179–183.

POULOS, C. X., & CAPPELL, H. An associative analysis of pretreatment effects in gustatory conditioning by amphetamine. *Psychopharmacology*, 1979, **64**: 201–207.

POUNDS, D., WILLIAMSON, P., & CHENEY, C. Interocular transfer of color aversion in pigeons. *Bulletin of the Psychonomic Society*, 1980, **15**: 178–180.

PRAKASH, I., & JAIN, A. P. Bait shyness of two gerbils *Tatera indica indica* Hardwicke and *Meriones hurrianae* Jerdon. *Annals of Applied Biology*, 1971, **69**: 169–172.

PRAKASH, I., & JAIN, A. Bait shyness and poison aversion in the hairy-footed gerbil (*Gerbillus gleadowi*). *Zeitschrift fur Angewandte Zoologie*, 1975, **62**: 89–97.

PRAKASH, I., RANA, B., & JAIN, A. Bait shyness in three species of rattus. *Zeitschrift fur Angewandte Zoologie*, in press.

PRATT, J. A., & STOLERMAN, I. P. Pharmacologically specific pretreatment effects on apomorphine-mediated conditioned taste aversions in rats. *Pharmacology, Biochemistry & Behavior*, 1984, **20**: 507–511.

PRESTON, K. L., WAGNER, G. C., SEIDEN, L. S., & SCHUSTER, C. R. Effects of methamphetamine on atropine-induced conditioned gustatory avoidance. *Pharmacology, Biochemistry & Behavior*, 1984, **20**: 601–607.

PRITCHARD, T. C., & SCOTT, T. R. Amino acids as taste stimuli. II. Quality coding. *Brain Research*, 1982, **253**: 93–104.

QUINN, J., & HENBEST, R. Partial failure of generalization in alcoholism following aversion therapy. *Quarterly Journal of Studies on Alcohol*, 1967, **28**: 70–75.

RABIN, B. M., & HUNT, W. A. Effects of antiemetics on the acquisition and recall of radiation- and lithium chloride–induced conditioned taste aversions. *Pharmacology, Biochemistry & Behavior*, 1983, **18**: 629–636.

RABIN, B. M., HUNT, W. A., & LEE, J. Studies on the role of central histamine in the acquisition of a radiation-induced conditioned taste aversion. *Radiation Research*, 1982, **90**: 609–620.

RABIN, B. M., HUNT, W. A., & LEE, J. State-dependent interactions in the antihistamine-induced disruption of a radiation-induced conditioned taste aversion. *Radiation Research*, 1982, **90**: 621–627.

RABIN, B. M., HUNT, W. A., & LEE, J. Acquisition of lithium chloride- and radiation-induced taste aversions in hypophysectomized rats. *Pharmacology, Biochemistry & Behavior*, 1983, **18**: 463–465.

RABIN, B. M., HUNT, W. A., & LEE, J. Attenuation of radiation and drug-induced conditioned taste aversions following area postrema lesions in the rat. *Radiation Research*, 1983, **93**: 388–394.

RABIN, B. M., HUNT, W. A., & LEE, J. Effects of dose and of partial body ionizing radiation on taste aversion learning in rats with lesions of the area postrema. *Physiology & Behavior*, 1984, **32**: 119–122.

RABIN, B. M., HUNT, W. A., & LEE, J. Recall of a previously acquired conditioned taste aversion in rats following lesions of the area postrema. *Physiology & Behavior*, 1984, **32**: 503–506.

RACHMAN, S. J. Aversion therapy: Chemical or electrical? *Behaviour Research and Therapy*, 1965, **2**: 289–299.

RACHMAN, S. J., & TEASDALE, J. (Eds.), *Aversion therapy and behavior disorders: An analysis*. Coral Gables, FL: University of Miami Press, 1969.

RALPH, T. L., & BALAGURA, S. Effect of intracranial electrical stimulation on the primary learned aversion to LiCl and the generalized aversion to NaCl. *Journal of Comparative and Physiological Psychology*, 1974, **86**: 664–669.

RAO, A., & RABAJAI, B. Bait shyness in two species of Mus. *Pest Control*, in press.

RAPPOLD, V. A., PORTER, J. H. & LLEWELLYN, G. C. Evaluation of the toxic effects of aflatoxin Bl with a taste aversion paradigm in rats. *Neurobehavioral Toxicology and Teratology*, 1984, **6**: 51–58.

RAYMOND, M. J. The treatment of addiction by aversion conditioning with apomorphine. *Behaviour Research and Therapy*, 1964, **1**: 287–291.

REICHER, M. A., & HOLMAN, E. W. Location preference and flavor aversion reinforced by amphetamine in rats. *Animal Learning & Behavior*, 1977, **5**: 343–346.

REININGER, R. F., JR., BEAUCHAMP, G. K., & BARTH, M. Conditioned aversion to a taste perceived while grooming. *Physiology & Behavior*, 1982, **28**: 715–723.

RENAULT, P. Alcohol aversion therapy. *HRST Assessment Report Series*, 1981, **1**: 1–9.

RESCORLA, R. A. Stimultaneous and successive associations in sensory preconditioning. *Journal of Experimental Psychology: Animal Behavior Processes*, 1980, **6**: 207–216.

RESCORLA, R. A. Simultaneous associations. In P. Harzem and M. Zeiler (Eds.), *Predictability, correlation and contiguity.* New York: Wiley, 1981.

RESCORLA, R. A., & CUNNINGHAM, C. L. Within-compound flavor associations. *Journal of Experimental Psychology: Animal Behavior Processes*, 1978, **4**: 267–275.

RESCORLA, R. A., & CUNNINGHAM, C. L. Recovery of the US representation over time during extinction. *Learning and Motivation*, 1978, **9**: 373–391.

RESCORLA, R. A., & FREBERG, L. The extinction of within-compound flavor associations. *Learning and Motivation*, 1978, **9**: 411–427.

REVUSKY, S. H. Aversion to sucrose produced by contingent x-irradiation: Temporal and dosage parameters. *Journal of Comparative and Physiological Psychology*, 1968, **65**: 17–22.

REVUSKY, S. The role of interference in association over a delay. In V. Honig and P. James (Eds.), *Animal memory.* New York: Academic Press, 1971.

REVUSKY, S. Some laboratory paradigms for chemical aversion treatment of alcoholism. *Journal of Behavior Therapy and Experimental Psychiatry*, 1973, **4**: 15–17.

REVUSKY, S. Correction of a paper by Mitchell, Scott, and Mitchell. *Animal Learning & Behavior*, 1977, **5**: 320.

REVUSKY, S. Learning as a general process with an emphasis on data from feeding experiments. In N. Milgram, L. Krames and T. Alloway (Eds.), *Food aversion learning.* New York: Plenum Press, 1977.

REVUSKY, S. Interference with progress by the scientific establishment: Examples from flavor aversion learning. In N. Milgram, L. Krames and T. Alloway (Eds.), *Food aversion learning.* New York: Plenum Press, 1977.

REVUSKY, S. The concurrent interference approach to delay learning. In L. Barker, M. Best and M. Domjan (Eds.), *Learning mechanisms in food selection.* Waco, Texas: Baylor University Press, 1977.

REVUSKY, S. Reply to Mitchell. *Animal Learning & Behavior*, 1978, **6**: 119–120.

REVUSKY, S. More about appropriate controls for taste aversion learning: A reply to Riley. *Animal Learning & Behavior*, 1979, **7**: 562–563.

REVUSKY, S. A sensory preconditioning effect after a single flavor-flavor pairing. *Bulletin of the Psychonomic Society*, 1980, **15**: 83–86.

REVUSKY, S. Drug-drug conditioning: A preliminary review. *Annals of The New York Academy of Sciences*, 1985, **443**: 250–270.

REVUSKY, S. H., & BEDARF, E. W. Association of illness with prior ingestion of novel foods. *Science*, 1967, **155**: 219–220.

REVUSKY, S., & COOMBES, S. Reacquisition of learned taste aversions. *Animal Learning & Behavior*, 1979, **7**: 377–382.

REVUSKY, S., & COOMBES, S. Long-delay associations between drug states produced in rats by injecting two drugs in sequence. *Journal of Comparative and Physiological Psychology*, 1982, **96**: 549-556.

REVUSKY, S., COOMBES, S., & POHL, R. W. Failure of albino guinea pigs to exhibit Lavin's poisoned partner effect. *Behavioral and Neural Biology*, 1981, **32**: 111–113.

REVUSKY, S., COOMBES, S., & POHL, R. W. US preexposure: Effects on flavor aversions produced by pairing a poisoned partner with ingestion. *Animal Learning & Behavior*, 1982, **10**: 83–90.

REVUSKY, S., COOMBES, S., & POHL, R. W. Pharmacological generality of the Avfail effect. *Behavioral and Neural Biology*, 1982, **34**: 240–260.

REVUSKY, S., COOMBES, S., & POHL, R. W. Drug states as discriminative stimuli in a flavor-aversion learning experiment. *Journal of Comparative and Physiological Psychology*, 1982, **96**: 200–211.

REVUSKY, S., & DEVENUTO, F. Attempt to transfer aversion to saccharin solution by injection of DNA from trained to naive rats. *Journal of Biological Psychology*, 1967, **18**: 18–22.

REVUSKY, S., & GARCIA, J. Learned associations over long delays. In G. Bower and J. Spence (Eds.), *Psychology of learning and motivation: Advances in research and theory* (*vol 4*). New York: Academic Press, 1970.

REVUSKY, S., & GORRY, T. Flavor aversions produced by contingent drug injection: Relative effectiveness of apomorphine, emetine, and lithium. *Behaviour Research and Therapy*, 1973, **11**: 403-409.

REVUSKY, S., & PARKER, L. A. Aversions to unflavored water and cup drinking produced by delayed sickness. *Journal of Experimental Psychology: Animal Behavior Processes*, 1976, **2**: 342–353.

Revusky, S., Parker, L. A., & Coombes, S. Flavor aversion learning: Extinction of the aversion to an interfering flavor after conditioning does not affect the aversion to the reference flavor. *Behavioral Biology*, 1977, **19**: 503–508.

Revusky, S., Parker, L. A., Coombes, J., & Coombes, S. Rat data which suggest alcoholic beverages should be swallowed during chemical aversion therapy, not just tasted. *Behaviour Research and Therapy*, 1976, **14**: 189–194.

Revusky, S., Pohl, R. W., & Coombes, S. Flavor aversions and deprivation state. *Animal Learning & Behavior*, 1980, **8**: 543–549.

Revusky, S., & Taukulis, H. Effects of alcohol and lithium habituation on the development of alcohol aversions through contingent lithium injection. *Behaviour Research and Therapy*, 1975, **13**: 163–166.

Revusky, S., Taukulis, H. K., & Coombes, S. Dependence of the Avfail effect of the sequence of training operations *Behavioral and Neural Biology*, 1980, **29**: 430–445.

Revusky, S., Taukulis, H. K., Parker, L. A., & Coombes, S. Chemical aversion therapy: Rat data suggest it may be countertherapeutic to pair an addictive drug state with sickness. *Behaviour Research and Therapy*, 1979, **17**: 177–188.

Revusky, S., Taukulis, H. K., & Peddle, C. Learned associations between drug states: Attempted analysis in Pavlovian terms. *Physiological Psychology*, 1979, **7**: 352–363.

Riccio, D. C., & Haroutunian, V. Failure to learn in a taste aversion paradigm: Associative or performance deficit? *Bulletin of the Psychonomic Society*, 1977, **10**: 219–222.

Richter, C. P. Experimentally produced behavior reactions to food poisoning in wild and domesticated rats. *Annals of the New York Academy of Sciences*, 1953, **56**: 225–239.

Riege, W. H. Possible olfactory transduction of radiation-induced aversion. *Psychonomic Science*, 1968, **12**: 303–304.

Riege, W. H. Disruption of radiation-induced aversion to saccharin by electroconvulsive shock. *Physiology & Behavior*, 1969, **4**: 157–161.

Rigter, H., & Popping, A. Hormonal influences on the extinction of conditioned taste aversion. *Psychopharmacologia*, 1976, **46**: 255–261.

Riley, A. L. In response to and in defense of Mitchell and Revusky: An analysis of nonassociative effects. *Animal Learning & Behavior*, 1978, **6**: 472–473.

Riley, A. L., & Baril, L. L. Conditioned taste aversions: A bibliography. *Animal Learning & Behavior*, 1976, **4**: 1S–13S.

Riley, A. L., & Clarke, C. M. Conditioned taste aversions: A bibliography. In L. Barker, M. Best and M. Domjan (Eds.), *Learning mechanisms in food selection*. Waco, Texas: Baylor University Press, 1977.

Riley, A. L., Dacanay, R. J., & Mastropaolo, J. P. The effects of trimethyltin chloride on long-delay taste aversion learning in the rat. *Neurotoxicology*, 1984, **5**: 291–296.

Riley, A. L., Dacanay, R. J., & Mastropaolo, J. P. The effect of morphine preexposure on the acquisition of morphine-induced taste aversions: A nonassociative effect. *Animal Learning & Behavior*, 1984, **12**: 157–162.

Riley, A. L., Hyson, R. L., Baker, C. S., & Kulkosky, P. J. The interaction of conditioned taste aversions and schedule-induced polydipsia: Effects of repeated conditioning trials. *Animal Learning & Behavior*, 1980, **8**: 211–217.

Riley, A. L., Jacobs, W. J., & LoLordo, V. M. Drug exposure and the acquisition and retention of a conditioned taste aversion. *Journal of Comparative and Physiological Psychology*, 1976, **90**: 799–807.

Riley, A. L., Jacobs, W. J., Jr., & LoLordo, V. M. Morphine-induced taste aversions: A consideration of parameters. *Physiological Psychology*, 1978, **6**: 96–100.

Riley, A. L., Jacobs, W. J., Jr., & Mastropoalo, J. P. The effects of extensive taste preexposure on the acquisition of conditioned taste aversions. *Bulletin of the Psychonomic Society*, 1983, **21**: 221–224.

Riley, A. L., Lotter, E. C., & Kulkosky, P. J. The effects of conditioned taste aversions on the acquisition and maintenance of scheduled-induced polydipsia. *Animal Learning & Behavior*, 1979, **7**: 3–12.

RILEY, A. L., & LOVELY, R. H. Chlordiazepoxide-induced reversal of an amphetamine-established aversion: Dipsogenic effects. *Physiological Psychology*, 1978, **6**: 488–492.

RILEY, A. L., PEELE, D. B., RICHARD, K. D., & KULKOSKY, P. J. The interaction of conditioned taste aversions and schedule-induced polydipsia: Availability of alternative behaviors. *Animal Learning & Behavior*, 1981, **9**: 287–290.

RILEY, A. L., & TUCK, D. L. Conditioned taste aversions: A behavioral index of toxicity. *Annals of The New York Academy of Sciences*, 1985, **443**: 272–292.

RILEY, A. L., & TUCK, D. L. Conditioned food aversions: A bibliography. *Annals of The New York Academy of Sciences*, 1985, **443**: 381–437.

RILEY, A. L., & WAXMAN, G. I. The social relevance of psychological research on animals: Conditioned taste aversion in the giant mutant rat. *The Worm Runner's Digest*, 1975, **17**: 121–122.

RILEY, A. L., & ZELLNER, D. A. Methylphenidate-induced conditioned taste aversion: An index of toxicity. *Physiological Psychology*, 1978, **6**: 354–358.

RILEY, A. L., ZELLNER, D. A., & DUNCAN, H. J. The role of endorphins in animal learning and behavior. *Neuroscience & Biobehavioral Reviews*, 1980, **4**: 69–76.

RILEY, E. P., LOCHRY, E. A., & SHAPIRO, N. R. Lack of response inhibition in rats prenatally exposed to alcohol. *Psychopharmacology*, 1979, **62**: 47–52.

RITTER, S., MCGLONE, J. J., & KELLY, K. W. Absence of lithium-induced taste aversion after area postrema lesions. *Brain Research*, 1980, **201**: 501–506.

ROBBINS, R. J. Poison-based taste aversion learning in deer mice (*Peromyscus maniculatus Bairdi*). *Journal of Comparative and Physiological Psychology*, 1978, **92**: 642–650.

ROBBINS, R. J. The effect of flavor preexposure upon the acquisition and retention of poison-based taste aversions in deer mice: Latent inhibition or partial reinforcement? *Behavioral and Neural Biology*, 1979, **25**: 387–397.

ROBBINS, R. J. Sex affects the initial strength but not the extinction of poison-based taste aversions in deer mice (*Peromyscus maniculatus Bairdi*). *Behavioral and Neural Biology*, 1980, **30**: 80–89.

ROBBINS, R. J. Learning and nonlearned neophobia enhancement both contribute to the formation of illness-induced taste aversions by deer mice (*Peromyscus maniculatus Bairdi*). *Animal Learning & Behavior*, 1980, **8**: 534–542.

ROBBINS, R. J. Considerations in the design of test methods for measuring bait shyness. In E. Schafer and C. Walker (Eds.), *Third conference for vetebrate pest control and management materials.* New York: American Society for Testing and Materials, 1981.

ROBBINS, R. J. Taste-aversion learning and its implications for rodent control. In J. Clark (Ed.), *Proceedings ninth vertebrate pest conference.* Fresno, California, 1980.

ROBERTS, D. C. S., & FIBIGER, H. C. Attenuation of amphetamine-induced conditioned taste aversion following intraventricular 6-hydroxydopamine. *Neuroscience Letters*, 1975, **1**: 343–347.

ROBERTS, D. C. S., & FIBIGER, H. C. Lesions of the dorsal noradrenergic projection attenuate morphine but not amphetamine-induced conditioned taste aversion. *Psychopharmacology*, 1977, **55**: 183–186.

ROBERTSON, D., & GARRUD, P. Variable processing of flavors in rat STM. *Animal Learning & Behavior*, 1983, **11**: 474–482.

ROGERS, J. G. Some characteristics of conditioned aversion in redwinged blackbirds. *The Auk*, 1978, **95**: 362–369.

ROGERS, M. P., REICH, P., STROM, T. B., & CARPENTER, C. B. Behaviorally conditioned immunosuppression: Replication of a recent study. *Psychosomatic Medicine*, 1976, **38**: 447–451.

ROGERS, Q. R., & LEUNG, P. M. B. The control of food intake: When and how are amino acids involved? In M. Kare and O. Maller (eds.), *The chemical senses and nutrition.* New York: Academic Press, 1977.

ROHAN, W. A. A comparison of two aversion conditioning procedures for problem drinking. *Newsletter for Research in Psychology*, 1970, **12**: 14–15.

ROHLES, F. H., OVERALL, J. E., & BROWN, W. L. Attempts to produce spatial avoidance as a result of exposure to x-radiation. *British Journal of Radiology*, 1959, **32**: 224–246.

ROLL, D., SCHAEFFER, R. W., & SMITH, J. C. Effects of a conditioned taste aversion on schedule-induced polydipsia. *Psychonomic Science*, 1969, **16**: 39–41.

ROLL, D., & SMITH, J. C. Conditioned taste aversion in anesthetized rats. In M. Seligman and J. Hager (Eds.), *Biological boundaries of learning*. New York: Appleton-Century-Crofts, 1972.

ROLLS, B. J., & ROLLS, E. T. Effects of lesions in the basolateral amygdala on fluid intake in the rat. *Journal of Comparative and Physiological Psychology*, 1973, **83**: 240–247.

RONDEAU, D. B., JOLICOEUR, F. B., KACHANOFF, R., SCHERZER, P., & WAYNER, M. J. Effects of phenobarbital on ethanol intake in fluid deprived rats. *Pharmacology, Biochemistry & Behavior*, 1975, **3**: 493–497.

RONDEAU, D. B., JOLICOEUR, F. B., MERKEL, A. D., & WAYNER, M. J. Drugs and taste aversion. *Neuroscience & Biobehavioral Reviews*, 1981, **5**: 279–294.

RONDEAU, D. B., WAYNER, M. J., & JOLICOEUR, F. B. Modification of ethanol preference in the rat by chronic administration of phenobarbital. In F. Seixas (Ed.), *Currents in alcoholism (vol. I)*. New York: Grune and Stratton, 1977.

ROOKE, I. J. Conditioned aversion by silvereyes *Zosterops lateralis* to food treated with methiocarb. *Bird Behaviour*, 1983, **4**: 86–89.

ROTH, S. R., SCHWARTZ, M., & TEITLEBAUM, P. Failure of recovered lateral hypothalamic rats to learn specific food aversions. *Journal of Comparative and Physiological Psychology*, 1973, **83**: 184–197.

ROY, M. A., & BRIZZEE, K. R. Motion sickness-induced food aversions in the squirrel monkey. *Physiology & Behavior*, 1979, **23**: 39–41.

ROYET, J-P., & PAGER, J. Olfactory bulb responsiveness to an aversive or novel food odor in the unrestrained rat. *Brain Research Bulletin*, 1981, **7**: 375–378.

ROYET, J-P., & PAGER, J. Lesions of the olfactory pathways affecting neophobia and learned aversion differentially. *Behavioural Brain Research*, 1982, **4**: 251–262.

ROZIN, P. Thiamine specific hunger. In C. Code (Ed.), *Handbook of physiology (section G): Alimentary canal (vol I): Control of food and water intake*. Washington, D.C.: American Physiological Society, 1967.

ROZIN, P. Specific aversions as a component of specific hungers. *Journal of Comparative and Physiological Psychology*, 1967, **64**: 237–242.

ROZIN, P. Specific aversions and neophobia resulting from vitamin deficiency or poisoning in half-wild and domestic rats. *Journal of Comparative and Physiological Psychology*, 1968, **66**: 82–88.

ROZIN, P. Central or peripheral mediation of learning with long CS-US intervals in the feeding system. *Journal of Comparative and Physiological Psychology*, 1969, **67**: 421–429.

ROZIN, P. Adaptive food sampling patterns in vitamin deficient rats. *Journal of Comparative and Physiological Psychology*, 1969, **69**: 126–132.

ROZIN, R. Psychobiological and cultural determinants of food choice. In T. Silverstone (Ed.), *Appetite and food intake*. Berlin: Dahlem Konferenzen, 1976.

ROZIN, P. The selection of foods by rats, humans, and other animals. In J. Rosenblatt, R. Hinde, E. Shaw and C. Beer (Eds.), *Advances in the study of behavior (vol 6)*. New York: Academic Press, 1976.

ROZIN, P. The significance of learning mechanisms in food selection: Some biology, psychology and sociology of science. In L. Barker, M. Best and M. Domjan (Eds.), *Learning mechanisms in food selection*. Waco, Texas: Baylor University Press, 1977.

ROZIN, P., & KALAT, J. W. Specific hungers and poison avoidance as adaptive specializations of learning. *Psychological Review*, 1971, **78**: 459–486.

ROZIN, P., & KALAT, J. Learning as a situation-specific adaptation. In M. Seligman and J. Hager (Eds.), *Biological boundaries of learning*. New York: Appleton-Century-Crofts, 1972.

ROZIN, P., & REE, P. Long extension of effective CS-US interval by anesthesia between CS and US. *Journal of Comparative and Physiological Psychology*, 1972, **80**: 43–48.

ROZIN, P., & RODGERS, W. Novel-diet preferences in vitamin-deficient rats and rats recovered from vitamin deficiency. *Journal of Comparative and Physiological Psychology*, 1967, **63**: 421–428.

ROZIN, P., & ZELLNER, D. The role of Pavlovian conditioning in the acquisition of food likes and dislikes. *Annals of The New York Academy of Sciences*, 1985, **443**: 189–202.

RUDY, J. W., & CHEATLE, M. D. Odor-aversion learning in neonatal rats. *Science*, 1977, **198**: 845–846.

RUDY, J. W., & CHEATLE, M. D. A role for conditioned stimulus duration in toxiphobia conditioning. *Journal of Experimental Psychology: Animal Behavior Processes*, 1978, **4**: 399–411.

RUDY, J. W., & CHEATLE, M. D. Ontogeny of associative learning: Acquisition of odor aversions by neonatal rats. In N. Spear and B. Campbell (Eds.), *Ontogeny of learning and memory.* Hillsdale, New Jersey: Lawrence Erlbaum Associates, 1980.

RUDY, J. W., & CHEATLE, M. D. Odor-aversion learning by rats following LiCl exposure: Ontogenetic influences. *Developmental Psychobiology,* 1983, **16**: 13–22.

RUDY, J. W., IWENS, J., & BEST, P. J. Pairing novel exteroceptive cues and illness reduces illness-induced taste aversions. *Journal of Experimental Psychology: Animal Behavior Processes,* 1977, **3**: 14–25.

RUDY, J. W., ROSENBERG, L., & SANDELL, J. H. Disruption of a taste familiarity effect by novel exteroceptive stimulation. *Journal of Experimental Psychology: Animal Behavior Processes,* 1977, **3**: 26–36.

RUSAK, B., & ZUCKER, I. Fluid intake of rats in constant light and during feeding restricted to the light or dark portion of the illumination cycle. *Physiology & Behavior,* 1974, **13**: 91–100.

RUSINIAK, K. W., GARCIA, J., & HANKINS, W. G. Bait shyness: Avoidance of the taste without escape from the illness in rats. *Journal of Comparative and Physiological Psychology,* 1976, **90**: 460–467.

RUSINIAK, K. W., GARCIA, J., PALMERINO, C. C., & CABRAL, R. J. Developmental flavor experience affects utilization of odor, not taste in toxiphobic conditioning. *Behavioral and Neural Biology,* 1983, **39**: 160–180.

RUSINIAK, K. W., GUSTAVSON, C. R., HANKINS, W. G., & GARCIA, J. Prey-lithium aversions. II: Laboratory rats and ferrets. *Behavioral Biology,* 1976, **17**: 73–85.

RUSINIAK, K. W., HANKINS, W. G., GARCIA, J., & BRETT, L. P. Flavor-illness aversions: Potentiation of odor by taste in rats. *Behavioral and Neural Biology,* 1979, **25**: 1–17.

RUSINIAK, K. W., PALMERINO, C. C., & GARCIA, J. Potentiation of odor by taste in rats: Tests of some nonassociative factors. *Journal of Comparative and Physiological Psychology,* 1982, **96**: 775–780.

RUSINIAK, K. W., PALMERINO, C. C., RICE, A. G., FORTHMAN, D. L., & GARCIA, J. Flavor-illness aversions: Potentiation of odor by taste with toxin but not shock in rats. *Journal of Comparative and Physiological Psychology,* 1982, **96**: 527–539.

RZOSKA, J. Bait shyness, a study in rat behaviour. *The British Journal of Animal Behaviour,* 1953, **1**: 128–135.

RZOSKA, J. The behavior of white rats towards poison baits. In D. Chitty (Ed.), *Control of rats and mice (vol 2).* Oxford: Clarendon Press, 1954.

SACKS, L. B., & INGRAM, G. L. Covert sensitization as a treatment for weight control. *Psychological Reports,* 1972, **30**: 971–974.

SANDERS, B., COLLINS, A. C., & WESLEY, V. H. Reduction of alcohol selection by pargyline in mice. *Psychopharmacologia,* 1976, **46**: 159–162.

SANDOR, G., & KNOLL, J. The selectivity of the anorectic effect of satietin. II. Ineffectiveness of satietin on the water intake in food deprived rats. Effect of satietin in "conditioned aversion" paradigm. *Polish Journal of Pharmacology and Pharmacy,* 1982, **34**: 25–32.

SANGER, D. J., GREENSHAW, A. J., THOMPSON, I. P., & MERCER, J. D. Learned taste aversion to saccharin produced by orally consumed d-amphetamine. *Pharmacology, Biochemistry & Behavior,* 1980, **13**: 31–36.

SCARBOROUGH, B. B., & MCLAURIN, W. A. The effect of intraperitoneal injection of aversive behavior conditioning with x-irradiation. *Radiation Research,* 1961, **15**: 829–835.

SCARBOROUGH, B. B., & MCLAURIN, W. A. Saccharin avoidance conditioning instigated immediately after the exposure period. *Radiation Research,* 1964, **21**: 299–307.

SCARBOROUGH, B. B., WHALEY, D. L., & ROGERS, J. G. Saccharin avoidance behavior instigated by x-irradiation in backward conditioning paradigms. *Psychological Reports,* 1964, **14**: 475–481.

SCHACHTMAN, T. R., KASPROW, W. J., & MILLER, R. R. Reminder treatments do not alleviate cue-to-consequence deficits. *Animal Learning & Behavior,* 1984, **12**: 97–105.

SCHAEFFER, A. A. Habit formation in frogs. *Journal of Animal Behavior,* 1911, **1**: 309–335.

SCHAEFFER, R. W., HUNT, E. L., & KIMELDORF, D. J. Application of Premack's theory to a classically conditioned sucrose aversion induced by x-ray exposure. *The Psychological Record,* 1967, **17**: 359–367.

SCHAEFFER, R. W., & SMITH, J. C. Lick rates in rats exposed to gamma-irradiation. *Psychonomic Science,* 1966, **6**: 201–202.

SCHMALTZ, G., & MARCANT, P. Transient aversion and long-lasting amnesia following cycloheximide injection in the rat. *Physiology & Behavior*, 1983, **30**: 845–852.

SCHNEIDER, K., & WOTHE, K. The contribution of naso-oral and postingestional factors in taste aversion learning in the rat. *Behavioral and Neural Biology*, 1979, **25**: 30–38.

SCHOENFELD, T. A., & HAMILTON, L. W. Disruption of appetite but not hunger or satiety following small lesions in the amygdala of rats. *Journal of Comparative and Physiological Psychology*, 1981, **95**: 565–587.

SCHWARTZ, M., & TEITELBAUM, P. Dissociation between learning and remembering in rats with lesions in the lateral hypothalamus. *Journal of Comparative and Physiological Psychology*, 1974, **87**: 384–398.

SCHWEITZER, L., & GREEN, L. Acquisition and extended retention of a conditioned taste aversion in preweanling rats. *Journal of Comparative and Physiological Psychology*, 1982, **96**: 791–806.

SCLAFANI, A., ARAVICH, P. F., & SCHWARTZ, J. Hypothalamic hyperphagic rats overeat bitter sucrose octa acetate diets but not quinine diets. *Physiology & Behavior*, 1979, **22**: 759–766.

SCLAFANI, A., & KOOPMANS, H. S. Intestinal bypass surgery produces conditioned taste aversion in rats. *International Journal of Obesity*, 1981, **5**: 497–500.

SCRIMA, L., COREY, D. T., & CHOO, A. F. Interanimal transferability of taste aversion learning for 0.1% saccharin. *International Journal of Neuroscience*, 1982, **16**: 135–142.

SELIGMAN, M. E. P., & HAGER, J. L. Biological boundaries of learning: The sauce-bearnaise syndrome. *Psychology Today*, 1972, **6**: 59–61.

SEMENOV, L., BURESOVA, O., & BURES, J. Conditioned taste aversion induced in rats by unilateral chemical blockade or electrical stimulation of vestibular nuclei. *Physiologia Bohemoslovaca*, 1982, **31**: 279–280.

SENGSTAKE, C. B., & CHAMBERS, K. C. Differential effects of fluid deprivation on the acquisition and extinction phases of a conditioned taste aversion. *Bulletin of the Psychonomic Society*, 1979, **14**: 85–87.

SENGSTAKE, C. B., CHAMBERS, K. C., & THROWER, J. H. Interactive effects of fluid deprivation and testosterone on the expression of a sexually dimorphic conditioned taste aversion. *Journal of Comparative and Physiological Psychology*, 1978, **92**: 1150–1155.

SESSIONS, G. R. Histamine and radiation-induced taste aversion conditioning. *Science*, 1975, **190**: 402–403.

SESSIONS, G. R., KANT, G. J., & KOOB, G. F. Locus coeruleus lesions and learning in the rat. *Physiology & Behavior*, 1976, **17**: 853–859.

SEWARD, J. P., & GREATHOUSE, S. R. Appetitive and aversive conditioning in thiamine-deficient rats. *Journal of Comparative and Physiological Psychology*, 1973, **83**: 157–167.

SHAW, N. Taste aversion learning: Simulation of interference with the gustatory cue during conditioning. *Behavioral and Neural Biology*, 1983, **38**: 307–312.

SHAW, N., & WEBSTER, D. M. Disruption of taste aversion learning by penthylenetetrazol. *Psychopharmacology*, 1979, **66**: 195–198.

SHAW, N., & WEBSTER, D. M. ECS and CO_2 anesthesia between tasting and illness: Effects on taste aversion learning. *Behavioral and Neural Biology*, 1980, **28**: 231–235.

SHAW, N., & WEBSTER, D. M. Disruption of conditioned taste aversion by the combined effects of LiCl and ECS. *Physiology & Behavior*, 1982, **29**: 755–757.

SHERMAN, J. E., HICKIS, C. F., RICE, A. G., RUSINIAK, K. W., & GARCIA, J. Preferences and aversions for stimuli paired with ethanol in hungry rats. *Animal Learning & Behavior*, 1983, **11**: 101–106.

SHERMAN, J. E., PICKMAN, C., RICE, A., LIEBESKIND, J. C., & HOLMAN, E. W. Rewarding and aversive effects of morphine: Temporal and pharmacological properties. *Pharmacology, Biochemistry & Behavior*, 1980, **13**: 501–505.

SHERMAN, J. E., ROBERTS, T., ROSKAM, S. E., & HOLMAN, E. W. Temporal properties of the rewarding and aversive effects of amphetamine in rats. *Pharmacology, Biochemistry & Behavior*, 1980, **13**: 597–599.

SHERMAN, J., RUSINIAK, K. W., & GARCIA, J. Alcohol-ingestive habits: The role of flavor and effect. In M. Galanter (Ed.), *Recent developments in alcoholism* (*vol. 2*). New York: Plenum Press, 1984.

SHETTLEWORTH, S. J. Stimulus relevance in the control of drinking and conditioned fear re-

sponses in domestic chicks (*Gallus gallus*). *Journal of Comparative and Physiological Psychology*, 1972, **80**: 175–198.
SHETTLEWORTH, S. J. The role of novelty in learned avoidance of unpalatable 'prey' by domestic chicks (*Gallus gallus*). *Animal Behaviour*, 1972, **20**: 29–35.
SHIMAI, S., & HOSHISHIMA, K. Effects of bilateral amygdala lesions on neophobia and conditioned taste aversion in mice. *Perception and Motor Skills*, 1982, **54**: 127–130.
SHIPLEY, J. E., & KOLB, B. Neural correlates of species-typical behavior in the Syrian golden hamster. *Journal of Comparative and Physiological Psychology*, 1977, **91**: 1056–1073.
SHORTEN, M. The reaction of the brown rat towards changes in its environment. In D. Chitty (Ed.), *Control of rats and mice* (*vol 2*). Oxford: Clarendon Press, 1954.
SHUMAKE, S. A., STERNER, R. T., GADDIS, S. E., & CRANE, K. A. Conditioned taste aversion in Philippine rice rats (*R. r. mindanensis*): Comparisons among drugs, dosages, modes of administration, and sexes. *Animal Learning & Behavior*, 1982, **10**: 499–504.
SIEGEL, J. L. Effect of medial septal lesions on conditioned taste aversion in the rat. *Physiology & Behavior*, 1976, **17**: 761–765.
SIEGEL, S. Flavor preexposure and "learned safety." *Journal of Comparative and Physiological Psychology*, 1974, **87**: 1073–1082.
SIEGEL, S. Pharmacological and toxicological assessments using conditioned food aversion methodology. *Annals of The New York Academy of Sciences*, 1985, **443**: 227–230.
SIMSON, P. C., & BOOTH, D. A. Olfactory conditioning by association with histidine-free or balanced amino acid loads in rats. *Quarterly Journal of Experimental Psychology*, 1973, **25**: 354–359.
SIMSON, P. C., & BOOTH, D. A. Dietary aversion established by a deficient load: Specificity to the amino acid omitted from a balanced mixture. *Pharmacology, Biochemistry & Behavior*, 1974, **2**: 481–485.
SIMSON, P. C., & BOOTH, D. A. The rejection of a diet which has been associated with a single administration of an histidine-free amino acid mixture. *British Journal of Nutrition*, 1974, **31**: 285–296.
SINYOR, D., SWITZMAN, L., & AMIT, Z. ACTH potentiates morphine-induced conditioned taste aversion. *Neuropharmacology*, 1980, **19**: 971–973.
SJODEN, P-O., & ARCHER, T. Conditioned taste aversion to saccharin induced by 2,4,5-trichlorophenoxyacetic acid in albino rats. *Physiology & Behavior*, 1977, **19**: 159–161.
SJODEN, P-O., & ARCHER, T. Associative and nonassociative effects of exteroceptive context in taste-aversion conditioning with rats. *Behavioral and Neural Biology*, 1981, **33**: 71–92.
SJODEN, P-O., & ARCHER, T. Potentiation of a bottle aversion by taste in compound conditioning with rats. *Experimental Animal Behaviour*, 1983, **2**: 1–18.
SJODEN, P-O., ARCHER, T., & CARTER, N. Conditioned taste aversion induced by 2,4,5-trichlorophenoxyacetic acid: Dose-response and preexposure effects. *Physiological Psychology*, 1979, **7**: 93–96.
SJODEN, P-O., & SODERBERG, T. Taste-aversion learning: An operant approach. In C. Bradshaw, E. Szabadi and C. Lowe (Eds.), *Quantification of steady-state operant behaviour*. Amsterdam: Elsevier North Holland Press, 1981.
SKLAR, L. S., & AMIT, Z. Manipulations of catecholamine systems block the conditioned taste aversion induced by self-administered drugs. *Neuropharmacology*, 1977, **16**: 649–655.
SLOTNICK, B. M., BROWN, D. L., & GELHARD, R. Contrasting effects of location and taste cues in illness-induced aversion. *Physiology & Behavior*, 1977, **18**: 333–335.
SLY, J., & BELL, F. R. Effect of lithium intake on sodium and lithium appetite in sodium deficient cattle. *Physiology & Behavior*, 1981, **27**: 147–152.
SMITH, D. F. Learned aversion and rearing movements in rats given LiCl, PbC12 or NaCl. *Experientia*, 1978, **34**: 1200–1201.
SMITH, D. F. Central and peripheral effects of lithium on conditioned taste aversions in rats. *Psychopharmacology*, 1980. **68**: 315–317.
SMITH, D. F. Lithium and carbamazepine: Effects on learned taste aversion and open field behavior in rats. *Pharmacology, Biochemistry & Behavior*, 1983, **18**: 483–488.
SMITH, D. F., & BALAGURA S. Role of oropharyngeal factors in LiCl aversion. *Journal of Comparative and Physiological Psychology*, 1969, **69**: 308–310.
SMITH, D. F., BALAGURA, S., & LUBRAN, M. Some effects of adrenalectomy on LiCl and excre-

tion in the rat. *American Journal of Physiology*, 1970, **218**: 751–754.

SMITH, D. V., TRAVERS, J. B., & VAN BUSKIRK, R. L. Brainstem correlates of gustatory similarity in the hamster. *Brain Research Bulletin*, 1979, **4**: 359–372.

SMITH, F. J., CHARNOCK, D. J., & WESTBROOK, R. F. Odor-aversion learning in neonate rat pups: The role of duration of exposure to an odor. *Behavioral and Neural Biology*, 1983, **37**: 284–301.

SMITH, G. P., GIBBS, J., & KULKOSKY, P. J. Relationships between brain-gut peptides and neurons in the control of food intake. In B. Hoebel and D. Novin (Eds.), *The neural basis of feeding and reward*. Brunswick, ME: Haer Institute, 1982.

SMITH, J. C., LEVIN, B. E., & ERVIN, G. N. Loss of active avoidance of responding after lateral hypothalamic injections of 6-hydroxydopamine. *Brain Research*, 1975, **88**: 483–498.

SMITH, J. C. Radiation: Its detection and its effects on taste preferences. In J. Sprague and A. Epstein (Eds.), *Progress in physiological psychology* (*vol. 4*). New York: Academic Press, 1971.

SMITH, J. C. Comment on paper by Mitchell, Scott, and Mitchell. *Animal Learning & Behavior*, 1978, **6**: 117–118.

SMITH, J. C., & BIRKLE, R. A. Conditioned aversion to sucrose in rats using x-rays as the unconditioned stimulus. *Psychonomic Science*, 1966, **5**: 271–272.

SMITH, J. C. & BLUMSACK, J. T. Learned taste aversion as a factor in cancer therapy. *Cancer Treatment Reports*, 1981, **65**: 37–42.

SMITH, J. C., BLUMSACK, J. T., BILEK, F. S., SPECTOR, A. C., HOLLANDER, G. R., & BAKER, D. L. Radiation-induced taste aversion as a factor in cancer therapy. *Cancer Treatment Reports*, in press.

SMITH, J. C., HOLLANDER, G. R., & SPECTOR, A. C. Taste aversions conditioned with partial body radiation exposures. *Physiology & Behavior*, 1981, **27**: 903–913.

SMITH, J. C., & MORRIS, D. D. Effects of atropine sulfate on the conditioned aversion to saccharin fluid with x-rays as the unconditioned stimulus. *Radiation Research*, 1963, **18**: 186–190.

SMITH, J. C., & MORRIS, D. D.The use of x rays as the unconditioned stimulus in five-hundred-day-old rats. *Journal of Comparative and Physiological Psychology*, 1963, **56**: 746–747.

SMITH, J. C., & MORRIS, D. D. The effects of atropine sulfate and physostigmine on the conditioned aversion to saccharin solution with x-rays as the unconditioned stimulus. In T. Haley and R. Snider (eds.), *Response of the nervous system to ionizing radiation*. New York: Little Brown, 1964.

SMITH, J. C., MORRIS, D. D., & HENDRICKS, J. Conditioned aversion to saccharin solution with high dose rates of x-rays as the unconditioned stimulus. *Radiation Research*, 1964, **22**: 507–510.

SMITH, J. C., & ROLL, D. L. Trace conditioning with x-rays as an aversive stimulus. *Psychonomic Science*, 1967, **9**: 11–12.

SMITH, J. C., & SCHAEFFER, R. W. Development of water and saccharin preferences after simultaneous exposures to saccharin solution and gamma rays. *Journal of Comparative and Physiological Psychology*, 1967, **63**: 434–438.

SMITH, J. C., TAYLOR, H. L., MORRIS, D. D., & HENDRICKS, J. Further studies of x-ray conditioned saccharin aversion during the postexposure period. *Radiation Research*, 1965, **24**: 423–431.

SMITH, R. G. The role of alimentary chemoreceptors in the development of taste aversions. *Communications in Behavioral Biology*, 1970, **5**: 199–204.

SMITH, R. G. Intake differentiation by rats of equimolar sodium chloride and lithium chloride solutions. *Psychonomic Science*, 1971, **23**: 11–12.

SMOTHERMAN, W. P. Odor aversion learning by the rat fetus. *Physiology & Behavior*, 1982, **29**: 769–771.

SMOTHERMAN, W. P. Glucocorticoid and other hormonal substrates of conditioned taste aversion. *Annals of The New York Academy of Sciences*, 1985, **443**: 126–144.

SMOTHERMAN, W. P., BURT, G., KIMBLE, D. P., STICKROD, G., BREMILLER, R., & LEVINE, S. Behavioral and corticosterone effects in conditioned taste aversions following hippocampal lesions. *Physiology & Behavior*, 1981, **27**: 569–574.

SMOTHERMAN, W. P., HENNESSY, J. W., & LEVINE, S. Plasma corticosterone levels during recovery from LiCl produced taste aversions. *Behavioral Biology*, 1976, **16**: 401–412.

SMOTHERMAN, W. P., HENNESSY, J. W., & LEVINE, S. Plasma corticosterone levels as an index of the strength of illness induced taste aversions. *Physiology & Behavior*, 1976, **17**: 903–908.

SMOTHERMAN, W. P., KOLP, L. A., COYLE, S., & LEVINE, S. Hippocampal lesion effects on conditioned taste aversion and pituitary-adrenal activity in rats. *Behavioural Brain Research*, 1981, **2**: 33–48.

SMOTHERMAN, W. P., & LEVINE, S. ACTH and ACTH4–10 modification of neophobia and taste aversion responses in the rat. *Journal of Comparative and Physiological Psychology*, 1978, **92**: 22–33.

SMOTHERMAN, W. P., & LEVINE, S. ACTH4–10 affects behavior but not plasma corticosterone levels in a conditioned taste aversion situation. *Peptides*, 1980, **1**: 207–210.

SMOTHERMAN, W. P., MARGOLIS, A., & LEVINE, S. Flavor preexposures in a conditioned taste aversion situation: A dissociation of behavioral and endocrine effects in rats. *Journal of Comparative and Physiological Psychology*, 1980, **94**: 25–35.

SNYDER, D. R., & BRAUN, J. J. Dissociation between behavioral and physiological indices of organomercurial ingestion. *Toxicology and Applied Pharmacology*, 1977, **41**: 277–284.

SOUTHERN, N. H. *Control of rats and mice* (*vol 3*). Oxford: Clarendon Press, 1954.

SPARENBORG, S. P., BUSKIST, W. F., MILLER, H. L., JR., FLEMING, D. E., & DUNCAN, P. C. Attenuation of taste aversion conditioning in rats recovered from thiamine deficiency: Atropine vs. lithium toxicosis. *Bulletin of the Psychonomic Society*, 1982, **17**: 237–239.

SPEAR, N. E., HAMBERG, J. M., & BRYAN, R. Forgetting of recently acquired or recently reactivated memories. *Learning and Motivation*, 1980, **11**: 456–475.

SPEAR, N. E., KUCHARSKI, D., & HOFFMAN, H. Contextual influences on conditioned taste aversions in the developing rat. *Annals of The New York Academy of Sciences*, 1985, **443**: 42–53.

SPECTOR, A. C., SMITH, J. C., & HOLLANDER, G. R. A comparison of dependent measures used to quantify radiation-induced taste aversion. *Physiology & Behavior*, 1981, **27**: 887–901.

SPECTOR, A. C., SMITH, J. C., & HOLLANDER, G. R. The effect of postconditioning CS experience on recovery from radiation-induced taste aversion. *Physiology & Behavior*, 1983, **30**: 647–649.

SPEERS, M. A., GILLAN, D. J., & RESCORLA, R. A. Within-compound associations in a variety of compound conditioning procedures. *Learning and Motivation*, 1980, **11**: 135–149.

SPIKER, V. A. Taste aversion: A procedural analysis and an alternative paradigmatic classification. *The Psychological Record*, 1977, **27**: 753–769.

SPRINGER, A. D., & FRALEY, S. M. Extinction of a conditioned taste aversion in young, midaged, and aged C57:BL6 mice. *Behavioral and Neural Biology*, 1981, **32**: 282–294.

SRIDHARA, S., & SRIDHARI, K. Bait shyness towards zinc phosphide & vacor in the larger bandicoot rat *Bandicota indica*. *Indian Journal of Experimental Biology*, 1980, **18**: 1029–1031.

STAPLETON, J. M., LIND, M. D., MERRIMAN, V. J., BOZARTH, M. A., & REID, L. D. Affective consequences and subsequent effects on morphine self-administration of d-ala^2-methionine enkephalin. *Physiological Psychology*, 1979, **7**: 146–152.

STEIN, J. M., WAYNER, M. J., & TILSON, H. A. The effect of parachlorphenylalanine on the intake of ethanol and saccharin solutions. *Pharmacology, Biochemistry & Behavior*, 1977, **6**: 117–122.

STEINBERG, H., & MCMILLAN, T. M. Lithium and reduced consumption of drugs of abuse. In F. Johnson and S. Johnson (Eds.), *Lithium in medical practice*. Lancaster: MTP Press Ltd., 1978.

STEINERT, P. A., INFURNA, R. N., JARDULA, M. F., & SPEAR, N. E. Effects of CS concentration on long-delay taste aversion learning in preweanling and adult rats. *Behavioral and Neural Biology*, 1979, **27**: 487–502.

STEINERT, P. A., INFURNA, R. N., & SPEAR, N. E. Long-term retention of a conditioned taste aversion in preweanling and adult rats. *Animal Learning & Behavior*, 1980, **8**: 375–381.

STERNER, R. T., & SHUMAKE, S. A. Bait-induced prey aversions in predators: Some methodological issues. *Behavioral Biology*, 1978, **22**: 565–566.

STEWART, J., & EIKELBOOM, R. Pre-exposure to morphine and the attenuation of conditioned taste aversion in rats. *Pharmacology, Biochemistry & Behavior*, 1978, **9**: 639–645.

STICKROD, G., KIMBLE, D. P., & SMOTHERMAN, W. P. Met-enkephalin effects on associations formed *in utero*. *Peptides*, 1982, **3**: 881–883.

STICKROD, G., KIMBLE, D. P., & SMOTHERMAN, W. P. In utero taste-odor aversion conditioning in the rat. *Physiology & Behavior*, 1982, **28**: 5–7.

STIERHOFF, K. A., & LAVIN, M. J. The influence of rendering rats anosmic on the poisoned-partner effect. *Behavioral and Neural Biology*, 1982, **34**: 180–189.

STOLERMAN, I. P., & D'MELLO, G. D. Amphetamine-induced taste aversions demonstrated with operant behaviour. *Pharmacology, Biochemistry & Behavior,* 1978, **8**: 107–111.

STOLERMAN, I. P., & D'MELLO, G. D. Amphetamine-induced hypodipsia and its implications for conditioned taste aversion in rats. *Pharmacology, Biochemistry & Behavior,* 1978, **8**: 333–338.

STOLERMAN, I. P., & D'MELLO, G. D. Conditioned taste aversion induced with apomorphine and an apomorphine analogue in rats. *Experimental Brain Research,* 1979, **36**: 22–23.

STOLERMAN, I. P., & D'MELLO, G. D. Oral self-administration and the relevance of conditioned taste aversions. In T. Thompson and P. Dews (Eds.), *Advances in behavioral pharmacology (vol. 3).* New York: Academic Press, 1981.

STOLERMAN, I. P., PILCHER, C. W. T., & D'MELLO, G. D. Aversive properties of narcotic antagonists in rats. *Neuropharmacology,* 1978, **17**: 427.

STOLERMAN, I. P., PILCHER, C. W. T., & D'MELLO, G. D. Stereospecific aversive property of narcotic antagonists in morphine-free rats. *Life Sciences,* 1978, **22**: 1755–1762.

ST. OMER, V. V., & KRAL, P. A. Electroconvulsive shock impedes the learning of taste aversions: Absence of blood-brain-barrier involvement. *Psychonomic Science,* 1971, **24**: 251–252.

STRICKER, E. M., & WILSON, N. E. Salt-seeking behavior in rats following acute sodium deficiency. *Journal of Comparative and Physiological Psychology,* 1970, **72**: 416–420.

STRICKER, E. M., & ZIGMOND, M. J. Effects on homeostasis of intraventricular injections of 6-hydroxydopamine in rats. *Journal of Comparative and Physiological Psychology,* 1974, **86**: 973–994.

STROM, C., LINGENFELTER, A., & BRODY, J. F. Discrimination of lithium and sodium chloride solutions by rats. *Pyschonomic Science,* 1970, **18**: 290–291.

STUNKARD, A. Presidential address-1974: From explanation to action in psychosomatic medicine: The case of obesity. *Psychosomatic Medicine,* 1975, **37**: 195–236.

STUNKARD, A. Satiety is a conditioned reflex. *Psychosomatic Medicine,* 1975, **37**: 383–387.

SUAREZ, E. M., & BARKER, L. M. Effects of water deprivation and prior LiCl exposure in conditioning taste aversions. *Physiology & Behavior,* 1976, **17**: 555–559.

SULLIVAN, L. G. Transfer of conditioning with an exteroceptive reinforcer to a new environment. *Australian Journal of Psychology,* 1981, **33**: 215–227.

SUPAK, T. D., MACRIDES, F., & CHOROVER, S. L. The bait-shyness effect extended to olfactory discrimination. *Communications in Behavioral Biology,* 1971, **5**: 321–324.

SUTKER, L. W. The effect of initial taste preference on subsequent radiation-induced aversive conditioning to saccharin solution. *Psychonomic Science,* 1971, **25**: 1–2.

SWITZMAN, L., AMIT, Z., WHITE, N., & FISHMAN, B. Novel-tasting food enhances morphine discrimination in rats. In F. Colpert and J. Rosecranz (Eds.), *Stimulus properties of drugs: Ten years of progress.* Amsterdam: Elsevier North Holland Press, 1978.

SWITZMAN, L., FISHMAN, B., & AMIT, Z. Pre-exposure effects of morphine, diazepam and delta-9-THC on the formation of conditioned taste aversions. *Psychopharmacology,* 1981, **74**: 149–157.

SWITZMAN, L., HUNT, T., & AMIT, Z. Heroin and morphine: Aversive and analgesic effects in rats. *Pharmacology, Biochemistry & Behavior,* 1981, **15**: 755–759.

TAPPER, D. N., & HALPERN, B. P. Taste stimuli: A behavioral categorization. *Science,* 1968, **161**: 708–710.

TARPY, R. M., & MACINTOSH, S. M. Generalized latent inhibition in taste-aversion learning. *Bulletin of the Psychonomic Society,* 1977, **10**: 379–381.

TAUKULIS, H. K. Thyrotropin-releasing hormone (TRH) potentiates pentobarbital-based flavor aversion learning. *Behavioral and Neural Biology,* 1983, **39**: 135–139.

TAUKULIS, H., & ST. GEORGE, S. Overshadowing of environmental cues by an odor in toxicosis-based conditioning in rats. *Animal Learning & Behavior,* 1982, **10**: 288–292.

TAUKULIS, H. K., & REVUSKY, S. Odor as a conditioned inhibitor: Applicability of the Rescorla-Wagner model to feeding behavior. *Learning and Motivation,* 1975, **6**: 11–27.

TERK, M. P., & GREEN, L. Taste aversion learning in the bat, *Carollia perspicillata. Behavioral and Neural Biology,* 1980, **28**: 236–242.

TERNES, J. W. Circadian cyclic sensitivity to gamma radiation as an unconditioned stimulus in taste aversion conditioning. In L. Sheving, F. Halberg and J. Pauly (Eds.), *Chronobiology.* Tokyo: Igaku Shoin, LTD, 1974.

TERNES, J. W. Conditioned aversion to morphine with naloxone. *Bulletin of the Psychonomic Society* 1975, **5**: 292–294.

TERNES, J. W. Resistance to extinction of a learned taste aversion varies with time of conditioning. *Animal Learning & Behavior*, 1976, **4**: 317–321.

TESTA, T. J., & TERNES, J. W. Specificity of conditioning mechanisms in the modification of food preferences. In L. Barker, M. Best and M. Domjan (Eds.), *Learning mechanisms in food selection*. Waco, Texas: Baylor University Press, 1977.

THIMANN, J. Conditioned reflex treatment of alcoholism. II. The risk of its application, its indications, contraindications and psychotherapeutic aspects. *New England Journal of Medicine*, 1949, **241**: 408–410.

THOMAS, J. B., & SMITH, D. A. VMH lesions facilitate baitshyness in the rat. *Physiology & Behavior*, 1975, **15**: 7–11.

THOMPSON, C. I., & ZAGON, I. S. 2-deoxy-d-glucose produces delayed hypophagia and conditioned taste aversion in rats. *Physiology & Behavior*, 1981, **27**: 1001–1004.

THOMKA, M. L., & BROWN, T. S. The effect of hippocampal lesions on the development and extinction of a learned taste aversion for a novel food. *Physiological Psychology*, 1975, **3**: 281–284.

TIMM, R., & CONNOLY, G. How coyotes kill sheep. *Rangeman's Journal*, 1977, **4**: 106–107.

TON, J. M., & AMIT, Z. Symmetrical effect of pre-exposure between alcohol and morphine on conditioned taste aversion. *Life Sciences*, 1983, **33**: 665–670.

TRENEER, C. M., & BERNSTEIN, I. L. Learned aversions in rats fed a tryptophan-free diet. *Physiology & Behavior*, 1981, **27**: 757–760.

TRISCARI, J., & SULLIVAN, A. Studies on the mechanism of action of a novel anorectic agent, (−)-threo-chlorocitric acid. *Pharmacology, Biochemistry & Behavior*, 1981, **15**: 311–318.

TUCKER, A., & GIBBS, M. Cycloheximide-induced amnesia for taste aversion memory in rats. *Pharmacology, Biochemistry & Behavior*, 1976, **4**: 181–184.

TUCKER, A. R., & GIBBS, M. E. Saccharin aversion memory in rats: Inhibition of cycloheximide-resistant memory by Ouabain. *Physiology & Behavior*, 1979, **23**: 341–346.

TUCKER, A. R., & OIE, T. P. Protein synthesis inhibition and amnesia for saccharin aversion memory in rats after intracisternal administration of cycloheximide. *Physiology & Behavior*, 1982, **28**: 1025–1028.

UNGERER, A., MARCHI, D., ROPARTZ, P., & WEIL, J. H. Aversive effects and retention impairment induced by acetoxycycloheximide in an instrumental task. *Physiology & Behavior*, 1975, **15**: 55–62.

VAN BUSKIRK, R. L. The role of odor in the maintenance of flavor aversion. *Physiology & Behavior*, 1981, **27**: 189–193.

VAN DER KOOY, D. Area postrema: Site where cholecystokinin acts to decrease food intake. *Brain Research*, 1984, **295**: 345–347.

VAN DER KOOY, D., O'SHAUGHNESSY, M., MUCHA, R. F., & KALANT, H. Motivational properties of ethanol in naive rats as studied by place conditioning. *Pharmacology, Biochemistry & Behavior*, 1983, **19**: 441–445.

VAN DER KOOY, D., & PHILLIPS, A. G. Temporal analysis of naloxone attenuation of morphine-induced taste aversion. *Pharmacology, Biochemistry & Behavior*, 1977, **6**: 637–641.

VAN DER KOOY, D., SWERDLOW, N. R., & KOOB, G. F. Paradoxical reinforcing properties of apomorphine: Effects of nucleus accumbens and area postrema lesions. *Brain Research*, 1983, **259**: 2087–2094.

VAWTER, M. P., & GREEN, K. F. Effects of desglycinamide-lysine vasopressin on a conditioned taste aversion in rats. *Physiology & Behavior*, 1980, **25**: 851–854.

VENKATAKRISHNA-BHATT, H., BURES, J., & BURESOVA, O. Differential effect of paradoxical sleep deprivation on acquisition and retrieval of conditioned taste aversion in rats. *Physiology & Behavior*, 1978, **20**: 101–107.

VENKATAKRISHNA-BHATT, H., BURES, J., & BURESOVA, O. Paradoxical sleep deprivation retards extinction of conditioned taste aversion. *Behavioral and Neural Biology*, 1979, **25**: 133–137.

VILA, J., & COLOTLA, V. A. Some stimulus properties of inhalants: Preliminary findings. *Neurobehavioral Toxicology and Teratology*, 1981, **3**: 477–480.

VITIELLO, M. V., & WOODS, S. C. Evidence for withdrawal from caffeine by rats. *Pharmacology, Biochemistry & Behavior*, 1977, **6**: 553–555.

VOEGTLIN, W. L. The treatment of alcoholism by establishing a conditioned reflex. *American Journal of the Medical Sciences*, 1940, **199**: 802–809.

VOEGTLIN, W. L. Conditioned reflex therapy of chronic alcoholism: Ten years experience with the method. *Rocky Mountain Medical Journal*, 1947, **44**: 807–812.

VOGEL, J. R. Antagonism of a learned taste aversion following repeated administrations of electroconvulsive shock. *Physiological Psychology*, 1974, **2**: 493–496.

VOGEL, J. R., & CLODY, D. E. Habituation and conditioned food aversion. *Psychonomic Science*, 1972, **28**: 275–276.

VOGEL, J. R., & NATHAN, B. A. Learned taste aversions induced by hypnotic drugs. *Pharmacology, Biochemistry & Behavior*, 1975, **3**: 189–194.

VOGEL, J. R., & NATHAN, B. A. Learned taste aversions induced by high doses of monosodium l-glutamate. *Pharmacology, Biochemistry & Behavior*, 1975, **3**: 935–937.

VOGEL, J. R., & NATHAN, B. A. Reduction of learned taste aversions by pre-exposure to drugs. *Psychopharmacology*, 1976, **49**: 167–172.

WAGNER, G. C., FOLTIN, R. W., SEIDEN, L. S., & SCHUSTER, C. R. Dopamine depletion by 6-hydroxydopamine prevents conditioned taste aversion induced by methylamphetamine but not lithium chloride. *Pharmacology, Biochemistry & Behavior*, 1981, **14**: 85–88.

WALLACE, P. Animal behavior: The puzzle of flavor aversion. *Science*, 1976, **193**: 989–991.

WALTERS, J. K. Effects of PCPA on the consumption of alcohol, water and other solutions. *Pharmacology, Biochemistry & Behavior*, 1977, **6**: 377–383.

WATSON, J. S. Control of the ship rat (*Rattus rattus*) in London. In D. Chitty (Ed.), *Control of rats and mice* (*vol 2*). Oxford: Clarendon Press, 1954.

WATSON, J. S., & PERRY, J. S. Experiments on rat control in Palestine and the Sudan. In D. Chitty (Ed.), *Control of rats and mice* (*vol 2*). Oxford: Clarendon Press, 1954.

WAYNER, E. A., FLANNERY, G. R., & SINGER, G. Effects of taste aversion conditioning on the primary antibody response to sheep red blood cells and *Brucella abortus* in the albino rat. *Physiology & Behavior*, 1978, **21**: 995–1000.

WAYNER, E. A., SINGER, G., WAYNER, M. J., & BARONE, F. The effects of several barbs on LiCl induced taste aversions. *Pharmacology, Biochemistry & Behavior*, 1980, **12**: 803–806.

WAYNER, E. A., SINGER, G., WAYNER, M. J., & BARONE, F. C. The taste aversion induction properties of two long duration barbiturates. *Pharmacology, Biochemistry & Behavior*, 1980, **12**: 807–810.

WAYNER, M. J., JOLICOEUR, F. B., RONDEAU, D. B., & MERKEL, A. D. The effect of sodium phenobarbitol on forced and voluntary consumption in the rat. In J. Sinclair and K. Kianmaa (Eds.), *The effects of centrally acting drugs on voluntary alcohol consumption*. Helsinki: The Finnish Foundation for Alcohol Studies, 1975.

WAYNER, M. J., RONDEAU, D. B., JOLICOEUR, F. B., & WAYNER, E. A. Effects of phenobarbitol on saccharin and citric acid intake in fluid deprived rats. *Pharmacology, Biochemistry & Behavior*, 1976, **4**: 335–337.

WEIJNEN, J. A. W. M. Current licking: Lick-contingent electrical stimulation of the tongue. In J. Weijnen and J. Mendelson (Eds.), *Drinking behavior: Oral stimulation, reinforcement and preference*. New York: Plenum Press, 1977.

WEINBERG, J., BRETT, L. P., LEVINE, S., & DALLMAN, P. R. Long-term effects of early iron deficiency on consummatory behavior in the rat. *Pharmacology, Biochemistry & Behavior*, 1981, **14**: 447–453.

WEINBERG, J., GUNNER, M. R., BRETT, L. P., GONZALES, C. A., & LEVINE, S. Sex differences in biobehavioral responses to conflict in a taste aversion paradigm. *Physiology & Behavior*, 1982, **29**: 201–210.

WEINBERG, J., SMOTHERMAN, W. P., & LEVINE, S. Early handling effects on neophobia and conditioned taste aversion. *Physiology & Behavior*, 1978, **20**: 589–596.

WEISINGER, R. S., PARKER, L. F., & SKORUPSKI, J. D. Conditioned taste aversions and specific need states in the rat. *Journal of Comparative and Physiological Psychology*, 1974, **87**: 655–660.

WEISMAN, R. N., HAMILTON, L. W., & CARLTON, P. L. Increased conditioned gustatory aversion following VMH lesions in rats. *Physiology & Behavior*, 1972, **9**: 801–804.

WELLMAN, P. J. Pre-exposure to flavor and conditioned taste aversion: Amphetamine and lithium reinforcers. *Neurobehavioral Toxicology and Teratology*, 1982, **4**: 609–620.

Wellman, P. J., & Boissard, C. G. Influence of fluid deprivation level on the extinction of conditioned taste aversion induced by amphetamine in female rats. *Physiological Psychology*, 1981, **9**: 281–284.

Wellman, P. J., Malpas, P. B., & Wikler, K. C. Conditioned taste aversion and unconditioned suppression of water intake induced by phenylpropanolamine in rats. *Physiological Psychology*, 1981, **9**: 203–207.

Wellman, P. J., McIntosh, P., & Guidi, E. Effects of dorsolateral tegmental lesions on amphetamine- and lithium-induced taste aversions. *Physiology & Behavior*, 1981, **26**: 341–344.

Wellman, P. J., Watkins, P. A., Nation, J. R., & Clark, D. Conditioned taste aversion in the adult rat induced by dietary ingestion of cadmium or cobalt. *Neurotoxicology*, 1984, **5**: 81–90.

West, D. B., Williams, R. H., Braget, D. J., & Woods, S. C. Bombesin reduces food intake of normal and hypothalamically obese rats and lowers body weight when given chronically. *Peptides*, 1982, **3**: 61–67.

Westbrook, R. F., Bond, N. W., & Feyer, A-M. Short- and long-term decrements in toxicosis-induced odor-aversion learning: The role of duration of exposure to an odor. *Journal of Experimental Psychology: Animal Behavior Processes*, 1981, **7**: 362–381.

Westbrook, R. F., & Homewood, J. The effects of a flavour-toxicosis pairing upon long-delay, flavour aversion learning. *Quarterly Journal of Experimental Psychology*, 1982, **34B**: 59–75.

Westbrook, R. F., Homewood, J., Horn, K., & Clarke, J. C. Flavour-odour compound conditioning: Odour-potentiation and flavour-attenuation. *Quarterly Journal of Experimental Psychology*, 1983, **35B**: 13–33.

Westbrook, R. F., Provost, S. C., & Homewood, J. Short-term flavour memory in the rat. *Quarterly Journal of Experimental Psychology*, 1982, **34B**, 235–256.

Westbrook, R. F., Provost, S. C., & Nagley, M. Lithium exposures interfere with a previously established taste aversion in the rat. *Australian Journal of Psychology*, 1982, **34**: 139–149.

Whaley, D. L., Scarborough, B. B., & Reichard, S. M. Traumatic shock, x-irradiation and avoidance behavior. *Physiology & Behavior*, 1966, **1**: 93–95.

White, N., Sklar, L., & Amit, Z. The reinforcing action of morphine and its paradoxical side effect. *Psychopharmacology*, 1977, **52**: 63–66.

Wiens, A. N., & Menustik, C. E. Treatment outcome and patient characteristics in an aversion therapy program for alcoholism. *American Psychologist*, 1983, **38**: 1089–1096.

Wiens, A. N., Montague, J. R., Manaugh, T. S., & English, C. J. Pharmacological aversive counterconditioning to alcohol in a private hospital: One year follow-up. *Journal of Studies on Alcohol*, 1976, **37**: 1320–1324.

Wilcoxon, H. C. Long-delay learning of ingestive aversions in quail. In L. Barker, M. Best and M. Domjan (Eds.), *Learning mechanisms in food selection*. Waco, Texas: Baylor University Press, 1977.

Wilcoxon, H. C., Dragoin, W. B., & Kral, P. A. Illness-induced aversions in rat and quail: Relative salience of visual and gustatory cues. *Science*, 1971, **171**: 826–828.

Wilkie, D. M., MacLennan, A. J., & Pinel, J. P. J. Rat defensive behavior: Burying noxious food. *Journal of the Experimental Analysis of Behavior*, 1979, **31**: 299–306.

Wilkin, L. D., Cunninhgam, C. L., & Fitzgerald, R. D. Pavlovian conditioning with ethanol and lithium: Effects on heart rate and taste aversion in rats. *Journal of Comparative and Physiological Psychology*, 1982, **96**: 781–790.

Williams, E. Y. Management of chronic alcoholism. *Psychiatric Quarterly*, 1947, **21**: 190–198.

Williamson, A. M., Ng, K. T., & Richdale, A. Changes in corticosterone levels in iron deficient rats. *Physiology & Behavior*, 1981, **27**: 1085–1088.

Willner, J. A. Blocking of a taste aversion by prior pairings of exteroceptive stimuli with illness. *Learning and Motivation*, 1978, **9**: 125–140.

Wilson, C. J., Sherman, J. E., & Holman, E. W. Aversion to the reinforcer differentially affects conditioned reinforcement and instrumental responding. *Journal of Experimental Psychology: Animal Behavior Processes*, 1981, **7**: 165–174.

Wilson, G. T. Alcoholism and aversion therapy: Issues, ethics and evidence. In G. Maflatt and D. Nathan (Eds.), *Behavioral approaches to alcoholism*. New Jersey: Rutgers Center for Alcohol Studies, 1978.

Wilson, G. T., & Davison, G. C. Aversion techniques in behavior therapy: Some theoretical and metatheoretical considerations. *Journal of Consulting and Clinical Psychology*, 1969, **33**: 327–329.

WILSON, G. T., & TRACEY, D. A. An experimental analysis of aversive imagery versus electrical aversive conditioning in the treatment of chronic alcoholics. *Behaviour Research and Therapy*, 1976, **14**: 41–51.

WING, J. F., & BIRCH, L. A. Relative cue properties of novel-tasting substances in avoidance conditioning. *Animal Learning & Behavior*, 1974, **2**: 63–65.

WINN, F. J., JR., KENT, M. A., & LIBKUMAN, T. M. Learned taste aversion induced by cortical spreading depression. *Physiology & Behavior*, 1975, **15**: 21–24.

WINN, F. J., JR., TODD, G. E., & ELIAS, J. W. Cortical spreading depression-induced aversion to saccharin at two levels of KCL: Electroencephalographic verification. *Behavioral Biology*, 1977, **19**: 55–63.

WISE, R. A., & ALBIN, J. Stimulation-induced eating disrupted by a conditioned taste aversion. *Behavioral Biology*, 1973, **9**: 289–297.

WISE, R. A., YOKEL, R. A., & DEWITT, H. Both positive reinforcement and conditioned aversion from amphetamine and from apomorphine in rats. *Science*, 1976, **191**: 1273–1275.

WITTLIN, W. A., & BROOKSHIRE, K. H. Apomorphine-induced conditioned aversion to a novel food. *Psychonomic Science*, 1968, **12**: 217–218.

WOODS, S. C., LAWSON, R., HADDAD, R. K., RABE, A., & LAWSON, W. E. Reversal of conditioned aversions in normal and microencephalic rats. *Journal of Comparative and Physiological Psychology*, 1974, **86**: 531–534.

WOODS, S. C., WEISINGER, R. S., & WALD, B. A. Conditioned aversions produced by subcutaneous injections of formalin in rats. *Journal of Comparative and Physiological Psychology*, 1971, **77**: 410–415.

WORSHAM, E. D., RILEY, E. P., ANANDAM, N., LISTER, P., FREED, E. X., & LESTER, D. Selective breeding of rats for differences in reactivity to alcohol: An approach to an animal model of alcoholism. III. Some physical and behavioral measures. *Advances in Experimental and Medical Biology*, 1977, **85A**: 71–81.

WRIGHT, W. E., FOSHEE, D. P., & MCCLEARY, G. E., Comparison of taste aversion with various delays and cyclophosphamide dose levels. *Psychonomic Science*, 1971, **22**: 55–56.

WU, M-F., CRUZ-MORALES, S. E., QUINAN, J. R., STAPLETON, J. M., & REID, L. D. Naloxone reduces fluid consumption: Relationship of this effect to conditioned taste aversion and morphine dependence. *Bulletin of the Psychonomic Society*, 1979, **14**: 323–325.

WYSOCKI, C. J., WHITNEY, G., & TUCKER, D. Specific anosmia in the laboratory mouse. *Behavior Genetics*, 1977, **7**: 171–188.

YAMAMOTO, T., AZUMA, S., & KAWAMURA, Y. Significance of cortical-amygdalar-hypothalamic connections in retention of conditional taste aversion in rats. *Experimental Neurology*, 1981, **74**: 758–768.

YAMAMOTO, B. K., & KUTSCHER, C. L. Using profiles of saccharin and water drinking to detect and discriminate actions of drugs and toxicants. *Pharmacology, Biochemistry & Behavior*, 1980, **13**: 507–512.

YAMAMOTO, T., MATSUO, R., & KAWAMURA, Y. Localization of cortical gustatory area in rats and its role in taste discrimination. *Journal of Neurophysiology*, 1980, **44**: 440–455.

YOKEL, R. A., & OGZEWALLA, C. D. Effects of plant ingestion in rats determined by the conditioned taste aversion procedure. *Toxicon.*, 1981, **19**: 223–232.

ZABIK, J. E., & ROACHE, J. B. 5-hydroxytryptophan-induced conditioned taste aversion to ethanol in the rat. *Pharmacology, Biochemistry & Behavior*, 1983, **18**: 785–790.

ZACHARKO, R. M., WISHART, T. B., & LOEW, F. M. Thiamin deprivation in ventromedial hypothalamic hyperphagic rats: Anorexia, specificity of food aversion, and a dietary consideration. *Journal of Comparative and Physiological Psychology*, 1979, **93**: 140–150.

ZAHLER, L. P., & HARPER, A. E. Effects of dietary amino acid pattern on food preference behavior of rats. *Journal of Comparative and Physiological Psychology*, 1972, **81**: 155–162.

ZAHORIK, D. M. Conditioned physiological changes associated with learned aversions to tastes paired with thiamine deficiency in the rat. *Journal of Comparative and Physiological Psychology*, 1972, **79**: 189–200.

ZAHORIK, D. M. The role of dietary history in the effects of novelty on taste aversions. *Bulletin of the Psychonomic Society*, 1976, **8**: 285–288.

ZAHORIK, D. M. Learned changes in preference for chemical stimuli: Asymmetrical effects of positive and negative consequences and species differences in learning. In E. Koster and J. Kroeze (Eds.), *The chemoreception of preference behavior.* London: ECRO Press, 1979.

ZAHORIK, D. M., & BEAN, C. A. Resistance of "recovery" flavors to later association with illness. *Bulletin of the Psychonomic Society*, 1975, **6**: 309–312.

ZAHORIK, D. M., & HOUPT, K. A. The concept of nutritional wisdom: Applicability of laboratory learning models to large herbivores. In L. Barker, M. Best and M. Domjan (Eds.), *Learning mechanisms in food selection*. Waco, Texas; Baylor University Press, 1977.

ZAHORIK, D. M., & HOUPT, K. A. Species differences in feeding strategies, food hazards, and the ability to learn food aversions. In A. Kamil and T. Sargent (Eds.), *Foraging behavior: Ecological, ethological and psychological approaches*. New York: Garland Press, 1980.

ZAHORIK, D. M., & JOHNSTON, R. E. Taste aversions to food flavors and vaginal secretion in golden hamsters. *Journal of Comparative and Physiological Psychology*, 1976, **90**: 57–66.

ZAHORIK, D. M., & MAIER, S. F. Appetitive conditioning with recovery from thiamine deficiency as the unconditioned stimulus. *Psychonomic Science*, 1969, **17**: 309–310.

ZELLNER, D. A., DACANAY, R. J., & RILEY, A. L. Opiate withdrawal: The result of conditioning or physiological mechanisms? *Pharmacology, Biochemistry & Behavior*, 1984, **20**: 175–180.

ZIEGLER, J. M., GUSTAVSON, C. R., HOLZER, G. A., & GRUBER, D. Anthelmintic-based taste aversions in wolves (*Canis lupus*). *Applied Animal Ethology*, 1983, **9**: 373–377.

ACKNOWLEDGMENTS

The authors would like to thank the many colleagues who generously contributed information for this bibliography. The authors would also like to thank Cora Lee Wetherington for helpful suggestions throughout the preparation of the article and Kathy Richard and Julie Sickel for their technical assistance. The preparation of this bibliography was supported by a faculty development grant from The American University.

Index of Contributors

Subject Index